Medical Radiology

Radiation Oncology

Series editors
Luther W. Brady
Jiade J. Lu

Honorary editors
Hans-Peter Heilmann
Michael Molls

For further volumes:
http://www.springer.com/series/4353

Carsten Nieder • Johannes Langendijk
Editors

Re-Irradiation: New Frontiers

Second Edition

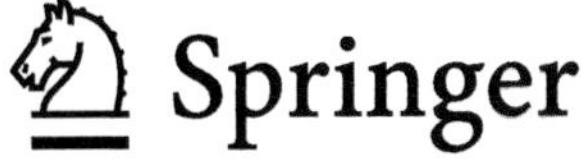

Editors
Carsten Nieder
Department of Oncology
University of Tromso and Nordland Hospital
Bodo
Norway

Johannes Langendijk
University Medical Center Groningen
Groningen
The Netherlands

ISSN 0942-5373 ISSN 2197-4187 (electronic)
Radiation Oncology
ISBN 978-3-319-82438-3 ISBN 978-3-319-41825-4 (eBook)
DOI 10.1007/978-3-319-41825-4

Softcover reprint of the hardcover 2nd edition 2016

Printed on acid-free paper

This Springer imprint is published by Springer Nature
The registered company is Springer International Publishing AG
The registered company address is Gewerbestrasse 11, 6330 Cham, Switzerland

Contents

Contributors

Sherif Abdel-Wahab Department of Clinical Oncology, Ain Shams University, Cairo, Egypt

Stefano Arcangeli Department of Radiation Oncology, S. Camillo and Forlanini Hospitals, Rome, Italy

Michael Baumann Department of Radiation Oncology, Faculty of Medicine and University Hospital Carl Gustav Carus, Technische Universität Dresden, Dresden, Germany

OncoRay – National Center for Radiation Research in Oncology, Faculty of Medicine and University Hospital Carl Gustav Carus, Technische Universität Dresden, Helmholtz-Zentrum Dresden – Rossendorf, Dresden, Germany

Helmholtz-Zentrum Dresden – Rossendorf, Institute od Radiooncology, Dresden, Germany

Deutsches Konsortium für Translationale Krebsforschung (DKTK), Dresden und Deutsches Krebsforschungszentrum (DKFZ), Heidelberg, Germany

National Center for Tumor Diseases (NCT), Partner Site Dresden, Dresden, Germany

Francesc Casas Department of Radiation Oncology, University Clinic, Barcelona, Spain

Colin Champ Department of Radiation Oncology, University of Pittsburgh Medical Center, Pittsburgh, PA, USA

Oscar S.H. Chan Department of Clinical Oncology, Pamela Youde Nethersole Eastern Hospital, Hong Kong, China

Nikola Cihoric Department of Radiation Oncology, Inselspital, Bern, Switzerland

Jennifer Croke Radiation Medicine Program, Princess Margaret Cancer Centre, Toronto, ON, Canada

Department of Radiation Oncology, University of Toronto, Toronto, ON, Canada

Vittorio Donato Department of Radiation Oncology, S. Camillo and Forlanini Hospitals, Rome, Italy

Pavol Dubinsky Department of Radiation Oncology, Eastern Slovakia University, Kosice, Slovakia

Avraham Eisbruch Department of Radiation Oncology, University of Michigan Medical Center, Ann Arbor, MI, USA

Shannon E. Fogh Department of Radiation Oncology, University of California, San Francisco, CA, USA

Steven Frank Department of Radiotherapy, University Medical Center Utrecht, Utrecht, The Netherlands

Anthony Fyles Radiation Medicine Program, Princess Margaret Cancer Centre, Toronto, ON, Canada

Department of Radiation Oncology, University of Toronto, Toronto, ON, Canada

Anca L. Grosu Department of Radiation Oncology, University Hospital Freiburg, Freiburg, Germany

Matthias Guckenberger Department of Radiation Oncology, University Hospital Zurich, Zurich, Switzerland

Peter Hoskin Department of Radiotherapy, Mount Vernon Hospital, London, UK

Daniel J. Indelicato Department of Radiation Oncology, University of Florida College of Medicine, Gainesville, FL, USA

University of Florida Proton Therapy Institute, Jacksonville, FL, USA

Branislav Jeremić Department of Radiation Oncology, Institute of Pulmonary Diseases, Sremska Kamenica, Serbia

BioIRC Centre for Biomedical Research, Kragujevac, Serbia

Chris R. Kelsey Department of Radiation Oncology, Duke University Medical Center, Durham, NC, USA

Grace J. Kim Department of Radiation Oncology, Duke University Medical Center, Durham, NC, USA

Johannes A. Langendijk Department of Radiation Oncology, University Medical Center Groningen, University of Groningen, Groningen, The Netherlands

Anne W.M. Lee Department of Clinical Oncology, The University of Hong Kong, Hong Kong, China

The University of Hong Kong – Shenzhen Hospital, Hong Kong, China

Eric Leung Department of Radiation Oncology, Odette Cancer Center, Toronto, ON, Canada

Department of Radiation Oncology, University of Toronto, Toronto, ON, Canada

Metha Maenhout Department of Radiotherapy, University Medical Center Utrecht, Utrecht, The Netherlands

Mariangela Massaccesi Radiation Oncology Department – Gemelli ART, Università Cattolica del Sacro Cuore, Rome, Italy

Mark W. McDonald Department of Radiation Oncology, Winship Cancer Institute of Emory University, Atlanta, GA, USA

Kevin P. McMullen Department of Radiation Oncology, The Cancer Center at Columbus Regional Health, Columbus, IN, USA

Minesh P. Mehta Department of Radiation Oncology, University of Maryland School of Medicine, Baltimore, MD, USA

Ana Mena Merino Department of Radiation Oncology, University of Palma de Majorca, Palma, Spain

John E. Munzenrider Department of Radiation Oncology, Massachusetts General Hospital, Boston, MA, USA

Wai Tong Ng Department of Clinical Oncology, Pamela Youde Nethersole Eastern Hospital, Hong Kong, China

Carsten Nieder Department of Oncology and Palliative Medicine, Nordland Hospital, Bodø, Norway

Oliver J. Ott Department of Radiation Oncology, University Hospital Erlangen, Erlangen, Germany

Joshua D. Palmer Department of Radiation Oncology, James Comprehensive Cancer Center, The Ohio State University, Columbus, Ohia, USA

Cedric Panje Department of Radiation Oncology, University Hospital Zurich, Zurich, Switzerland

Max Peters Department of Radiotherapy, University Medical Center Utrecht, Utrecht, The Netherlands

Michael S. Rutenberg Department of Radiation Oncology, University of Florida College of Medicine, Gainesville, FL, USA

University of Florida Proton Therapy Institute, Jacksonville, FL, USA

Manfred Schmidt Department of Radiation Oncology, University Hospital Erlangen, Erlangen, Germany

Helen A. Shih Central Nervous System and Eye Services, Department of Radiation Oncology, Massachusetts General Hospital, Boston, MA, USA

Susan C. Short UCL Cancer Institute, London, UK

William Small Jr. Department of Radiation Oncology, Loyola University, Cardinal Bernardin Cancer Center, Maywood, IL, USA

Puma Sundaresan Department of Radiation Oncology, Crown Princess Mary Cancer Centre, Westmead Hospital, Westmead, NSW, Australia

University of Sydney, Sydney, NSW, Australia

Reinhart A. Sweeney Department of Radiation Oncology, Leopoldina Hospital Schweinfurt, Schweinfurt, Germany

Henry C.K. Sze Department of Clinical Oncology, Pamela Youde Nethersole Eastern Hospital, Hong Kong, China

Stephanie Tanadini-Lang Department of Radiation Oncology, University Hospital Zurich, Zurich, Switzerland

Alexei V. Trofimov Physics Division, Department of Radiation Oncology, Massachusetts General Hospital, Boston, MA, USA

Vincenzo Valentini Radiation Oncology Department – Gemelli ART, Università Cattolica del Sacro Cuore, Rome, Italy

Marco van Vulpen Department of Radiotherapy, University Medical Center Utrecht, Utrecht, The Netherlands

Yvette van der Linden Department of Radiotherapy, Leiden University Medical Centre, Leiden, The Netherlands

Michael J. Veness Department of Radiation Oncology, Crown Princess Mary Cancer Centre, Westmead Hospital, Westmead, NSW, Australia

University of Sydney, Sydney, NSW, Australia

Andrew O. Wahl Department of Radiation Oncology, University of Nebraska Medical Center, Buffett Cancer Center, Omaha, NE, USA

Luhua Wang Department of Radiation Oncology, Chinese Medical Academy of Science, Beijing, China

The original version of this book was revised. An erratum to this book can be found at DOI 10.1007/978-3-319-41825-4_78.

Normal Tissue Tolerance to Reirradiation

Carsten Nieder and Johannes A. Langendijk

Contents

The original version of this chapter was revised. An erratum to this chapter can be found at 10.1007/978-3-319-41825-4_78.

C. Nieder, MD (✉)
Department of Oncology and Palliative Medicine, Nordland Hospital, Bodø, Norway
e-mail: Carsten.Nieder@nordlandssykehuset.no

J.A. Langendijk, MD
Department of Radiation Oncology, University Medical Center Groningen/University of Groningen, Groningen, The Netherlands

Abstract

As a result of longer survival times, even among patients with incurable malignancies, the prevalence of patients at risk of developing second primary tumours and/or locoregional recurrences in previously irradiated areas might increase. Consequently, the need for additional therapeutic measures providing local control and/or symptom palliation along different lines of treatment has emerged. This has resulted in increasing requests for delivering a second and sometimes even third course of radiation to target volumes within or close to previously irradiated anatomical areas. On the one hand, improved imaging and delivery techniques including image-guided and intensity-modulated radiotherapy might facilitate reirradiation of previously exposed regions of the body. On the other hand, late toxicity is of concern because it often causes serious impact on health-related quality of life. Therefore, knowledge about long-term recovery of occult radiation injury is of utmost importance. This chapter summarises available experimental and clinical data on the effects of reirradiation to various organs.

1 Introduction

The increasing number of publications on reirradiation demonstrates that many clinicians seriously consider this treatment modality in selected

Med Radiol Radiat Oncol (2016)
DOI 10.1007/174_2016_59, © Springer International Publishing Switzerland
Published Online: 21 Apr 2016

patients with favourable risk/benefit ratio. A large variety of regimens exists, which might be associated with quite different risks of toxicity, e.g. 2 fractions of 2 Gy for relapsed follicular lymphoma (Heinzelmann et al. 2010) as compared to repeat radiosurgery for intracranial targets (Raza et al. 2007; Holt et al. 2015) or brachytherapy for previously irradiated prostate cancer (Moman et al. 2009). Even radiation-induced tumours such as glioma might be considered for reirradiation (Paulino et al. 2008). Increasing the distance between organs at risk and the high-dose region, e.g. by injectable or implanted spacers, is an interesting approach (Kishi et al. 2009), but only feasible in certain anatomical sites and in a limited proportion of patients. Both experimental and clinical data have shown that a variety of normal tissues recover from occult radiation injury. However, decision-making on whether to reirradiate a patient is, indeed, a complex process. Factors to be taken into account include the type of tissue at risk for injury, the total dose, fractionation and interval from previous irradiation, observable normal tissue changes resulting from previous irradiation, the patient's prognosis, disease extent and so forth. The following paragraphs on experimental and clinical data on reirradiation tolerance of various tissues summarise our current knowledge and provide a basis for better understanding of the challenges associated with reirradiation to higher cumulative total doses.

2 Acute Reactions

2.1 Skin and Mucosa

In 1989, Terry et al. reported that the acute reactions of mouse foot skin receiving reirradiation 2 months or more after receiving a single dose of 15–30 Gy were indistinguishable from those of unirradiated skin. They also found that the tolerance to a second course of irradiation decreased and the latency to manifestation of acute reactions shortened when reirradiation was given 1 month after a previous course or when a single dose of 34.5–37.5 Gy was given, which was sufficient to produce a near-complete breakdown of the skin. Simmonds et al. (1989) reported comparable results for reirradiation of pig skin at intervals of 17, 35 or 52 weeks after single priming doses below the threshold for inducing moist desquamation. The regain in the acute tolerance of the skin to reirradiation is likely a result of the ability of the epidermis to respond to radiation-induced damage by accelerated repopulation and stem cell migration into the irradiated tissue leading to restoration of the original cell number and tissue integrity. Published clinical data on reirradiation of head and neck tumours, breast cancer, non-small cell lung cancer and others summarised in other chapters of this book also showed that acute skin and mucosal reactions after reirradiation were well within the range observed after the first course of radiotherapy (De Crevoisier et al. 1998; Montebello et al. 1993; Harms et al. 2004; Tada et al. 2005; Langendijk et al. 2006; Würschmidt et al. 2008; Tian et al. 2014). If the previous treatment has caused persistent severe mucosal damage, reirradiation might be poorly tolerated.

2.2 Intestine

There is only a single study on experimental reirradiation tolerance of the intestine (Reynaud and Travis 1984). Mice received 9 or 11.5 Gy whole abdominal irradiation, which did not cause acute mortality but reduced the jejunal crypt number by about 10% and caused 10% late mortality from intestinal damage within 1 year. Single graded doses of total body irradiation were then given after 2, 6 or 12 months. Assessment of crypt survival 3.5 days after reirradiation showed that very little, if any, of the initial abdominal radiation dose was remembered by the surviving crypts, indicating a remarkable tolerance to reirradiation. In the clinic, Haque et al. (2009) observed only one case of acute high-grade toxicity (grade 3 or higher) in 13 patients treated with reirradiation to the abdomen for gastrointestinal malignancies. These authors administered a hyperfractionated-accelerated regimen, using 1.5 Gy fractions twice daily, with a median dose of 30 Gy (range 24–48 Gy) and in most cases concurrent chemotherapy.

3 Late Side Effects

3.1 Epithelial and Mesenchymal Tissues

Simmonds et al. (1989) found in a pig model that there was no or little residual injury retained for late ischaemic dermal necrosis (corresponding to at most 2–7 % of the initial dose). Moreover, the latency for development of necrosis was not different. The exact mechanism underlying such recovery is not yet clearly understood. However, clinical data related to many cancer types revealed that late complications were more frequent than anticipated after reirradiation to high cumulative doses. For patients with mycosis fungoides ($n=14$) receiving a second course of total skin electron beam therapy (18–24 Gy after an initial dose of about 30 Gy), late skin toxicities included generalised xerosis, toenail and fingernail dystrophy and scattered telangiectasia (Ysebaert et al. 2004). The majority of data is derived from head and neck cancer retreatment. For example, the authors of a large series of 169 patients reirradiated for recurrent unresectable head and neck tumours after a median time of 33 months to a median cumulative dose of 130 Gy (some with concurrent chemotherapy) found 21 % and 8 % incidences of mucosal necrosis and osteoradionecrosis, respectively (De Crevoisier et al. 1998). Moderate late morbidity, such as trismus and cervical fibrosis, developed in up to 41 % of patients. Within their respective ranges, the reirradiation dose, cumulative dose, reirradiated volume or interval between the two treatment courses did not predict the risk of severe late injury. Other factors, such as perfusion disturbance after previous surgery or pre-existing cardiovascular diseases, might also impact on the eventual development of epithelial and connective tissue complications. Lee et al. (1997) reported the data of 654 patients with recurrent nasopharyngeal carcinoma receiving reirradiation to median initial and reirradiation doses of 60 Gy and 46 Gy, respectively, with a median interval of 2 years. The actuarial incidence of symptomatic late sequelae (for all complications combined) was approximately 50 % at 5 years. They found that the biologically effective dose (BED) of the first radiation course affected the risk of late injury significantly, the BED of reirradiation was of borderline significance, but the interval between both treatments was not significant. The potential effects of volume were not evaluated. In a later analysis, the same group found that the major determinant of post-retreatment complications was the severity of damage during the initial course (Lee et al. 2000). A study by Xiao et al. (2015) included 291 patients and found that gross tumour volume was predictive not only for the prognosis and risk of distant metastases, but also for toxicity-related death, e.g. resulting from massive haemorrhage. The prospective study by Tian et al. (2014) also showed that tumour volume significantly influenced the risk of mucosal necrosis (53 % if volume >26 cc vs. 23 % in smaller tumours). A small study of 16 patients who received amifostine together with postoperative reirradiation and chemotherapy for head and neck cancer did not suggest reduced late toxicity rates with this strategy (Machtay et al. 2004). Severe toxicity occurred also after intensity-modulated radiotherapy (IMRT) but no prospective head to head comparison of IMRT versus 3-D conformal RT is available (Sulman et al. 2009). In the IMRT study reported by Duprez et al. (2009), 84 patients were reirradiated to a median cumulative total dose of 130 Gy (median time interval 49.5 months, median reirradiation dose 69 Gy, 17 patients received concurrent chemotherapy). Late toxicity was scored in 52 patients with at least 6 months of follow-up. Eight patients developed grade 3 or 4 late dysphagia and three developed osteoradionecrosis. Overall, 30 different grade 3 or 4 late complications were recorded. Osteoradionecrosis might even develop in the cervical vertebrae, though the most common location is the mandible (Kosaka et al. 2010). Clearly, it is unrealistic to expect absence of any severe late toxicity after IMRT or other highly conformal techniques since certain parts of the mucosal and/or connective tissues will always be part of the planning target volume and receive high cumulative doses. This issue is further addressed in other chapters of this book. Overall, the available data indicate that the mesenchymal tissues recover from radiation injury less than rapidly reacting tissues like the epidermis and mucosa, at least in the head and neck region.

3.2 Thoracic Aorta and Carotid Arteries

Reports of high-dose reirradiation have identified the large arteries as critical organs at risk. Evans et al. (2013) analysed the end point of grade 5 aortic toxicity in 35 patients with lung cancer. The median prescribed dose was 54 Gy in 1.8-Gy fractions and 60 Gy in 2-Gy fractions, respectively. The median interval between the two courses was 32 months. The median raw composite dose to 1 cc of the aorta was 110 Gy. Toxicity developed in 25% of patients who received ≥120 Gy but not in patients irradiated to lower cumulative doses. The issue of carotid blowout syndrome (CBOS) has been studied by Yamazaki et al. (2013). They pooled data from 7 Japanese CyberKnife institutions and analysed 381 patients. Of these 32 (8.4%) developed CBOS after a median of 5 months from reirradiation. Twenty-two patients died (69%). Later, a predictive model (CBOS index) was developed, which includes carotid invasion of >180°, presence of ulceration and lymph node area irradiation (0–3 points) (Yamazaki et al. 2015). A larger pooled series included 1554 patients who received head and neck reirradiation (McDonald et al. 2012). There were 41 reported CBOS, for a rate of 2.6, and 76% were fatal. The median time to CBOS was 7.5 months. In patients treated in a continuous course with 1.8–2 Gy daily fractions or 1.2 Gy twice-daily fractions, 36% of whom received concurrent chemotherapy, the rate of CBOS was 1.3%, compared with 4.5% in patients treated with 1.5 Gy twice daily in alternating weeks or with delayed accelerated hyperfractionation, all of whom received concurrent chemotherapy ($p=0.002$).

3.3 Intestine

Late toxicity data are available from a study of palliative reirradiation for recurrent rectal cancer (Lingareddy et al. 1997). In this study, 52 patients were reirradiated to approximately 30 Gy (once daily 1.8 or 2 Gy in 30 patients and bid 1.2 Gy daily in 22 patients) after an initial course of median 50.4 Gy. The median interval was 24 months. Twenty patients received an additional boost dose to a maximum of 40.8 Gy. Most patients ($n=47$) also had concurrent 5-fluorouracil chemotherapy with reirradiation. Grade 3 or 4 (by Radiation Therapy Oncology Group (RTOG) criteria) small bowel obstruction occurred in nine patients (17%), cystitis in three patients (6%) and non-tumour-related fistulas in four patients (8%). The cumulative dose, reirradiation dose and time interval were not significantly related to late toxicity. However, conventional fractionation with 1.8–2 Gy resulted in more toxicity as compared to hyperfractionation (hazard ratio 3.9). The latter finding was confirmed in a follow-up publication that included 103 patients (Mohiuddin et al. 2002). In this study, interval to reirradiation >24 months was also associated with significantly lower late toxicity rates. Fifteen percent of patients developed small bowel obstruction and 2% colo-anal stricture. Persistent severe diarrhoea was recorded in 17% of patients. As with many other studies discussed in this chapter, actuarial rates of late adverse events and detailed dose-volume histogram analyses were not provided. Another group performed reirradiation after omental flap transposition (OFT) in 12 patients with locoregional recurrent rectal cancers (Kim et al. 2010). No severe complications of grade 3 or higher involving the small bowel or bladder occurred. It was suggested that OFT effectively excluded small bowel from the radiation field. Intestinal complications also hampered the benefits of high-dose reirradiation of tumours in the female genital tract with combined external beam RT and brachytherapy (Russell et al. 1987). They were uncommon (one case of gastrointestinal bleeding classified as grade 4 late toxicity, no grade 3 adverse events among 13 patients) after palliative abdominal reirradiation to a median dose of 30 Gy given after an initial course of median 45 Gy (Haque et al. 2009). Abusaris et al. (2011, 2012) reported institutional dose constraints that also resulted in low rates of grade 3–4 toxicities, albeit in small groups of patients.

3.4 Lung

Terry et al. (1988) assessed the risk of pneumonitis after reirradiation in a mouse model. The whole thorax was irradiated with a priming dose of 6, 8 or 10 Gy, which did not cause changes in breathing rate or lethality. One to six months later, reirradiation was given (over a full range of doses). The end point of this experiment was radiation pneumonitis within 196 days after reirradiation. Both the size of the priming dose and the interval had a significant impact on the response to reirradiation. After a low priming dose of 6 Gy, the lungs could tolerate reirradiation as if they had not received previous radiation exposure. Some occult injury remained at 1 month after an 8-Gy priming dose. Residual damage in the order of 25–70 % persisted at all time intervals after a 10-Gy priming dose. The experimental set-up is different from the clinical situation where only limited parts of the lung receive irradiation. Moreover, the radiation dose to the heart might also impact on lung toxicity and late pulmonary function. Our own unpublished clinical experience with palliative reirradiation of lung cancer is consistent with published data, which suggest that pneumonitis is rarely observed (Montebello et al. 1993). For example, Jackson and Ball (1987) observed no symptomatic radiation pneumonitis among 22 patients with non-small cell lung cancer reirradiated to 20–30 Gy in 2-Gy fractions after having received a median dose of 55 Gy (median interval 15 months). A Japanese study with 15 patients (median reirradiation dose 50 Gy in 25 fractions, median interval 16 months) reported one case of grade 3 radiation pneumonitis and three cases of grade 2 esophagitis (Tada et al. 2005). After brachytherapy, severe toxicity was uncommon too (Hauswald et al. 2010). Apparently, the lungs recover at least partially from occult injury. Experimental data on trachea, bronchi or oesophagus are lacking. Most clinical series did not describe particular problems with these critical structures, except for stereotactic treatment of central lesions. Also after proton beam reirradiation, oesophageal fistula (raw dose 136 Gy) and tracheal necrosis (raw dose 147 Gy) have been reported (McAvoy et al. 2013). Of note, however, is that the median survival after moderate-dose reirradiation was only 5–7 months and, hence, was too short for assessment of true late damage to the lungs and other thoracic structures. As shown in Fig. 1, lung fibrosis might develop in patients with longer survival. Experience with higher reirradiation doses is still limited and typically derived from small-field stereotactic radiotherapy series (Peulen et al. 2011; Liu et al. 2012; Meijneke et al. 2013).

3.5 Spinal Cord

Reirradiation tolerance of the spinal cord has been most extensively studied in animal models using paresis, predominantly resulting from white matter necrosis that manifests in 10–12 months in rodents, as the end point and the median paresis dose (ED_{50}) for computation. Results of two reirradiation experiments revealed that the fractionation sensitivity of reirradiation was similar to that of single-course irradiation (Ruifrok et al. 1992a; Wong et al. 1993). Lower spine reirradiation experiments (T10-L2 in adult mice, L3–5 in adult rats, L2–6 in young guinea pigs) showed remarkable long-term recovery if the initial dose was limited to 50–75 % of the ED_{50} (Hornsey et al. 1982; Lavey et al. 1994; Knowles 1983; Mason et al. 1993). The extent of injury retained was highest after initial irradiation to 75 % of the ED_{50}, but even under this condition, only 30 % of injury was retained. A series of reirradiation experiments of rat cervical spinal cord showed that the initial dose, the interval to reirradiation and the reirradiation dose influenced the latency to myelopathy (Wong et al. 1993; Wong and Han 1997). Beyond an 8-week interval, there was a progressive increase in recovery with an increasing time interval to reirradiation, but recovery was never complete. In adult rats main long-term recovery occurred between 2 and 6 months. For 3-week-old rats, partial recovery took place during the first month, which increased only slightly between 1 and 6 months (Ruifrok et al. 1992b). In a different study, an initial single dose of 15 Gy was administered, followed 8 or

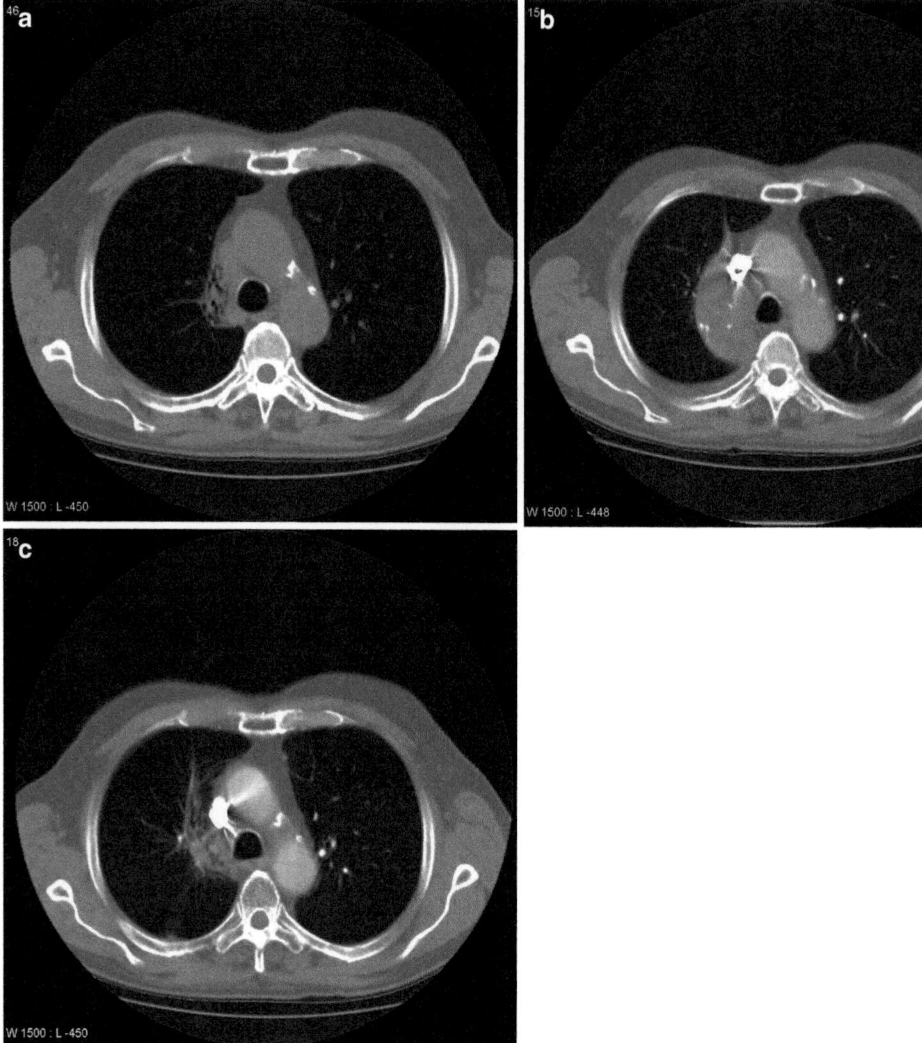

Fig. 1 In 1995, a 58-year-old gentleman received combined chemoradiation for small cell lung cancer of the right lung (limited disease) resulting in a cure. (**a**) Shows a follow-up computed tomography (CT) scan from 2008 demonstrating slight paramediastinal radiation fibrosis. In January 2009, the patient was diagnosed with stage IIIB adenocarcinoma of the right lung (**b**). He received two cycles of platinum-based chemotherapy and achieved a partial response. He went on to simultaneous chemotherapy and 3D-conformal reirradiation (15 fractions of 2.8 Gy). He developed grade III acute esophagitis but no pulmonary toxicity. (**c**) Shows the most recent CT scan taken 1 year after reirradiation demonstrating increasing radiation fibrosis in the reirradiated region (clinically asymptomatic). At that time the patient was diagnosed with multiple brain metastases and started palliative whole-brain irradiation (no previous prophylactic whole-brain radiotherapy had been given)

16 weeks later by additional graded doses (van der Kogel 1979). In contrast to all other studies, separate dose-response curves were obtained for white matter necrosis (latent period <7 months) and vascular damage (latent period up to 18 months). Recovery between 8 and 16 weeks was significant for the white matter necrosis end point but was much less for vascular damage. It has also been shown that modification of the reirradiation tolerance of the spinal cord can be obtained (Nieder et al. 2005a). In these experiments, a combination of systemically administered insulin-like growth factor-1 and intrathecal amifostine resulted in lower incidence of myelop-

athy after cervical spinal cord reirradiation in rats. Such strategies were not pursued further because of increasing availability of equipment and software, which allows for spinal cord sparing (IMRT, stereotactic RT etc.). Other pharmacologic strategies aiming at radioprotection in different tissues and organs typically were examined in previously untreated animals (Greenberger 2009) although the reirradiation setting appears attractive for studying radioprotectors.

As compared to rodent experiments, more clinically applicable data were generated in adult rhesus monkeys at MD Anderson Cancer Center, Houston, USA, by Ang et al. (1995). The cervical spinal cord of these primates was irradiated with 2.2 Gy per fraction. The control group received a single radiation course to total doses of 70.4, 77 or 83.6 Gy. The number of animals developing myelopathy in these 3 dose groups was 3 of 15, 3 of 6 and 7 of 8, respectively. Twelve asymptomatic animals in the 70.4 Gy group were retreated 2 years later to cumulative doses of 83.6, 92.4 or 101.2 Gy (four animals each). Only two developed paresis at 11 (83.6 Gy) and 8 (92.4 Gy) months after reirradiation. Subsequently, 16 monkeys received 44 Gy in 20 fractions and 2 years later were reirradiated to cumulative doses of 83.6, 92.4, 101.2 or 110 Gy. Only two (one received 101.2 Gy and the other 110 Gy) developed myelopathy. These data indicate that a substantial amount of the occult injury induced by the priming dose decayed within 2 years. As published in 2001, Ang et al. confirmed their initial observations in a group of 56 rhesus monkeys. The dose of the initial course was 44 Gy in all monkeys. Reirradiation dose was 57.2 Gy, given after 1-year ($n=16$) or 2-year ($n=20$) intervals, or 66 Gy, given after 2-year ($n=4$) or 3-year ($n=14$) intervals. Only 4 of 45 monkeys completing the required observation period (2–2.5 years after reirradiation, 3–5.5 years total) developed myelopathy. Fitting the data with a model, assuming that all (single course and reirradiation) dose-response curves were parallel, yielded recovery estimates of 33.6 Gy (76 %), 37.6 Gy (85 %) and 44.6 Gy (101 %) of the initial dose, after 1, 2 and 3 years, respectively, at the 5 % incidence level. Another way to look at these results is to estimate the total cumulative dose that can be tolerated, expressed in EQD_2 that is equivalent dose in 2-Gy fractions calculated using the linear-quadratic approach. For a time interval of 1, 2 and 3 years between the treatment courses, cumulative doses of 150, 156 and 167 % of the first-line setting's tolerance dose appear possible.

If true in humans, an initial exposure equivalent to 46 Gy in 2-Gy fractions (arbitrarily selected to represent 100 % of the tolerance dose at the 5 % myelopathy risk level because many institutions limit the spinal cord dose to lower levels than true tolerance (Kirkpatrick et al. 2010)) might be followed by an additional 23–24 Gy in 2-Gy fractions (50 % of the tolerance dose) 1 or 2 years later. Clinical data from different institutions supporting this interpretation have been published (Schiff et al. 1995; Grosu et al. 2002). Most patients were treated with palliative reirradiation and therefore follow-up was often limited. In patients with better prognosis, the cumulative spinal cord dose often was kept at very low levels, e.g. in the RTOG head and neck cancer reirradiation protocols (Langer et al. 2007). Nevertheless, data from patients with longer follow-up have been published, e.g. five patients with recurrent Hodgkin's disease who were followed for more than 5 years after reirradiation (Magrini et al. 1990). The first spinal cord dose was 30 Gy in 1.7 Gy fractions (plus chemotherapy) and 1–3 years later up to 40 Gy in 2-Gy fractions was administered (two to three vertebral segments) without causing myelopathy. The cumulative EQD_2 of this treatment is slightly lower than 150 %. All available data from different published series including those reporting on myelopathy (Wong et al. 1994) were analysed by Nieder et al. (2005b, 2006a). Seventy-eight patients were included and a risk prediction model was developed, based on time interval, cumulative dose and presence or absence of any treatment course resulting in quite high spinal cord exposure. Besides cumulative dose, interval <6 months and total dose equivalent to >50 Gy in 2-Gy fractions in one of the two courses increases the risk of myelopathy. Low-risk patients had <5 % risk of myelopathy and intermediate risk patients approximately 25 %. However, unpublished cases treated after 2006 in the author's institution in Bodø, Norway, all remained free from myelopathy, suggesting that the actual risk might be lower than previously anticipated. Chapter "Fractionation Concepts" of this book contains a table showing calculations of the myelopathy risk based on this model (Table 3).

The introduction of stereotactic body radiotherapy has resulted in new challenges as such treatment typically is administered with few high-dose fractions or even single doses. Rather than irradiating complete spinal cord cross sections with homogeneous doses, small areas are exposed and steep dose gradients achieved. Medin et al. (2012) developed a swine model where a 10-cm length of the spinal cord (C3-T1) was uniformly irradiated to 30 Gy in 10 fractions and reirradiated 1 year later with a single radiosurgery dose centred within the previously irradiated segment. Radiosurgery was delivered to a cylindrical volume approximately 5 cm in length and 2 cm in diameter, which was positioned laterally to the cervical spinal cord, resulting in a dose distribution with the 90 %, 50 % and 10 % isodose lines traversing the ipsilateral, central and contralateral spinal cord, respectively. Follow-up after reirradiation was 1 year. Summarised briefly, pigs receiving radiosurgery 1 year following 30 Gy in 10 fractions were not at significantly higher risk of developing motor deficits than pigs that received radiosurgery alone. Limited data on reirradiated patients are available. Damast et al. (2011) reviewed the records of patients with in-field recurrence after previous spine radiation (median dose 30 Gy) that received salvage IMRT with either five 4-Gy (20-Gy group, $n=42$) or five 6-Gy (30-Gy group, $n=55$) daily fractions. The median follow-up was 12 months (range, 0.2–63.6 months). Maximal point dose to the spinal cord and cauda equina were limited to 14 Gy and 16 Gy, respectively. Neither previous cord dose from first radiotherapy nor interval between first and second course had bearing on these dose constraints. There was no incidence of myelopathy. Notably, there were nine vertebral body fractures and one benign oesophageal stricture after IMRT, which was potentially attributable to radiation. In 36 patients treated with helical tomotherapy, radiation myelopathy was not observed (Sterzing et al. 2010). The most common initial regimen was 10 fractions of 3 Gy. All patients had low cumulative EQD_2 and thus belonged to the low-risk group. Choi et al. (2010) retrospectively reviewed 51 lesions in 42 patients whose spinal metastases recurred in a previous radiation field (median previous spinal cord dose of 40 Gy) and were subsequently treated with stereotactic radiosurgery to a median marginal dose of 20 Gy (range, 10–30 Gy) in 1–5 fractions (median, 2). The median follow-up was 7 months (range, 2–47 months). The median spinal cord maximum total dose and dose per fraction from reirradiation were 19.3 Gy (range, 5.1–31.3 Gy) and 7.2 Gy (range, 2.9–19.3 Gy), respectively. One patient (2 %) experienced grade 4 neurotoxicity. Having received 39.6 Gy in 1.8 Gy fractions (total spinal cord dose of 40 Gy) to the T4 to L1 vertebral bodies 81 months before receiving reirradiation, she received 20 Gy in 2 fractions to treat a T5 recurrence. Treatment was prescribed to the 80 % isodose line. The maximal spinal cord dose from reirradiation was 19.25 Gy, which is equivalent to 56 Gy in 2-Gy fractions. Therefore, this patient would be predicted to have a high likelihood of myelopathy by the aforementioned risk score (Nieder et al. 2006a). A case with comparably high reirradiation dose (maximum 20.9 Gy in 2 fractions to the thecal sac at T1) resulting in myelopathy 5 months after retreatment has been reported by Sahgal et al. (2012). Previous treatment was only 25 Gy in 28 fractions (interval 70 months). A third case was also reported in the same paper. Here, initial treatment was close to tolerance, i.e. equivalent to 52 Gy in 2-Gy fractions. The maximum reirradiation dose to the thecal sac was 14.7 Gy in one single fraction (level T10, interval 12 months). Myelopathy developed after 3 months. In a fourth case, initial treatment was equivalent to 50 Gy in 2-Gy fractions and reirradiation dose maximum to the thecal sac was 32.6 Gy in 3 fractions (level C1/C2, interval 18 months). Myelopathy developed after 8 months. In their report, Sahgal et al. (2012) provided a recommendation of reasonable stereotactic reirradiation doses after initial conventional radiotherapy (interval at least

5 months). A thecal sac point maximum $P(\max)$ EQD_2 of 20–25 Gy appears to be safe provided the total $P(\max)$ EQD_2 does not exceed approximately 70 Gy, and the SBRT thecal sac $P(\max)$ EQD_2 comprises no more than approximately 50% of the total normalised biologically equivalent dose. The feasibility of salvaging spinal metastases initially irradiated with SBRT, who subsequently progressed with imaging-confirmed local tumour progression, with a second SBRT course to the same level has recently been confirmed (Thibault et al. 2015).

3.6 Brain

Reirradiation of brain tumours is often performed on an individual case-by-case basis and not yet based on the highest level of evidence (Veninga et al. 2001; Schwartz et al. 2015). In fact, no large randomised phase 3 trials have been published so far. It seems, however, that the selection criteria employed by experienced clinicians allow for retreatment, e.g. of glioblastoma with fractionated stereotactic radiotherapy, with low to moderate risk of late toxicity and encouraging median survival (Nieder et al. 2006b, 2008; Fogh et al. 2010). True long-term survival after reirradiation of brain tumours is unlikely and differentiation between tumour- and treatment-related deficits might be challenging. Therefore the actual rates of toxicity are difficult to estimate (Mayer and Sminia 2008; Sminia and Mayer 2012). In fact, toxicity risk might differ between brain regions with highly collateralised blood supply and those perfused by only few small branches. Importantly and in contrast to spinal cord and other organs, no animal experiments on reirradiation of the brain are available. Flickinger et al. (1989) published a series of nine patients with suprasellar or pituitary tumours having more than 5 years of follow-up after receiving two series of radiotherapy. Doses varied between 36 and 54 Gy for the first and 35–50 Gy for the second course. The median interval was as long as 7.5 years. The cumulative dose varied from 70 to 89 Gy in 2-Gy fractions with three patients receiving at least 86 Gy. Only one patient who was treated to 86 Gy developed a severe complication, namely, optic neuropathy. Of 32 patients treated by Dritschilo et al. (1981), 11 were alive at the time of analysis. Eight were experiencing productive lives and three were suffering from severe neurological damage including two cases of radionecrosis. Temporal lobe injury after treatment of nasopharynx cancer is not uncommon (Liu et al. 2014), and more details about this topic can be found in the chapter reviewing this particular tumour type.

Reirradiation of glioma with fractionated stereotactic radiotherapy (5 fractions per week, 5 Gy per fraction) after a median dose of 55 Gy was reported by Shepherd et al. (1997). All patients treated with more than 40 Gy developed late toxicity whereas only 25% of those who received 30–40 Gy developed such adverse events. Several institutions have used reirradiation doses of 30–40 Gy with fraction sizes below 4 Gy with acceptable rates of toxicity (Combs et al. 2005; Fogh et al. 2010), and there is now also a prospective trial in progress (Combs et al. 2010). Radiosurgery was systematically studied by the RTOG (Shaw et al. 1996, 2000). Adults with cerebral or cerebellar solitary non-brainstem tumours ≤40 mm in maximum diameter were eligible. Initial radiosurgical doses were 18 Gy for tumours ≤20 mm, 15 Gy for that 21–30 mm and 12 Gy for that 31–40 mm in maximum diameter. Dose was prescribed to the 50–90% isodose line. Doses were escalated in 3-Gy increments providing the incidence of irreversible grade 3 or any grade 4 or 5 RTOG central nervous system toxicity was <20% within 3 months of radiosurgery. Between 1990 and 1994, 156 analysable patients were entered, 36% of whom had recurrent primary brain tumours (median prior dose 60 Gy) and 64% recurrent brain metastases (median prior dose 30 Gy). The median interval was 11 months, minimum 3 months. The maximum tolerated doses were 24 Gy, 18 Gy and 15 Gy for tumours ≤20 mm, 21–30 mm and 31–40 mm in maximum diameter, respectively. However, for tumours <20 mm, investigators' reluctance to escalate to 27 Gy, rather than excessive toxicity, determined the maximum tolerated dose. The actuarial incidence of radionecrosis was 5%, 8%, 9% and 11% at 6, 12, 18 and 24 months following radiosurgery, respectively. Unacceptable toxicity was more likely in patients with larger tumours. Sneed et al. (2015) reported that radiosurgery followed by a second radiosurgery for recurrent brain metastases resulted in a 20% 1-year cumulative incidence of symptomatic adverse radiation effect (median reirradiation dose 18 Gy, $n=72$, crude risk 14%). Compared to patients who had not received prior radiosurgery to the same lesion, the hazard ratio for any adverse radiation effect was 5.05 (95% confidence interval 1.9–13.2).

3.7 Heart

Wondergem et al. (1996) assessed reirradiation tolerance of the heart at intervals of up to 9 months in a rat model by measuring cardiac function ex vivo 6 months after reirradiation. The cardiac tolerance dose was arbitrarily defined as the dose causing at least a 50% function loss in one-half of the treated animals (ED_{50}). Up to a 6-month interval, the reirradiation ED_{50} was close to the single-course ED_{50} but dropped significantly when the interval was longer than 6 months. The reirradiation tolerance also decreased with an increasing priming dose. A slow progression of damage induced by the priming dose is a plausible explanation for the decrease in tolerance with increasing time from the initial course. Systematic clinical data are not available.

3.8 Bladder

Stewart et al. (1990) studied whole bladder irradiation in mice. Priming doses were 8 Gy, which did not induce any observable functional bladder damage, and 16 Gy, which corresponded to 60% of a full tolerance dose and produced a moderate level of damage starting from about 30 weeks. Reirradiation was given after approximately 13 or 39 weeks. Acute toxicity, manifesting as increased urination frequency, was mild when reirradiation was delivered 13 weeks after both priming dose levels but was amplified in the group receiving reirradiation 39 weeks after a priming dose of 16 Gy. However, with respect to late bladder damage (end point defined as >50% reduction in bladder volume, increased urination frequency at ≥27 weeks after reirradiation), no long-term recovery was observed in up to a 9-month interval. Unfortunately, neither experimental data for partial organ reirradiation nor larger clinical studies on bladder re-exposure are available.

3.9 Kidney

Studies on mouse, rat and pig kidney suggested that radiation-induced toxicity progresses rather than recovers with time (Robbins et al. 1991; Stewart et al. 1994). For example, mouse experiments performed by Stewart et al. (1994) showed that reirradiation tolerance was inversely related to the priming dose, and tolerance decreased rather than increased significantly with increasing time interval. Analysis of the data on reirradiation at 26 weeks after lower priming doses using the linear-quadratic model gave an alpha/beta value of 1.4 Gy, which was significantly lower than the 3.3 Gy obtained for a single radiation course, indicating a larger fractionation-sparing effect for the reirradiation setting. Of clinical interest is also the finding in a rat model that single-dose cisplatin (5 mg/kg) administered 1 year after unilateral kidney irradiation progressively deteriorated the function of the irradiated kidney measured at 5 and 11 weeks after drug treatment (Landuyt et al. 1988). Compared with the contralateral kidney, the irradiated kidney showed a larger sensitivity to cisplatin-induced injury, even at subclinical doses of both drug and radiation.

4 Liver

The increasing numbers of patients with primary and secondary liver tumours receiving radiotherapy have led to occasional situations where the feasibility and potential of reirradiation for in-field or marginal progression or adjacent new lesions has to be discussed. Data are still very limited. Lee et al. (2016) treated 12 patients with hepatocellular carcinoma (median initial dose 50 Gy, range 36–60; median dose per fraction 1.8 Gy). Minimum interval to reirradiation was 5 months (median 20). The median dose was 50 Gy, range 36–58, with a median dose per fraction of 2.5 Gy. They aimed at a mean remaining liver dose ≤30 Gy with at least 700 cc of remaining liver volume. After reirradiation, 6 of 12 patients showed deterioration of liver function, and severe worsening of liver function (Child-Pugh score elevation ≥3 points) was also observed in four patients. The causal relationship was difficult to judge because several other local and systemic therapies were administered in most cases.

5 Discussion

Reirradiation should only be considered if the radiation tolerance of critical tissues or organs has not been exceeded during the first treatment, i.e. after careful review of the initial dose distribution and fields and assessment of organ status and side effects after the first treatment. Moreover, reasonable performance status and absence of other, less toxic treatment alternatives are prerequisites. It is important to weigh the expected benefits against morbidity and compromised quality of life. Solid preclinical evidence of recovery from occult radiation injury has been obtained for a variety of end points in several tissues and organs. However, these animal experiments cannot completely resemble the clinical situation, e.g. with regard to complexity of host factors. Cancer patients vary in biological and chronological age, cardiovascular and other comorbidity, organ reserve capacity and extent of multimodal therapies (additional surgery or even repeat surgeries, different types of anticancer drugs). It is also challenging to achieve dose distributions in partial organ irradiation of laboratory animals that are comparable to human IMRT and stereotactic RT. The majority of animal experiments were performed before such technology became available. It is therefore of utmost importance to collect clinical data on reirradiation tolerance. For many tissues and organs, an increasing body of data is now becoming available. Nevertheless, little is known for a number of end points such as neurocognitive function, damage to endocrine organs or the reirradiation tolerance of paediatric patients. Acutely responding tissues, in general, recover radiation changes practically completely within a few months and, therefore, can tolerate a repeat treatment course. For late injury end points, the heart, bladder and kidney did not exhibit long-term recovery (Fig. 2), whereas the skin, mucosa and spinal cord did. However, long-term recovery occurs within a defined time period that depends on the size of the priming dose and differs among tissues, species and age. Importantly, clinical evidence suggests that fibrosis, impaired blood perfusion and, in general, late normal tissue injury in humans continues to progress for many years and even decades. Lee et al. (1992) analysed more than 4,500 patients irradiated for nasopharyngeal cancer and found that the incidence of all types of late radiation toxicity, except of myelopathy, continued to rise even more than 10 years after treatment. Of course, individual prediction of toxicity risk would be a major step towards optimal choice of treatment intensity. Several reviews have summarised the current research efforts in this field (Coates et al. 2015; Jentsch et al. 2015; Kerns et al. 2014, 2015), which will not be discussed in any detail in this overview on reirradiation. The following book chapters provide both literature synopsis and exemplary cases that hopefully guide the choice of reirradiation regimens with acceptable complication probabilities. The paucity of data for many scenarios clinicians might face should encourage our community to embark on additional prospective clinical trials.

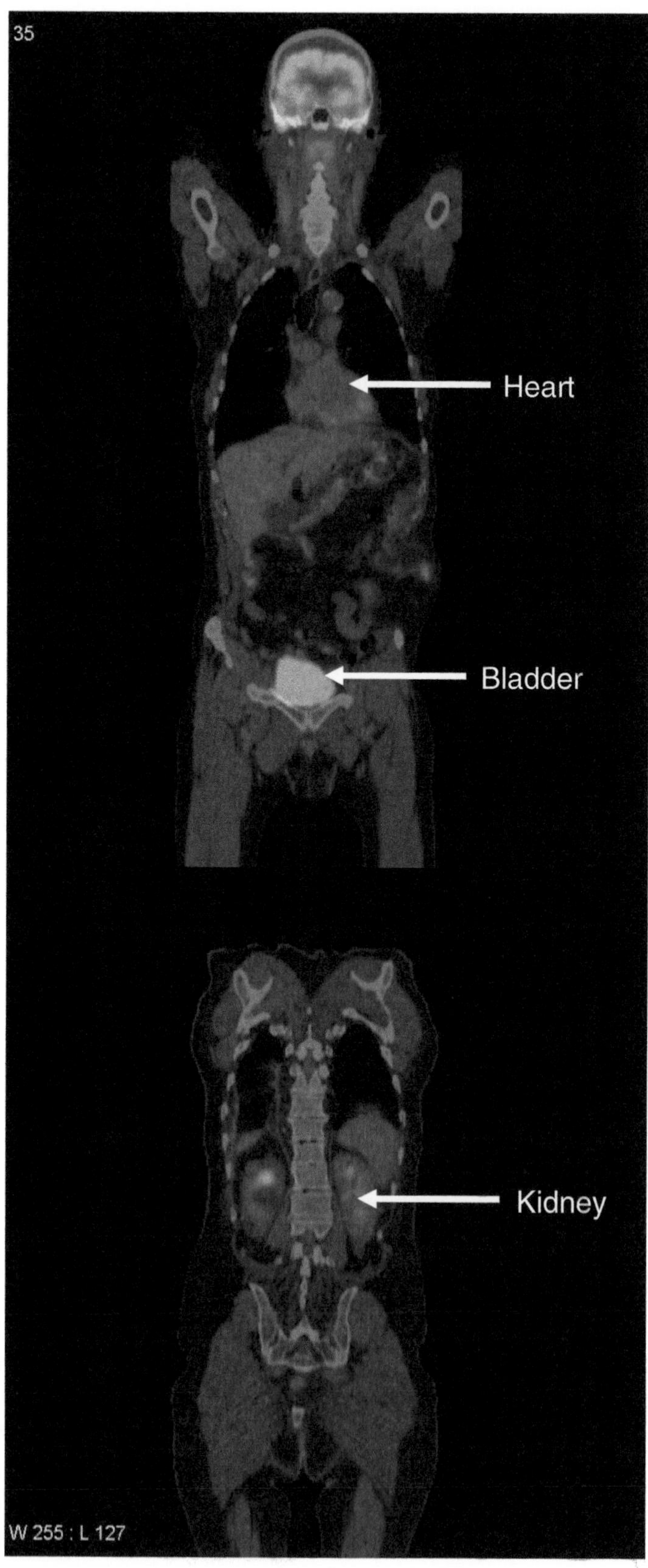

Fig. 2 Animal experiments suggest that radiation-induced toxicity progresses rather than recovers with time in the organs indicated by arrows (heart, kidney, bladder). Therefore, reirradiation of these organs might cause considerable late side effects

References

Abusaris H, Storchi PR, Brandwijk RP et al (2011) Second re-irradiation: efficacy, dose and toxicity in patients who received three courses of radiotherapy with overlapping fields. Radiother Oncol 99:235–239

Abusaris H, Hoogeman M, Nuyttens JJ (2012) Re-irradiation: outcome, cumulative dose and toxicity in patients retreated with stereotactic radiotherapy in the abdominal or pelvic region. Technol Cancer Res Treat 11:591–597

Ang KK, Price RE, Stephens LC et al (1995) The tolerance of primate spinal cord to re-irradiation. Int J Radiat Oncol Biol Phys 25:459–464

Ang KK, Jiang GL, Feng Y et al (2001) Extent and kinetics of recovery of occult spinal cord injury. Int J Radiat Oncol Biol Phys 50:1013–1020

Choi CY, Adler JR, Gibbs IC et al (2010) Stereotactic radiosurgery for treatment of spinal metastases recurring in close proximity to previously irradiated spinal cord. Int J Radiat Oncol Biol Phys 78:499–506

Coates J, Jeyaseelan AK, Ybarra N et al (2015) Contrasting analytical and data-driven frameworks for radiogenomic modeling of normal tissue toxicities in prostate cancer. Radiother Oncol 115:107–113

Combs SE, Thilmann C, Edler L et al (2005) Efficacy of fractionated stereotactic reirradiation in recurrent gliomas: long-term results in 172 patients treated in a single institution. J Clin Oncol 23:8863–8869

Combs SE, Burkholder I, Edler L et al (2010) Randomised phase I/II study to evaluate carbon ion radiotherapy versus fractionated stereotactic radiotherapy in patients with recurrent or progressive gliomas: the CINDERELLA trial. BMC Cancer 10:533

Damast S, Wright J, Bilsky M et al (2011) Impact of dose on local failure rates after image-guided reirradiation of recurrent paraspinal metastases. Int J Radiat Oncol Biol Phys 81:819–826

De Crevoisier R, Bourhis J, Domenge C et al (1998) Full-dose reirradiation for unresectable head and neck carcinoma: experience at the Gustave-Roussy Institute in a series of 169 patients. J Clin Oncol 16:3556–3562

Dritschilo A, Bruckman JE, Cassady JR, Belli JA (1981) Tolerance of brain to multiple courses of radiation therapy. I. Clinical experiences. Br J Radiol 54:782–786

Duprez F, Madani I, Bonte K et al (2009) Intensity-modulated radiotherapy for recurrent and second primary head and neck cancer in previously irradiated territory. Radiother Oncol 93:563–569

Evans JD, Gomez DR, Amini A et al (2013) Aortic dose constraints when reirradiating thoracic tumors. Radiother Oncol 106:327–332

Flickinger JC, Deutsch M, Lunsford LD (1989) Repeat megavoltage irradiation of pituitary and suprasellar tumours. Int J Radiat Oncol Biol Phys 17:171–175

Fogh SE, Andrews DW, Glass J et al (2010) Hypofractionated stereotactic radiation therapy: an effective therapy for recurrent high-grade gliomas. J Clin Oncol 28:3048–3053

Greenberger JS. (2009) Radioprotection. In Vivo. 23(2):323–36

Grosu AL, Andratschke N, Nieder C, Molls M (2002) Retreatment of the spinal cord with palliative radiotherapy. Int J Radiat Oncol Biol Phys 52:1288–1292

Haque W, Crane CH, Krishnan S et al (2009) Reirradiation to the abdomen for gastrointestinal malignancies. Radiat Oncol 4:55

Harms W, Krempien R, Grehn C et al (2004) Reirradiation of chest wall local recurrences from breast cancer. Zentralbl Gynakol 126:19–23

Hauswald H, Stoiber E, Rochet N et al (2010) Treatment of recurrent bronchial carcinoma: the role of high-dose-rate endoluminal brachytherapy. Int J Radiat Oncol Biol Phys 77:373–377

Heinzelmann F, Ottinger H, Engelhard M et al (2010) Advanced-stage III/IV follicular lymphoma: treatment strategies for individual patients. Strahlenther Onkol 186:247–254

Holt DE, Gill BS, Clump DA et al (2015) Tumor bed radiosurgery following resection and prior stereotactic radiosurgery for locally persistent brain metastasis. Front Oncol 5:84

Hornsey S, Myers R, Warren P (1982) Residual injury in the spinal cord after treatment with X-rays or neutrons. Br J Radiol 55:516–519

Jackson MA, Ball DL (1987) Palliative retreatment of locally recurrent lung cancer after radical radiotherapy. Med J Aust 147:391–394

Jentsch C, Beuthien-Baumann B, Troost EG et al (2015) Validation of functional imaging as a biomarker for radiation treatment response. Br J Radiol 88:20150014

Kerns SL, West CM, Andreassen CN et al (2014) Radiogenomics: the search for genetic predictors of radiotherapy response. Future Oncol 10:2391–2406

Kerns SL, Kundu S, Oh JH et al (2015) The prediction of radiotherapy toxicity using single nucleotide polymorphism-based models: a step toward prevention. Semin Radiat Oncol 25:281–291

Kim TH, Kim DY, Jung KH et al (2010) The role of omental flap transposition in patients with locoregional recurrent rectal cancer treated with reirradiation. J Surg Oncol 102:789–795

Kirkpatrick JP, van der Kogel AJ, Schultheiss TE (2010) Radiation dose-volume effects in the spinal cord. Int J Radiat Oncol Biol Phys. 1;76(3 Suppl):S42–9

Kishi K, Sonomura T, Shirai S et al (2009) Critical organ preservation in reirradiation brachytherapy by injectable spacer. Int J Radiat Oncol Biol Phys 75:587–594

Knowles JW (1983) The radiosensitivity of the guinea pig spinal cord to x-rays: the effect of retreatment at one year and the effect of age at the time of irradiation. Int J Radiat Biol 44:433–442

Kosaka Y, Okuno Y, Tagawa Y et al (2010) Osteoradionecrosis of the cervical vertebrae in patients irradiated for head and neck cancers. Jpn J Radiol 28:388–394

Landuyt W, van der Kogel AJ, de Roo M et al (1988) Unilateral kidney irradiation and late retreatment with cis-dichlorodiammineplatinum (II): functional measurements with 99m technetium-dimercaptosuccinic acid. Int J Radiat Oncol Biol Phys 14:95–101

Langendijk JA, Kasperts N, Leemans CR et al (2006) A phase II study of primary reirradiation in squamous cell carcinoma of head and neck. Radiother Oncol 78:306–312

Langer CJ, Harris J, Horwitz EM et al (2007) Phase II study of low-dose paclitaxel and cisplatin in combination with split-course concomitant twice-daily reirradiation in recurrent squamous cell carcinoma of the head and neck: results of Radiation Therapy Oncology Group Protocol 9911. J Clin Oncol 25:4800–4805

Lavey RS, Taylor J, Tward JD et al (1994) The extent, time course, and fraction size dependence of mouse spinal cord recovery from radiation injury. Int J Radiat Oncol Biol Phys 30:609–617

Lee AW, Law SC, Ng SH et al (1992) Retrospective analysis of nasopharyngeal carcinoma treated during 1976-1985: late complications following megavoltage irradiation. Br J Radiol 65:918–928

Lee AW, Foo W, Law SC (1997) Reirradiation for recurrent nasopharyngeal carcinoma: factors affecting the therapeutic ratio and ways for improvement. Int J Radiat Oncol Biol Phys 38:43–52

Lee AW, Foo W, Law SC et al (2000) Total biological effect on late reactive tissues following reirradiation for recurrent nasopharyngeal carcinoma. Int J Radiat Oncol Biol Phys 46:865–872

Lee DS, Woo JY, Kim JW et al (2016) Re-irradiation of hepatocellular carcinoma: clinical applicability of deformable image registration. Yonsei Med J 57:41–49

Lingareddy V, Ahmad NR, Mohiuddin M (1997) Palliative reirradiation for recurrent rectal cancer. Int J Radiat Oncol Biol Phys 38:785–790

Liu H, Zhang X, Vinogradskiy YY et al (2012) Predicting radiation pneumonitis after stereotactic ablative radiation therapy in patients previously treated with conventional thoracic radiation therapy. Int J Radiat Oncol Biol Phys 84:1017–1023

Liu S, Lu T, Zhao C et al (2014) Temporal lobe injury after re-irradiation of locally recurrent nasopharyngeal carcinoma using intensity modulated radiotherapy: clinical characteristics and prognostic factors. J Neurooncol 119:421–428

Machtay M, Rosenthal DI, Chalian AA et al (2004) Pilot study of postoperative reirradiation, chemotherapy, and amifostine after surgical salvage for recurrent head-and-neck cancer. Int J Radiat Oncol Biol Phys 59:72–77

Magrini SM, Biti GP, de Scisciolo G et al (1990) Neurological damage in patients irradiated twice on the spinal cord: a morphologic and electrophysiological study. Radiother Oncol 17:209–218

Mason KA, Withers HR, Chiang CS (1993) Late effects of radiation on the lumbar spinal cord of guinea pigs: re-treatment tolerance. Int J Radiat Oncol Biol Phys 26:643–648

Mayer R, Sminia P (2008) Reirradiation tolerance of the human brain. Int J Radiat Oncol Biol Phys 70:1350–1360

McAvoy SA, Ciura KT, Rineer JM et al (2013) Feasibility of proton beam therapy for reirradiation of locoregionally recurrent non-small cell lung cancer. Radiother Oncol 109:38–44

McDonald MW, Moore MG, Johnstone PA (2012) Risk of carotid blowout after reirradiation of the head and neck: a systematic review. Int J Radiat Oncol Biol Phys 82:1083–1089

Medin PM, Foster RD, van der Kogel AJ et al (2012) Spinal cord tolerance to reirradiation with single-fraction radiosurgery: a swine model. Int J Radiat Oncol Biol Phys 83:1031–1037

Meijneke TR, Petit SF, Wentzler D et al (2013) Reirradiation and stereotactic radiotherapy for tumors in the lung: dose summation and toxicity. Radiother Oncol 107:423–427

Mohiuddin M, Marks G, Marks J (2002) Long-term results of reirradiation for patients with recurrent rectal carcinoma. Cancer 95:1144–1150

Moman MR, Van der Poel HG, Battermann JJ et al (2009) Treatment outcome and toxicity after salvage 125-I implantation for prostate cancer recurrences after primary 125-I implantation and external beam radiotherapy. Brachytherapy 9:119–125

Montebello JF, Aron BS, Manatunga AK et al (1993) The reirradiation of recurrent bronchogenic carcinoma with external beam irradiation. Am J Clin Oncol 16:482–488

Nieder C, Price RE, Rivera B et al (2005a) Effects of insulin-like growth factor-1 (IGF-1) and amifostine in spinal cord reirradiation. Strahlenther Onkol 181:691–695

Nieder C, Grosu AL, Andratschke NH, Molls M (2005b) Proposal of human spinal cord reirradiation dose based on collection of data from 40 patients. Int J Radiat Oncol Biol Phys 61:851–855

Nieder C, Grosu AL, Andratschke NH, Molls M (2006a) Update of human spinal cord reirradiation tolerance based on additional data from 38 patients. Int J Radiat Oncol Biol Phys 66:1446–1449

Nieder C, Adam M, Molls M, Grosu AL (2006b) Therapeutic options for recurrent high-grade glioma in adult patients: recent advances. Crit Rev Oncol Hematol 60:181–193

Nieder C, Astner ST, Mehta MP et al (2008) Improvement, clinical course, and quality of life after palliative radiotherapy for recurrent glioblastoma. Am J Clin Oncol 31:300–305

Paulino AC, Mai WY, Chintagumpala M et al (2008) Radiation-induced malignant gliomas: is there a role for reirradiation? Int J Radiat Oncol Biol Phys 71:1381–1387

Peulen H, Karlsson K, Lindberg K et al (2011) Toxicity after reirradiation of pulmonary tumours with stereotactic body radiotherapy. Radiother Oncol 101:260–266

Raza SM, Jabbour S, Thai QA et al (2007) Repeat stereotactic radiosurgery for high-grade and large intracranial arteriovenous malformations. Surg Neurol 68:24–34

Reynaud A, Travis EL (1984) Late effects of irradiation in mouse jejunum. Int J Radiat Biol 46:125–134

Robbins ME, Bywaters T, Rezvani M et al (1991) Residual radiation-induced damage to the kidney of the pig as assayed by retreatment. Int J Radiat Biol 60:917–928

Ruifrok ACC, Kleiboer BJ, van der Kogel AJ (1992a) Fractionation sensitivity of the rat cervical spinal cord during radiation retreatment. Radiother Oncol 25:295–300

Ruifrok ACC, Kleiboer BJ, van der Kogel AJ (1992b) Reirradiation tolerance of the immature rat spinal cord. Radiother Oncol 23:249–256

Russell AH, Koh WJ, Markette K et al (1987) Radical reirradiation for recurrent or second primary carcinoma of the female reproductive tract. Gynecol Oncol 27:226–232

Sahgal A, Ma L, Weinberg V et al (2012) Reirradiation human spinal cord tolerance for stereotactic body radiotherapy. Int J Radiat Oncol Biol Phys 82:107–116

Schiff D, Shaw E, Cascino TL (1995) Outcome after spinal reirradiation for malignant epidural spinal cord compression. Ann Neurol 37:583–589

Schwartz C, Romagna A, Thon N et al (2015) Outcome and toxicity profile of salvage low-dose-rate iodine-125 stereotactic brachytherapy in recurrent high-grade gliomas. Acta Neurochir (Wien) 157:1757–1764

Shaw E, Scott C, Souhami L et al (1996) Radiosurgery for the treatment of previously irradiated recurrent primary brain tumours and brain metastases: initial report of radiation therapy oncology group protocol (90-05). Int J Radiat Oncol Biol Phys 34:647–654

Shaw E, Scott C, Souhami L et al (2000) Single dose radiosurgical treatment of recurrent previously irradiated primary brain tumours and brain metastases: final report of RTOG protocol 90-05. Int J Radiat Oncol Biol Phys 47:291–298

Shepherd SF, Laing RW, Cosgrove VP et al (1997) Hypofractionated stereotactic radiotherapy in the management of recurrent glioma. Int J Radiat Oncol Biol Phys 37:393–398

Simmonds RH, Hopewell JW, Robbins MEC (1989) Residual radiation-induced injury in dermal tissue: implications for retreatment. Br J Radiol 62:915–920

Sminia P, Mayer R (2012) External beam radiotherapy of recurrent glioma: radiation tolerance of the human brain. Cancers (Basel) 4:379–399

Sneed PK, Mendez J, Vemer-van den Hoek JG et al (2015) Adverse radiation effect after stereotactic radiosurgery for brain metastases: incidence, time course, and risk factors. J Neurosurg 123:373–386

Sterzing F, Hauswald H, Uhl M et al (2010) Spinal cord sparing reirradiation with helical tomotherapy. Cancer 116:3961–3968

Stewart FA, Oussoren Y, Luts A (1990) Long-term recovery and reirradiation tolerance of mouse bladder. Int J Radiat Oncol Biol Phys 18:1399–1406

Stewart FA, Oussoren Y, van Tinteren H et al (1994) Loss of reirradiation tolerance in the kidney with increasing time after single or fractionated partial tolerance doses. Int J Radiat Biol 66:169–179

Sulman EP, Schwartz DL, Le TT et al (2009) IMRT reirradiation of head and neck cancer-disease control and morbidity outcomes. Int J Radiat Oncol Biol Phys 73:399–409

Tada T, Fukuda H, Matsui K et al (2005) Non-small-cell lung cancer: reirradiation for loco-regional relapse previously treated with radiation therapy. Int J Clin Oncol 10:247–250

Terry NHA, Tucker SL, Travis EL (1988) Residual radiation damage in murine lung assessed by pneumonitis. Int J Radiat Oncol Biol Phys 14:929–938

Terry NHA, Tucker SL, Travis EL (1989) Time course of loss of residual radiation damage in murine skin assessed by retreatment. Int J Radiat Biol 55:271–283

Thibault I, Campbell M, Tseng CL et al (2015) Salvage stereotactic body radiotherapy (SBRT) following in-field failure of initial SBRT for spinal metastases. Int J Radiat Oncol Biol Phys 93:353–360

Tian YM, Zhao C, Guo Y et al (2014) Effect of total dose and fraction size on survival of patients with locally recurrent nasopharyngeal carcinoma treated with intensity-modulated radiotherapy: a phase 2, single-center, randomized controlled trial. Cancer 120:3502–3509

Van der Kogel AJ (1979) Late effects of radiation on the spinal cord. PhD thesis, University of Amsterdam, Amsterdam

Veninga T, Langendijk HA, Slotman BJ et al (2001) Reirradiation of primary brain tumours: survival, clinical response and prognostic factors. Radiother Oncol 59:127–137

Wondergem J, van Ravels FJ, Reijnart IW et al (1996) Reirradiation tolerance of the rat heart. Int J Radiat Oncol Biol Phys 36:811–819

Wong CS, Han Y (1997) Long-term recovery kinetics of radiation damage in rat spinal cord. Int J Radiat Oncol Biol Phys 37:171–179

Wong CS, Minkin S, Hill RP (1993) Re-irradiation tolerance of rat spinal cord to fractionated X-ray doses. Radiother Oncol 28:197–202

Wong CS, van Dyk J, Milosevic M et al (1994) Radiation myelopathy following single courses of radiotherapy and retreatment. Int J Radiat Oncol Biol Phys 30:575–581

Würschmidt F, Dahle J, Petersen C et al (2008) Reirradiation of recurrent breast cancer with and without concurrent chemotherapy. Radiat Oncol 3:28

Xiao W, Liu S, Tian Y et al (2015) Prognostic significance of tumor volume in locally recurrent nasopharyngeal carcinoma treated with salvage intensity-modulated radiotherapy. PLoS One 10:e0125351

Yamazaki H, Ogita M, Kodani N et al (2013) Frequency, outcome and prognostic factors of carotid blowout syndrome after hypofractionated re-irradiation of head and neck cancer using CyberKnife: a multi-institutional study. Radiother Oncol 107:305–309

Yamazaki H, Ogita M, Himei K et al (2015) Carotid blowout syndrome in pharyngeal cancer patients treated by hypofractionated stereotactic re-irradiation using CyberKnife: a multi-institutional matched-cohort analysis. Radiother Oncol 115:67–71

Ysebaert L, Truc G, Dalac S et al (2004) Ultimate results of radiation therapy for T1-T2 mycosis fungoides (including reirradiation). Int J Radiat Oncol Biol Phys 58:1128–1134

Fractionation Concepts

Carsten Nieder and Michael Baumann

Contents

The original version of this chapter was revised. An erratum to this chapter can be found at 10.1007/978-3-319-41825-4_78.

C. Nieder, MD (✉)
Department of Oncology and Palliative Medicine, Nordland Hospital, Prinsensgate 164, Bodø 8092, Norway
e-mail: carsten.nieder@nordlandssykehuset.no

M. Baumann, MD
Department of Radiation Oncology, Faculty of Medicine and University Hospital Carl Gustav Carus, Technische Universität Dresden, Fetscherstr. 74, Dresden 01307, Germany

OncoRay – National Center for Radiation Research in Oncology, Faculty of Medicine and University Hospital Carl Gustav Carus, Technische Universität Dresden, Helmholtz-Zentrum Dresden – Rossendorf, Fetscherstr. 74, Dresden 01307, Germany

Helmholtz-Zentrum Dresden – Rossendorf, Institute od Radiooncology, Dresden, Germany

Deutsches Konsortium für Translationale Krebsforschung (DKTK), Dresden und Deutsches Krebsforschungszentrum (DKFZ), Heidelberg, Germany

National Center for Tumor Diseases (NCT), Partner Site Dresden, Dresden, Germany

Abstract

This chapter summarizes the principles of fractionated radiotherapy and altered fractionation approaches. We also provide clinical reirradiation examples and isoeffect calculations. The vast majority of published reirradiation series consist of retrospective data or small prospective studies with limited statistical power. In addition, the typical patient populations are more heterogeneous than in first-line radiotherapy studies. For example, patients with local relapse, regional relapse, or second primary tumors might be included. Therefore, the level of evidence is not comparable to that of first-line radiotherapy, where many treatment recommendations and guidelines rely on large and well-designed prospective randomized trials or meta-analyses of several trials. Reirradiation is often used to palliative symptoms, but occasionally a curative approach, which requires high cumulative radiation

Med Radiol Radiat Oncol (2016)
DOI 10.1007/174_2016_60, © Springer International Publishing Switzerland
Published Online: 07 May 2016

doses, is possible and should be offered. A key consideration is to apply high precision radiotherapy techniques. Hyperfractionated reirradiation might theoretically improve the therapeutic ratio, but prospective trials are required to confirm this hypothesis. Many recent studies actually relied on more convenient hypofractionated regimens.

1 Background

Radiobiological research during the twentieth century has indicated that fractionation of the total radiation dose often produces better tumor control for a given level of normal tissue toxicity than a single large dose. Better normal tissue sparing might result from repair of sublethal radiation damage between dose fractions. Beneficial effects such as reoxygenation of tumor cells and reassortment of cells into radiosensitive phases of the cell cycle may contribute to better tumor control for the same level of normal tissue damage when compared to single-dose application. However, it was also realized that prolonged overall treatment time may result in repopulation of cancer cells and thus be disadvantageous. In many clinical instances, regimens consisting of administration of 1.8–2 Gy once daily five times per week were considered standard (Hellman 1975; Greenberg et al. 1976; Holsti et al. 1978; Dörr et al. 1996; Beck-Bornholdt et al. 1997; Baumann and Gregoire 2009; Baumann and Krause 2009; Mauguen et al. 2012). Clinical interest in the use of more and smaller dose fractions in radical radiotherapy was stimulated by experimental normal tissue studies (Stewart et al. 1984). It has been found that if the dose per fraction is reduced (i.e., in hyperfractionation where a higher number of fractions of less than 1.8 Gy is given, usually two fractions per day) there is sparing of late responding normal tissues relative to those which respond early (Withers et al. 1982; Withers 1985; Niewald et al. 1998). This phenomenon can be understood in terms of the shapes of the underlying dose-effect relationships, which can be described using the linear-quadratic equation. The ratio (alpha/beta) of the linear (alpha) and quadratic (beta) terms is a useful measure of the curviness of such dose-effect curves. Low alpha/beta values (1.5–5 Gy) have been observed for late responding normal tissues and indicate that radiation damage should be greatly spared by the use of dose fractions smaller than the 1.8–2 Gy used in conventional radiotherapy. By contrast, the high alpha/beta values (6–14 Gy) observed for acutely responding normal tissues indicate that the response is relatively linear over the dose range of clinical interest. Hence, less extra sparing effect is to be expected if lower doses per fraction are administered (Hermann et al. 2006; Baumann and Gregoire 2009; Bentzen and Joiner 2009; Joiner and Bentzen 2009). If tumors respond in the same way as acutely responding normal tissues, then hyperfractionation might confer a therapeutic gain relative to late responding normal tissues. Basically, this effect is caused by differences in repair capability. Clinical studies of hyperfractionation assumed that moderate escalation of the total dose would improve tumor control rates without causing excess late complications (Fig. 1). However, the radiation fractions should not be given too close together, certainly not closer than 6 h, because of incomplete damage repair (Joiner 1993; Baumann and Gregoire 2009; Joiner and Bentzen 2009).

In the context of reirradiation, the issue of normal tissue toxicity is of utmost importance. While acute toxicity largely is comparable to that of first-line treatment, late toxicity resulting from high cumulative radiation doses has often been observed (Simmonds et al. 1989; Stewart 1999). Chronically progressive fibrosis, stenosis, and perfusion deficits resulting in tissue necrosis have been described. Their impact on quality of life and organ function might be severe. With regard to palliative reirradiation, late toxicity might not become clinically apparent during the limited life span of most patients. However, the situation might be different in patients treated with curative intent (Nieder et al. 2000). It is therefore necessary to assess the biologically effective dose (BED) and late effects of the initial course of radiotherapy and to exclude patients who

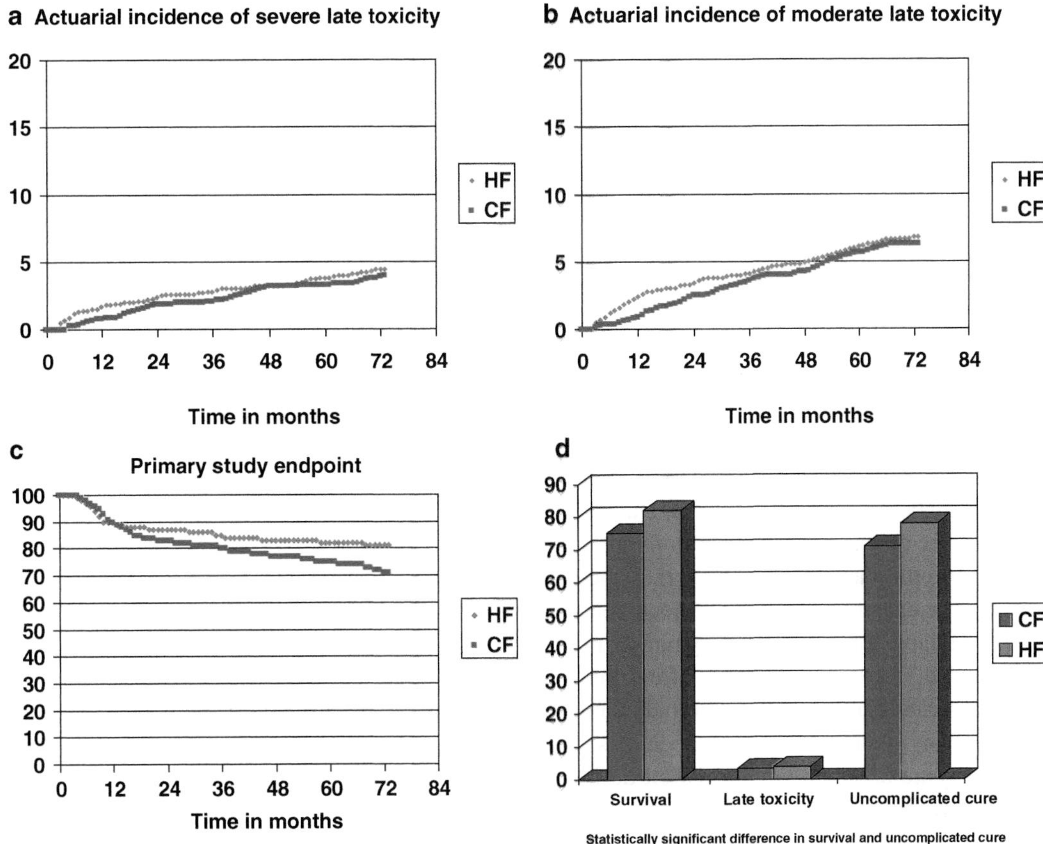

Fig. 1 (**a–d**) Hypothetical outcome of hyperfractionated (*HF*) as compared to conventional radiotherapy (*CF*), e.g., in head and neck squamous cell carcinoma. Actuarial curves displaying the primary study endpoint, e.g., overall survival and development of late toxicity. Hyperfractionated radiotherapy results in a therapeutic gain and increased rate of uncomplicated cure, i.e., survival without serious side effects

tolerated their previous treatment poorly. In addition, efforts must be made to limit the volume of reirradiated normal tissues. Today's improved target volume imaging and definition approaches as well as image-guided high precision techniques contribute to volume reduction and improved dose distribution. Proton radiotherapy may in the future add to current options for high conformity reirradiation techniques. Harnessing high precision technology might even allow for hypofractionated short-course reirradiation as demonstrated, e.g., in palliative treatment of head and neck cancer (Heron et al. 2011), recurrent high-grade gliomas (Grosu et al. 2005; Nieder et al. 2008; Fogh et al. 2010), stereotactic irradiation of lung (Peulen et al. 2011; Meijneke et al. 2013; Kilburn et al. 2014) and stereotactic radiosurgery of vestibular schwannomas (Yomo et al. 2009), spinal metastases (Choi et al. 2010), or brain metastases (Maranzano et al. 2012). Single doses were also given with intraoperative approaches, e.g., in rectal cancer (Haddock et al. 2001). In addition, several brachytherapy regimens have been used, e.g., in prostate and head and neck cancer (Burri et al. 2010). Intraoperative radiotherapy and single fraction radiosurgery are not the focus of this chapter. The disease-specific chapters provide details on such approaches. In a Canadian survey on reirradiation, many respondents recommended brachytherapy or highly conformal external irradiation techniques (Joseph et al. 2008). Hyperfractionated schedules were suggested as a means of limiting retreatment toxicity. Obviously, hyperfractionation was among the few strategies available in the past and also utilized by one of the authors of this chapter in the 1990s (Nieder et al. 1999) before positron emission tomography (PET), intensity-modulated radiotherapy (IMRT), proton beams, and other tools became a part of our armamentarium.

Reirradiation is not a new idea, some clinical studies were published already more than 40 years ago and some of these included patients treated as early as 1940 (Shehata et al. 1974; Fu et al. 1975; Hunter and Stewart 1977; Laramore et al. 1978; Dritschilo et al. 1981). The same holds true for accompanying experimental studies (Brown and Probert 1975). The vast majority of published reirradiation series consist of retrospective data or small prospective studies. In addition, the typical patient populations are more heterogeneous than in first-line radiotherapy studies. For example, patients with local relapse, regional relapse, or second primary tumors might be included. Therefore, the level of evidence is not comparable to that of first-line radiotherapy, where many treatment recommendations and guidelines are based on large and well-designed prospective randomized trials or meta-analyses of several trials. However, it appears that reirradiation not only palliates cancer-related symptoms but, under certain circumstances, might contribute to improved survival, especially in diseases where local control determines survival (Jereczek-Fossa et al. 2008). One example is a study of 108 children with relapsed ependymoma where 66 % received radiotherapy at relapse and 50 % of older children were reirradiated, and where reirradiation was associated with better outcome (Messahel et al. 2009). In a smaller study, which included 25 patients with previously irradiated recurrent medulloblastoma, a trend towards better event-free survival was seen in patients who received additional radiotherapy as part of their retrieval therapy (Dunkel et al. 2010). Limited evidence is also available from reirradiation of benign tumors such as pituitary adenoma (Schoenthaler et al. 1992). In a randomized trial, 130 patients with head and neck cancer were treated with salvage surgery and randomly assigned to full-dose reirradiation combined with chemotherapy or to observation. Full-dose reirradiation combined with chemotherapy after salvage surgery significantly improved disease-free survival, but had no significant impact on overall survival (Janot et al. 2008).

2 Hyperfractionation in First-Line Radiotherapy

The clinical evaluation of hyperfractionated radiotherapy in patients with advanced squamous cell carcinoma of the head and neck started in the 1970s (Meoz et al. 1984). EORTC protocol 22791 compared once-daily fractionation of 70 Gy in 35–40 fractions in 7–8 weeks, to pure hyperfractionation of 80.5 Gy in 70 fractions in 7 weeks using 2 fractions of 1.15 Gy per day (i.e., same conventional overall treatment time), in T2-T3 oropharyngeal carcinoma (excluding base of tongue), node negative, or N1 of less than 3 cm (Horiot et al. 1992). From 1980 to 1987, 356 patients were randomized. As published in 1992, the local control was significantly higher ($p=0.02$) after hyperfractionation. The multivariate Cox model confirmed that the treatment regimen was an independent significant prognostic factor for locoregional control ($p=0.007$). This improvement of locoregional control was responsible for a trend to an improved survival ($p=0.08$). There was no difference in late normal tissue damage between the two treatment modalities, although some controversy exists about the certainty to which differences in normal tissue damage may be excluded by this and other trials (Baumann et al. 1998; Baumann and Beck-Bornholdt 1999; Bentzen et al. 1999). Several trials of unconventional fractionated radiotherapy in head and neck squamous cell carcinoma followed, e.g., by the RTOG (Fu et al. 2000), but the effect of such treatment on survival remained unclear. A meta-analysis of updated individual patient data was performed (Bourhis et al. 2006). Trials were grouped in three prespecified categories: hyperfractionated, accelerated, and accelerated with total dose reduction. Tumor sites were mostly oropharynx and larynx; 74 % of patients had stage III-IV disease. There was a significant survival benefit with altered fractionated radiotherapy, corresponding to an absolute benefit of 3.4 % at 5 years (hazard ratio 0.92, 95 % CI 0.86–0.97; $p = 0.003$). The benefit was significantly higher with hyperfractionated radiotherapy (8 % at 5 years) than with accelerated radiotherapy (2 % with accelerated fractionation without total dose reduction and 1.7 % with total dose reduction at 5 years, $p = 0.02$). There was a benefit on locoregional control in favor of altered fractionation versus conventional radiotherapy (6.4 % at 5 years; $p < 0.0001$), which was particularly efficient in reducing local failure, whereas the benefit on nodal control was less pronounced.

Certain side effects such as development of radiation retinopathy might also be less likely in patients with head and neck cancer treated with hyperfractionated radiotherapy. In a study by Monroe et al. (Monroe et al. 2005), 186 patients received a significant dose to the retina as part of curative radiotherapy. Primary sites included nasopharynx, paranasal sinus, nasal cavity, and palate. Hyperfractionated radiation was delivered to 42 % of the patients in the study, typically at 1.1–1.2 Gy per fraction. The remainder were treated once daily. Thirty-one eyes in 30 patients developed radiation retinopathy, resulting in monocular blindness in 25, bilateral blindness in one, and decreased visual acuity in four. The actuarial incidence of developing radiation retinopathy was 20 % at both 5 and 10 years. Higher retinal doses resulted in a steady increase in the incidence of retinopathy, with 25 of the 30 cases occurring after 60 Gy or more. Of the patients receiving more than 50 Gy to the retina, hyperfractionation was associated with a significantly lower incidence of radiation retinopathy (37 % vs. 13 %; $p = 0.0037$). On multivariate analysis, retinal dose ($p < 0.0001$) and fractionation schedule ($p = 0.0003$) were significant predictors of radiation retinopathy.

Patients with localized unresectable non-small cell carcinoma of the lung were also treated with hyperfractionated regimens, e.g. 1.2 Gy twice daily (Seydel et al. 1985). Of 120 eligible patients, 10 received a dose of 50.4 Gy, 20 received 60.0 Gy, 79 received 69.6 Gy, and 11 patients received 74.4 Gy. Complete regression occurred in 19 % of T1-T3, N0-N2 patients. There were six cases of severe and two of life-threatening toxicity, but there were no fatalities attributable to the treatment. Toxicity consisted mainly of pneumonitis and pulmonary fibrosis as well as esophagitis. Median survival of the entire group was 7.2 months, which was consistent with previous experience at that time. It was later found that all five of the 5-year survivors came from the 79 patients assigned to receive 69.6 Gy (Cox et al. 1991). Combined stage II and III 5-year survival rates were 8 % for 69.6 Gy compared to 6 % for standard once-a-day irradiation in concurrent RTOG trials. A randomized phase III trial shed more light on the issue of hyperfractionation (Sause et al. 1995). Three arms were evaluated (1) standard radiation therapy, (2) induction chemotherapy followed by standard radiation therapy, and (3) twice-daily radiation therapy. Patients were required to have a Karnofsky performance status of 70 or more and weight loss less than 5 % for 3 months prior to entry into the trial. Of the 490 patients registered in the trial, 452 were eligible. The disease in 95 % of the patients was stage IIIA or IIIB. Patients were randomly assigned to receive either 60 Gy of radiation therapy delivered at 2 Gy per fraction, 5 days a week, over a 6-week period (standard radiation therapy), induction chemotherapy consisting of cisplatin and vinblastine followed by standard radiation therapy starting on day 50, or 69.6 Gy delivered at 1.2 Gy per fraction twice daily. One-year survival (%) and median survival (months) were as follows: standard radiation therapy – 46 %, 11.4 months; chemotherapy plus radiotherapy – 60 %, 13.8 months; and hyperfractionated radiation therapy – 51 %, 12.3 months. The chemotherapy plus radiotherapy arm was statistically superior to the other two treatment arms ($p = 0.03$). This was confirmed in a later analysis of the trial (Sause et al. 2000). Other groups explored hyperfractionation in non-randomized studies of early stage non-small cell lung cancer (Jeremić and Milicić 2008, Jeremic et al. 1997). However, other developments (accelerated radiotherapy (Mauguen et al. 2012), concomitant chemoradiation (Aupérin et al. 2010, stereotactic body radiotherapy (Zhang et al. 2014)) outperformed classical hyperfractionation, which has not evolved into a standard of care in non-small cell lung cancer.

Hyperfractionated radiotherapy was studied in a large variety of other cancer types, but no general benefit was found. One of the unsuccessful examples is high-grade gliomas (Nieder et al. 2004). None of the glioma studies reviewed in 2004 reported a significant improvement in survival by altered fractionation in comparison to either institutional historical controls or their respective randomized control arm.

3 Hyperfractionated Reirradiation

In contrast to first-line radiotherapy where systematic efforts were undertaken to compare different fractionation regimens, no such randomized comparisons are available. The retrospective series reported by Bauman et al. (Bauman et al. 1996) included 17 patients with primary CNS tumors who received hyperfractionated reirradiation and 17 patients treated with once-daily fractionation (Table 1). Some children, e.g., with medulloblastoma were included in this heterogeneous population. Median overall survival was 8.3 months in all 34 patients. The actuarial risk of necrosis was 22 % at 1 year following retreatment. Fractionation had no statistically significant influence on overall survival, progression-free survival, or increased complications in this study with limited statistical power. A retrospective comparison in patients with rectal cancer was reported in 1997 (Lingareddy et al. 1997). The study included 52 patients, 22 of whom opted for hyperfractionated radiotherapy, while the others preferred conventional once-daily treatment, mainly for logistical reasons. Ninety percent received concomitant 5-FU. Fractionation had no statistically significant influence on overall survival, but late toxicity was significantly reduced in patients who had received hyperfractionated treatment (relative risk 3.9, 95 % confidence limit 1.1–14.4). No such correlation was found in the retrospective study of reirradiation for rectal cancer patients who underwent resection after reirradiation with concurrent 5-FU (Mohiuddin et al. 1997). Another study in rectal cancer where all patients received hyperfractionated reirradiation reported relatively moderate rates of late toxicity (necessitating surgery in only one patient, Table 1), but 15 % serious postoperative complications in those patients who eventually underwent tumor resection after chemoradiation (Valentini et al. 2006). The other studies summarized in Table 1 were not designed to evaluate the impact of hyperfractionation on outcome. In patients reirradiated for head and neck cancer and analyzed for development of carotid blowout syndrome (CBOS), the rate of CBOS was 1.3 % in those treated in a continuous course with 1.8–2 Gy daily fractions or 1.2 Gy twice-daily fractions (McDonald et al. 2012). However, the rate was 4.5 % in patients treated with 1.5 Gy twice daily in alternating weeks or with delayed accelerated hyperfractionation ($p=0.002$). Another retrospective study on reirradiation of head and neck cancer patients treated with hyperfractionated radiotherapy with 1.2 Gy up to 66 Gy showed that 56 % of the surviving patients will develop grade 3 or higher toxicity (Lohaus et al. 2013). Thus, there is very limited evidence supporting the hypothesis that hyperfractionated reirradiation, which is challenging with regard to logistics and resource utilization, would improve the therapeutic index by reducing late toxicity. On the other hand, the regimens evaluated so far were often administered with treatment planning approaches and technology that are no longer in use, resulting in unnecessary large volumes of irradiated normal tissues. This leads us to conclude that a randomized trial of conventional versus hyperfractionated reirradiation utilizing, e.g., image-guided IMRT or IMPT would be of interest.

Table 2 summarizes the results of hyperfractionated-accelerated reirradiation. In these studies, the typical dose per fraction was 1.5 Gy. If one intends to administer a total dose of 45 Gy in a hyperfractionated accelerated fashion, i.e., 1.5 Gy b.i.d., 15 treatment days are needed. This compares to 25 treatment days when once-daily treatment with 1.8 Gy per fraction is chosen. As with hyperfractionated reirradition, no randomized trials have been published. Given the design and size of the available studies, no

Table 1 Hyperfractionated reirradiation: study overview

Reference	Study type	Disease site	Number of patients	Interval between series	Reirradiation	Side effects	Median survival
Lingareddy et al. (1997)	Retrospective	Locally recurrent rectal cancer	22 out of 52 in the study	Minimum 3 months, median 24 months[a]	30 Gy with or without additional boost, varying total doses, 1.2 Gy b.i.d., typically with concurrent 5-FU	Acute grade III toxicity in 31 %[a]. Late grade III-IV toxicity in 33%[a]	12 months[a]
Mohiuddin et al. (1997)	Retrospective	Locally recurrent rectal cancer	21 out of 39 in the study	Minimum 3 months, median 18 months[a]	30 Gy with or without additional boost, varying total doses, 1.2 Gy b.i.d., typically with concurrent 5-FU, resection 8–12 weeks later	Treatment break or termination in 18 %[a]. Delayed wound healing in 7 %[a]. Severe late toxicity in 28 %[a].	45 months[a]
Valentini et al. (2006)	Multicenter phase II	Locally recurrent rectal cancer	59	Minimum 9 months, median 27 months	30 Gy + 10.8 Gy boost, 1.2 Gy b.i.d., concurrent 5-FU, resection 6–8 weeks later, then chemotherapy	12 % of patients developed late toxicity	42 months
Karam et al. (2015)	Retrospective	Recurrent nasopharyngeal carcinoma	32 out of 42 in the study	Minimum not reported, median 4.6 years	Total dose 40–60 Gy, 1.1–1.4 Gy b.i.d., typically with chemotherapy, IMRT in 27 patients	Late grade III-IV toxicity rate 37 % at 3 years[a]	3-year survival 49%[a]
Popovtzer et al. (2009)	Retrospective	Recurrent squamous cell head and neck cancer	31 out of 66 in the study	Minimum 6 months, median 37 months[a]	Total dose 70 Gy at 1.25 Gy b.i.d. with concurrent cisplatin and 5-FU	Acute grade III-V in 10 %. Late grade III-V in 29 %	Approximately 19 months (estimated from the published graph)[a]
Benchalal et al. (1995)	Pilot study	Head and neck cancer	19	Minimum 9 months, median 30 months	Total dose 60 Gy at 1.2 Gy b.i.d.	Acute grade III toxicity in 47 %. Late grade III toxicity in 11 %	Approximately 18 months (estimated from the published graph)
Bauman et al. (1996)	Retrospective	Primary central nervous system tumors	17	Minimum 3.7 months, median 17.5 months	Total dose 30–44 Gy, in some cases over 60 Gy at 1.0 Gy b.i.d.	1 case of necrosis, 1 of cognitive decline, 1 of increased tumor cyst	Not reported
Lohaus et al. (2013)	Retrospective	Recurrent squamous cell head and neck cancer	34 out of 40 in the study	Minimum 6 months, median 12 months	Total dose 60–66 Gy at 1.2 Gy b.i.d. with concurrent cisplatin and 5-FU	Late grade III-IV toxicity in 56 %	18 months

[a]Relates to all patients including those treated with conventional fractionation

Table 2 Hyperfractionated-accelerated reirradiation: study overview (not all head and neck cancer studies are shown)

Reference	Study type	Disease site	Number of patients	Interval between series	Reirradiation	Side effects	Median survival
Abdel-Wahab et al. (1997)	Pilot study	Relapsed brain metastases	15	Minimum 8 weeks, median 10 months	Limited brain fields after previous WBRT; 1.5 Gy b.i.d., median 30 Gy	No serious toxicity	3.2 months
Nieder et al. (1999)	Retrospective	Relapsed high-grade gliomas	32	Minimum 8 weeks, median 20 months	Limited brain fields; 1.3 Gy b.i.d., total dose 45.5 Gy (during the later part of the study 1.5 Gy b.i.d., total dose 45 Gy)	16 % late toxicity including 2 patients with radionecrosis	8.5 months
Spencer et al. (2008)	Multi-institutional prospective trial RTOG 9610	Unresectable recurrent squamous cell carcinoma of the head and neck	79	Minimum 0.6 years, median 2.5 years	4 weekly cycles of chemoradiotherapy separated by 1 week of rest; 1.5 Gy b.i.d., total dose 60 Gy	6 deaths in acute period, acute grade IV in 18 %, late grade III and IV in 22 %, feeding tube at last follow-up in 70 %	8.5 months
Watkins et al. (2009)	Retrospective	Locoregionally recurrent head and neck tumors	39	Minimum 0.5 years, median 2.3 years	4 weekly cycles of chemoradiotherapy separated by 1 week of rest; 1.5 Gy b.i.d., total dose 60 Gy	4 deaths in acute period, acute grade IV in 10 %, late grade III-V in 56 %	19 months
Haque et al. (2009)	Retrospective	Gastrointestinal tumors (pancreas, bile duct, colon etc.)	13	Minimum 5 months, median 26 months	Typically 30–39 Gy total dose, 1.5 Gy b.i.d.	Late grade III toxicity: 0, late grade IV toxicity: 1 (8 %)	14 months
Das et al. (2010)	Retrospective	Rectal cancer	50	Minimum 0.4 years, median 2.3 years	If interval <1 year: 30 Gy If interval ≥ 1 year: 39 Gy 1.5 Gy b.i.d. Typically with concurrent capecitabine	Late grade III or IV toxicity: 13 (26 %)	26 months

WBRT whole brain radiotherapy, *RTOG* Radiation Therapy Oncology Group definitive conclusions can be drawn. However, comparison with studies where conventional fractionation was employed in the same cancer types does not provide strong indications for improved efficacy or therapeutic ratio. This should be considered in clinical decision making, as illustrated in the example provided in Fig. 2. Figure 3 elaborates on the usefulness of isoeffect calculations in reirradiation scenarios. The BED obtained with different fractionation regimens is calculated in Table 3A and 3B.

4 Low-Dose Ultrafractionation

The principles of this unconventional approach including a historical perspective will be reviewed briefly. In an early clinical trial, 168 patients with carcinoma of the bladder, T2-T4, were randomized to one of two treatments, 1.0 Gy 3 times a day to a total dose of 84 or 2 Gy once a day to a total dose of 64 Gy (Edsmyr et al. 1985). Both treatments were given over 8 weeks with a rest interval of 2 weeks in the middle of the treatment period. This is different from current chemoradiation approaches in bladder cancer. Local eradication of the tumor in the bladder cystoscopically and cytologically at 6 months after completion of treatment and patient survival were analyzed. The results favored significantly for the patients treated with 84 Gy. A report from 1994 included all patients after a follow-up period of at least 10 years (Näslund et al. 1994). The survival benefit from dose-escalated hyperfractionation initially reported after 5 years was still evident after 10 years. The effect was detectable in all three stages (T2, T3, and T4) and in the pooled data. However, it only reached statistical significance in the T3 subset and in the total pooled data set. An improvement in local control was seen, but the differences were not statistically significant. Complications in the bowel requiring surgical treatment were more common in the hyperfractionated group, but with the statistical power (number of events) of this trial the difference was not significant. During the same era, comparable fractionation regimens were studied in breast cancer patients, but they never entered clinical routine (Notter and Turesson 1984). It was then shown in tumor cell lines, many of them considered radioresistant, that low-dose hyperradiosensitivity at fraction doses ≤0.5 Gy might exist and several radiobiological explanations for this phenomenon were discussed (Joiner et al. 2001; Short et al. 2001; Tomé and Howard 2007; Simonsson et al. 2008). However, studies on tumor models in vivo, including those generated from cell lines showing low-dose hyperradiosensitivity in vitro, failed to show any advantage of ultrafractionated radiotherapy with 3 doses of 0.4 Gy per day of 6 weeks compared to conventional fractionation to the same dose (Krause et al. 2003; Krause et al. 2005a, b).

A clinical reirradiation study included 11 highly selected adult patients (Pulkkanen et al. 2007). Three-dimensional conformal beam radiotherapy was used. Three fractions of 0.5 Gy (nine patients) or 0.6–0.66 Gy were given daily 4 h apart. The total dose was 30–51 Gy (median 45 Gy) with treatment times of 28–46 days. The minimum interval was 1 year, median 6 years. Previous radiotherapy typically had been given with 50–60 Gy. Favorable local control was observed in patients with grade II and III gliomas. Three patients with rectal cancer progressed locally after 3–12 months. One patient with lung metastasis from rectal cancer progressed locally after 10 months. However, palliation of symptoms could be achieved. Neither acute nor late toxicity was observed. In this small series, it is difficult to estimate with regard to efficacy the impact of favorable tumor biology, as indicated by the long time interval from initial radiotherapy to relapse. The time interval might also explain the toxicity results. It is thus not clear whether comparable outcome might have been obtained with other fractionation regimens, which demand less resources and are more convenient to patients.

5 Pulse-Reduced Dose Rate (PRDR) Reirradiation

This technique was used for large-volume glioma recurrences by Magnuson et al. (2014). An apparent dose rate of 0.067 Gy/min is achieved

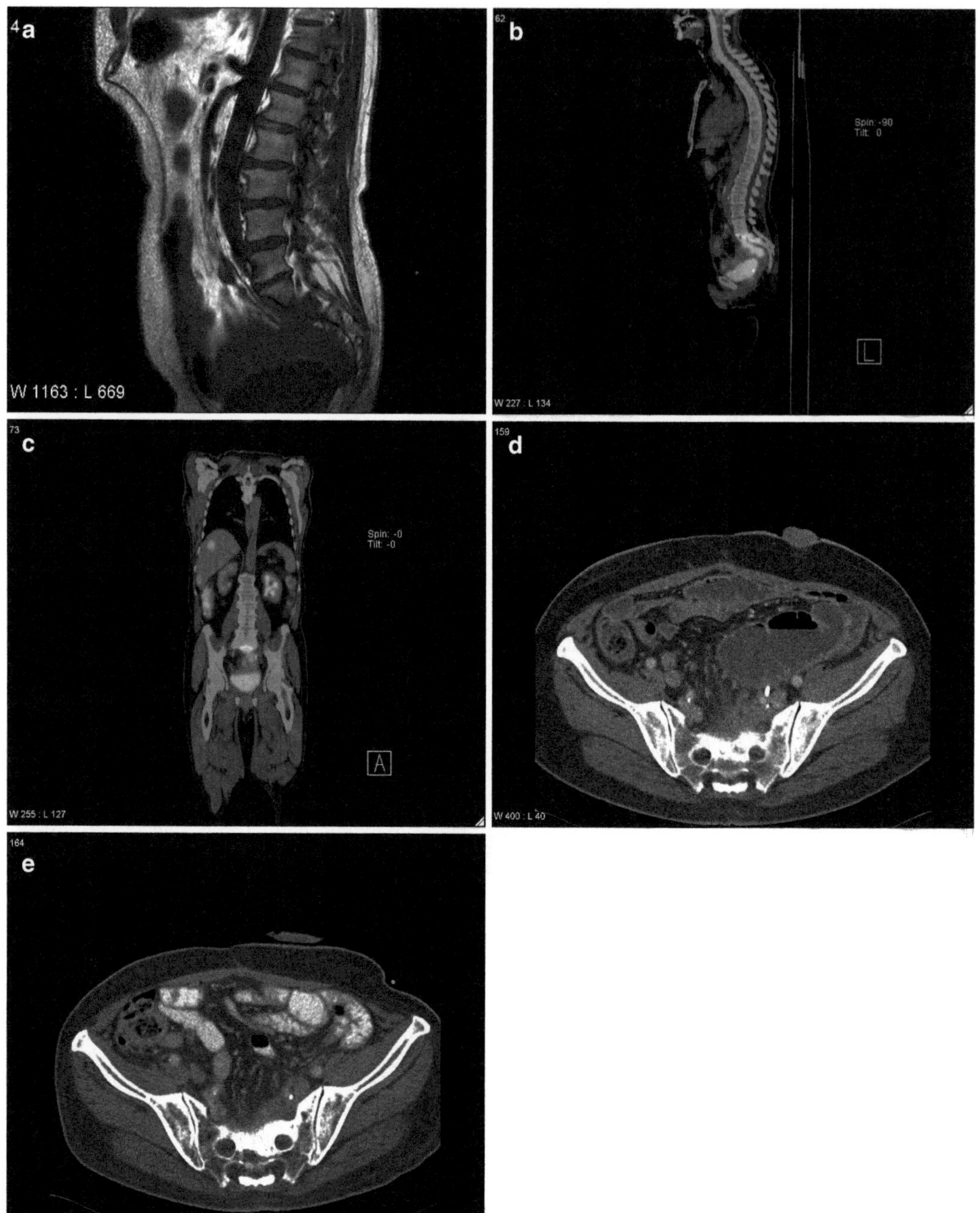
4a
W 1163 : L 669
62
b
Spin: -90
Tilt: 0
L
W 227 : L 134
73
c
Spin: -0
Tilt: -0
A
W 255 : L 127
159
d
W 400 : L 40
164
e
W 400 : L 40

by giving 0.2 Gy pulses separated by 3-min intervals. Their study included 23 patients with glioblastoma after progression on bevacizumab and earlier standard radiotherapy plus temozolomide. Within 7–14 days of progression on bevacizumab, patients initiated reirradiation to a dose of 54 Gy in 27 fractions using PRDR radiotherapy. The median planning target volume was 424 cm^3. At the start of reirradiation, bevacizumab (10 mg/kg) was given every 4 weeks for two additional cycles. The median survival and 6-month survival after bevacizumab failure was 6.9 months and 65 %, respectively. Reirradiation was well tolerated with no symptomatic grade 3–4 toxicities. Additional studies are needed to fully understand the clinical role of this approach.

6 Hypofractionation in Randomized Clinical Reirradiation Studies

Chow et al. (2014) performed a large multicenter randomized trial in patients who had radiologically confirmed painful bone metastases. Patients were randomly assigned (1:1) to receive either 8 Gy in a single fraction or 20 Gy in multiple fractions (most often five), stratified by previous radiation fraction schedule, response to initial radiation, and treatment center. The primary endpoint was overall pain response at 2 months. The most frequently reported acute radiation-related toxicities at 14 days were lack of appetite (201 [56 %] of 358 assessable patients who received 8 Gy vs. 229

Fig. 2 An illustrative case from one of the authors' institutions (Nordland Hospital Bodø, Norway). A 56-year-old male patient was diagnosed with anal cancer stage T3 N0 M0 in 1997. He received radiotherapy (40 Gy plus 10 Gy boost in 2-Gy fractions) with concomitant 5-FU and mitomycin-C. In 2001, the patient developed local relapse and was salvaged surgically. In 2007, both local relapse in the presacral region and liver metastases were detected. Palliative chemotherapy was initiated, first cisplatin and 5-FU, then 5-FU and mitomycin-C. Because of increasing pelvic pain, the patient was referred for palliative reirradiation in December 2008. The liver metastases were stable. No obvious late toxicity from the initial course of radiotherapy was present. The patients Karnofsky performance status (KPS) at that time was 70. We considered the following key questions. Is the patient's performance status at a level that justifies initiation of radiation therapy? Yes, the KPS was 70. Do laboratory tests point to advanced hepatic disease and/or poor tolerability/efficacy of the planned therapy? No, the only abnormal finding was slight anemia and elevated alkaline phosphatase. Are other disease sites absent or controlled and if so, does one expect continued disease control? The liver metastases were stable. Will systemic treatment be offered or are there no more options left? Taxane-based chemotherapy was an option. Will local control impact on the survival of the patient or is treatment focused on palliation of symptoms? The aim was palliation of pelvic pain. Might the cumulative radiation dose to critical normal tissue structures result in serious toxicity in patients with expect prolonged survival? The probability of bowel or bladder toxicity, insufficiency fracture, or nerve damage was considered low and the same holds true for the probability of long-term survival. How did the tumor respond to initial radiotherapy and how long is the interval? Complete remission was obtained in 1997 and the interval of 11 years did permit reirradiation. The magnetic resonance, positron emission tomography (PET), and computed tomography (CT) images above show the presacral tumor mass, its bony extension, two liver metastases, and a ureteral stent. Tables 1 and 2 provide an overview on rectal cancer reirradiation studies, which might guide decision making. When deciding between hyperfractionated, conventional, and hypofractionated three-dimensional conformal radiotherapy in this case, the following facts were considered. The planning target volume resulting from the PET-CT-defined gross tumor volume did not include large volumes of bowel or bladder. The interval from initial treatment was very long. No concomitant chemotherapy would be added because the patient had previous heavy exposure to the standard drugs. Because of a lack of clinical data in the reirradiation setting, taxanes or oxaliplatin were not considered. Thus, we decided that hypofractionated reirradiation appeared feasible in this palliative setting. The patient received 12 fractions of 3 Gy in January 2009. He developed urinary infection and received antibiotics and a new stent. No other acute complications or toxicity was registered. Pelvic pain improved, though not completely. No additional systemic treatment was given. At the last follow-up in February 2010, the presacral tumor was stable (CT image panel **e**), and the patient was without obvious late toxicity

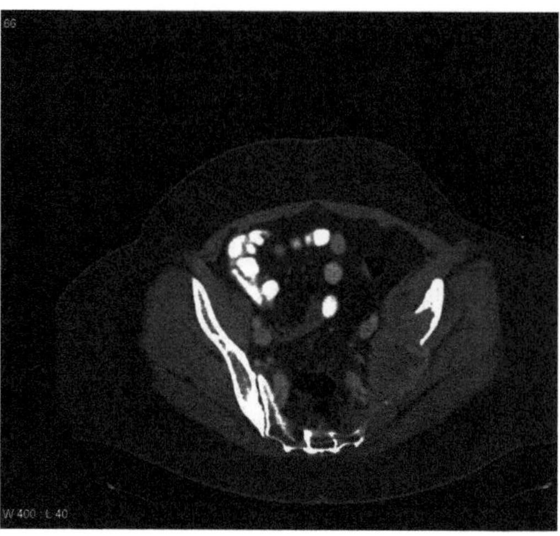

Fig. 3 An illustrative case from one of the authors' institutions (Nordland Hospital Bodø, Norway). A 49-year-old female patient was diagnosed with metastasized high-grade leiomyosarcoma of the uterus with multiple lung metastases and two bone metastases in 2005. After hysterectomy, she received three cycles of adriamycin without objective response. Palliative radiotherapy to a large painful pelvic bone metastasis (computed tomography (CT) image below) was given in May 2006, and the total dose was 39 Gy in 13 fractions of 3 Gy. Two anterior-posterior opposing fields were used. The lesion diminished in size (<50 % reduction) and then remained stable until February 2008 when the patient presented with increasing pain and bone destruction and was referred for reirradiation. She had not received second-line chemotherapy. With regard to potential side effects and fractionation of reirradiation, the following considerations are important. On a planning CT scan with empty bladder, the amount of reirradiated bladder was judged to be minimal. Bony structures had to be reirradiated to full dose as they were part of the clinical target volume. The same holds true for certain muscles and soft tissue. The skin could be spared to a large degree with three-dimensional treatment planning. The major organs at risk were small and large bowel and the sacral and presacral nerve roots and nerves. When calculating the biologically effective dose (BED) of the first irradiation course, one has to keep in mind that two opposing fields were used resulting in a maximum dose to parts of the bowel of 105 % of the prescribed dose, which was 3 Gy. Thus, these parts had received 13 fractions of 3.15 Gy. We will use an alpha/beta value of 3 Gy in this example. The resulting BED is 13 × 3.15 × (1 + 3.15÷3), i.e., 84 Gy_3, according to the formula $n \times d \times$ (1+ d÷alpha/beta value) where n is the number of fractions and d the dose per fraction. This dose is actually equivalent to 50 Gy in 25 fractions of 2 Gy (BED 83 Gy_3). If one wishes to limit the reirradiation BED to the equivalent of 40 Gy in 20 fractions of 2 Gy (BED 67 Gy_3), the following alternatives result: 40 Gy in 20 fractions of 2 Gy, 35 Gy in 14 fractions of 2.5 Gy (BED 64 Gy_3), 30 Gy in 10 fractions of 3 Gy (BED 60 Gy_3), 28 Gy in 7 fractions of 4 Gy (BED 65 Gy_3) and, of course, lower doses such as 20 Gy in 5 fractions of 4 Gy. For an alpha/beta value of 4 Gy, the same reirradiation schedules would be feasible. The previous regimen of 39 Gy in 13 fractions had resulted in a quite long palliative benefit and no obvious late toxicity. The choice will now depend on the patient's life expectation and willingness to accept the possible consequences of bowel, soft tissue, and nerve toxicity. Other factors such as travel distance might also impact on the patient's preference

[66 %] of 349 assessable patients who received 20 Gy; $p = 0.01$) and diarrhea (81 [23 %] of 357 vs. 108 [31 %] of 349; $p = 0.02$). Treatment with 8 Gy in a single fraction seemed to be non-inferior and less toxic than 20 Gy in multiple fractions; however, as findings were not robust in a per-protocol analysis, trade-offs between efficacy and toxicity might exist. This issue is discussed further in the chapter on bone metastases. Patients with bone metastases receive moderate cumulative total doses, even if reirradiated. Therefore, clinically significant late toxicity is usually not anticipated.

The study on nasopharyngeal carcinoma by Tian et al. (2014) is much more informative for late toxicity endpoints. This group randomized 117 patients, whereof 85 % had initial 2-D radiotherapy (median dose 70 Gy). The median time interval was 2 years. The median recurrent tumor volume was 31 vs. 36.5 cc (79 % had T3 or T4

Table 3A Isoeffect calculations: the biologically effective dose (BED) of different fractionation regimens is shown (formula $n \times d \times (1+ d \div \text{alpha/beta ratio})$ where n is the number of fractions and d the dose per fraction as described in Baumann and Gregoire 2009)

	Tumor cells and acute responding normal tissues Alpha/beta ratio 10 Gy	Spinal cord Alpha/beta ratio 2 Gy	Other late responding normal tissue Alpha/beta ratio 3 Gy	Other late responding normal tissue Alpha/beta ratio 4 Gy
First course, 60 Gy in 30 fractions of 2 Gy, once daily	72 Gy_{10}	Exceeds commonly accepted constraints	100 Gy_3	90 Gy_4
Same fractionation, but normal tissue sparing[a]		79 Gy_2[a] Equivalent to 40 Gy in 2-Gy fractions	67.5 Gy_3[a] Equivalent to 40 Gy in 2-Gy fractions	62 Gy_4[a] Equivalent to 42 Gy in 2-Gy fractions

It is assumed that acute responding tissues react to reirradiation in the same manner as to first-line radiotherapy. Regarding late responding tissues, it has been demonstrated that the fractionation sensitivity of the rat cervical spinal cord during reirradiation was not significantly different from the fractionation sensitivity of not previously irradiated control rats, with an alpha/beta ratio of 2.3 Gy in control rats and 1.9 Gy during reirradiation of the spinal cord (Ruifrok et al. 1992). The alpha/beta ratio of tumors might vary. A second primary squamous cell carcinoma in the aerodigestive tract might have the same alpha/beta ratio as a squamous cell carcinoma treated several years earlier in the same patient. However, that might not necessarily be true for a locally recurrent squamous cell carcinoma arising from malignant cells that survived a radical course of radiotherapy and where the surviving clonogens might be biologically different from the ones that could be eradicated

[a]The maximum normal tissue dose in this example is 30 fractions of 1.5 Gy, i.e., 75 % of the prescription dose of 2 Gy

tumors). IMRT to 68 Gy in 34 fractions was compared to a moderately hypofractionated regimen of 60 Gy in 27 fractions (2.22 Gy), 5 fractions per week. Both regimens were equivalent according to the time-corrected LQ model with $\alpha/\beta = 10$ Gy for tumor cells. For normal tissue with $\alpha/\beta = 3$ Gy (no time factor), BED is reduced from 113 to 104 Gy_3 (minus 8 %) in the 60-Gy arm. No significant differences in survival nor different types of failure-free survival were detected, but the study was not designed as an equivalence study. Significantly more mucosal necrosis occurred after 68 Gy (51 vs. 29 %, hazard ratio 2.3, 95 % CI 1.1–5.0, $p = 0.02$). There was also a numerically greater risk of massive hemorrhage resulting from necrosis (31 vs. 19 %, hazard ratio 1.7, 95 % CI 0.7–4.3, $p = 0.12$). No significant differences were found regarding temporal lobe necrosis (21 %), cranial nerve palsy (13 %), trismus, and other toxicities. Besides dose/fractionation, tumor volume influenced the risk of mucosal necrosis. The authors classified 51 % of deaths in the 68-Gy arm as treatment related, as compared to 40 % in the 60-Gy arm. Their results suggest that moderately hypofractionated reirradiation is feasible.

7 A Small Randomized Study of Conventionally Fractionated External Beam Radiotherapy Versus High-Dose-Rate (HDR) Brachytherapy

In this study conducted between 2008 and 2011, 64 patients with head and neck cancer recurrence were randomly assigned at a 1:1 ratio to receive either 3-D conformal radiotherapy (25 fractions of 2 Gy) or HDR brachytherapy (30 Gy, 2.5 Gy twice daily, at least 6-h interval) (Rudžianskas et al. 2014). Unfortunately, the authors failed to state the primary endpoint and underlying statistical assumptions for their study. The median initial dose was 66 Gy (minimum 50 Gy), and the median interval to reirradiation 15 months. Absence of grade 3 or higher late toxicity after the first course was required. More than 70 % of the patients were node positive when entering the study. Surgery before reirradiation was permitted. Despite randomization, a statistically significant difference regarding size of the PTV was observed (median 177 cm^3 in the external beam arm vs. 35 cm^3 in the brachytherapy arm). Therefore, the

Table 3B The hypothetical patient from Table 3A is considered for different reirradiation scenarios where the spinal cord is the major dose-limiting organ

Dose to tumor	Dose to spinal cord	Spinal cord BED Alpha/beta ratio 2 Gy	Comment on cumulative spinal cord BED[a], interval >6 months	Comment on cumulative spinal cord BED[a], shorter interval
First course, 60 Gy in 30 fractions of 2 Gy, once daily	30 fractions of 1.5 Gy	79 Gy_2 Equivalent to 40 Gy in 2-Gy fractions		
Reirradiation 8 Gy in 1 fraction	1 fraction of 8 Gy	40 Gy_2 Equivalent to 20 Gy in 2-Gy fractions	119 Gy_2 Equivalent to 60 Gy in 2-Gy fractions Myelopathy risk score 0	119 Gy_2 Equivalent to 60 Gy in 2-Gy fractions Myelopathy risk score 4.5
Reirradiation 30 Gy in 10 fractions of 3 Gy, once daily	10 fractions of 3 Gy	75 Gy_2 Equivalent to 38 Gy in 2-Gy fractions	154 Gy_2 Equivalent to 76 Gy in 2-Gy fractions Myelopathy risk score 4	154 Gy_2 Equivalent to 76 Gy in 2-Gy fractions Myelopathy risk score 8.5
Reirradiation 30 Gy in 15 fractions of 2 Gy, once daily	15 fractions of 2 Gy	60 Gy_2 Equivalent to 30 Gy in 2-Gy fractions	139 Gy_2 Equivalent to 70 Gy in 2-Gy fractions Myelopathy risk score 2	139 Gy_2 Equivalent to 70 Gy in 2-Gy fractions Myelopathy risk score 6.5
Reirradiation 60 Gy in 30 fractions of 2 Gy, once daily	30 fractions of 1.4 Gy	71 Gy_2 Equivalent to 36 Gy in 2-Gy fractions	150 Gy_2 Equivalent to 74 Gy in 2-Gy fractions Myelopathy risk score 3	150 Gy_2 Equivalent to 74 Gy in 2-Gy fractions Myelopathy risk score 7.5
Reirradiation 60 Gy in 30 fractions of 2 Gy, once daily	30 fractions of 1.0 Gy	45 Gy_2 Equivalent to 22 Gy in 2-Gy fractions	124 Gy_2 Equivalent to 62 Gy in 2-Gy fractions Myelopathy risk score 1	124 Gy_2 Equivalent to 62 Gy in 2-Gy fractions Myelopathy risk score 5.5

A risk score of ≤3 points suggests a myelopathy risk of <5 %, i.e., comparable to that of previously unirradiated patients
A risk score of 4–6 points suggests a myelopathy risk of approximately 25 %
A risk score of >6 points suggests a myelopathy risk of approximately 90 %
[a]Myelopathy risk derived from Nieder et al. (2006) (based on cumulative BED, interval between the two radiotherapy courses <6 months and BED of one course ≥102 Gy_2, i.e., the equivalent of more than 50 Gy in 2-Gy fractions)

observed differences in outcome might result from the small study size and imbalances in baseline characteristics. No attempts were made to adjust for the effects of the reirradiation regimen in a multivariate model. The difference in grade 3–4 acute toxicity was not significant (34 % after brachytherapy vs. 55 % in the other arm). However, the difference in late toxicity was ($p=0.001$; one case of osteoradionecrosis after brachytherapy vs. two such cases plus three pharyngeal strictures, one skin ulceration, one severe laryngeal edema, and other complications in the other arm). Survival (2-year rate 67 vs. 32 %) and local control (2-year rate 63 vs. 25 %) were also significantly better after brachytherapy.

References

Abdel-Wahab MM, Wolfson AH, Raub W et al (1997) The role of hyperfractionated re-irradiation in metastatic brain disease: a single institutional trial. Am J Clin Oncol 20:158–160

Aupérin A, Le Péchoux C, Rolland E et al (2010) Meta-analysis of concomitant versus sequential radiochemotherapy in locally advanced non-small-cell lung cancer. J Clin Oncol 28:2181–2190

Bauman GS, Sneed PK, Wara WM et al (1996) Reirradiation of primary CNS tumors. Int J Radiat Oncol Biol Phys 36:433–441

Baumann M, Beck-Bornholdt HP (1999) Hyperfractionated radiotherapy: tops or flops. Med Pediat Oncol 33:399–402

Baumann M, Gregoire V (2009) Modified fractionation. In: Joiner M, van der Kogel A (eds) Basic clinical radiobiology. London, Hodder Arnold, pp 135–148

Baumann M, Krause M (2009) Linear-quadratisches Modell und Fraktionierung. In: Bamberg M, Molls M, Sack H (eds) Radioonkologie Band 1 Grundlagen, 2nd edn. W. Zuckschwerdt Verlag GmbH, München, pp 251–267

Baumann M, Bentzen S, Ang KK (1998) Hyperfractionated radiotherapy in head and neck cancer: a second look at the clinical data. Radiother Oncol 46:127–130

Beck-Bornholdt HP, Dubben HH, Liertz-Petersen C, Willers H (1997) Hyperfractionation: where do we stand? Radiother Oncol 43:1–21

Benchalal M, Bachaud JM, François P et al (1995) Hyperfractionation in the reirradiation of head and neck cancers. Result of a pilot study. Radiother Oncol 36:203–210

Bentzen SM, Joiner MC (2009) The linear-quadratic approach in clinical practice. In: Joiner M, van der Kogel A (eds) Basic clinical radiobiology, 4th edn. Hodder Education, London, pp 120–134

Bentzen SM, Saunders MI, Dische S (1999) Repair halftimes estimated from observations of treatment-related morbidity after CHART or conventional radiotherapy in head and neck cancer. Radiother Oncol 53: 219–226

Bourhis J, Overgaard J, Audry H et al (2006) Hyperfractionated or accelerated radiotherapy in head and neck cancer: a meta-analysis. Lancet 368: 843–854

Brown JM, Probert JC (1975) Early and late radiation changes following a second course of irradiation. Radiology 115:711–716

Burri RJ, Stone NN, Unger P et al (2010) Long-term outcome and toxicity of salvage brachytherapy for local failure after initial radiotherapy for prostate cancer. Int J Radiat Oncol Biol Phys 77:1338–1344

Choi CY, Adler JR, Gibbs IC et al (2010) Stereotactic radiosurgery for treatment of spinal metastases recurring in close proximity to previously irradiated spinal cord. Int J Radiat Oncol Biol Phys 78:499–506

Chow E, van der Linden YM, Roos D et al (2014) Single versus multiple fractions of repeat radiation for painful bone metastases: a randomised, controlled, noninferiority trial. Lancet Oncol 15:164–171

Cox JD, Pajak TF, Herskovic A et al (1991) Five-year survival after hyperfractionated radiation therapy for non-small-cell carcinoma of the lung (NSCCL): results of RTOG protocol 81-08. Am J Clin Oncol 14:280–284

Das P, Delclos ME, Skibber JM et al (2010) Hyperfractionated accelerated radiotherapy for rectal cancer in patients with prior pelvic irradiation. Int J Radiat Oncol Biol Phys 77:60–65

Dörr W, Baumann M, Herrmann T (1996) Nomenclature of modified fractionation protocols in radiotherapy. Strahlenther Onkol 172:353–355

Dritschilo A, Bruckman JE, Cassady JR, Belli JA (1981) Tolerance of brain to multiple courses of radiation therapy. Br J Radiol 54:782–786

Dunkel IJ, Gardner SL, Garvin JH Jr et al (2010) High-dose carboplatin, thiotepa, and etoposide with autologous stem cell rescue for patients with previously irradiated recurrent medulloblastoma. Neuro Oncol 12:297–303

Edsmyr F, Andersson L, Esposti PL et al (1985) Irradiation therapy with multiple small fractions per day in urinary bladder cancer. Radiother Oncol 4:197–203

Fogh SE, Andrews DW, Glass J et al (2010) Hypofrationated stereotactic radiation therapy: an effective therapy for recurrent high-grade gliomas. J Clin Oncol 28:3048–3053

Fu KK, Newman H, Phillips TL (1975) Treatment of locally recurrent carcinoma of the nasopharynx. Radiology 117:425–431

Fu KK, Pajak TF, Trotti A et al (2000) A Radiation Therapy Oncology Group (RTOG) phase III randomized study to compare hyperfractionation and two variants of accelerated fractionation to standard fractionation radiotherapy for head and neck squamous cell carcinomas: first report of RTOG 9003. Int J Radiat Oncol Biol Phys 48:7–16

Greenberg M, Eisert DR, Cox JD (1976) Initial evaluation of reduced fractionation in the irradiation of malignant epithelial tumors. AJR Am J Roentgenol 126: 268–278

Grosu AL, Weber WA, Franz M et al (2005) Reirradiation of recurrent high-grade gliomas using amino acid PET (SPECT)/CT/MRI image fusion to determine gross tumor volume for stereotactic fractionated radiotherapy. Int J Radiat Oncol Biol Phys 63:511–519

Haddock MG, Gunderson LL, Nelson H et al (2001) Intraoperative irradiation for locally recurrent colorectal cancer in previously irradiated patients. Int J Radiat Oncol Biol Phys 49:1267–1274

Haque W, Crane CH, Krishnan S et al (2009) Reirradiation to the abdomen for gastrointestinal malignancies. Radiat Oncol 4:55

Hellman S (1975) Cell kinetics, models, and cancer treatment – some principles for the radiation oncologist. Radiology 114:219–223

Hermann T, Baumann M, Dörr W (2006) Klinische Strahlenbiologie: kurz und bündig, 4th edn. Elsevier GmbH/Urban & Fischer Verlag, München

Heron DE, Rwigema JC, Gibson MK et al (2011) Concurrent cetuximab with stereotactic body radiotherapy for recurrent squamous cell carcinoma of the head and neck: a single institution matched case-control study. Am J Clin Oncol 34:165–172

Holsti LR, Salmo M, Elkind MM (1978) Unconventional fractionation in clinical radiotherapy. Br J Cancer Suppl 3:307–310

Horiot JC, Le Fur R, N'Guyen T et al (1992) Hyperfractionation versus conventional fractionation in oropharyngeal carcinoma: final analysis of a randomized trial of the EORTC cooperative group of radiotherapy. Radiother Oncol 25:231–241

Hunter RD, Stewart JG (1977) The tolerance of re-irradiation of heavily irradiated human skin. Br J Radiol 50:573–575

Janot F, de Raucourt D, Benhamou E et al (2008) Radomized trial of postoperative reirradiation combined with chemotherapy after salvage surgery compared with salvage surgery alone in head and neck carcinoma. J Clin Oncol 26:5518–5523

Jereczek-Fossa BA, Kowalczyk A, D'Onofrio A (2008) Three-dimensional conformal or stereotactic reirradiation of recurrent, metastatic or new primary tumors. Analysis of 108 patients. Strahlenther Onkol 184:36–40

Jeremić B, Milicić B (2008) From conventionally fractionated radiation therapy to hyperfractionated radiation therapy alone and with concurrent chemotherapy in patients with early-stage nonsmall cell lung cancer. Cancer 112:876–884

Jeremic B, Shibamoto Y, Acimovic L et al (1997) Hyperfractionated radiotherapy alone for clinical stage I nonsmall cell lung cancer. Int J Radiat Oncol Biol Phys 38(3):521–525

Joiner MC (1993) Hyperfractionation and accelerated radiotherapy. In: Steel GG (ed) Basic clinical radiobiology. London, Arnold Publishers, pp 65–71

Joiner MC, Bentzen SM (2009) Fractionation: the linear-quadratic approach. In: Joiner M, van der Kogel A (eds) Basic clinical radiobiology, 4th edn. Hodder Education, London, pp 102–119

Joiner MC, Marples B, Lambin P et al (2001) Low-dose hypersensitivity: current status and possible mechanisms. Int J Radiat Oncol Biol Phys 49:379–389

Joseph KJ, Al-Mandhari Z, Pervez N et al (2008) Reirradiation after radical radiation therapy: a survey of patterns of practice among Canadian radiation oncologists. Int J Radiat Oncol Biol Phys 72:1523–1529

Karam I, Huang SH, McNiven A et al (2015) Outcomes after reirradiation for recurrent nasopharyngeal carcinoma: North American experience. Head Neck doi: 10.1002/hed.24166

Kilburn JM, Kuremsky JG, Blackstock AW et al (2014) Thoracic re-irradiation using stereotactic body radiotherapy (SBRT) techniques as first or second course of treatment. Radiother Oncol 110:505–510

Krause M, Hessel F, Wohlfarth J et al (2003) Ultrafractionation in A7 human malignant glioma in nude mice. Int J Radiat Biol 79:377–383

Krause M, Prager J, Wohlfarth J et al (2005a) Ultrafractionation dose not improve the results of radiotherapy in radioresistant murine DDL1 lymphoma. Strahlenther Onkol 181:440–444

Krause M, Wohlfarth J, Georgi B et al (2005b) Low-dose hyperradiosensitivity of human glioblastoma cell lines in vitro does not translate into improved outcome of ultrafractionated radiotherapy in vivo. Int J Radiat Biol 81:751–758

Laramore GE, Griffin TW, Parker RG et al (1978) The use of electron beams in treating local recurrence of breast cancer in previously irradiated fields. Cancer 41:991–995

Lingareddy V, Ahmad NR, Mohiuddin M (1997) Palliative reirradiation for recurrent rectal cancer. Int J Radiat Oncol Biol Phys 38:785–790

Lohaus F, Appold S, Krause M, Baumann M (2013) Local recurrence rate and toxicities after curative reirradiation of HNSCC. Strahlenther Onkol Suppl 1:P24

Magnuson W, Ian Robins H, Mohindra P, Howard S (2014) Large volume reirradiation as salvage therapy for glioblastoma after progression on bevacizumab. J Neurooncol 117:133–139

Maranzano E, Trippa F, Casale M et al (2012) Reirradiation of brain metatases with radiosurgery. Radiother Oncol 102:192–197

Mauguen A, Péchoux L, Saunders MI et al (2012) Hyperfractionated or accelerated radiotherapy in lung cancer: an individual patient data meta-analysis. J Clin Oncol 30:2788–2797

McDonald MW, Moore MG, Johnstone PA (2012) Risk of carotid blowout after reirradiation of the head and neck: a systematic review. Int J Radiat Oncol Biol Phys 82:1083–1089

Meijneke TR, Petit SF, Wentzler D, Hoogeman M, Nuyttens JJ (2013) Reirradiation and stereotactic radiotherapy for tumors in the lung: dose summation and toxicity. Radiother Oncol 107:423–427

Meoz RT, Fletcher GH, Peters LJ et al (1984) Twice-daily fractionation schemes for advanced head and neck cancer. Int J Radiat Oncol Biol Phys 10:831–836
Messahel B, Ashley S, Saran F et al (2009) Relapsed intracranial ependymoma in children in the UK: patterns of relapse, survival and therapeutic outcome. Eur J Cancer 45:1815–1823
Mohiuddin M, Marks GM, Lingareddy V, Marks J (1997) Curative surgical resection following reirradiation for recurrent rectal cancer. Int J Radiat Oncol Biol Phys 39:643–649
Monroe AT, Bhandare N, Morris CG, Mendenhall WM (2005) Preventing radiation retinopathy with hyperfractionation. Int J Radiat Oncol Biol Phys 61: 856–864
Näslund I, Nilsson B, Littbrand B (1994) Hyperfractionated radiotherapy of bladder cancer. A ten-year follow-up of a randomized clinical trial. Acta Oncol 33: 397–402
Nieder C, Nestle U, Niewald M et al (1999) Hyperfractionated reirradiation for malignant glioma. Front Radiat Ther Oncol 33:150–157
Nieder C, Milas L, Ang KK (2000) Tissue tolerance to reirradiation. Semin Radiat Oncol 10:200–209
Nieder C, Andratschke N, Wiedenmann N et al (2004) Radiotherapy for high-grade gliomas. Does altered fractionation improve the outcome? Strahlenther Onkol 180:401–407
Nieder C, Grosu AL, Andratschke NH, Molls M (2006) Update of human spinal cord reirradiation tolerance based on additional data from 38 patients. Int J Radiat Oncol Biol Phys 66:1446–1449
Nieder C, Astner ST, Mehta MP et al (2008) Improvement, clinical course, and quality of life after palliative radiotherapy for recurrent glioblastoma. Am J Clin Oncol 31:300–305
Niewald M, Feldmann U, Feiden W et al (1998) Multivariate logistic analysis of dose-effect relationship and latency of radiomyelopathy after hyperfractionated and conventionally fractionated radiotherapy in animal experiments. Int J Radiat Oncol Biol Phys 41:681–688
Notter G, Turesson I (1984) Multiple small fractions per day versus conventional fractionation. Comparison of normal tissue reactions and effect on breast carcinoma. Radiother Oncol 1:299–308
Peulen H, Karlsson K, Lindberg K et al (2011) Toxicity after reirradiation of pulmonary tumours with stereotactic body radiotherapy. Radiother Oncol 101:260–266
Popovtzer A, Gluck I, Chepeha DB et al (2009) The pattern of failure after reirradiation of recurrent squamous cell head and neck cancer: implications for defining the targets. Int J Radiat Oncol Biol Phys 74:1342–1347
Pulkkanen K, Lahtinen T, Lehtimäki A et al (2007) Effective palliation without normal tissue toxicity using low-dose ultrafractionated re-irradiation for tumor recurrence after radical or adjuvant radiotherapy. Acta Oncol 46:1037–1041
Rudžianskas V, Inčiūra A, Vaitkus S et al (2014) Reirradiation for patients with recurrence head and neck squamous cell carcinoma: a single-institution comparative study. Medicina (Kaunas) 50:92–99
Ruifrok AC, Kleiboer BJ, van der Kogel AJ (1992) Fractionation sensitivity of the rat cervical spinal cord during radiation retreatment. Radiother Oncol 25:295–300
Sause WT, Scott C, Taylor S et al (1995) Radiation Therapy Oncology Group (RTOG) 88-08 and Eastern Cooperative Oncology Group (ECOG) 4588: preliminary results of a phase III trial in regionally advanced, unresectable non-small-cell lung cancer. J Natl Cancer Inst 87:198–205
Sause W, Kolesar P, Taylor S IV et al (2000) Final results of phase III trial in regionally advanced unresectable non-small cell lung cancer: Radiation Therapy Oncology Group, Eastern Cooperative Oncology Group, and Southwest Oncology Group. Chest 117:358–364
Schoenthaler R, Albright NW, Wara WM et al (1992) Reirradiation of pituitary adenoma. Int J Radiat Oncol Biol Phys 24:307–314
Seydel HG, Diener-West M, Urtasun R et al (1985) Hyperfractionation in the radiation therapy of unresectable non-oat cell carcinoma of the lung: preliminary report of a RTOG Pilot Study. Int J Radiat Oncol Biol Phys 11:1841–1847
Shehata WM, Hendrickson FR, Hindo WA (1974) Rapid fractionation technique and re-treatment of cerebral metastases by irradiation. Cancer 34:257–261
Short SC, Kelly J, Mayes CR et al (2001) Low-dose hypersensitivity after fractionated low-dose irradiation in vitro. Int J Radiat Biol 77:655–664
Simmonds RH, Hopewell JW, Robbins ME (1989) Residual radiation-induced injury in dermal tissue: implications for retreatment. Br J Radiol 62:915–920
Simonsson M, Qvarnström F, Nyman J et al (2008) Low-dose hypersensitive gammaH2AX response and infrequent apoptosis in epidermis from radiotherapy patients. Radiother Oncol 88:388–397
Spencer SA, Harris J, Wheeler RH et al (2008) Final report of RTOG 9610, a multi-institutional trial of reirradiation and chemotherapy for unresectable recurrent squamous cell carcinoma of the head and neck. Head Neck 30:281–288
Stewart FA (1999) Re-treatment after full-course radiotherapy: is it a viable option? Acta Oncol 38:855–862
Stewart FA, Soranson JA, Alpen EL et al (1984) Radiation-induced renal damage: the effects of hyperfractionation. Radiat Res 98:407–420
Tian YM, Zhao C, Guo Y et al (2014) Effect of total dose and fraction size on survival of patients with locally recurrent nasopharyngeal carcinoma treated with intensity-modulated radiotherapy: a phase 2, single-center, randomized controlled trial. Cancer 120:3502–3509
Tomé WA, Howard SP (2007) On the possible increase in local tumour control probability for gliomas exhibiting low dose hyper-radiosensitivity using a pulsed schedule. Br J Radiol 80:32–37
Valentini V, Morganti AG, Gambacorta MA et al (2006) Preoperative hyperfractionated chemoradiation for

locally recurrent rectal cancer in patients previously irradiated to the pelvis: a multicentric phase II study. Int J Radiat Oncol Biol Phys 64:1129–1139

Watkins JM, Shirai KS, Wahlquist AE et al (2009) Toxicity and survival outcomes of hyperfractionated split-course reirradiation and daily concurrent chemotherapy in locoregionally recurrent, previously irradiated head and neck cancers. Head Neck 31:493–502

Withers HR (1985) Biological basis for altered fractionation schemes. Cancer 55:2086–2095

Withers HR, Peters LJ, Thames HD, Fletcher GH (1982) Hyperfractionation. Int J Radiat Oncol Biol Phys 8:1807–1809

Yomo S, Arkha Y, Delsanti C et al (2009) Repeat gamma knife surgery for regrowth of vestibular schwannomas. Neurosurgery 64:48–54

Zhang B, Zhu F, Ma X et al (2014) Matched-pair comparisons of stereotactic body radiotherapy (SBRT) versus surgery for the treatment of early stage non-small cell lung cancer: a systematic review and meta-analysis. Radiother Oncol 112:250–255

Hyperthermia and Reirradiation

Oliver J. Ott and Manfred Schmidt

Contents

Abstract

Quality-assured local and regional hyperthermia procedures have been proven to enhance the clinical benefits of oncological standard treatments in several clinical settings without a substantial increase of late toxicity. This makes hyperthermia an attractive sensitizer for both radiotherapy and chemotherapy. It is no longer the question whether hyperthermia is an effective oncological treatment at all. Currently, the question is which patient, which tumor entity, and which clinical stage of disease benefit most from additional hyperthermia as integral part of current multimodality oncological standard treatment schedules. This remains particularly true for patients with recurrent malignant diseases and a previous irradiation series in the involved area.

1 Hyperthermia in Clinical Oncology

Currently, local and regional hyperthermia treatments undergo quite a revival in clinical oncology as part of multimodality therapy approaches for several malignant diseases. In several prospective clinical trials, systematic reviews, and large retrospective analyses, concurrent local and regional hyperthermia has been proven to enhance the efficacy of standard radiotherapy and chemotherapy protocols, e.g., in the treatment of chest

The original version of this chapter was revised. An erratum to this chapter can be found at 10.1007/978-3-319-41825-4_78.

O.J. Ott (✉) • M. Schmidt
Department of Radiation Oncology, University Hospital Erlangen, Universitätsstraße 27, Erlangen D-91054, Germany
e-mail: oliver.ott@uk-erlangen.de

Med Radiol Radiat Oncol (2016)
DOI 10.1007/174_2016_34, © Springer International Publishing Switzerland
Published Online: 30 Mar 2016

wall recurrences after breast cancer (Vernon et al. 1996; Jones et al. 2005; Kouloulias et al. 2015; Linthorst et al. 2013 and 2015; Oldenborg et al. 2015), locally advanced cervical cancer (van der Zee et al. 2000; Franckena et al. 2008 and 2009; Lutgens et al. 2010), rectal cancer (Berdov and Menteshashvili 1990; De Haas-Kock et al. 2009; Schroeder et al. 2012; Gani et al. 2016), high-risk soft tissue sarcoma (Issels 2008; Issels et al. 2010; Angele et al. 2014), malignant melanoma (Overgaard et al. 1995), anal carcinoma (Kouloulias et al. 2005), and bladder cancer (Colombo et al. 2003; Ott et al. 2009; Wittlinger et al. 2009). New applicator systems enable better temperature distributions, also in deeper sited regions, and offer more comfort for the patient. Systems including magnetic resonance imaging (MRI) scanners allow noninvasive 3D thermometry in the treatment region (Gellermann et al. 2005 and 2006; Winter et al. 2015). Planning systems on the basis of computed tomography (CT) or MRI data sets can support the selection of appropriate treatment parameters. These technical advances and standardized quality assurance programs (Bruggmoser et al. 2012) are opening the door to better treatment quality.

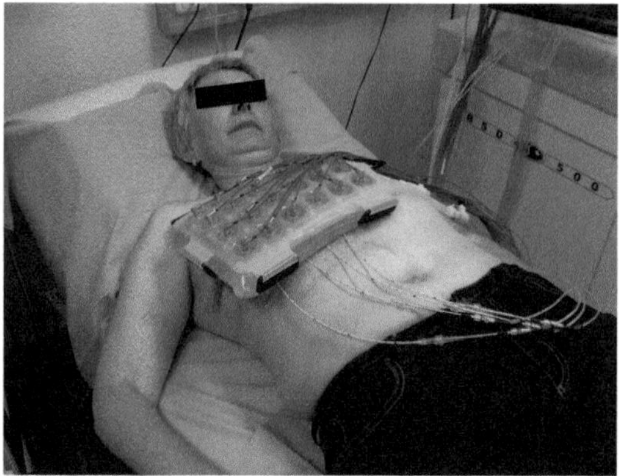

Fig. 1 Superficial hyperthermia of recurrent breast cancer

1.1 Classical Hyperthermia Treatment Techniques

In classical hyperthermia, tissue is temporarily exposed to elevated temperatures to damage and kill cancer cells. It is always used combined with standard radio- and/or chemotherapy. Several methods of hyperthermia are currently in use, including local (LHT), interstitial (IHT), deep regional (RHT), and whole-body hyperthermia (WBHT). Targeted tumor temperatures for local and regional hyperthermia applications are 40–44 °C, for WBHT usually 41.5–42 °C, respectively.

1.1.1 Superficial Hyperthermia

Superficial hyperthermia (LHT) devices are using various techniques that deliver energy to heat the tumor. Different types of energy may be used to apply heat, including microwave, radiofrequency, and ultrasound. An external applicator is positioned exactly over a localized tumor formation growing in the skin or the adjacent subcutaneous tissue, and energy is deposit to the tumor to raise its temperature (Fig. 1). Generally, the penetration depth of therapeutic heat levels amounts few centimeters. Typical clinical examples for the beneficial use of LHT in combination with radiotherapy are, e.g., non-resectable chest wall recurrences of breast cancer after mastectomy (Vernon et al. 1996; Jones et al. 2005; Kouloulias et al. 2015; Linthorst et al. 2013 and 2015; Oldenborg et al. 2015), local recurrences and in-transit metastases of malignant melanoma (Overgaard et al. 1995), and macroscopic cervical tumor in locally advanced head and neck cancer (Datta et al. 1990; Valdagni and Amichetti 1994). In a couple of randomized trials, additional LHT significantly improved local tumor control compared to irradiation alone (Valdagni and Amichetti 1994; Overgaard et al. 1995; Vernon et al. 1996; Jones et al. 2005).

1.1.2 Interstitial and Endocavitary/Intraluminal Hyperthermia

Interstitial and endocavitary/intraluminal hyperthermia (IHT) methods may be used to treat tumors within or near body cavities, such as the head and neck area (Datta et al. 1990; Geiger et al. 2002; Strnad et al. 2015), the esophagus, or the anal canal (Kouloulias et al. 2005). Probes are placed inside the cavity or inserted into the tumor to deliver energy and heat the area directly. IHT is also often combined with interstitial brachytherapy (Fig. 2). Before and/or

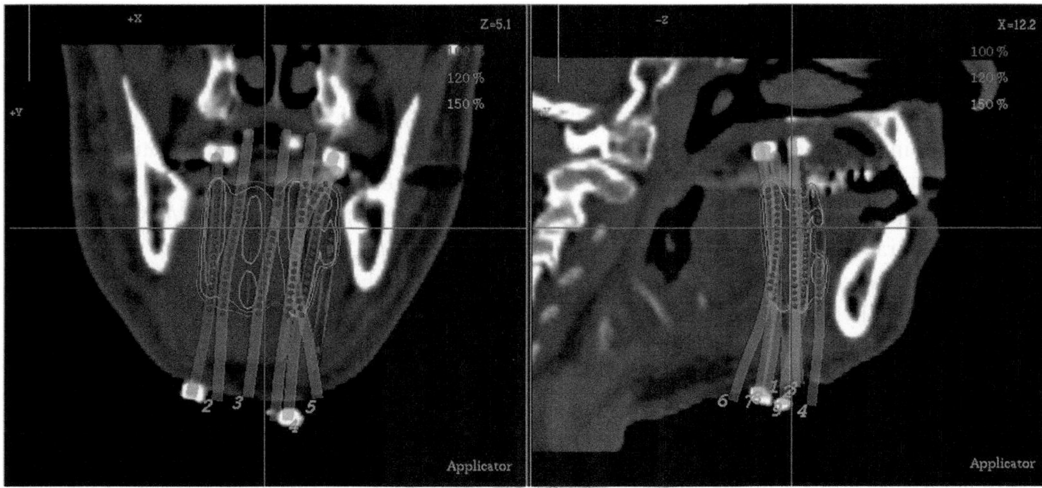

Fig. 2 Interstitial brachytherapy and hyperthermia of pre-irradiated recurrent tongue tumor

after high-dose-rate or pulsed-dose-rate afterloading irradiation, dedicated applicators (e.g., microwave antennas) are placed, e.g., within the brachytherapy tubes to additionally heat the target lesion. In clinical trials, additional IHT had been shown to improve overall survival and/or local recurrence rates of patients with bladder cancer (Colombo et al. 2003) as well as glioblastoma (Sneed et al. 1998).

1.1.3 Deep Regional Hyperthermia

For locally advanced carcinomas of the abdomen, pelvis, and extremities, deep regional hyperthermia (RHT) is recommended. External applicators are positioned around the body cavity or organ to be treated, and microwave or radiofrequency radiation is focused on the area to raise its temperature (Fig. 3). The clinical efficacy of RHT has been proven in randomized trials, e.g., in locally advanced cervical carcinoma (van der Zee et al. 2000; Franckena et al. 2008), rectal cancer (Rau et al. 2002), and soft tissue sarcoma (Issels et al. 2010; Angele et al. 2014). Further indications for the additional use of RHT in combination with radiotherapy, chemotherapy, and chemoradiation are locally recurrent rectal (Juffermans et al. 2003), bladder (Ott et al. 2009; Wittlinger et al. 2009), prostate (Tilly et al. 2005), anal (Kouloulias et al. 2005), pancreatic (Schlemmer et al. 2004), and gastric cancer (Mochiki et al. 2007). Other regional hyperthermia approaches, for example, comprise perfusion techniques (Cornett et al. 2006) that can be used to treat cancers in the arms and legs, such as melanoma, or cancer in some organs, such as the liver or lung. In this procedure, some of the patient's blood is removed, heated, and then perfused back into the limb or organ. Anticancer drugs are usually combined with this kind of hyperthermia treatment. Continuous hyperthermic peritoneal perfusion (HIPEC) is a technique used to treat disseminated cancers within the peritoneal cavity, including primary peritoneal mesothelioma and stomach cancer (Verwaal et al. 2008).

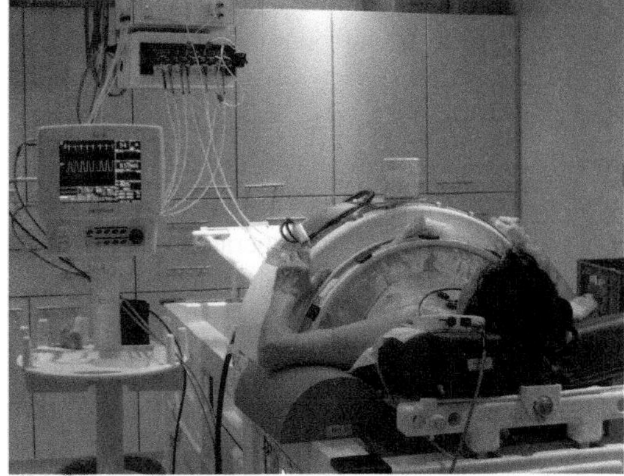

Fig. 3 Deep regional hyperthermia of recurrent rectal cancer

1.1.4 Noninvasive Thermometry

The combination of deep regional hyperthermia systems with MRI systems has been established for clinical use in some major oncological departments in Europe during the past few years. Controlling the effect of hyperthermia during patient treatment is essential for quality-controlled therapy. Using the combination of a deep regional hyperthermia system with a dedicated MRI, the physician obtains detailed, three-dimensional information about temperature and perfusion during RHT (Gellermann et al. 2005 and 2006; Winter et al. 2015). After short MRI measuring sequences, color-coded temperature distribution images covering the whole region of interest are available for review and optimization of treatment parameters. With the introduction of noninvasive MRI thermometry techniques, RHT treatment quality is expected to further improve effective heating of tumors and avoidance of painful hot spots in the surrounding normal tissues.

1.1.5 Whole-Body Hyperthermia

Whole-body hyperthermia (WBHT) is usually used in the intention to treat systemically disseminated cancer. The body temperature is artificially raised to 41.5–42 °C, by the use of incubators or hot water blankets. Combined WBHT and chemotherapy was predominantly used in patients with incurable metastasized malignancies who developed progressive disease after first- or second-line systemic treatment. Some phase II trials proved the feasibility of WBHT with chemotherapy for metastasized rectal, prostate, and ovarian cancer, but an explicit benefit for the additional use of WBHT could not be shown because of the lack of randomized trials (Hildebrandt et al. 2005). In evidence-based medicine, WBHT currently receives limited attention.

1.2 Hyperthermia: Not an Alternative but Additive Treatment Option

In the perception of many cancer patients, hyperthermia is a treatment comparable to surgery and radio- and chemotherapy. Suffering from a malignant disease and confronted with radical therapeutic approaches in established evidence-based oncology scenarios, some of them are desperately searching for an alternative way to be cured. A heat treatment in the temperature range of 40–44 °C seems to be a quite attractive choice to avoid surgery and chemo- and/or radiotherapy. But, up to date, there is no data for the beneficial use of hyperthermia as sole modality in the treatment of any malignancy, neither for whole body nor local and regional hyperthermia techniques. This fact remains true despite of many contradictory advertisements in the Internet. The German Society of Radiation Oncology (DEGRO) published a guideline for the proper use of local and regional hyperthermia in the year 2000. It emphasizes that hyperthermia must be used exclusively in combination with radio- and/or chemotherapy for sensitization of the tumor tissue for the established anticancer treatment. Therefore, local and regional hyperthermia techniques are *not alternative but additive* options in the treatment of specific cancer diseases and have to fulfill quality criteria (Bruggmoser et al. 2012).

2 The Rationale to Integrate Hyperthermia into Multimodality Approaches for the Treatment of Recurrent Malignancies

The treatment of patients with locally recurrent malignant diseases is very often a difficult task due to heavy pretreatment including surgery, radiotherapy, and systemic therapies. In many cases, primary surgery for the recurrent tumor is not feasible because of the extent of disease (e.g., inflammatory chest wall recurrence of breast cancer after mastectomy) or infiltration of indispensable anatomic structures (e.g., substantial infiltration of the first sacral vertebra in case of recurrent rectal cancer or vessel infiltration in pancreatic cancer). Frequently, breast cancer patients already received the most effective chemotherapeutics like taxanes and anthracyclines during the treatment of the primary tumor, and a large number of patients with breast and rectal cancer have had adjuvant radiotherapy. All these preconditions have to be considered for an individualized treatment schedule of a locally relapsed tumor.

In case of previous irradiation doses of ≥50 Gy, many radiation oncologists prefer to prescribe a palliative dose of another 30 Gy to a nonresectable local recurrence of rectal cancer to avoid serious side effects, especially to the bladder and small intestine. However, it is well known that a pathologically confirmed complete resection of the local recurrence of a rectal cancer opens a curative perspective for up to 50 % of the patients (Dresen et al. 2008; Tanis et al. 2013). For these cases, the intensification of neoadjuvant treatment may lead to a higher rate of cure. Local and regional hyperthermia applications have been proven to be effective radio- and/or chemosensitizers in various tumor entities, usually with no significant contribution to late toxicity. In the treatment of locally recurrent breast cancer, one trial even found that the beneficial effects of additional hyperthermia were most pronounced in pre-irradiated patients (Vernon et al. 1996). This makes hyperthermia a very attractive partner for multimodality treatment approaches, especially for patients with recurrent disease and limited treatment options due to pretreatment.

3 Clinical Data

Whereas clinical data on the use and the effects of local and regional hyperthermia for the treatment of primary tumors is easy to find, data on the individualized treatment of locally recurrent tumors are sparse. The available data are summarized below.

3.1 Breast Cancer

A total of six randomized trials analyzed the effects of combined radiotherapy and LHT in breast cancer patients. Five of them were started between 1988 and 1991 by the UK Medical Research Council, the European Society of Hyperthermic Oncology (ESHO), the Dutch Hyperthermia Group, and the Princess Margaret Hospital/Ontario Cancer Institute (Vernon et al. 1996). Patients were eligible if they had locally advanced primary or recurrent breast cancer, and local radiotherapy was indicated in preference to surgery. The primary endpoint of all trials was local complete response. Slow recruitment led to a decision to collaborate and combine the trial results in one meta-analysis and report them in one publication. A total of 306 patients were analyzed: 44 % (135/306) received radiotherapy alone, and 56 % (171/306) received combined treatment. The biologically effective radiation doses ranged between 40 and 70 Gy, the single fraction doses between 1.8 and 4 Gy, and the overall treatment time between 2 and 5 weeks. In the five trials, heat was applied with different devices for superficial hyperthermia. Depending on the protocol, 2–8 hyperthermia treatments were scheduled during the radiation course. The duration of a single hyperthermia fraction ranged between 45 and 70 min and the target temperature aimed at 42.5–43 °C. The overall complete remission rate for radiotherapy alone was 41 % and for the combined treatment 59 % ($p<0.001$). The most pronounced effect was observed in patients with recurrent lesions in previously irradiated areas, where further irradiation was limited to low doses. Of all patients who achieved a complete remission, 17 % of those having received combined treatment and 31 % of the radiotherapy only patients developed a local relapse during further follow-up ($p=0.007$). The majority of the patients (227/306) showed progression of disease outside the treatment area during follow-up. The authors discussed this finding as the reason for the fact that overall survival was not improved by additional hyperthermia despite a significantly better local control. Hyperthermia was well tolerated and did not add to the clinically relevant acute or long-term toxicity compared to irradiation alone, even in those patients who had received prior radiotherapy. The authors concluded that the combined analysis of the five trials demonstrated the efficacy of hyperthermia as an adjunct to radiotherapy for the treatment of recurrent breast cancer.

The sixth randomized trial evaluating the role in the treatment of breast cancer was published in 2005 by Jones et al. of the Duke University, North Carolina (Jones et al. 2005). A total of 108 patients with superficially located tumors with different origins was analyzed in detail. The patients received either radiation alone ($n=52$) or radiation combined with LHT ($n=56$). Of the patients who received radiation alone, 63 % (33/52) had breast cancer or chest wall recurrences after a history of breast cancer, 12 % (6/52) had head and neck cancer, 12 % (6/52) had malignant melanoma, and 13 % (7/52) had other tumor histologies. In the combined group, the distribution was 66 % (37/56), 14 % (8/56), 9 % (5/56), and 11 % (6/56), respectively. A separate analysis for the breast cancer patients only was not performed. Among patients in both arms, the median radiation dose if prior radiation had been given was 41 Gy (range 18–66 Gy), and the median dose if no prior radiation had been given was 60 Gy (range, 24–70 Gy). Patients were randomly assigned to receive no further treatment (no-LHT arm) or additional hyperthermia (LHT arm) throughout the course of radiation, delivered twice a week for a maximum of 10 treatments, 1–2 h duration, separated by at least 48 h. Microwave spiral strip applicators, operating at 433 MHz, were used for external heating. Temperature was measured invasively. Maximally allowed temperatures in the adjacent normal tissue and tumor tissue were 43 °C and 50 °C, respectively. The complete remission rate in the LHT arm was 66 %; the CR rate in the no-HT arm was 42 % ($p=0.02$). There was no significant difference in the proportion of patients in each arm who received additional systemic therapy. The improved local response in the LHT arm resulted in a significant difference in duration of local control between the two arms ($p=0.02$). Local control at death or last follow-up was 48 % vs. 25 %, respectively. The improvement in complete response rate and local control was most pronounced for patients who were previously irradiated. Overall survival was not significantly different between the two groups. Recently published retrospective series concentrating exclusively on irresectable chest wall recurrence after breast cancer underline the value of additional superficial hyperthermia in combination with reirradiation for these patients (Oldenborg et al. 2015; Linthorst et al. 2013 and 2015).

3.2 Rectal Cancer

For patients with locally recurrent rectal cancer, there is no standardized treatment regimen, especially for the subgroup with a history of prior pelvic radiotherapy. The curative potential of surgery and radio- and chemotherapy as sole treatment option is very limited (Tanis et al. 2013). Therefore, a combined modality treatment approach is mandatory. Surgery as well as radiochemotherapy is established in the treatment of recurrent rectal cancer. But treatment results are still not satisfying. RHT has proved to be feasible in combination with radio- and/or chemotherapy (Juffermans et al. 2003; Schaffer et al. 2003; Milani et al. 2008). Two randomized trials for locally advanced primary rectal cancer showed the effectiveness of additional hyperthermia in increasing the response rate and prolonging the time to progression (Berdov and Menteshashvili 1990; Gani et al. 2016). Only few reports exist on combined modality treatment regimens including hyperthermia for recurrent rectal cancer. Endpoints of the following studies were feasibility and palliation.

Juffermans et al. (2003) evaluated the palliative effect of reirradiation and hyperthermia in patients with non-resectable, recurrent colorectal carcinoma in 54 patients. The total reirradiation dose varied from 24 to 32 Gy given in fractions of 4 Gy twice weekly. Three or four hyperthermia treatments were given once weekly during the radiation course. The combined treatment was feasible and well tolerated. Comparison of results from radiotherapy plus hyperthermia with results after radiotherapy alone suggested that additional hyperthermia prolonged the duration of palliation.

Schaffer et al. (2003) analyzed treatment and follow-up data of 14 patients with local recurrence of rectal cancer that were treated with radiotherapy, chemotherapy, and RHT. Nine patients had received previous irradiation and chemotherapy. These pretreated patients received a total irradiation dose of 30.6–39.6 Gy and 5-fluorouracil (5-FU) as a continuous infusion over 5 days per week (350 mg/m^2/24 h) combined with RHT twice weekly. The 5 remaining not pretreated patients received irradiation of 45 Gy with an additional boost between 9 and 14.4 Gy, combined with continuous infusion of 5-FU on days 1–4, and 29–33 (500 mg/m^2/24 h), and RHT twice a week. Among 13 evaluated cases, the overall objective response rate was 54 % (5 complete responses, 2 partial responses). At a mean follow-up of 13.9 months (range 5–32 months), 7 patients were alive. The therapeutic regimen appeared to be active in the treatment of local recurrences of rectal cancer.

Hildebrandt et al. (2004) reported on a pilot study of nine previously irradiated patients with local recurrence of rectal cancer treated with chemotherapy and hyperthermia. Hyperthermic chemotherapy was applied with weekly infusions of 43 mg/m^2 of oxaliplatin (i.v., 120 min), 500 mg/m^2 of folinic acid (i.v., 120 min), and 2.6 g/m^2 of continuous infusion 5-FU (24 h) for 6 consecutive weeks. Oxaliplatin was started in parallel to pelvic RHT. A total of 67 applications were administered to nine patients and were well tolerated. A total of 55/67 (82 %) chemotherapy courses were applied without dose reduction. In 62/67 (93 %) hyperthermia sessions, a treatment time of more than 60 min was maintained. Eight out of 10 episodes of severe (WHO grade III) toxicity represented typical side effects of the chemotherapy given (nausea $n=4$, diarrhea $n=3$, neuropathy $n=1$). Two severe adverse events were mainly attributable to hyperthermia (hematuria, $n=1$; deterioration of a decubital ulcer, $n=1$). No patient suffered disease progression according to WHO criteria during the treatment period. Two patients achieved a partial remission. It is concluded that hyperthermic chemotherapy with oxaliplatin, folinic acid, and 5-FU is feasible. Overall toxicity was moderate. Results, moreover, suggest a relevant palliative effect in patients with previously irradiated pelvic recurrence of rectal cancer.

Wiig et al. (2005) studied the clinical outcome in patients with complete pathologic response (pT0) to preoperative irradiation/chemo-irradiation operated for locally advanced or locally recurrent rectal cancer. Four hundred and nineteen patients had preoperative irradiation (46–50 Gy, 2 Gy per fraction) for primary locally advanced (PLA) or locally recurrent (LR) rectal cancer. Pathologically proven complete response (pT0) was achieved in 7 % of PLA ($n=229$) and 8 % of LR ($n=190$) patients. For the PLA group, actuarial 5-year survival of pT0 was 90 % versus 53 % for the pT>0 group. The difference was statistically significant. At 5 years local recurrence was 0 % in pT0 patients versus 23 % in pT>0. For the LR group, 5-year survival was 62 % for pT0 versus 45 % for the other pT stages; local recurrence rates were 17 % and 35 %, respectively.

In summary, there is some evidence that radiochemotherapy combined with deep regional hyperthermia can improve response, local control, and survival rates in patients with recurrent rectal cancer. A phase I/II study of neoadjuvant chemoradiation with 5-FU (or capecitabine) and oxaliplatin combined with deep regional hyperthermia in locally recurrent rectal cancer (HyRec Trial) was started in 2011 at the Erlangen University Medical Center, Germany (Figs. 4 and 5). As already described above, it is well known that patients with a local relapse of rectal cancer have a much better prognosis in case of complete resection of the recurrence. The intensified neoadjuvant treatment schedule (addition of oxaliplatin and RHT two times per week up to a total of 10 treatments) of the HyRec Trial is aiming to maximize the complete resection rates in these patients. This trial recruited about 60 patients and is still open for both pre-irradiated and previously not irradiated patients. Primary endpoints are the feasibility and the complete remission rate. To date, final results are not available. The HyRec trial is planned to provide the basis for a randomized trial, evaluating the role of additional deep regional hyperthermia in patients with locally recurrent rectal cancer.

3.3 Head and Neck Cancer

A total of 104 patients with recurrent head and neck cancer were treated with pulsed-dose-rate

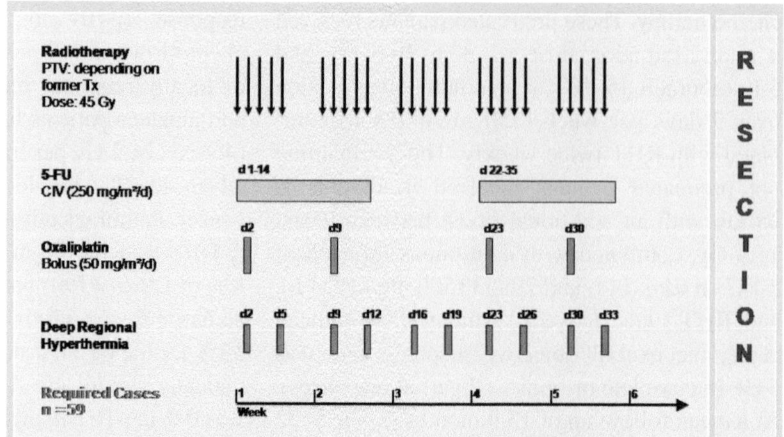

Fig. 4 Flowchart of the HyRec Trial for the treatment of recurrent rectal cancer

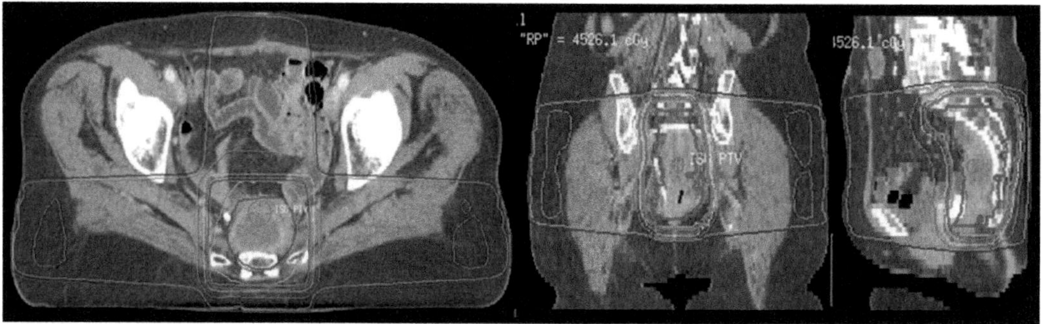

Fig. 5 Example of a reirradiation of a recurrent rectal cancer with 5-FU and oxaliplatin and RHT

(PDR) interstitial brachytherapy combined with external beam irradiation ($n=23$), platinum-based chemotherapy ($n=58$), and IHT ($n=33$) within an institutional protocol at the Erlangen University Medical Center, Germany (Strnad et al. 2015). All patients had received prior radiotherapy. A dose per pulse of 0.46–0.55 Gy was given up to a median total dose of 56.7 Gy. Simultaneously to the PDR brachytherapy, in a subgroup chemotherapy was given with cisplatin (20 mg/m^2, bolus i.v., days 1–5) and 5-FU (800 mg/m^2, CIV, days 1–5). After the PDR brachytherapy was finished, one third of the patients received a single session of interstitial hyperthermia. Soft tissue necrosis or bone necrosis developed in 18/104 (17.3 %) and 11/104 (9.6 %) patients, respectively, but only 3 % of patients required surgical treatment. Local tumor control rates after 2, 5, and 10 years were 92.5, 82.4, and 58.9 %, respectively. Simultaneous chemotherapy improved the clinical results. The impact of a single session of IHT remained unclear.

3.4 Cervical Cancer

Data on reirradiation combined with hyperthermia for the treatment of recurrent pelvic or para-aortic cervical carcinoma is not available at the moment, but several working groups are currently using a trimodality schedule of reirradiation combined with cisplatin chemotherapy (40 mg/m^2, weekly bolus) and RHT during cisplatin application. Patients with recurrent cervical carcinoma within a previously irradiated area usually respond poorly to chemotherapy alone.

There are some data on the combination of concurrent cisplatin and RHT. Franckena et al. (2007) treated these patients with simultaneous cisplatin and hyperthermia and investigated response, toxicity, palliative effect, and survival. Between 1992 and 2005, 47 patients had been treated. Response was evaluated by gynecologic examination and CT scan. The objective response rate was 55 %; palliation was achieved in 74 %

and operability in 19 % of patients. Two patients were disease-free at 9 years and 18 months following treatment, and 2 remained disease-free until death by non-cervical carcinoma-related causes. The median survival was 8 months and was influenced by duration of disease-free interval and tumor diameter. Grade 3–4 hematological toxicity was observed in 36 % of patients, and renal toxicity was maximum grade 2. The authors concluded that the combination of concurrent cisplatin and RHT resulted in a high response rate and acceptable toxicity in patients with recurrent cervical cancer. An updated study with 38 patients who experienced recurrence after simultaneous chemoradiation did not find a benefit from combined chemotherapy and hyperthermia (Heijkoop et al. 2014).

Rietbroek et al. (1997) reported on 23 patients with a pelvic recurrence of cervical carcinoma and a history of previous pelvic irradiation. Patients were treated with weekly cycles of RHT and cisplatin (50 mg/m^2 i.v.) for a maximum of 12 cycles. A total of 169 cycles were given. Responses were observed in 12/23 (52 %) of patients (95 % confidence interval, 31–73 %). Salvage surgery became possible in 3 of 12 responding patients, whose tumors were previously considered non-resectable. The median duration of response was 9.5 months, the median overall survival was 8 months, and the 1-year survival was 42 %. Overall toxicity was moderate. Weekly RHT and cisplatin have been shown to be an effective treatment in patients with a previously irradiated recurrent carcinoma of the uterine cervix. A more recent phase I study evaluated the combination of cisplatin, hyperthermia, and lapatinib for recurrent cervical carcinoma, but clinical results are preliminary (van Meerten et al. 2015).

4 Summary

Quality-assured local and regional hyperthermia procedures have been proven to enhance the clinical benefits of oncological standard treatments in several clinical settings without a substantial increase of late toxicity. This makes hyperthermia an attractive sensitizer for both radiotherapy and chemotherapy. It is no longer the question whether hyperthermia is an effective oncological treatment at all. Today, the question is which patient, which tumor entity, and which clinical stage of disease benefit most from additional hyperthermia as integral part of current multimodality oncological treatment schedules. Significant advances have been made during the past decade, e.g., in the treatment of cervical cancer, soft tissue sarcoma, breast cancer, etc., but still there is a lot of work to do to develop proper patient selection guidelines for other entities in the context of clinical trials. This remains particularly true for patients with recurrent malignant diseases and a previous irradiation series in the involved area.

References

Angele MK, Albertsmeier M, Prix NJ, Hohenberger P, Abdel-Rahman S, Dieterle N et al (2014) Effectiveness of regional hyperthermia with chemotherapy for high-risk retroperitoneal and abdominal soft-tissue sarcoma after complete surgical resection: a subgroup analysis of a randomized phase-III multicenter study. Ann Surg 260:749–754; discussion 54–6

Berdov BA, Menteshashvili GZ (1990) Thermoradiotherapy of patients with locally advanced carcinoma of the rectum. Int J Hyperthermia 6:881–890

Bruggmoser G, Bauchowitz S, Canters R, Crezee H, Ehmann M, Gellermann J et al (2012) Guideline for the clinical application, documentation and analysis of clinical studies for regional deep hyperthermia: quality management in regional deep hyperthermia. Strahlenther Onkol 188(Suppl 2):198–211

Colombo R, Da Pozzo LF, Salonia A, Rigatti P, Leib Z, Baniel J et al (2003) Multicentric study comparing intravesical chemotherapy alone and with local microwave hyperthermia for prophylaxis of recurrence of superficial transitional cell carcinoma. J Clin Oncol 21:4270–4276

Cornett WR, McCall LM, Petersen RP, Ross MI, Briele HA, Noyes RD et al (2006) Randomized multicenter trial of hyperthermic isolated limb perfusion with melphalan alone compared with melphalan plus tumor necrosis factor: American College of Surgeons Oncology Group Trial Z0020. J Clin Oncol 24:4196–4201

Datta NR, Bose AK, Kapoor HK, Gupta S (1990) Head and neck cancers: results of thermoradiotherapy versus radiotherapy. Int J Hyperthermia 6:479–486

De Haas-Kock DF, Buijsen J, Pijls-Johannesma M, Lutgens L, Lammering G, van Mastrigt GA et al (2009) Concomitant hyperthermia and radiation therapy for treating locally advanced rectal cancer. Cochrane Database Syst Rev (3):CD006269

Dresen RC, Gosens MJ, Martijn H, Nieuwenhuijzen GA, Creemers GJ, Daniels-Gooszen AW et al (2008) Radical resection after IORT-containing multimodality treatment is the most important determinant for outcome in patients treated for locally recurrent rectal cancer. Ann Surg Oncol 15:1937–1947

Franckena M, De Wit R, Ansink AC, Notenboom A, Canters RA, Fatehi D et al (2007) Weekly systemic cisplatin plus locoregional hyperthermia: an effective treatment for patients with recurrent cervical carcinoma in a previously irradiated area. Int J Hyperthermia 23:443–450

Franckena M, Stalpers LJ, Koper PC, Wiggenraad RG, Hoogenraad WJ, van Dijk JD et al (2008) Long-term improvement in treatment outcome after radiotherapy and hyperthermia in locoregionally advanced cervix cancer: an update of the Dutch Deep Hyperthermia Trial. Int J Radiat Oncol Biol Phys 70:1176–1182

Franckena M, Lutgens LC, Koper PC, Kleynen CE, van der Steen-Banasik EM, Jobsen JJ et al (2009) Radiotherapy and hyperthermia for treatment of primary locally advanced cervix cancer: results in 378 patients. Int J Radiat Oncol Biol Phys 73:242–250

Gani C, Schroeder C, Heinrich V, Spillner P, Lamprecht U, Berger B et al (2016) Long-term local control and survival after preoperative radiochemotherapy in combination with deep regional hyperthermia in locally advanced rectal cancer. Int J Hyperthermia 1–6

Geiger M, Strnad V, Lotter M, Sauer R (2002) Pulsed-dose rate brachytherapy with concomitant chemotherapy and interstitial hyperthermia in patients with recurrent head-and-neck cancer. Brachytherapy 1:149–153

Gellermann J, Wlodarczyk W, Hildebrandt B, Ganter H, Nicolau A, Rau B et al (2005) Noninvasive magnetic resonance thermography of recurrent rectal carcinoma in a 1.5 Tesla hybrid system. Cancer Res 65:5872–5880

Gellermann J, Hildebrandt B, Issels R, Ganter H, Wlodarczyk W, Budach V et al (2006) Noninvasive magnetic resonance thermography of soft tissue sarcomas during regional hyperthermia: correlation with response and direct thermometry. Cancer 107: 1373–1382

Heijkoop ST, van Doorn HC, Stalpers LJ, Boere IA, van der Velden J, Franckena M et al (2014) Results of concurrent chemotherapy and hyperthermia in patients with recurrent cervical cancer after previous chemoradiation. Int J Hyperthermia 30:6–10

Hildebrandt B, Wust P, Drager J, Ludemann L, Sreenivasa G, Tullius SG et al (2004) Regional pelvic hyperthermia as an adjunct to chemotherapy (oxaliplatin, folinic acid, 5-fluorouracil) in pre-irradiated patients with locally recurrent rectal cancer: a pilot study. Int J Hyperthermia 20:359–369

Hildebrandt B, Hegewisch-Becker S, Kerner T, Nierhaus A, Bakhshandeh-Bath A, Janni W et al (2005) Current status of radiant whole-body hyperthermia at temperatures >41.5 degrees C and practical guidelines for the treatment of adults. The German 'Interdisciplinary Working Group on Hyperthermia'. Int J Hyperthermia 21:169–183

Issels RD (2008) Regional hyperthermia in high-risk soft tissue sarcomas. Curr Opin Oncol 20:438–443

Issels RD, Lindner LH, Verweij J, Wust P, Reichardt P, Schem BC et al (2010) Neo-adjuvant chemotherapy alone or with regional hyperthermia for localised high-risk soft-tissue sarcoma: a randomised phase 3 multicentre study. Lancet Oncol 11:561–570

Jones EL, Oleson JR, Prosnitz LR, Samulski TV, Vujaskovic Z, Yu D et al (2005) Randomized trial of hyperthermia and radiation for superficial tumors. J Clin Oncol 23:3079–3085

Juffermans JH, Hanssens PE, van Putten WL, van Rhoon GC, van Der Zee J (2003) Reirradiation and hyperthermia in rectal carcinoma: a retrospective study on palliative effect. Cancer 98:1759–1766

Kouloulias V, Plataniotis G, Kouvaris J, Dardoufas C, Gennatas C, Uzunoglu N et al (2005) Chemoradiotherapy combined with intracavitary hyperthermia for anal cancer: feasibility and long-term results from a phase II randomized trial. Am J Clin Oncol 28:91–99

Kouloulias V, Triantopoulou S, Uzunoglou N, Pistevou-Gompaki K, Barich A, Zygogianni A et al (2015) Hyperthermia is now included in the NCCN clinical practice guidelines for breast cancer recurrences: an analysis of existing data. Breast Care 10:109–116

Linthorst M, van Geel AN, Baaijens M, Ameziane A, Ghidey W, van Rhoon GC et al (2013) Re-irradiation and hyperthermia after surgery for recurrent breast cancer. Radiother Oncol 109:188–193

Linthorst M, Baaijens M, Wiggenraad R, Creutzberg C, Ghidey W, van Rhoon GC et al (2015) Local control rate after the combination of re-irradiation and hyperthermia for irresectable recurrent breast cancer: results in 248 patients. Radiother Oncol 117:217–222

Lutgens L, van der Zee J, Pijls-Johannesma M, De Haas-Kock DF, Buijsen J, Mastrigt GA et al (2010) Combined use of hyperthermia and radiation therapy for treating locally advanced cervix carcinoma. Cochrane Database Syst Rev (3):CD006377

Milani V, Pazos M, Issels RD, Buecklein V, Rahman S, Tschoep K et al (2008) Radiochemotherapy in combination with regional hyperthermia in preirradiated patients with recurrent rectal cancer. Strahlenther Onkol 184:163–168

Mochiki E, Shioya M, Sakurai H, Andoh H, Ohno T, Aihara R et al (2007) Feasibility study of postoperative intraperitoneal hyperthermochemotherapy by radiofrequency capacitive heating system for advanced gastric cancer with peritoneal seeding. Int J Hyperthermia 23:493–500

Oldenborg S, Griesdoorn V, van Os R, Kusumanto YH, Oei BS, Venselaar JL et al (2015) Reirradiation and hyperthermia for irresectable locoregional recurrent breast cancer in previously irradiated area: size matters. Radiother Oncol 117:223–228

Ott OJ, Rodel C, Weiss C, Wittlinger M, Krause FS, Dunst J et al (2009) Radiochemotherapy for bladder cancer. Clin Oncol (R Coll Radiol) 21:557–565

Overgaard J, Gonzalez Gonzalez D, Hulshof MC, Arcangeli G, Dahl O, Mella O et al (1995) Randomised trial of hyperthermia as adjuvant to radiotherapy for recurrent or metastatic malignant melanoma. Eur Soc Hyperther Oncol Lancet 345:540–543

Rau B, Benhidjeb T, Wust P, Schlag PM (2002) Stellenwert der hyperthermie für die chirurgische onkologie (German). Viszeralchirurgie 37:379–384

Rietbroek RC, Schilthuis MS, Bakker PJ, van Dijk JD, Postma AJ, Gonzalez Gonzalez D et al (1997) Phase II trial of weekly locoregional hyperthermia and cisplatin in patients with a previously irradiated recurrent carcinoma of the uterine cervix. Cancer 79:935–943

Schaffer M, Krych M, Pachmann S, Abdel-Rahman S, Schaffer PM, Ertl-Wagner B et al (2003) Feasibility and morbidity of combined hyperthermia and radiochemotherapy in recurrent rectal cancer – preliminary results. Onkologie 26:120–124

Schlemmer M, Lindner LH, Abdel-Rahman S, Issels RD (2004) Principles, technology and indication of hyperthermia and part body hyperthermia. Radiologe 44:301–309

Schroeder C, Gani C, Lamprecht U, von Weyhern CH, Weinmann M, Bamberg M et al (2012) Pathological complete response and sphincter-sparing surgery after neoadjuvant radiochemotherapy with regional hyperthermia for locally advanced rectal cancer compared with radiochemotherapy alone. Int J Hyperthermia 28:707–714

Sneed PK, Stauffer PR, McDermott MW, Diederich CJ, Lamborn KR, Prados MD et al (1998) Survival benefit of hyperthermia in a prospective randomized trial of brachytherapy boost +/- hyperthermia for glioblastoma multiforme. Int J Radiat Oncol Biol Phys 40:287–295

Strnad V, Lotter M, Kreppner S, Fietkau R (2015) Reirradiation for recurrent head and neck cancer with salvage interstitial pulsed-dose-rate brachytherapy: long-term results. Strahlenther Onkol 191:495–500

Tanis PJ, Doeksen A, van Lanschot JJ (2013) Intentionally curative treatment of locally recurrent rectal cancer: a systematic review. Can J Surg 56:135–144

Tilly W, Gellermann J, Graf R, Hildebrandt B, Weissbach L, Budach V et al (2005) Regional hyperthermia in conjunction with definitive radiotherapy against recurrent or locally advanced prostate cancer T3 pN0 M0. Strahlenther Onkol 181:35–41

Valdagni R, Amichetti M (1994) Report of long-term follow-up in a randomized trial comparing radiation therapy and radiation therapy plus hyperthermia to metastatic lymph nodes in stage IV head and neck patients. Int J Radiat Oncol Biol Phys 28:163–169

van der Zee J, Gonzalez Gonzalez D, van Rhoon GC, van Dijk JD, van Putten WL, Hart AA (2000) Comparison of radiotherapy alone with radiotherapy plus hyperthermia in locally advanced pelvic tumours: a prospective, randomised, multicentre trial. Dutch Deep Hyperthermia Group. Lancet 355:1119–1125

van Meerten E, Franckena M, Wiemer E, van Doorn L, Kraan J, Westermann A et al (2015) Phase I study of cisplatin, hyperthermia, and lapatinib in patients with recurrent carcinoma of the uterine cervix in a previously irradiated area. Oncologist 20:241–242

Vernon CC, Hand JW, Field SB, Machin D, Whaley JB, van der Zee J et al (1996) Radiotherapy with or without hyperthermia in the treatment of superficial localized breast cancer: results from five randomized controlled trials. International Collaborative Hyperthermia Group. Int J Radiat Oncol Biol Phys 35:731–744

Verwaal VJ, Bruin S, Boot H, van Slooten G, van Tinteren H (2008) 8-year follow-up of randomized trial: cytoreduction and hyperthermic intraperitoneal chemotherapy versus systemic chemotherapy in patients with peritoneal carcinomatosis of colorectal cancer. Ann Surg Oncol 15:2426–2432

Wiig JN, Larsen SG, Dueland S, Giercksky KE (2005) Clinical outcome in patients with complete pathologic response (pT0) to preoperative irradiation/chemo-irradiation operated for locally advanced or locally recurrent rectal cancer. J Surg Oncol 92:70–75

Winter L, Oberacker E, Paul K, Ji Y, Oezerdem C, Ghadjar P et al (2015) Magnetic resonance thermometry: methodology, pitfalls and practical solutions. Int J Hyperthermia 1–13

Wittlinger M, Rodel CM, Weiss C, Krause SF, Kuhn R, Fietkau R et al (2009) Quadrimodal treatment of high-risk T1 and T2 bladder cancer: transurethral tumor resection followed by concurrent radiochemotherapy and regional deep hyperthermia. Radiother Oncol 93:358–363

Therapeutic Ratio of Reirradiation with Cytotoxic Drugs and Other Response-Modifying Agents

Carsten Nieder and Avraham Eisbruch

Contents

The original version of this chapter was revised. An erratum to this chapter can be found at 10.1007/978-3-319-41825-4_78.

C. Nieder, MD (✉)
Department of Oncology and Palliative Medicine, Nordland Hospital, Prinsensgate 164, Bodo 8092, Norway
e-mail: Carsten.Nieder@nordlandssykehuset.no

A. Eisbruch, MD
Department of Radiation Oncology, University of Michigan Medical Center, Ann Arbor, MI 48109-5010, USA

Abstract

The introduction of combined modality approaches was a highly significant step in the evolution of curative radiation treatment. Achieving a favorable balance between tumor cell kill and normal tissue toxicity is important, especially in the context of reirradiation. As a result of previous treatments, which often include surgery and chemotherapy, function and reserve capacity of tissues and organs are impaired. Therefore, strategies that could increase the tumor cell kill of reirradiation without increasing serious toxicities would improve the therapeutic index. Two major examples where reirradiation often is combined with concomitant chemotherapy are head and neck tumors and rectal cancer. Compared with the systematic experimental models used for development of first-line combinations and their evaluation through a classic series of clinical trials including randomized phase III studies, development of sound combination regimens for reirradiation is still in its infancy. The clinical situation is complicated by more heterogeneous tumors with changes in physiological and microenvironmental parameters over time and quite variable pretreatment approaches, time intervals, irradiated volumes, etc. This chapter summarizes the principles of combined modality treatment and studies performed in the reirradiation setting.

Med Radiol Radiat Oncol (2016)
DOI 10.1007/174_2016_62, © Springer International Publishing Switzerland
Published Online: 01 May 2016

1 Introduction

The combination of radiation therapy and chemotherapy has been shown to be superior to radiation alone in both tumor response and patient survival for a number of malignancies. New classes of agents are being developed and rapidly introduced to clinical use. These agents target one or more of the processes that play important roles in the malignant phenotype. These new drugs include specific antibodies against growth factors or their receptors and small molecules that interfere with signal transduction pathways regulating the cell cycle, gene transcription, and survival in cancer cells. Some of the drugs have a single specific target, whereas others may have multiple targets. Because the targets of this therapy are processes that are dysregulated only in cancer cells, these agents do not share the same side effects in normal tissues of the conventional cytotoxic chemotherapy and radiation, their combination with radiation therapy has attracted significant interest (Nieder et al. 2003). More recently, immunologic mechanisms have also attracted considerable attention (Pilones et al. 2015).

Achieving a favorable balance between tumor cell kill and normal tissue toxicity is important, especially in the context of reirradiation. As a result of previous treatments, which often include surgery and chemotherapy, function and reserve capacity of tissues and organs are impaired. Even if patients with severe morbidity from first-line therapy are not offered reirradiation, the therapeutic ratio is different from typical first-line settings. In other words, strategies that could increase the tumor cell kill of reirradiation without increasing serious toxicities would improve the therapeutic index (Fig. 1a–c). As has been suggested from the data of patients with glioblastoma who received radiotherapy alone or radiotherapy plus temozolomide (Stupp et al. 2005), the effect of the drug in combined modality treatment corresponds to the equivalent of 9.1 Gy in 2-Gy fractions (Jones and Sanghera 2007). In patients treated with neoadjuvant combined chemotherapy and radiotherapy for esophagus cancer (data from 26 trials combined), it was estimated that 1 g/m^2 of 5-fluorouracil (5-FU) was equivalent to a radiation dose of 1.9 Gy and that 100 mg/m^2 cisplatin was equivalent to a radiation dose of 7.2 Gy (Geh et al. 2006). A combined analysis of 14 head and neck cancer trials confirms these data (Kasibhatla et al. 2007). With 2–3 cycles of cisplatin, carboplatin, and/or 5-FU containing radiochemotherapy regimens, the additional dose corresponds to 12 Gy in 2 Gy per fraction daily. In many reirradiation scenarios, radiation dose escalation by 9–12 Gy would

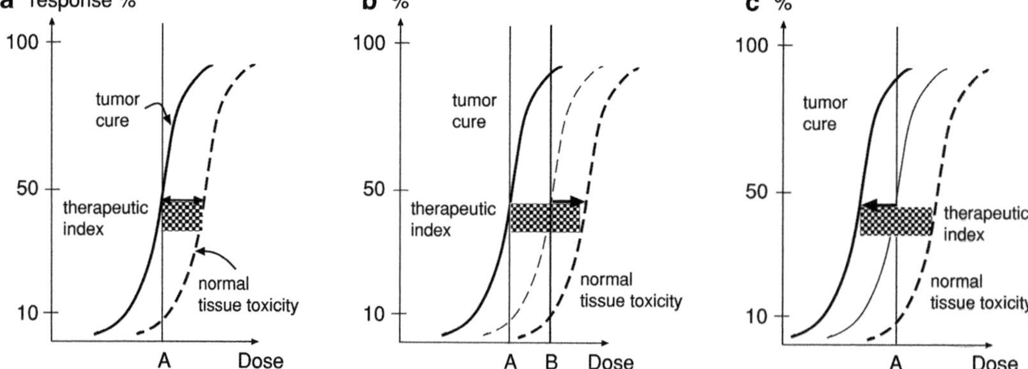

Fig. 1 The therapeutic index. (**a**) Therapeutic index for treatment with radiation alone. Radiation with *dose A* implies specific probabilities for tumor cure and normal tissue toxicity (e.g., 50 % cure vs <10 % toxicity). (**b**) If radiation is combined with radioprotectors, the radiation dose can be increased (*dose B*) because normal tissue toxicity is reduced (curve for normal tissue toxicity shifted to the right). (**c**) If radiation is combined with radiosensitizers, the probability for tumor cure increases (curve for tumor cure shifted to the left). Radioprotectors and radiosensitizers both increase the therapeutic index

result in increased late toxicity risk. Under these circumstances, combining radiotherapy and chemotherapy theoretically increases the therapeutic window.

Many studies on reirradiation of different cancer types report on combinations of radiation and various drugs (Haraf et al. 1996; Arcicasa et al. 1999; Schaefer et al. 2000; Mohiuddin et al. 2002; Wurm et al. 2006; Biagioli et al. 2007; Combs et al. 2008; Spencer et al. 2008; VanderSpek et al. 2008; Würschmidt et al. 2008; Dornoff et al. 2015; Minniti et al. 2015). Nevertheless, there is limited evidence from systematic, prospective clinical trials addressing reirradiation with or without response-modifying agents. This results in considerable uncertainty with regard to current clinical practice. In a Canadian survey, 28 % of respondents would use concurrent chemotherapy along with reirradiation in cases of chemosensitive tumors, 43 % would not recommend concurrent chemotherapy, and 30 % were uncertain (Joseph et al. 2008). This chapter provides an overview on the principles of combined modality treatment and reirradiation with classical chemotherapy or other response modifiers.

2 Clinical Relevance of Combined Modality Approaches

The introduction of combined modality approaches was a highly significant step in the evolution of curative radiation treatment. Parallel to analysis of altered fractionation schedules, combined treatment has actively been investigated in recent decades in both preclinical and clinical studies around the world. When judged at this time, the most pronounced increase in therapeutic gain was probably seen by combining radiation with chemotherapy and few other response modifiers.

Meanwhile, a huge body of evidence supports the use of combined modality approaches based on the combination of ionizing radiation with cytostatic drugs. In this regard, several randomized phase III trials for many relevant cancer sites provide a sound basis for level one evidence-based decision. This holds true especially for glioblastoma multiforme (Stupp et al. 2005), head and neck cancers including nasopharyngeal cancer and laryngeal cancer (Brizel et al. 1998; Forastiere et al. 2003; Budach et al. 2005), esophageal cancer (Minsky et al. 2002), colorectal and anal cancer (Sauer et al. 2004; Bartelink et al. 1997), cervical cancer (Green et al. 2001), as well as lung cancer (Schaake-Koning et al. 1992).

The most important aim of curative cancer treatment is to eradicate all clonogenic tumor cells or stem cells, which are able to give rise to a recurrence. With regard to the amount of quantitative cell kill, it has to be emphasized that important differences exist between ionizing radiation and chemotherapy (Fig. 2). In principle, radiation treatment can be designed to cover the whole tumor with a homogeneously distributed full radiation dose, maybe including a biology-driven boost, capable of inactivation of all tumor cells (Belka 2006). In contrast, pharmacotherapy is limited by the fact that the dose of the active, cell killing form of the compound is variable within the tumor and its cells. This results from problems in the delivery of drugs (perfusion, interstitial fluid pressure, tissue pH, etc.), cellular uptake, efflux, inactivation, and resistance. In many instances, the agent does not reach the relevant therapeutic targets in the required concentration and for a sufficient time period (Tannock et al. 2002; Primeau et al. 2005; Minchinton and Tannock 2006). In fact, the pharmacokinetic profile of anticancer drugs is characterized by substantial inter-patient variability where two- to threefold variation is not uncommon (Brunsvig et al. 2007). These issues gain complexity with simultaneous administration of two or more drugs and in the context of reirradiation because of the heterogeneity of reirradiated tumors (Fig. 3). As illustrated in Fig. 2, the quantitative cell kill of ionizing radiation is significantly larger than that of chemotherapy (Tannock 1992, 1998). The magnitude of this effect might vary with cell type, culture conditions, drug, exposure time, etc. Experimental evidence suggests, however, that single radiation doses result in 1 % or less cell survival compared with 10–50 % with

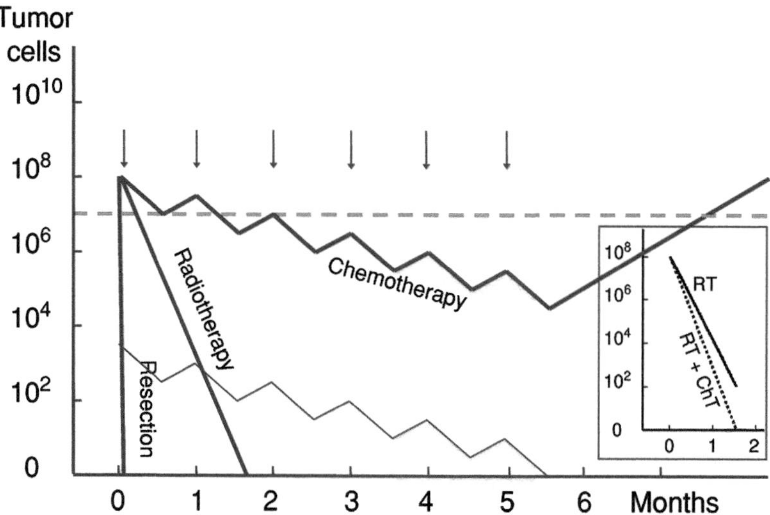

Fig. 2 Differences in quantitative cell kill and time course. Influence of different therapeutic modalities on number of tumor cells during a course of treatment, based on the models by Tannock (1989, 1992) and Minchinton and Tannock (2006). The *dashed line* represents the border between microscopic and macroscopic tumors, defined as a size of approximately 5 mm. Compared with surgical resection and fractionated radiotherapy, multiple courses of chemotherapy (in this case six, indicated by *arrows*) are less efficient in cell kill. While microscopic disease might be eradicated (*lower chemotherapy curve*), clinical evidence suggests that most macroscopic solid tumors (exception: more sensitive testicular cancers) will shrink temporarily but eventually regrow from surviving residues (*upper chemotherapy curve*). As shown in the *inset*, the strength of chemotherapy in combination with radiation treatment (besides of spatial cooperation) is the modification of the slope of the curve

cytotoxic drugs (Epstein 1990; Kim et al. 1992; Simoens et al. 2003; Eliaz et al. 2004). Although clinically impressive remissions of solid tumors might occur after chemotherapy, the underlying cell kill is often not larger than 1–2 log and pathological examination of tissue specimens reveals residual viable tumor cells.

In most clinical situations, chemotherapy augments the radiation-induced cell kill within the irradiated volume and may improve distant control. To maximize augmentation of cell kill, optimization of parameters of drug exposure is necessary. It has been shown, for example, that continuous infusion is better than bolus administration of 5-FU. The following example illustrates the efficacy of chemotherapy as a radiation enhancer. In the large randomized FFCD 9203 trial in rectal cancer, preoperative radiotherapy (45 Gy in 25 fractions) resulted in pathological complete remission (pCR) in 4%, whereas the addition of 5-FU and folinic acid improved this figure to 12% (Gerard et al. 2005). While radiation alone can be considered as a curative treatment in a variety of early-stage solid tumors (especially T1-2 N0 M0, e.g., skin, anal, cervix, larynx, lung, and prostate cancers), long-term control with chemotherapy alone is rarely observed. Current concepts of cancer biology suggest that most traditional chemotherapy approaches fail to eradicate cancer stem cells, which are slow-cycling cells that often express multidrug resistance (MDR) proteins (Miller et al. 2005; Prince and Ailles 2008; Moitra 2015; Yoshida and Saya 2015).

3 Basic Considerations

3.1 Therapeutic Gain

Therapeutic gain is defined by an increase of tumor control and finally survival without a parallel increase in the severity of specific side effects (Fig. 1). A very nice preclinical example is the comprehensive studies with cisplatin and 5-FU in different tumors transplanted into mice,

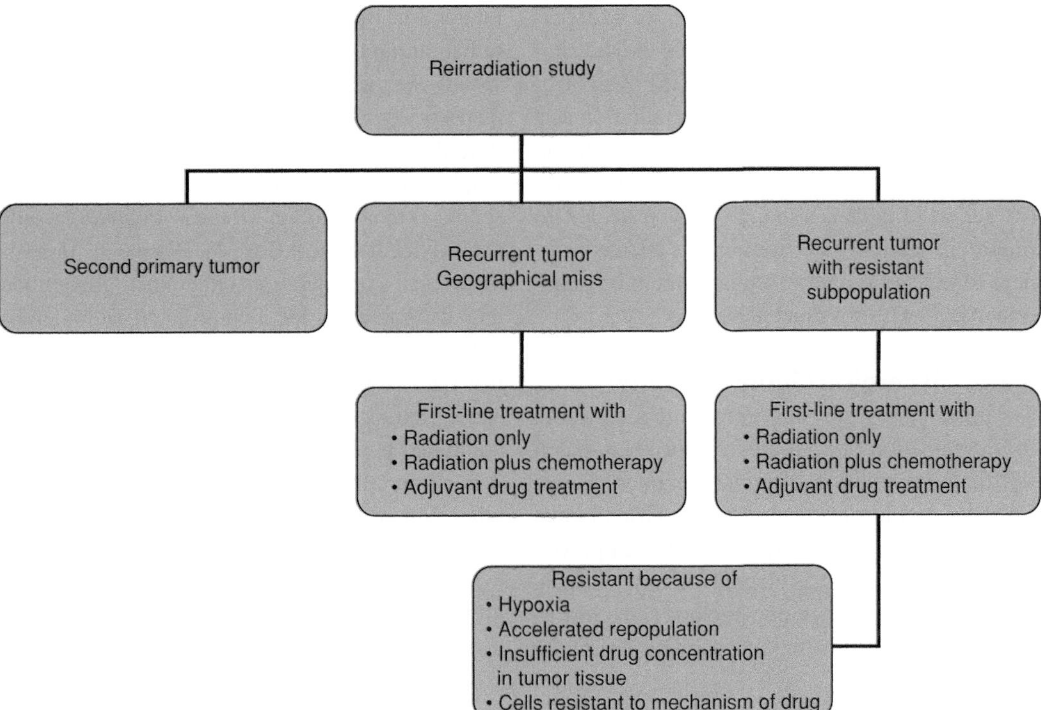

Fig. 3 In clinical reirradiation studies, the situation is complicated by very complex and heterogeneous tumor biology and changes in physiological and microenvironmental parameters resulting from the first course of radiotherapy, for example, fibrosis and impaired tissue perfusion. It has been suggested that human tumor cells derived from radiotherapy failures (head and neck carcinomas) are relatively radioresistant (Weichselbaum et al. 1988). Among radioresistant cell lines, those from previously irradiated patients were significantly more resistant than those from non-irradiated patients (Grenman et al. 1991). Importantly, some radiosensitive tumors from previously irradiated patients were also found in the latter study (three of seven examined cases)

which were reported by Kallman et al. (1992). Independently of the term "therapeutic gain," the interaction of radiation with chemotherapy follows a precise nomenclature based on some groundbreaking theoretical considerations published in the late 1970s (Steel 1979; Steel and Peckham 1979). In every case of a scientific description and quantification of the effects of combined modality therapy in appropriate models, it is highly recommended to adhere to the proposed nomenclature. The complexity of effects increases with each step of investigation, that is, from cell culture to tumor-bearing animal to cancer patient. A thorough examination of all possible treatment combinations and administration schedules for a given drug plus radiation is very challenging, as can be seen in the publication by Kallman et al. (1992), who studied in depth the radiosensitizing effects of cisplatin. Although extensive discussion of radiobiological principles is beyond the scope of this chapter, a few definitions shall be mentioned. Since the introduction of mammalian cell survival curves, the parameters D_0 and N have been used as quantitative measures of inherent radiation sensitivity, as was the shoulder width Dq (Thames and Suit 1986). The ratio alpha/beta is a measure of fractionation sensitivity.

3.2 Additivity, Synergism, and Subadditivity

When combining two treatment modalities the resulting net effect on cell killing is mainly described by the terms "additivity, synergism, and subadditivity," which are derived from experimental work. They are not applicable to the clinical situation and do not reflect the results of clinical trials, where changes from radiation as a monotherapy to multimodal treatment usually do not result in extraordinarily favorable cure rates (or supraadditivity), although they have led to important gradual improvement. It appears prudent to refer to the term "enhancement of radiation effect" within a clinical context.

3.2.1 Synergism (Supraadditivity)

The term "synergism" describes a situation where the combination of both drugs induces more cell kill than the addition of either treatment alone. The term "radiosensitization" is also used in this regard; however, it should only be employed when the drug used is devoid of any intrinsic potential. Regardless of nomenclature, the resulting effect is a shift of the tumor control curve to the left.

3.2.2 Additivity

The term "additivity" is used to describe situations where both triggers act completely independent of each other resulting in a net kill not larger than expected from the calculated additive combinatory effect.

3.2.3 Infra (Sub)-additivity (Protection)

This term describes situations where the drug interferes negatively with the efficacy of ionizing radiation, or vice versa.

4 Interaction of Radiation and Chemotherapy

4.1 Spatial Interaction

On a large scale, chemotherapy and radiation may be effective on several levels. The concept of spatial interaction was devised to mean that chemotherapy and radiation act on spatially distinct compartments of the body, resulting in a net gain in tumor control. The concept of spatial interaction does not take into account any drug-radiation interaction on the level of the tumor itself, but rather assumes that radiation or chemotherapy would be active in different compartments, respectively. In a narrow sense, this concept describes the fact that chemotherapy would be employed for the sterilization of distant microscopic tumor seeding, whereas radiation would achieve local control (Fig. 4). Obviously, this is a theoretical consideration only, since chemotherapy also increases local control and radiotherapy reduces distant metastasis via increased local control rates; thus, when integrating the concept of spatial interaction into a more complete view on combined modality, spatial cooperation is still of major importance. Next to spatial effects, several other important mechanisms may increase the efficacy of a combined treatment approach. In this regard, inhibition of repopulation and effective killing of hypoxic radioresistant cells may contribute to the efficacy of a combined treatment.

4.2 Role of Repopulation

The fractionated treatment of tumors with ionizing radiation is associated with the phenomenon of repopulation (Kim and Tannock 2005). Speaking simply, a certain amount of tumor cells repair the induced damage in between two fractions and proliferate. Repopulation may neutralize around 0.5 Gy/day; however, the range of repopulation is considerably large and may reach levels exceeding 4 Gy (Trott 1990; Baumann et al. 1994; Budach et al. 1997). Based on these findings, radiation biologists advocated the use of accelerated radiation schedules. The phenomenon of repopulation must also be taken into account when trying to design combined modality regimens. In theoretical models, cell loss from neoadjuvant chemotherapy preceding fractionated radiation treatment might trigger accelerated repopulation. Then, a certain percentage of the daily radiation dose is wasted to counteract increased tumor cell proliferation. Under such conditions, despite of a response to chemotherapy, cell survival after radiotherapy is not better than after the same course of radiotherapy alone (yet toxicity results from both

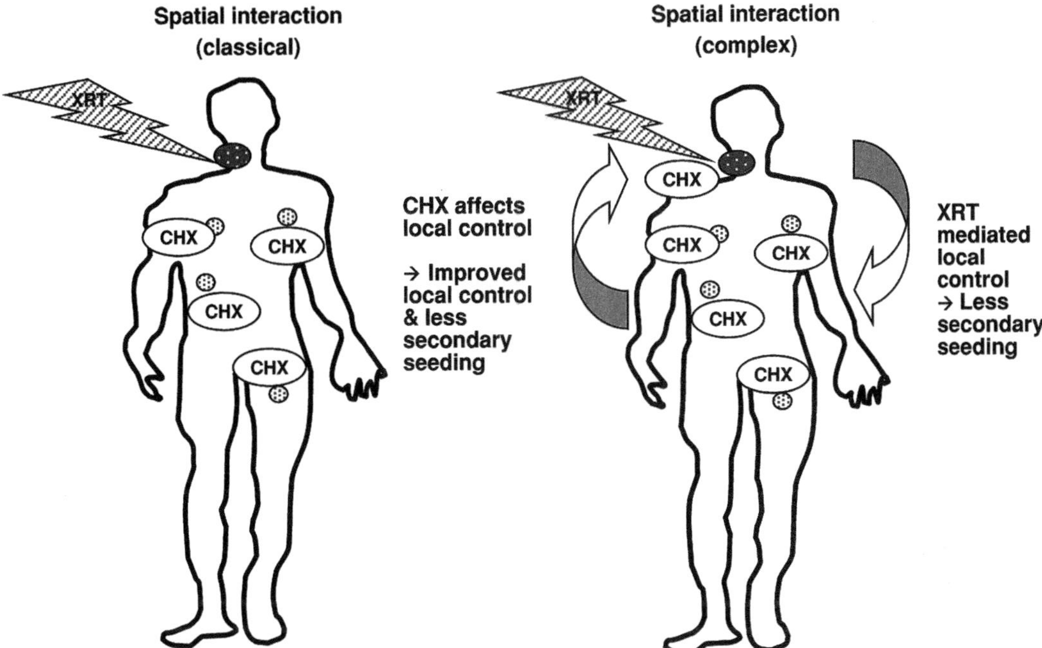

Fig. 4 Spatial interaction. In a classical interpretation (*left panel*), the term "spatial interaction" refers to the fact that chemotherapy is effective on tumor compartments where radiation has no efficacy, and vice versa, resulting in a generally increased control rate. In a more complex view, spatial interaction is relevant on multiple interacting levels: increased local control by radiation reduces the risk of a secondary seeding. Furthermore, the interaction of radiation with chemotherapy increases local control; thus, in addition to the classical spatial interaction, several levels of interacting feedback loops exist, which increase efficacy of spatial interactions

modalities). Whether such effects are more important than reduced interstitial fluid pressure (IFP) and improved oxygenation might depend on tumor type.

The clinical observation that the combination of 5-FU, mitomycin C, or cisplatin with radiation is of value in rapidly proliferating squamous cell cancers has led to the suspicion that the addition of drugs may influence the potential of cancer cells to repopulate. At least for mitomycin C, this effect was documented precisely using a xenograft model (Budach et al. 2002). In this model, transplanted tumors were treated with 11 fractions of 4.5 Gy under ambient conditions with or without mitomycin C followed by a graded top-up dose on days 16, 23, 30, or 37 given under hypoxic conditions. Repopulation in the interval between the fractionated treatment and the top-up dose accounted for 1.33 Gy top-up dose per day in animals not receiving mitomycin C, but only 0.68 Gy in animals receiving the drug. Thus, at least mitomycin C may increase the efficacy of radiation by the inhibition of repopulation.

4.3 Role of Hypoxia

As known for years, radiation-induced cell kill is strongly dependent on the presence of adequate oxygen tensions. With increasing tumors, for example, in head and neck cancer, areas of hypoxia and even anoxia are present leading to an increased radiation resistance of clonogenic tumor cells within such areas (Molls and Vaupel 1998; Nordsmark et al. 2005; Molls et al. 2009). It has been speculated that chemotherapeutic agents especially those which kill even hypoxic cells (mitomycin C) may overcome global radiation resistance simply by killing radioresistant hypoxic cells, thereby being of special value in highly hypoxic tumors (Teicher et al. 1981; Rockwell 1982).

Comparing the effects of several cytostatic drugs in combination with radiation on the growth of a C3H mammary carcinoma, it turned out that cyclophosphamide, adriamycin, and mitomycin C had the most significant effect on the proportional cell kill of hypoxic cells. In contrast, bleomycin and cisplatin did not exert strong effects on hypoxic cells (Grau and Overgaard 1988). In addition, it has clearly been shown that tumor blood flow in xenografts is increased after mitomycin C treatment (Durand and LePard 1994). Using two different squamous cell carcinomas, the latter authors tested the drug's influence on outcome of radiation treatment with or without hypoxia (Durand and LePard 2000). The authors did not report an increased killing of hypoxic cell by mitomycin C, nor a consistent increase in tumor blood flow rates; however, mitomycin C in combination with radiation was associated with a slight increase in cell killing of hypoxic subpopulations of the xenograft system. Based on this observation it was concluded that the efficacy of a combined treatment with mitomycin C and radiation cannot be rationalized on either a complementary cytotoxicity or on drug-induced improvement in tumor oxygenation secondary to an increased blood flow.

In the case of paclitaxel, it has been tested whether the enhanced killing by the combination of paclitaxel and radiation is connected to the presence of oxygen. Using a MCA-4 xenograft system, the authors could show that in the absence of oxygen the paclitaxel-mediated change of the TCD50 value is strikingly less prominent (Milas et al. 1994, 1995); thus, it can be concluded that at least in part the influence of paclitaxel on the radiation response is mediated via an optimized oxygenation. In conclusion, several sets of data indicate that the efficacy of chemotherapy in combination with radiation may be related to an increased oxygenation of hypoxic tumors; however, it still remains speculative whether or to what amount the efficacy of a combined treatment is strictly related to specific influences on the hypoxic cell compartment.

5 Molecular Interactions

5.1 DNA Damage

One of the underlying molecular aspects of the efficacy of the combination of radiation and chemotherapy, which has been understood in some more detail, is influence on DNA repair. The induction of DNA damage is probably one of the most crucial events after irradiation of cells. In this regard, ionizing radiation triggers a wide array of lesions including base damage, single-strand breaks, and notably, double-strand breaks (DSBs). After irradiation, different molecular systems are involved in recognition and repair of the damage. Whereas most of the induced damage is quickly repaired, DSB repair is slow and unrepaired DSBs are considerably important for the final induction of cell death.

Many chemotherapeutic agents, especially those known to be of value in combination with radiation, also induce considerable DNA damage or interfere with effective DNA repair; therefore, two general patterns of interactions may be separated: (a) the combination of the drug with radiation directly leads to more damage; (b) the drug may interact with DNA repair pathway thus increasing the level of DNA damage more indirectly; however, none of the potential mechanisms acts without the other in real settings. Cisplatin, for example, acts by complex formation with guanosine residues and subsequent adduct formation ultimately resulting in intra- and interstrand cross-links. This type of damage is mostly removed by base excision repair and mismatch repair. Several sets of data suggest that single-strand damage induced by radiation in close vicinity to DNA damage triggered by cisplatin results in a mutual inhibition of the damage-specific repair system; thus, the amount of resulting damage leads to an increased net cell kill (Begg 1990; Yang et al. 1995). Similarly, etoposide, which is a strong topoisomerase-IIa-directed toxin, exerts DSB mostly during the S-phase of the cell cycle (Berrios et al. 1985; Earnshaw and Heck 1985). Again, several lines of evidence show that the combination of both agents results in a strongly increased level of damage (Giocanti et al. 1993; Yu et al. 2000).

The biochemical pathways implicated in DNA repair and DNA synthesis overlap in several regards; thus, drugs acting on the synthesis of DNA putatively also interfere with the repair of DNA damage induced by ionizing radiation. Several prototypical radiation sensitizers, including 5-FU, fludarabine, and gemcitabine, may act via these mechanisms. Besides cisplatin, 5-FU is probably the most commonly employed drug in clinical combined modality settings. Basically, 5-FU inhibits thymidilate synthase thereby reducing the intracellular pool of nucleoside triphosphates (Pinedo and Peters 1988; Miller and Kinsella 1992). In addition, the drug is integrated into DNA via fluorodeoxyuridine, also contributing to its anti-neoplastic effects. Several lines of evidence suggest that the amount of 5-FU integrated into DNA directly correlates with the radiosensitizing effect. In addition, the complementation of the cell culture medium with higher levels of thymidine reverses the effects of 5-FU on the radiation sensitivity (McGinn et al. 1996; Lawrence et al. 1994).

5.2 Radiation Sensitization via Cell Cycle Synchronization

The fact that striking differences in the radiation sensitivity occur as cells move through the different phases of the cell cycle has stimulated the speculation that the efficacy of a combined treatment may also be related to possible effects on the reassortment of cells in more vulnerable cell cycle phases.

Several experimental settings provide evidence that cell cycle effects are involved in the modulation of the efficacy of combined modality approaches. In this regard, the use of a temperature-sensitive p53 mutant allows the analysis of cell cycle effects very nicely. The underlying hypothesis was that fluoropyrimidine-mediated radiosensitization occurs only in tumor cells that inappropriately enter S-phase in the presence of drug resulting in a subsequent repair defect of the radiation-induced damage. The use of the mutated p53 allowed p21-mediated arrest prior to S-phase entry when cells are grown under 32 °C, in contrast to no arrest in cells grown at the nonpermissive temperatures of 38 °C. The radiation-sensitizing effect of fluoropyrimidine was directly connected to the lacking G1 arrest when cells were grown under nonpermissive temperatures; thus, the fluoropyrimidine-mediated radiosensitization clearly requires progression into S-phase (Naida et al. 1998).

In an extension of these findings, Naida et al. (1998) analyzed the effects of fluorodeoxyuridine on the radiation sensitivity in HT29 and SW620 human colon cancer cells under nearly complete inhibition of thymidylate synthase (both cell lines harbor a similar p53 mutation). Interestingly, only the HT29 cells were sensitized. As an underlying feature, the authors found that only the HT29 cells progressed into S-phase and demonstrated increased cyclin E-dependent kinase activity. In contrast, SW620 cells were found to be arrested just past the G1-S boundary and an increase in kinase activity was not detectable; thus, the findings underline the requirement of an S-phase transition for the efficacy of halogenated fluoropyrimidines in combination with radiation. These findings also highlight the role of molecules involved in cell cycle regulation as key players for the modulation of a combined modality approach (McGinn et al. 1994; Lawrence et al. 1996a, b, c). In addition to the fact that the S-phase transition is required for the radiosensitization effect, it has also been shown that fluoropyrimidines under defined dosage conditions facilitate the accumulation of cells in S-phase (Miller and Kinsella 1992).

In addition to the findings on halogenated fluoropyrimidines, several other sets of data obtained with paclitaxel suggest that an increased radiation sensitivity occurred at the time of a taxane-induced G2-M block; however, the situation for taxane combinations is highly complex in so far as other data provide evidence that the mitotic arrest is not sufficient for the effects of paclitaxel (Geard and Jones 1994; Hennequin et al. 1996). The picture becomes even more complicated when taking into account that radiation was shown to decrease the net killing of taxanes (Sauer et al. 2004). In this regard, it has been shown that the combination of paclitaxel and gamma radiation did not produce a synergistic or additive effect in a breast cancer and epidermoid cancer cell model. Instead, the overall cytotoxicity of the combination was lower than that of the drug treatment alone. Especially apoptosis induction was found to be strikingly reduced. A detailed analysis revealed that radiation resulted in cell cycle arrest at G2 phase preventing the G1-M transition-dependent cytotoxic effects of paclitaxel. Furthermore, radiation inhibited paclitaxel-induced IkappaBalpha degradation and bcl-2 phosphorylation and increased the protein levels of cyclin B1 and inhibitory phosphorylation of p34 (cdc2).

Taken together, the impact of chemotherapy-induced cell cycle alterations as major mechanism for the efficacy of the combined action is still questionable. In clinical settings, the importance of an adequate cell cycle progression for the efficacy of radiochemotherapy approaches has been impressively documented. In the case of a neoadjuvant 5-FU-based radiochemotherapy for rectal cancer, it has been shown that a decrease of the cell cycle inhibitory protein p21 during neoadjuvant treatment is strongly associated with an improved disease-specific survival. This finding has been corroborated by the observation that a parallel increase of the expression level of the proliferation marker Ki-67 is similarly associated with an improved outcome (Rau et al. 2003); thus, preclinical findings on the action of 5-FU in combination with radiation are clearly reflected by clinical observations.

6 Radiation and Platinum-Based Drugs: Example of Clinically Established Combined Modality Treatments

Contemporary clinical concepts include combined administration of radiation and three different platinum compounds (cisplatin, carboplatin, and oxaliplatin) in a variety of common solid tumors. Examples are sites such as head and neck, esophagus, lung, cervix uteri, rectum, and bladder. All these platinum drugs have demonstrated efficacy against a variety of cell lines, tumor xenografts, and human tumors. Yet, their effects vary with several molecular features of the cells, for example, p53 status and expression of drug resistance proteins. Resistance also results from increased expression of the *ERCC1* gene (excision repair cross-complementing 1), which is involved in nucleotide excision repair and the removal of DNA interstrand cross-links, and other repair genes (ALTAHA et al. 2004). Both intrinsic and acquired drug resistance have been described. The simultaneous administration of platinum agents can be used to enhance the effects of radiation treatment, aiming either at additive cell kill or true radiosensitization ("radiopotentiation") within the target volume, or to treat distant, out-of-field tumor sites based on the principle of spatial cooperation. Thereby, it is hoped to achieve a therapeutic gain.

6.1 Cisplatin

Discovered 50 years ago and initially recognized for its bacteriostatic effects (Rosenberg et al. 1965), cis-dichlorodiammine-platinum (II) or cisplatin was found in 1969 to cause antitumor effects. In 1971, the drug was, for the first time, combined with radiation in mice (Zak and Drobnik 1971) and subsequently was the first platinum-based drug entering the clinical practice of radiation oncology. Positive randomized trials were published for cervical cancer and non-small cell lung cancer (Choo et al. 1986, Schaake-Koning et al. 1990). Today, a large variety of administration schedules are in clinical use, including daily dosing with 6 mg/m^2, 20 mg/m^2/day on day 1–5 and 29–33 of fractionated radiotherapy, 40 mg/m^2/day on day 1, 8, 15, 22, 29, and 36, 100 mg/m^2/day on day 1, 22, and 43, etc. Heterogeneity of tissue concentration has been examined in various tumor models, for example, in mouse B16 melanoma, human non-small cell lung cancer xenografts (Zamboni et al. 2002), and the human prostate cancer cell line PC-3 M grown in nude mice, where the tumor concentrations ranged from 478 to 937 ppb (Coughlin et al. 1994). A prerequisite for drug efficacy is cellular uptake and avoidance of either efflux or inactivation, for example, by glutathione or other sulfur-containing molecules (Ekshyyan et al. 2009).

After transport into the cell, which appears to be linked to the copper metabolic pathway, but can also take place by passive diffusion, the chloride ligands are replaced by hydroxyl groups. This aquated the reactive form of the drug reacts with several proteins and DNA binding sites, as reviewed by Dewit (1987), and causes DNA-protein linkage and DNA interstrand and intrastrand cross-links interfering with DNA replication and repair, including repair of double-strand breaks (Taylor et al. 1976; Richmond and Powers 1976; Begg 1990; Amorino et al. 1999). The cellular responses include replication arrest, transcription inhibition, cell cycle arrest, and DNA repair via several signal transduction pathways (AKT, p53, MAPK/JNK/ERK, etc.). Cisplatin adducts might be removed by nucleotide excision repair mechanisms, following first-order kinetics. In cell culture, knockout of the nonhomologous endjoining (NHEJ) repair pathway did not change the response to cisplatin, whereas mutation of the homologous recombination repair pathway through XRCC3 resulted in increased radiation and cisplatin sensitivity (Raaphorst et al. 2005). Other data also demonstrate that yeast mutants in double-strand break repair by NHEJ and mutants in base excision repair showed no sensitivity to cis- or oxaliplatin (Wu et al. 2004). Other authors suggest that the cellular responses to cisplatin depend on DNA-activated protein kinase and DNA polymerase eta (Turchi et al. 1997; Albertella et al. 2005). It has been postulated that the loss of DNA mismatch repair is linked to the failure in detecting the DNA damage caused by cisplatin and to the lack of signal triggering the cell death mechanisms (Fink et al. 1996). Putative defective repair of oxidative damage also resulted in sensitivity to cis- and oxaliplatin in yeast (Wu et al. 2004). Cell killing after higher drug doses appears apoptosis-related, whereas after lower drug doses failure to overcome a G_2 block is more important (Ormerod et al. 1994). In p53-mutated 9 L rat gliosarcoma, intraperitoneal cisplatin (1 mg/kg) led to an increase in micronuclei formation, most likely indicating induction of mitotic catastrophe, but produced little or no apoptosis (Driessens et al. 2003). The drug is not cell cycle specific.

Concomitant application with radiation might reduce the likelihood of acquired resistance compared to induction chemotherapy and reduces the overall time from initiation of any treatment to completion of local radiotherapy. In early experiments, cisplatin reduced the repair of sublethal radiation-induced damage, as defined by split-dose recovery, in exponentially growing rat hepatoma cells. In plateau phase, radiation sensitization was found (Carde and Laval 1981). Later on, Dolling et al. reported inhibition of DNA double-strand break repair when cisplatin was administered prior to radiation (Dolling et al. 1998). When cis- or carboplatin were present at the time of irradiation, higher enhancement ratios were observed compared to administration 24 h prior to or 3 h after irradiation (Schwachöfer et al. 1991). Overgaard and Khan examined mouse mammary tumors exposed to radiotherapy with or without 6 mg/kg cisplatin administered intraperitoneally 30 min before irradiation (Overgaard and Khan 1981). The dose modification factor in these TCD_{50} experiments was 1.8, compared to 1.3 if the drug was given 30 min or 4 h after irradiation. Kallman reported a large set of animal experiments where fractionated radiotherapy was combined with cisplatin (Kallman et al. 1992). Tumor growth inhibition (RIF-1 and SCCVII tumors) and three normal tissue endpoints (duodenal crypt cell survival, lung toxicity after 5 and 10 months, respectively) were assessed. With few exceptions, the greatest therapeutic gain was achieved with multiple doses of cisplatin administered simultaneously with 5 daily fractions of radiotherapy.

6.2 Carboplatin

In chronological order, cis-diammine (1,1-cyclobutanedicarboxylate) platinum (II) (carboplatin) was the second compound that became part of clinical treatment protocols. In 20 cervical cancer cell lines, 30 % of the tumors resistant to cisplatin were also resistant to carboplatin (Monk et al. 1998). However, the toxicity profile is advantageous. Carboplatin has greater chemical stability than cisplatin and longer half-lives of ultrafilterable platinum. The terminal half-lives are comparable (5–6 days). It forms a similar spectrum of DNA adducts as cisplatin with slightly different sequence preferences (Blommaert et al. 1995). In order to obtain equivalent DNA platination levels, higher concentrations of carboplatin are needed. The sensitivity of squamous cell carcinoma cell lines to carboplatin differs at least by a factor of 4 (pekkola-Heino et al. 1992). In these experiments, no cross-resistance was observed between inherent radiosensitivity and chemosensitivity. When administered 1 h before irradiation to carboplatin-sensitive cell lines, additive effects were observed.

Carboplatin enhances the production and persistence of radiation-induced DNA single-strand breaks (Yang et al. 1995) and reduces cell survival after radiation treatment measured by clonogenic assays (supraadditive effect) (Scalliet et al. 1999). In two cell lines proficient in both excision repair and DNA double-strand break repair, and in a cell line deficient in nucleotide excision repair, carboplatin before and during irradiation enhanced radiation-induced cell killing (Yang et al. 1995). In air and under hypoxic conditions, the enhancement was characterized as both a reduction in the shoulder region of the survival curves (reduced Dq) and a reduction in D0 in the terminal region of the survival curves. Only the latter effect was observed in a cell line deficient in DNA double-strand break repair. Enhancement ratios ranged from 1.3 to 1.7, irrespective of oxygenation. Drug levels sufficient to produce cytotoxicity by themselves were required for the effect of radiation enhancement. In the extreme case, only 1/30 of the drug concentration required for other cell lines produced enhanced cell killing, as seen in the intrinsically sensitive UV41 cells. In a mouse model of Ehrlich ascites tumors, combined treatment was compared to a single dose of carboplatin alone and a single dose of radiation alone. Tumor growth delay was better with simultaneous combined treatment than each modality alone (Aratani et al. 1997). In mouse lip mucosa there was no influence of carboplatin on the response to single-dose irradiation, the capacity to repair sublethal radiation damage, and the ability to repopulate (Landuyt et al. 1987).

6.3 Oxaliplatin

Oxaliplatin (1,2-diaminocyclohexaneoxalato platinum (II)) is a third-generation lipophil platinum drug. The drug has less hematological toxicity and lacks nephrotoxicity. The dose-limiting side effect is peripheral neurotoxicity. The parent compound undergoes hydrolysis to form the effective reactive species. Cisplatin-resistant cell lines tend not to be resistant to oxaliplatin. Furthermore, oxaliplatin was more effective in several animal tumor models. Despite the fact that oxaliplatin forms covalent adducts with DNA that have similar sequence and region specificity to those formed by cisplatin, they are more cytotoxic (Pendyala and Creaven 1993; Woynarowski et al. 1998). It has been shown that cellular proteins, for example, mismatch repair proteins, recognize oxaliplatin adducts differentially and that the effects of oxaliplatin when compared to cisplatin are less dependent on intact mismatch repair (Raymond et al. 2002). Further differences exist regarding postreplicative bypass mechanisms. DNA polymerase beta and eta catalyze translesion synthesis past certain oxaliplatin adducts with greater efficiency than past cisplatin adducts. Further data provide a link between oxaliplatin sensitivity and DNA repair involving DNA polymerase beta, the major DNA polymerase involved in base excision repair (Yang et al. 2010). Like cisplatin, interstrand cross-links appear to be important toxic lesions caused by oxaliplatin (Wu et al. 2004).

Oxaliplatin showed synergistic effects with 5-FU as well as radiosensitization in human colon cancer cells (Kjellstrom et al. 2005; Folkvord et al. 2008). Additional data suggest that these effects might vary with p53 status of the colon cancer cell line (Magne et al. 2003). In p53 wild type SW403 cells, additive-synergistic effects were observed when the best sequence was administered, that is, irradiation 2 h before or at mid-drug application. Oxaliplatin was given over 2 h followed by 5-FU/folinic acid over 24 h. In p53-mutated WiDr cells, additive-antagonistic effects were seen, irrespective of sequence. Radiosensitization was also found in head and neck cancer cell lines (Espinosa et al. 2005). Oxaliplatin sensitized human HeLa and SiHa cells to ionizing radiation (Yang et al. 2009). In this model, drug pretreatment enhanced the cell cycle arrest in the G2/M phase and the radiation-induced mitotic catastrophe. Oxaliplatin modulated radiation-induced DNA double-strand breaks, as indicated by delayed abrogation of gamma-H2AX, attenuation of radiation-induced phosphorylation of ataxia telangiectasia-mutated kinase, and checkpoint kinase 2. In vivo data generated with transplanted mammary adenocarcinoma, but with the disputable endpoint of tumor growth delay rather than cure, suggest that sequence and time interval of radiation treatment and oxaliplatin do not influence the results for single-dose treatments (10 Gy and 6 or 10 mg/kg) (Cividalli et al. 2002). With 10 daily fractions of 2 Gy, however, the drug increased the efficacy of radiation treatment better when administered only twice during the treatment course as compared to daily.

7 Combined Modality Reirradiation

Two major examples where reirradiation often is combined with concomitant chemotherapy are head and neck tumors and rectal cancer. As already discussed, a therapeutic gain is expected on the basis of different models and extrapolation of results from first-line treatment approaches. With regard to the latter, there have been several meta-analyses of randomized trials performed suggesting a survival benefit with use of concurrent chemotherapy with external beam radiotherapy in head and neck cancer (Munro 1995; El-Sayed and Nelson 1996; Pignon et al. 2000, 2009). Among these meta-analyses, one was based on the collection of updated individual patient data. This Meta-Analysis of Chemotherapy in Head and Neck Cancer (MACH-NC) previously confirmed a survival benefit for concurrent radiochemotherapy and was later updated to include 24 new trials. This update reconfirmed the benefit of concurrent treatment for patients with locoregionally advanced disease, yielding an HR of 0.81 ($p<0.001$), with an absolute survival benefit of 8 % at 5 years. The 5-year absolute benefits associated with concomitant chemotherapy were 8.9 %, 8.1 %, 5.4 %, and 4 % for oral cavity, oropharynx, larynx, and hypopharynx tumors, respectively (Blanchard et al. 2011). The investigators found no significant difference between mono- and poly-chemotherapy regimens used concurrently. The benefit was found to be more pronounced for platinum-based combinations with or without 5-FU. In addition, the benefit of adding chemotherapy was more significant in younger patients and progressively decreased to become non-detectable beyond the age of 70. Together, these data support the use of concurrent radiochemotherapy as a standard of care first-line treatment option for stage III and IV head and neck cancer patients who can tolerate systemic chemotherapy.

Table 1 Agents that have been used in published reirradiation studies

Cisplatin, carboplatin
Docetaxel, paclitaxel
Lomustine, fotemustine
Temozolomide
Gemcitabine
Hydroxyurea
5-Fluorouracil, capecitabine
Topotecan

In the reirradiation setting, such high-quality randomized trials or even meta-analyses of randomized trials comparing reirradiation with reirradiation and chemotherapy are lacking. Therefore, the question arises whether or not the theoretical advantages of combined modality treatment are detectable in the published literature. Table 1 summarizes the recently published head and neck cancer reirradiation trials that might shed some light on this question. The trials are basically retrospective in nature, of limited size and thus underpowered, included heterogeneous patient groups with tremendous variation in tumor biology and size, and applied quite individual treatment. Often, second primary tumors and locoregional relapses are lumped together. Between 20 and 92% of the patients received chemotherapy along with reirradiation, the others reirradiation alone. Unexpectedly, no major impact of the combined approach is obvious, regardless of endpoint. However, none of the trials was really designed to prove the superiority of radiochemotherapy in this setting. The lack of efficacy might just reflect selection bias. More favorable patient groups might have received reirradiation alone, the others combined treatment. Alternatively, chemotherapy might not have improved the outcome, for example, because many patients were reexposed to platinum-based regimens, which they already had received during previous treatment, or because the drugs did not gain sufficient access to the tumor cells (altered perfusion and microenvironment after previous therapy, increased fibrosis, see Fig. 5).

A small study in squamous cell head and neck cancer with 29 patients (no second primaries included) who received reirradiation with platinum-based chemotherapy was published by Nagar et al. (2004). The median dose was only 34 Gy. This study suggested better efficacy in patients previously, that is, in first line, treated with radiation alone as compared to radiochemotherapy and that rechallenge with platinum-based combination treatment might not work very well. Theoretically, agents with different modes of action might be preferable (Table 2). The highest level of evidence results from a small phase II randomized trial in patients with recurrent nasopharyngeal cancer (Guan et al. 2016). These relatively young patients were required to have KPS ≥70 and minimum time interval of 6 months. All 69 patients received IMRT (27 fractions of 2.2 Gy, total dose 60 Gy, inclusion between 2002 and 2008). The investigational arm also received weekly cisplatin 30 mg/m^2. Despite the small sample size, overall survival was the primary endpoint. Median follow-up was 35 months.

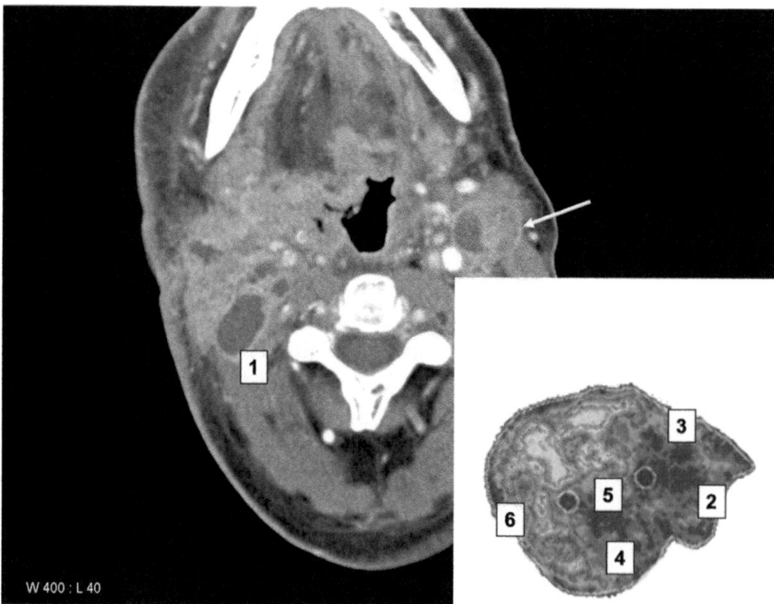

Fig. 5 Computed tomography scan of a patient with recurrent squamous cell carcinoma of the oropharynx. Note the large lymph node metastasis which contains necrotic areas (*white arrow*). The inserted cartoon is an example of histological and molecular heterogeneity within a recurrent tumor. *1* tumor subvolume with insufficient blood perfusion resulting, for example, in hypoxia or poor access of systemically administered drugs. *2* cells that are primarily resistant to the mechanism of a given drug. *3* cells with acquired resistance. *4* cells that can be killed by drug treatment. *5* cells that can be killed by radiation. *6* cells that can be killed by combined radiation and drug

Table 2 Overview of clinical reirradiation studies addressing the added value of concomitant chemotherapy (Ctx), some studies included cases with additional induction and/or adjuvant Ctx

Reference	Study type, patient number	Cancer type	Treatment details	Results
Strnad et al. (2015)	Retrospective, 104	Squamous cell and other head and neck cancer including second primaries	Interstitial PDR brachytherapy, 22 % combined with EBRT, 32 % hyperthermia, 56 % received Ctx (mostly cisplatin/5-FU)	Simultaneous Ctx improved 10-year local control (76 vs. 39 %, $p = 0.014$)
Hoebers et al. (2011)	Retrospective, 58	Squamous cell and other head and neck cancer including second primaries	3-D or IMRT, median 66 Gy, 57 % received concurrent Ctx, often daily low-dose cisplatin	Ctx increased the risk of serious toxicity and was associated with shorter survival. However, patients managed without Ctx typically were irradiated after salvage surgery (smaller volumes, lower doses, better prognosis)
Unger et al. (2010)	Retrospective, 65	Squamous cell and other head and neck cancer including second primaries	SFRT, e.g., 30 Gy in five fractions of 6 Gy, 51 % received Ctx (no standard regimen)	The impact of Ctx on severe toxicity, locoregional failure rate, progression-free survival, and overall survival was evaluated. No significant difference was observed
Popovtzer et al. (2009)	Retrospective, 66	Squamous cell head and neck cancer including second primaries	3-D or IMRT, median 68 Gy, 71 % received Ctx (no standard regimen)	The impact of Ctx on locoregional failure rate was evaluated. No significant difference was observed
Sulman et al. (2009)	Retrospective, 74	Squamous cell and other head and neck cancer including second primaries	IMRT, median 60 Gy, 49 % received Ctx (no standard regimen)	The impact of Ctx on locoregional failure rate and overall survival was evaluated. No significant difference was observed
Duprez et al. (2009)	Retrospective, 84	Squamous cell and other head and neck cancer including second primaries	IMRT, median 69 Gy, 20 % received induction or concurrent Ctx (no standard regimen)	The impact of Ctx on locoregional failure rate and overall survival was evaluated. No significant difference was observed. However, Ctx significantly increased acute non-hematological toxicity $\geq$ grade III
Tanvetyanom et al. (2009)	Retrospective, 103	Squamous cell and other head and neck cancer including second primaries	Different approaches, median 60 Gy, 70 % received concurrent Ctx (no standard regimen)	The impact of Ctx on overall survival was evaluated. No significant difference was observed
Iseli et al. (2009)	Retrospective, 87	Squamous cell head and neck cancer including second primaries	Different approaches, median >58 Gy, 92 % received Ctx (no standard regimen)	The impact of Ctx on overall survival and toxicity was evaluated. No significant difference was observed
Lee et al. (2007)	Retrospective, 105	Squamous cell and other head and neck cancer including 1 s primary	3-D or IMRT, median 59.4 Gy, 71 % received Ctx (no standard regimen)	Ctx was associated with improved locoregional progression-free survival and overall survival, but not statistically significant

(continued)

Table 2 (continued)

Reference	Study type, patient number	Cancer type	Treatment details	Results
Ohizumi et al. (2002)	Retrospective, 44	Recurrent squamous cell head and neck cancer	Different approaches, mean 53 Gy, 23 % received Ctx (no standard regimen)	Ctx was associated with borderline significant increase in complete response. There was no significant impact on relapse-free and overall survival
Guan et al. (2016)	Prospective randomized phase II, 69	Recurrent nasopharyngeal carcinoma	IMRT, 60 Gy in 27 fractions, with or without weekly cisplatin 30 mg/m^2	Ctx was associated with significantly better survival. Acute toxicity was increased too
Karam et al. (2015)	Retrospective, 42	Recurrent nasopharyngeal carcinoma	IMRT or other technique, 74 % received concurrent Ctx (no standard regimen)	Ctx did not significantly impact on overall survival, local control, or locoregional control; however, late toxicities were significantly increased
Chen et al. (2013)	Retrospective, 54	Recurrent nasopharyngeal carcinoma	IMRT, average 70 Gy, 33 % received concurrent CTx (no standard regimen)	Ctx given concurrently was associated with significantly worse local progression-free survival; however, an imbalance in T-stage was present
Wahl et al. (2008)	Retrospective, 81	Recurrent breast cancer	Different approaches, median 48 Gy, 54 % received Ctx (no standard regimen)	Ctx did not significantly impact on complete remission rate, local disease-free survival, and toxicity

3-D three-dimensional conformal, *EBRT* external beam radiotherapy, *IMRT* intensity-modulated radiotherapy, *PDR* pulsed dose rate, *SFRT* stereotactic fractionated radiotherapy

Most patients had rT3-4 N0 tumors and median volume was 28 and 29 cm^3, respectively. Initial treatment was mostly 2-D radiotherapy alone, but 29 % had received radiochemotherapy before (regimens not reported in detail). In the investigational arm, more patients developed mucositis and grade 3–4 hematological toxicity. Late toxicity was not significantly increased. Survival was significantly better in the combined modality arm. In multivariate analysis, survival was associated with age, rT stage, clinical stage, and treatment arm. These analyses did not include comparisons of initial radiotherapy alone vs. radiochemotherapy.

Overall, it is desirable to perform sufficiently large prospective randomized trials that confirm many institutions' current clinical practice of reirradiation and chemotherapy. Such trials will also have to address another hypothesis derived from a previous study (Salama et al. 2006). In that study, seven consecutive phase I–II studies at the University of Chicago were compared. A total of 115 patients with squamous cell carcinoma of the head and neck including some patients with second primary tumors were included. The protocols mandated that each patient be treated on 14-day cycles. During each cycle, radiochemotherapy was delivered on days 1–5, followed by a 9-day break. The study suggested a potential benefit from triple-agent chemotherapy as compared to 5-FU and hydroxyurea combination. The third agent was either cisplatin, gemcitabine, or paclitaxel. Obviously, toxicity of triple-agent chemotherapy might limit the applicability of this strategy in a considerable number of patients. Less toxic alternatives are therefore desirable. Ideally, future research will include phase I trials examining combinations with new agents such as the trial by Van Waes et al. (2005), which found that reirradiation with concurrent twice weekly bortezomib in patients with recurrent head and neck squamous cell carcinoma was not feasible at the drug doses studied. Given the limited efficacy and at least in part considerable toxicity of reirradiation with chemotherapy, the examination of new and hopefully less toxic agents in such trials is warranted.

Cetuximab, a drug interfering with the epidermal growth factor receptor (EGFR) pathway, has shown encouraging results in first-line head and neck cancer radiotherapy (Bonner et al. 2010). This has led several investigators to explore the drug in the setting of reirradiation (Tanvetyanom et al. 2009; Unger et al. 2010; Heron et al. 2011), albeit without formal prospective trials. More details on reirradiation and cetuximab have recently been reported (Dornoff et al. 2015). The authors retrospectively compared 3-D conformal external beam reirradiation combined with cetuximab for patients with inoperable and recurrent squamous cell carcinoma of the head and neck in 33 patients to another group of 33 patients who received cisplatin ± 5-FU. Overall, 62 patients were eligible for both compounds. The decision for or against cisplatin was based on patient or physician preference. The median radiation dose was 50.4 Gy in 1.8-Gy fractions. Baseline characteristics were similar, except for a trend toward younger age in the cisplatin group. Seventy-six percent had previously been exposed to simultaneous chemotherapy for their primary tumors, but none to cetuximab. Previous chemotherapy was not associated with any survival difference. Both compounds resulted in similar overall survival, local control, and freedom from metastases. Hematological toxicity $\geq$ grade 3 occurred more often in the cisplatin group, pain $\geq$ grade 3 in the cetuximab group, $p < 0.05$ for both. Hypofractionated stereotactic radiotherapy (mostly 40–44 Gy in five fractions) has also been used in conjunction with cetuximab (Heron et al. 2011). This matched case-control study suggests that cetuximab might improve local control and survival as compared to radiotherapy alone, but includes only 35 patients treated with combined modality. From July 2007 to March 2013, Vargo et al. (2015) treated 50 patients with inoperable locoregionally confined recurrent squamous cell carcinoma of the head and neck in the context of a phase II protocol. All tumors were located within a previously irradiated field receiving $\geq$60 Gy. Concurrent cetuximab plus stereotactic radiotherapy was given (40–44 Gy in five fractions on alternating days over 1–2 weeks). Primary endpoints were 1-year locoregional progression-free survival (PFS) and toxicity. Median follow-up for surviving patients was 18 months. The 1-year local PFS rate was 60 %, locoregional PFS was 37 %, distant PFS was 71 %, and PFS was 33 %. The median overall survival was 10 months, with a 1-year overall survival of 40 %. Acute and late grade 3 toxicity was observed in 6 % of patients respectively. Another phase II study was reported by Lartigau et al. (2013). Patients with inoperable recurrent, or new primary tumor in a previously irradiated area, were included. Reirradiation dose was 36 Gy in six fractions of 6 Gy to the 85 % isodose line covering 95 % of the planning target volume with concomitant cetuximab. Forty-eight percent had previous chemotherapy. The study included 60 patients (three were not treated and one received only cetuximab). Mean time between previous radiotherapy and reirradiation was 38 months. There was one toxic death from hemorrhage and malnutrition. Median follow-up was 11.4 months. The 1-year survival rate was 47.5 %, comparable to the results reported by Vargo et al. (2015). These single-arm studies did not provide compelling evidence for combined modality therapy. Other authors reported similar 1-year survival rates with reirradiation alone (Yamazaki et al. 2015) or no impact of systemic therapy in mixed patient groups (Kress et al. 2015).

Erlotinib has also been examined in the phase I setting (Rusthoven et al. 2010). This tyrosine kinase inhibitor interacts with the EGFR pathway. Six of 14 patients had new primary tumors, the others recurrent disease. Erlotinib treatment started 7 days before reirradiation (66 Gy in 2.2 Gy fractions in the final patient cohort). The median time for administration of the drug was 4.1 months. Acute grade 3 radiation-associated toxicity developed in 85 % of patients. Nevertheless, the authors reported that concurrent and maintenance erlotinib (150 mg daily) was feasible. Median survival and progression-free survival was 15 months and 7.8 months, respectively.

A phase I study examined bevacizumab, an inhibitor of the vascular endothelial growth factor (VEGF) pathway, added to 5-FU and hydroxyurea concomitant to radiotherapy (1.8–2 Gy per fraction) in poor prognosis head and neck cancer (Seiwert et al. 2008). Dose escalation of bevacizumab and 5-FU/hydroxyurea were performed sequentially. Cohorts of 3–6 patients were enrolled at each dose level. Treatment was administered as described by Salama et al. (2006), that is, 14-day cycles. During each cycle, radiochemotherapy was delivered on days 1–5, followed by a 9-day break. Bevacizumab was given on day 1. The trial enrolled 43 patients including an expanded cohort after closure of phase I. The expanded cohort was treated with 10 mg/kg bevacizumab, 600 mg/m^2 5-FU, and 500 mg hydroxyurea. Twenty-nine patients had received prior radiation. The median time interval was 18.4 months (minimum 4 months). The median initial radiation dose was 63 Gy. The median reirradiation dose was 70 Gy. Overall, 7 of 43 patients died during or shortly after therapy (5 in the expansion cohort), of which some events were possibly treatment related. The rate, timing, and severity of fistulas reported with this regimen were of concern. Median survival in the reirradiated patients was 9.2 months. However, some patients had known distant metastases. After exclusion of these patients, median survival was 10.3 months (2-year survival 17 %). Fourteen reirradiated patients experienced recurrence (eight distally, four locoregionally, two both). It is therefore unclear whether antiangiogenic agents improve the therapeutic ratio of reirradiation. The role of bevacizumab in recurrent brain tumors is discussed elsewhere in this book.

Regarding rectal cancer, 5-FU has been the most commonly used single chemotherapeutic agent during the last five decades. Since its synthesis in 1957 by Heidelberger (Heidelberger et al. 1957), the metabolism and mechanism of action of 5-FU have been studied in detail. 5-FU enters a complex anabolic process that accounts for cytotoxicity at the cellular level by interfering with normal DNA and RNA function. Heidelberger et al. also initially discovered that the addition of 5-FU to radiation in rodent tumors markedly enhanced the effects of radiation therapy (Heidelberger et al. 1958). Based on these early preclinical data, Moertel et al. administered 5-FU with radiation to patients with gastrointestinal cancers and noted significant activity (Moertel et al. 1969). The pioneering contribution to the use of combined radiotherapy and 5-FU was made by Byfield et al., who demonstrated that 5-FU radiosensitization resulted from specific time and concentration factors. The sensitizing effects of 5-FU in vitro are maximal when its exposure occurs for at least 24 h and up to 48 h after the radiation exposure, thus supporting a prolonged 5-FU exposure approach when given with fractionated irradiation (Byfield et al. 1982). Historically, the combination of postoperative radiotherapy and 5-FU-based chemotherapy has been shown in several randomized trials to reduce local recurrence rates and to improve overall survival compared with surgery alone or surgery plus postoperative radiotherapy. The NCI Consensus Conference concluded in 1990 that combined radiochemotherapy was the standard adjuvant treatment for patients with TNM stages II and III rectal cancer (NIH consensus conference 1990). NCCTG trial 864751 tested the best method of administering 5-FU during radiotherapy: Bolus 5-FU (500 mg/m^2 for 3 days during weeks 1 and 5 of radiation therapy) was compared with continuous infusion (225 mg/m^2 during the whole course of radiotherapy). A 10% disease-free and overall survival advantage was achieved with continuous infusion 5-FU (O'Connell et al. 1994). The interest in preoperative radiochemotherapy for resectable tumors of the rectum is based not only on the success of the combined modality approach in the postoperative setting, but also on many radio- and tumorbiological advantages of the preoperative approach. Among those are downsizing effects that possibly enhance curative surgery in locally advanced disease, and sphincter preservation in low-lying tumors. Prospective randomized trials comparing the efficacy of preoperative with standard postoperative radiochemotherapy in stage II and III rectal cancer were initiated both in the United States through the Radiation Therapy Oncology Group (RTOG 94-01) and the NSABP (R-03) as well as in Germany (Protocol CAO/ARO/AIO-94). Unfortunately, both US trials suffered from lack of accrual and were closed prematurely. The German study has been completed with more than 820 patients included. Compared with postoperative radiochemotherapy, the preoperative combined modality approach was superior in terms of local control, downstaging, acute and chronic toxicity, and sphincter preservation in those patients judged by the surgeon to require an abdominoperineal resection (Sauer et al. 2004). Reirradiation of rectal cancer is typically performed with concomitant continuous infusion 5-FU or the newer alternative capecitabine. Treatment might be performed preoperatively or with palliative intent. The current practice is extrapolated from first-line experience. As with head and neck cancer, it is unclear whether combined modality treatment is superior because adequate prospective clinical trials are lacking in the reirradiation setting. The integration of new agents (or agents that have not been used during first-line treatment) such as oxaliplatin, EGFR inhibitors, and angiogenesis inhibitors is at the beginning. Systematic data are not available yet.

As shown in Table 3, several small studies suggest a potential advantage of reirradiation together with sequential chemotherapy in different types of central nervous system tumors. The data from the Japanese germinoma study are corroborated by another small series (eight patients) of platinum-based chemotherapy followed by focal, reduced-dose irradiation (Douglas et al. 2006). Two patients suffered marginal (at field edge) failures and both were salvaged using reinduction platinum-based chemotherapy followed by cranial spinal irradiation and a boost to the primary tumor. The 5-year actuarial overall survival was 100%. Nevertheless, due to concerns about study size and design, no firm conclusion about the role of reirradiation and sequential chemotherapy can be drawn.

In a study of reirradiation and hyperthermia for irresectable recurrent breast cancer, which included 248 patients, local control was not associated with receipt of prior chemotherapy or hormonal therapy or continuation of hormonal therapy during local treatment (Linthorst et al. 2015).

There has been a long-lasting interest in prediction of individual response and this interest is of particular importance in the reirradiation setting, where certain proportions of patients fail to respond and the toxicity risk might be higher than in first-line treatment. Treatment monitoring

Table 3 Overview of clinical reirradiation studies addressing the added value of sequential chemotherapy (Ctx)

Reference	Study type, patient number	Cancer type	Treatment details	Results
Kamoshima et al. (2008)	Retrospective, 25	CNS germinoma[a]	Different approaches, 14 patients had reirradiation and Ctx, often 24–25.2 Gy and platinum-based Ctx	7 of 11 patients treated with reirradiation alone died due to further recurrences, while 10 of the combined modality patients were salvaged successfully (Kaplan-Meier curves and p value were not published)
Fokas et al. (2009)	Retrospective, 53	Glioblastoma	SFRT (no standard fractionation), 47 % received Ctx (no standard regimen)	Ctx was associated with numerically improved survival, but not statistically significant
Grosu et al. (2005)	Prospective non-randomized single institution, 44	High-grade glioma	SFRT, six fractions of 5 Gy, 66 % received temozolomide	Ctx was associated with significantly improved survival
Fogh et al. (2010)	Retrospective, 147	High-grade glioma	SFRT, median 35 Gy in 3.5-Gy fractions, 33 % received Ctx (no standard regimen)	Ctx had no significant impact on survival (no trend toward improvement either)
Chua et al. (2005)	Phase II, 31	Nasopharyngeal carcinoma	IMRT (no standard fractionation), 68 % received 2–3 cycles of Ctx before reirradiation (advanced stage tumors)	Ctx had no significant impact on locoregional control and survival

CNS central nervous system, *SFRT* stereotactic fractionated radiotherapy, *IMRT* intensity-modulated radiotherapy
[a]All patients had achieved complete remission after initial therapy and were tumor-free for at least 6 months

early during a course of chemotherapy or radiochemotherapy by means of positron emission tomography, diffusion magnetic resonance imaging, and other biological imaging methods has shown promising results (Weber 2005; Schöder and Ong 2008; de Geus-Oei et al. 2009; Kim et al. 2009; Joye et al. 2014; Jentsch et al. 2015). Nevertheless, treatment individualization, also with regard to normal tissue toxicity and drug metabolism, for example, based on single nucleotide polymorphisms, continues to be an area of active investigation (Nuyten and van de Vijver 2008; Hummel et al. 2010; Kang et al. 2015; Volm and Efferth 2015). Complexity is added to this area by tissue changes resulting from previous treatment.

Conclusion

Although the combination of chemotherapeutic agents and ionizing radiation is of high relevance in diverse clinical settings, its role in reirradiation regimens and the underlying cellular and molecular mechanisms are only understood to a limited degree. Compared with the systematic experimental models used for development of first-line combinations and their evaluation through a classic series of clinical trials including randomized phase III studies, development of sound combination regimens for reirradiation is in its infancy. The clinical situation is complicated by more heterogeneous tumors with changes in physiological and microenvironmental parameters over time and quite variable pretreatment approaches, time intervals, irradiated volumes, etc. A gradual refinement of commonly administered regimens was achieved in subsequent small clinical trials rather than preclinical studies. While drug treatment evolved over time, the same holds true for advances in radiation treatment, for example, increasing use of IMRT. In addition, various fractionation schedules are in use. The impact of fraction size on radiosensitizing effects in the reirradiation setting is quite unclear. Thus, the ultimate goal of feasible and effective regimens in all patients treated with curative aim requires further substantial advances. In the palliative setting, systematic research is also needed, although the aim of treatment often might be achieved without adding drugs to reirradiation.

References

Albertella MR, Green CM, Lehmann AR et al (2005) A role for polymerase eta in the cellular tolerance to cisplatin-induced damage. Cancer Res 65:9799–9806

Altaha R, Liang X, Yu JJ et al (2004) Excision repair cross complementing-group 1: gene expression and platinum resistance. Int J Mol Med 14:959–970

Amorino GP, Freeman ML, Carbone DP et al (1999) Radiopotentiation by the oral platinum agent, JM216: role of repair inhibition. Int J Radiat Oncol Biol Phys 44:399–405

Aratani Y, Yoshiga K, Mizuuchi H et al (1997) Antitumor effect of carboplatin combined with radiation on tumors in mice. Anticancer Res 17:2535–2538

Arcicasa M, Roncadin M, Bidoli E et al (1999) Reirradiation and lomustine in patients with relapsed high-grade gliomas. Int J Radiat Oncol Biol Phys 43:789–793

Bartelink H, Roelofsen F, Eschwege F et al (1997) Concomitant radiotherapy and chemotherapy is superior to radiotherapy alone in the treatment of locally advanced anal cancer: results of a phase III randomized trial of the European Organization for Research and Treatment of Cancer Radiotherapy and Gastrointestinal Cooperative Groups. J Clin Oncol 15: 2040–2049

Baumann M, Liertz C, Baisch H et al (1994) Impact of overall treatment time of fractionated irradiation on local control of human FaDu squamous cell carcinoma in nude mice. Radiother Oncol 32:137–143

Begg AC (1990) Cisplatin and radiation: interaction probabilities and therapeutic possibilities. Int J Radiat Oncol Biol Phys 19:1183–1189

Belka C (2006) The fate of irradiated tumor cells. Oncogene 25:969–971

Berrios M, Osheroff N, Fisher PA (1985) In situ localization of DNA topoisomerase II, a major polypeptide component of the Drosophila nuclear matrix fraction. Proc Natl Acad Sci U S A 82:4142–4146

Biagioli MC, Narvey M, Roman E et al (2007) Intensity-modulated radiotherapy with concurrent chemotherapy for previously irradiated, recurrent head and neck cancer. Int J Radiat Oncol Biol Phys 69:1067–1073

Blanchard P, Baujat B, Holostenco V et al (2011) Meta-analysis of chemotherapy in head and neck cancer (MACH-NC): a comprehensive analysis by tumour site. Radiother Oncol 100:33–40

Blommaert FA, van Dijk-Knijnenburg HCM, Dijt FJ et al (1995) Formation of DNA adducts by the anticancer drug carboplatin: different nucleotide sequence preferences in vitro and in cells. Biochemistry 34:8474–8480

Bonner JA, Harari PM, Giralt J et al (2010) Radiotherapy plus cetuximab for locoregionally advanced head and neck cancer: 5-year survival data from a phase 3 randomised trial, and relation between cetuximab-induced rash and survival. Lancet Oncol 11:21–28

Brizel DM, Albers ME, Fisher SR et al (1998) Hyperfractionated irradiation with or without concurrent chemotherapy for locally advanced head and neck cancer. N Engl J Med 338:1798–1804

Brunsvig PF, Andersen A, Aamdal S et al (2007) Pharmacokinetic analysis of two different docetaxel dose levels in patients with non-small cell lung cancer treated with docetaxel as monotherapy or with concurrent radiotherapy. BMC Cancer 7:197

Budach W, Gioioso D, Taghian A et al (1997) Repopulation capacity during fractionated irradiation of squamous cell carcinomas and glioblastomas in vitro. Int J Radiat Oncol Biol Phys 39:743–750

Budach W, Paulsen F, Welz S et al (2002) Mitomycin C in combination with radiotherapy as a potent inhibitor of tumour cell repopulation in a human squamous cell carcinoma. Br J Cancer 86:470–476

Budach V, Stuschke M, Budach W et al (2005) Hyperfractionated accelerated chemoradiation with concurrent fluorouracil-mitomycin is more effective than dose-escalated hyperfractionated accelerated radiation therapy alone in locally advanced head and neck cancer: final results of the radiotherapy cooperative clinical trials group of the German Cancer Society 95-06 Prospective Randomized Trial. J Clin Oncol 23:1125–1135

Byfield JE, Calabro-Jones P, Klisak I et al (1982) Pharmacologic requirements for obtaining sensitization of human tumor cells in vitro to combined 5-Fluorouracil or ftorafur and X rays. Int J Radiat Oncol Biol Phys 8:1923–1933

Carde P, Laval F (1981) Effects of cis-dichlorodiammine platinum II and x rays on mammalian cell survival. Int J Radiat Oncol Biol Phys 7:929–933

Chen HY, Ma XM, Ye M et al (2013) Effectiveness and toxicities of intensity-modulated radiotherapy for patients with locally recurrent nasopharyngeal carcinoma. PLoS One 8:e73918

Choo YC, Choy TK, Wong LC, et al (1986) Potentiation of radiotherapy by cis-dichlorodiammine platinum (II) in advanced cervical carcinoma. Gynecol Oncol. 23(1):94–100.

Chua DT, Sham JS, Leung LH et al (2005) Re-irradiation of nasopharyngeal carcinoma with intensity-modulated radiotherapy. Radiother Oncol 77:290–294

Cividalli A, Ceciarelli F, Livdi E et al (2002) Radiosensitization by oxaliplatin in a mouse adenocarcinoma: influence of treatment schedule. Int J Radiat Oncol Biol Phys 52:1092–1098

Combs SE, Bischof M, Welzel T et al (2008) Radiochemotherapy with temozolomide as re-irradiation using high precision fractionated stereotactic radiotherapy (SFRT) in patients with recurrent gliomas. J Neurooncol 89:205–210

Coughlin CT, Richmond RC, Page RL (1994) Platinum drug delivery and radiation for locally advanced prostate cancer. Int J Radiat Oncol Biol Phys 28: 1029–1038

de Geus-Oei LF, Vriens D, van Laarhoven HW et al (2009) Monitoring and predicting response to therapy with 18F-FDG PET in colorectal cancer: a systematic review. J Nucl Med 50(Suppl 1):43S–54S

Dewit L (1987) Combined treatment of radiation and cis-diamminedichloroplatinum (II): a review of experimental and clinical data. Int J Radiat Oncol Biol Phys 13:403–426

Dolling JA, Boreham DR et al (1998) Modulation of radiation-induced strand break repair by cisplatin in mammalian cells. Int J Radiat Biol 74:61–69

Dornoff N, Weiss C, Rödel F et al (2015) Re-irradiation with cetuximab or cisplatin-based chemotherapy for recurrent squamous cell carcinoma of the head and neck. Strahlenther Onkol 191:656–664

Douglas JG, Rockhill JK, Olson JM et al (2006) Cisplatin-based chemotherapy followed by focal, reduced-dose irradiation for pediatric primary central nervous system germinomas. J Pediatr Hematol Oncol 28:36–39

Driessens G, Harsan L, Browaeys P et al (2003) Assessment of in vivo chemotherapy-induced DNA damage in a p53-mutated rat tumor by micronuclei assay. Ann N Y Acad Sci 1010:775–779

Duprez F, Madani I, Bonte K et al (2009) Intensity-modulated radiotherapy for recurrent and second primary head and neck cancer in previously irradiated territory. Radiother Oncol 93:563–569

Durand RE, LePard NE (1994) Modulation of tumor hypoxia by conventional chemotherapeutic agents. Int J Radiat Oncol Biol Phys 29:481–486

Durand RE, LePard NE (2000) Effects of mitomycin C on the oxygenation and radiosensitivity of murine and human tumours in mice. Radiother Oncol 56: 245–252

Earnshaw WC, Heck MM (1985) Localization of topoisomerase II in mitotic chromosomes. J Cell Biol 100:1716–1725

Ekshyyan O, Rong Y, Rong X et al (2009) Comparison of radiosensitizing effects of the mammalian target of rapamycin inhibitor CCI-779 to cisplatin in experimental models of head and neck squamous cell carcinoma. Mol Cancer Ther 8:2255–2265

Eliaz RE, Nir S, Marty C, Szoka FC Jr (2004) Determination and modeling of kinetics of cancer cell killing by doxorubicin and doxorubicin encapsulated in targeted liposomes. Cancer Res 64:711–718

El-Sayed S, Nelson N (1996) Adjuvant and adjunctive chemotherapy in the management of squamous cell carcinoma of the head and neck region. A meta-analysis of prospective and randomized trials. J Clin Oncol 14:838–847

Epstein RJ (1990) Drug-induced DNA damage and tumor chemosensitivity. J Clin Oncol 8:2062–2084

Espinosa M, Martinez M, Aguilar JL et al (2005) Oxaliplatin activity in head and neck cancer cell lines. Cancer Chemother Pharmacol 55:301–305

Fink D, Zheng H, Nebel S et al (1996) The role of DNA mismatch repair in platinum drug resistance. Cancer Res 56:4881–4886

Fogh SE, Andrews DW, Glass J et al (2010) Hypofrationated stereotactic radiation therapy: an effective therapy for recurrent high-grade gliomas. J Clin Oncol 28:3048–3053

Fokas E, Wacker U, Gross MW et al (2009) Hypofractionated stereotactic reirradiation of recurrent glioblastomas: a beneficial treatment option after high-dose radiotherapy? Strahlenther Onkol 185: 235–240

Folkvord S, Flatmark K, Seierstad T et al (2008) Inhibitory effects of oxaliplatin in experimental radiation treatment of colorectal carcinoma: does oxaliplatin improve 5-fluorouracil-dependent radiosensitivity? Radiother Oncol 86:428–434

Forastiere AA, Goepfert H, Maor M et al (2003) Concurrent chemotherapy and radiotherapy for organ preservation in advanced laryngeal cancer. N Engl J Med 349:2091–2098

Geard CR, Jones JM (1994) Radiation and taxol effects on synchronized human cervical carcinoma cells. Int J Radiat Oncol Biol Phys 29:565–569

Geh JI, Bond SJ, Bentzen SM et al (2006) Systemic overview of preoperative (neoadjuvant) chemoradiotherapy in patients with oesophageal cancer: evidence of a radiation and chemotherapy dose response. Radiother Oncol 78:236–244

Gerard J, Romestaing P, Bonnetain F et al (2005) Preoperative chemoradiotherapy (CT-RT) improves local control in T3-4 rectal cancers: results of the FFCD 9203 randomized trial (Abstract). Int J Radiat Oncol Biol Phys 63(Suppl 1):S2–S3

Giocanti N, Hennequin C, Balosso J et al (1993) DNA repair and cell cycle interactions in radiation sensitization by the topoisomerase II poison etoposide. Cancer Res 53:2105–2111

Grau C, Overgaard J (1988) Effect of cancer chemotherapy on the hypoxic fraction of a solid tumor measured using a local tumor control assay. Radiother Oncol 13:301–309

Green JA, Kirwan JM, Tierney JF et al (2001) Survival and recurrence after concomitant chemotherapy and radiotherapy for cancer of the uterine cervix: a systematic review and meta-analysis. Lancet 358:781–786

Grenman R, Carey TE, McClatchey KD et al (1991) In vitro radiation resistance among cell lines established from patients with squamous cell carcinoma of the head and neck. Cancer 67:2741–2747

Grosu AL, Weber WA, Franz M et al (2005) Reirradiation of recurrent high-grade gliomas using amino acid PET (SPECT)/CT/MRI image fusion to determine gross tumor volume for stereotactic fractionated radiotherapy. Int J Radiat Oncol Biol Phys 63:511–519

Guan Y, Liu S, Wang HY et al (2016) Long-term outcomes of a phase II randomized controlled trial comparing intensity-modulated radiotherapy with or without weekly cisplatin for the treatment of locally recurrent nasopharyngeal carcinoma. Chin J Cancer 35:20

Haraf DJ, Weichselbaum RR, Vokes EE (1996) Re-irradiation with concomitant chemotherapy of unresectable recurrent head and neck cancer: a potentially curable disease. Ann Oncol 7:913–918

Heidelberger C, Chaudhuri NK, Danneberg P et al (1957) Fluorinated pyrimidines, a new class of tumour-inhibitory compounds. Nature 179:663–666

Heidelberger C, Griesbach L, Montag BJ et al (1958) Studies on fluorinated pyrimidines. II. Effects on transplanted tumors. Cancer Res 18:305–317

Hennequin C, Giocanti N, Favaudon V (1996) Interaction of ionizing radiation with paclitaxel (taxol) and docetaxel (taxotere) in HeLa and SQ20B cells. Cancer Res 56:1842–1850

Heron DE, Rwigema JC, Gibson MK et al (2011) Concurrent cetuximab with stereotactic body radiotherapy for recurrent squamous cell carcinoma of the head and neck: a single institution matched case-control study. Am J Clin Oncol 34(2):165–172

Hoebers F, Heemsbergen W, Moor S et al (2011) Reirradiation for head-and-neck cancer: delicate balance between effectiveness and toxicity. Int J Radiat Oncol Biol Phys 81:e111–e118

Hummel R, Hussey DJ, Haier J (2010) MicroRNAs: predictors and modifiers of chemo- and radiotherapy in different tumour types. Eur J Cancer 46:298–311

Iseli TA, Iseli CE, Rosenthal EL et al (2009) Postoperative reirradiation for mucosal head and neck squamous cell carcinomas. Arch Otolaryngol Head Neck Surg 135:1158–1164

Jentsch C, Beuthien-Baumann B, Troost EG et al (2015) Validation of functional imaging as a biomarker for radiation treatment response. Br J Radiol 88:20150014

Jones B, Sanghera P (2007) Estimation of radiobiologic parameters and equivalent radiation dose of cytotoxic chemotherapy in malignant glioma. Int J Radiat Oncol Biol Phys 68:441–448

Joseph KJ, Al-Mandhari Z, Pervez N et al (2008) Reirradiation after radical radiation therapy: a survey of patterns of practice among Canadian radiation oncologists. Int J Radiat Oncol Biol Phys 72:1523–1529

Joye I, Deroose CM, Vandecaveye V et al (2014) The role of diffusion-weighted MRI and (18)F-FDG PET/CT in the prediction of pathologic complete response after radiochemotherapy for rectal cancer: a systematic review. Radiother Oncol 113:158–165

Kallman RF, Bedarida G, Rapacchietta D (1992) Experimental studies on schedule dependence in the treatment of cancer with combinations of chemotherapy and radiotherapy. Front Radiat Ther Oncol 26:31–44

Kamoshima Y, Sawamura Y, Ikeda J et al (2008) Late recurrence and salvage therapy of CNS germinomas. J Neurooncol 90:205–211

Kang H, Kiess A, Chung CH (2015) Emerging biomarkers in head and neck cancer in the era of genomics. Nat Rev Clin Oncol 12:11–26

Karam I, Huang SH, McNiven A et al (2015) Outcomes after reirradiation for recurrent nasopharyngeal carcinoma: North American experience. Head Neck. doi:10.1002/hed.24166

Kasibhatla M, Kirkpatrick JP, Brizel DM (2007) How much radiation is the chemotherapy worth in advanced head and neck cancer? Int J Radiat Oncol Biol Phys 68:1491–1495

Kim JJ, Tannock IF (2005) Repopulation of cancer cells during therapy: an important cause of treatment failure. Nat Rev Cancer 5:516–525

Kim JH, Kim SH, Kolozsvary A, Khil MS (1992) Potentiation of radiation response in human carcinoma cells in vitro and murine fibrosarcoma in vivo by topotecan, an inhibitor of DNA topoisomerase I. Int J Radiat Oncol Biol Phys 22:515–518

Kim S, Loevner L, Quon H et al (2009) Diffusion-weighted magnetic resonance imaging for predicting and detecting early response to chemoradiation therapy of squamous cell carcinomas of the head and neck. Clin Cancer Res 15:986–994

Kjellstrom J, Kjellen E, Johnsson A (2005) In vitro radiosensitization by oxaliplatin and 5-fluorouracil in a human colon cancer cell line. Acta Oncol 44:687–693

Kress MA, Sen N, Unger KR et al (2015) Safety and efficacy of hypofractionated stereotactic body reirradiation in head and neck cancer: long-term follow-up of a large series. Head Neck 37:1403–1409

Landuyt W, Keizer J, Chin A et al (1987) Evaluation of mouse lip mucosa reactions after combinations of cis-diammine-1,1-cyclobutanedicarboxylate platinum (II) (CBDCA) and irradiation: single and fractionated treatments. Int J Radiat Oncol Biol Phys 13: 1367–1370

Lartigau EF, Tresch E, Thariat J et al (2013) Multi institutional phase II study of concomitant stereotactic reirradiation and cetuximab for recurrent head and neck cancer. Radiother Oncol 109:281–285

Lawrence TS, Davis MA, Maybaum J (1994) Dependence of 5-fluorouracil-mediated radiosensitization on DNA-directed effects. Int J Radiat Oncol Biol Phys 29:519–523

Lawrence TS, Davis MA, Tang HY, Maybaum J (1996a) Fluorodeoxyuridine-mediated cytotoxicity and radiosensitization require S phase progression. Int J Radiat Biol 70:273–280

Lawrence TS, Davis MA, Loney TL (1996b) Fluoropyrimidine-mediated radiosensitization depends on cyclin E-dependent kinase activation. Cancer Res 56:3203–3206

Lawrence TS, Chang EY, Hahn TM (1996c) Radiosensitization of pancreatic cancer cells by 2',2'-difluoro-2'-deoxycytidine. Int J Radiat Oncol Biol Phys 34:867–872

Lee N, Chan K, Bekelman JE et al (2007) Salvage re-irradiation for recurrent head and neck cancer. Int J Radiat Oncol Biol Phys 68:731–740

Linthorst M, Baaijens M, Wiggenraad R et al (2015) Local control rate after the combination of re-irradiation and hyperthermia for irresectable recurrent breast cancer: Results in 248 patients. Radiother Oncol 117:217–222

Magne N, Fischel JL, Formento P et al (2003) Oxaliplatin-5-fluorouracil and ionizing radiation. Importance of the sequence and influence of p53 status. Oncology 64:280–287

McGinn CJ, Miller EM, Lindstrom MJ et al (1994) The role of cell cycle redistribution in radiosensitization: implications regarding the mechanism of fluorodeoxyuridine radiosensitization. Int J Radiat Oncol Biol Phys 30:851–859

McGinn CJ, Shewach DS, Lawrence TS (1996) Radiosensitizing nucleosides. J Natl Cancer Inst 88:1193–1203

Milas L, Hunter NR, Mason KA et al (1994) Enhancement of tumor radioresponse of a murine mammary carcinoma by paclitaxel. Cancer Res 54:3506–3510

Milas L, Hunter NR, Mason KA et al (1995) Role of reoxygenation in induction of enhancement of tumor radioresponse by paclitaxel. Cancer Res 55:3564–3568

Miller EM, Kinsella TJ (1992) Radiosensitization by fluorodeoxyuridine: effects of thymidylate synthase inhibition and cell synchronization. Cancer Res 52: 1687–1694

Miller SJ, Lavker RM, Sun TT (2005) Interpreting epithelial cancer biology in the context of stem cells: tumor properties and therapeutic implications. Biochim Biophys Acta 1756:25–52

Minchinton AI, Tannock IF (2006) Drug penetration in solid tumours. Nat Rev Cancer 2006:583–592

Minniti G, Agolli L, Falco T et al (2015) Hypofractionated stereotactic radiotherapy in combination with bevacizumab or fotemustine for patients with progressive malignant gliomas. J Neurooncol 122:559–566

Minsky BD, Pajak TF, Ginsberg RJ et al (2002) INT 0123 (Radiation Therapy Oncology Group 94-05) phase III trial of combined-modality therapy for esophageal cancer: high-dose versus standard-dose radiation therapy. J Clin Oncol 20:1167–1174

Moertel CG, Childs DS Jr, Reitemeier RJ et al (1969) Combined 5-fluorouracil and supervoltage radiation therapy of locally unresectable gastrointestinal cancer. Lancet 2:865–867

Mohiuddin M, Marks G, Marks J (2002) Long-term results of reirradiation for patients with recurrent rectal cancer. Cancer 95:1144–1150

Moitra K (2015) Overcoming multidrug resistance in cancer stem cells. Biomed Res Int 2015:635745. doi:10.1155/2015/635745

Molls M, Vaupel P (1998) Blood perfusion and microenvironment of human tumors. Springer, Berlin/Heidelberg/New York

Molls M, Vaupel P, Nieder C et al (2009) The impact of tumor biology on cancer treatment and multidisciplinary strategies. Springer, Berlin/Heidelberg/New York

Monk BJ, Alberts DS, Burger RA et al (1998) In vitro phase II comparison of the cytotoxicity of a novel platinum analog, nedaplatin (254-S), with that of cisplatin and carboplatin against fresh, human cervical cancers. Gynecol Oncol 71:308–312

Munro AJ (1995) An overview of randomised controlled trials of adjuvant chemotherapy in head and neck cancer. Br J Cancer 71:83–91

Nagar YS, Singh S, Datta NR (2004) Chemo-reirradiation in persistent/recurrent head and neck cancers. Jpn J Clin Oncol 34:61–68

Naida JD, Davis MA, Lawrence TS (1998) The effect of activation of wild-type p53 function on fluoropyrimidine-mediated radiosensitization. Int J Radiat Oncol Biol Phys 41:675–680

Nieder C, Milas L, Ang KK (2003) Modification of radiation response: cytokines, growth factors, and other biological targets. Springer, Berlin/Heidelberg/New York

NIH consensus conference (1990) Adjuvant therapy for patients with colon and rectal cancer. JAMA 264:1444–1450

Nordsmark M, Bentzen SM, Rudat V et al (2005) Prognostic value of tumor oxygenation in 397 head and neck tumors after primary radiotherapy. An international multicenter study. Radiother Oncol 77:18–24

Nuyten DS, van de Vijver MJ (2008) Using microarray analysis as a prognostic and predictive tool in oncology: focus on breast cancer and normal tissue toxicity. Semin Radiat Oncol 18:105–114

O'Connell MJ, Martenson JA, Wieand HS et al (1994) Improving adjuvant therapy for rectal cancer by combining protracted-infusion fluorouracil with radiation therapy after curative surgery. N Engl J Med 331:502–507

Ohizumi Y, Tamai Y, Imamiya S et al (2002) Prognostic factors of reirradiation for recurrent head and neck cancer. Am J Clin Oncol 25:408–413

Ormerod MG, Orr RM, Peacock JH (1994) The role of apoptosis in cell killing by cisplatin: a flow cytometric study. Br J Cancer 69:93–100

Overgaard J, Khan AR (1981) Selective enhancement of radiation response in a C3H mammary carcinoma by cisplatin. Cancer Treat Rep. 65(5–6):501–503

Pekkola-Heino K, Kulmala J, Grenman R (1992) Carboplatin-radiation interaction in squamous cell carcinoma cell lines. Arch Otolaryngol Head Neck Surg 118:1312–1315

Pendyala L, Creaven PJ (1993) In vitro cytotoxicity, protein binding, red blood cell partitioning, and biotransformation of oxaliplatin. Cancer Res 53:5970–5976

Pignon JP, Bourhis J, Domenge C et al (2000) Chemotherapy added to locoregional treatment for head and neck squamous-cell carcinoma: three meta-analyses of updated individual data. MACH-NC Collaborative Group Meta-Analysis of Chemotherapy on Head and Neck Cancer. Lancet 355:949–955

Pignon JP, le Maître A, Maillard E et al (2009) Meta-analysis of chemotherapy in head and neck cancer (MACH-NC): an update on 93 randomised trials and 17,346 patients. Radiother Oncol 92:4–14

Pilones KA, Vanpouille-Box C, Demaria S (2015) Combination of radiotherapy and immune checkpoint inhibitors. Semin Radiat Oncol 25:28–33

Pinedo HM, Peters GF (1988) Fluorouracil: biochemistry and pharmacology. J Clin Oncol 6:1653–1664

Popovtzer A, Gluck I, Chepeha DB et al (2009) The pattern of failure after reirradiation of recurrent squamous cell head and neck cancer: implications for defining the targets. Int J Radiat Oncol Biol Phys 74:1342–1347

Primeau AJ, Rendon A, Hedley D et al (2005) The distribution of the anticancer drug doxorubicin in relation to blood vessels in solid tumors. Clin Cancer Res 11:8782–8788

Prince ME, Ailles LE (2008) Cancer stem cells in head and neck squamous cell cancer. J Clin Oncol 26:2871–2875

Raaphorst GP, Leblanc M, Li LF (2005) A comparison of response to cisplatin, radiation and combined treatment for cells deficient in recombination repair pathways. Anticancer Res 25:53–58

Rau B, Sturm I, Lage H et al (2003) Dynamic expression profile of p21WAF1/CIP1 and Ki-67 predicts survival in rectal carcinoma treated with preoperative radiochemotherapy. J Clin Oncol 21:3391–3401

Raymond E, Faivre S, Chaney S et al (2002) Cellular and molecular pharmacology of oxaliplatin. Mol Cancer Ther 1:227–235

Richmond RC, Powers EL (1976) Radiation sensitization of bacterial spores by cis-dichlorodaimmineplatinum (II). Radiat Res 68:251

Rockwell S (1982) Cytotoxicities of mitomycin C and X rays to aerobic and hypoxic cells in vitro. Int J Radiat Oncol Biol Phys 8:1035–1039

Rosenberg B, van Camp L, Krigas T (1965) Inhibition of cell division in Escherichia coli by electrolysis products from a platinum electrode. Nature 205:698–699

Rusthoven KE, Feigenberg SJ, Raben D et al (2010) Initial results of a phase I dose-escalation trial of concurrent and maintenance erlotinib and reirradiation for recurrent and new primary head-and-neck cancer. Int J Radiat Oncol Biol Phys 78(4):1020–5

Salama JK, Vokes EE, Chmura SJ et al (2006) Long-term outcome of concurrent chemotherapy and reirradiation for recurrent and second primary head-and-neck squamous cell carcinoma. Int J Radiat Oncol Biol Phys 64:382–391

Sauer R, Becker H, Hohenberger W et al (2004) Preoperative versus postoperative chemoradiotherapy for rectal cancer. N Engl J Med 351:1731–1740

Scalliet P, De Pooter C, Hellemans PW et al (1999) Interactions of carboplatin, cisplatin, and ionizing radiation on a human cell line of ovarian cancer (French). Cancer Radiother 3:30–38

Schaake-Koning C, van den Bogaert W, Dalesio O et al (1992) Effects of concomitant cisplatin and radiotherapy on inoperable non-small-cell lung cancer. N Engl J Med 326:524–530

Schaefer U, Micke O, Schueller P et al (2000) Recurrent head and neck cancer: retreatment of previously irradiated areas with combined chemotherapy and radiation therapy-results of a prospective study. Radiology 216:371–376

Schöder H, Ong SC (2008) Fundamentals of molecular imaging: rationale and applications with relevance for radiation oncology. Semin Nucl Med 38:119–128

Schwachöfer JHM, Crooijmans RP, Hoogenhout J et al (1991) Effectiveness in inhibition of recovery of cell survival by cisplatin and carboplatin: influence of treatment sequence. Int J Radiat Oncol Biol Phys 20:1235–1241

Schaake-Koning C, Maat B, van Houtte P, van den Bogaert W, Dalesio O, Kirkpatrick A, Bartelink H (1990) Radiotherapy combined with low-dose cis-diammine dichloroplatinum (II) (CDDP) in inoperable nonmetastatic non-small cell lung cancer (NSCLC): a randomized three arm phase II study of the EORTC Lung Cancer and Radiotherapy Cooperative Groups. Int J Radiat Oncol Biol Phys.19(4):967–972

Seiwert TY, Haraf DJ, Cohen EE et al (2008) Phase I study of bevacizumab added to fluorouracil- and hydroxyurea-based oncomitant chemoradiotherapy for poor-prognosis head and neck cancer. J Clin Oncol 26:1732–1741

Simoens C, Korst AE, De Pooter CM et al (2003) In vitro interaction between ecteinascidin 743 (ET-743) and radiation, in relation to its cell cycle effects. Br J Cancer 89:2305–2311

Spencer SA, Harris J, Wheeler RH et al (2008) Final report of RTOG 9610, a multi-institutional trial of reirradiation and chemotherapy for unresectable recurrent squamous cell carcinoma of the head and neck. Head Neck 30:281–288

Steel GG (1979) Terminology in the description of drug-radiation interactions. Int J Radiat Oncol Biol Phys 5:1145–1150

Steel GG, Peckham MJ (1979) Exploitable mechanisms in combined radiotherapy–chemotherapy: the concept of additivity. Int J Radiat Oncol Biol Phys 5:85–91

Strnad V, Lotter M, Kreppner S et al (2015) Reirradiation for recurrent head and neck cancer with salvage interstitial pulsed-dose-rate brachytherapy. Strahlenther Onkol 191:495–500

Stupp R, Mason WP, van den Bent MJ et al (2005) Radiotherapy plus concomitant and adjuvant temozolomide for glioblastoma. N Engl J Med 352: 987–996

Sulman EP, Schwartz DL, Le TT et al (2009) IMRT reirradiation of head and neck cancer – disease control and morbidity outcomes. Int J Radiat Oncol Biol Phys 73:399–409

Tannock IF (1989) Combined modality treatment with radiotherapy and chemotherapy. Radiother Oncol 16: 83–101

Tannock IF (1992) Potential for therapeutic gain from combined-modality treatment. Front Radiat Ther Oncol 26:1–15

Tannock IF (1998) Conventional cancer therapy: promise broken or promise delayed? Lancet 351(Suppl 2): SII9–SII16

Tannock IF, Lee CM, Tunggal JK et al (2002) Limited penetration of anticancer drugs through tumor tissue: a potential cause of resistance of solid tumors to chemotherapy. Clin Cancer Res 8:878–884

Tanvetyanom T, Padhya T, McCaffrey J et al (2009) Prognostic factors for survival after salvage reirradiation of head and neck cancer. J Clin Oncol 27:1983–1991

Taylor DM, Tew KD, Jones JD (1976) Effects of cis-dichlorodiammine platinum (II) on DNA synthesis in kidney and other tissues of normal and tumoour-bearing rats. Eur J Cancer 12:249–254

Teicher BA, Lazo JS, Sartorelli AC (1981) Classification of antineoplastic agents by their selective toxicities toward oxygenated and hypoxic tumor cells. Cancer Res 41:73–81

Thames HD, Suit HD (1986) Tumor radioresponsiveness versus fractionation sensitivity. Int J Radiat Oncol Biol Phys 12:687–691

Trott KR (1990) Cell repopulation and overall treatment time. Int J Radiat Oncol Biol Phys 19:1071–1075

Turchi JJ, Patrick SM, Henkels KM (1997) Mechanism of DNA-dependent protein kinase inhibition by cis-diamminedichloro-platinum(II)-damaged DNA. Biochemistry 36:7586–7593

Unger KR, Lominska CE, Deeken JF et al (2010) Fractionated stereotactic radiosurgery for reirradiation of head-and-neck cancer. Int J Radiat Oncol Biol Phys 77:1411–1419

Van Waes C, Chang AA, Lebowitz PF et al (2005) Inhibition of nuclear factor-kappaB and target genes during combined therapy with proteasome inhibitor bortezomib and reirradiation in patients with recurrent head-and-neck squamous cell carcinoma. Int J Radiat Oncol Biol Phys 63:1400–1412

VanderSpek L, Fisher B, Bauman G et al (2008) 3D conformal radiotherapy and cisplatin for recurrent malignant glioma. Can J Neurol Sci 35:57–64

Vargo JA, Ferris RL, Ohr J et al (2015) A prospective phase 2 trial of reirradiation with stereotactic body radiation therapy plus cetuximab in patients with previously irradiated recurrent squamous cell carcinoma of the head and neck. Int J Radiat Oncol Biol Phys 91:480–488

Volm M, Efferth T (2015) Prediction of cancer drug resistance and implications for personalized medicine. Front Oncol 5:282

Wahl AO, Rademaker A, Kiel KD et al (2008) Multi-institutional review of repeat irradiation of chest wall and breast for recurrent breast cancer. Int J Radiat Oncol Biol Phys 70:477–484

Weber WA (2005) Use of PET for monitoring cancer therapy and for predicting outcome. J Nucl Med 46:983–995

Weichselbaum RR, Beckett MA, Schwartz JL et al (1988) Radioresistant tumor cells are present in head and neck carcinomas that recur after radiotherapy. Int J Radiat Oncol Biol Phys 15:575–579

Woynarowski JM, Chapman WG, Napier C et al (1998) Sequence- and region-specificity of oxaliplatin adducts in naked and cellular DNA. Mol Pharmacol 54:770–777

Wu HI, Brown JA, Dorie MJ et al (2004) Genome-wide identification of genes conferring resistance to the anticancer agents cisplatin, oxaliplatin, and mitomycin C. Cancer Res 64:3940–3948

Wurm RE, Kuczer DA, Schlenger L et al (2006) Hypofractionated stereotactic radiotherapy combined with topotecan in recurrent malignant glioma. Int J Radiat Oncol Biol Phys 66:S26–S32

Würschmidt F, Dahle J, Petersen C et al (2008) Reirradiation of recurrent breast cancer with and without concurrent chemotherapy. Radiat Oncol 3:28

Yamazaki H, Ogita M, Himei K et al (2015) Predictive value of skin invasion in recurrent head and neck cancer patients treated by hypofractionated stereotactic re-irradiation using a cyberknife. Radiat Oncol 10:210

Yang LX, Douple EB, O'Hara JA, Wang HJ (1995) Production of DNA double-strand breaks by interactions between carboplatin and radiation: a potential mechanism for radiopotentiation. Radiat Res 143: 309–315

Yang YC, Chao KS, Lin CP et al (2009) Oxaliplatin regulates DNA repair responding to ionizing radiation and enhances radiosensitivity of human cervical cancer cells. Int J Gynecol Cancer 19:782–786

Yang J, Parsons J, Nicolay NH et al (2010) Cells deficient in the base excision repair protein, DNA polymerase beta, are hypersensitive to oxaliplatin chemotherapy. Oncogene 29:463–468

Yoshida GJ, Saya H (2015) Therapeutic strategies targeting cancer stem cells. Cancer Sci. doi:10.1111/cas.12817

Yu YQ, Giocanti N, Averbeck D et al (2000) Radiation-induced arrest of cells in G2 phase elicits hypersensitivity to DNA double-strand break inducers and an altered pattern of DNA cleavage upon re-irradiation. Int J Radiat Biol 76:901–912

Zak M, Drobnik J (1971) Effects of cis-dichlorodiammineplatinum (II) on the post irradiation lethality in mice after irradiation with X-rays. Strahlentherapie 142:112–115

Zamboni WC, Gervais AC, Egorin MJ et al (2002) Inter- and intratumoral disposition of platinum in solid tumors after administration of cisplatin. Clin Cancer Res 8:2992–2999

Reduced Normal Tissue Doses Through Advanced Technology

Matthias Guckenberger, Reinhart A. Sweeney, Cedric Panje, and Stephanie Tanadini-Lang

Contents

Abstract

Re-irradiation is probably the most challenging situation in radiotherapy because the radiation tolerance of the normal tissue is significantly reduced compared with the first treatment series. Results with traditional radiotherapy techniques have been disappointing because of the poor conformality of the dose distributions: radiation doses were either insufficiently low resulting in poor rates of tumor control or substantial toxicity was the consequence of high-dose re-irradiation. This chapter will focus on modern techniques of radiation treatment planning and delivery, which make improved sparing of the normal tissue possible. All techniques will be discussed in the context of re-irradiation and theoretical and clinical data supporting the use of these technologies will be presented. Palliative reirradiation to moderate doses might be feasible without using advanced technology. However, under many circumstances 2D or 3D conformal approaches cannot fulfill the required normal tissue constraints. The present chapter discusses the advantages and challenges associated with more complex planning and delivery methods.

The original version of this chapter was revised. An erratum to this chapter can be found at 10.1007/978-3-319-41825-4_78.

M. Guckenberger (✉) • C. Panje • S. Tanadini-Lang
Department of Radiation Oncology, University Hospital Zurich, Zurich, Switzerland
e-mail: guckenberger_m@klinik.uni-wuerzburg.de

R.A. Sweeney
Department of Radiation Oncology, Leopoldina Hospital Schweinfurt, Schweinfurt, Germany

Med Radiol Radiat Oncol (2016)
DOI 10.1007/174_2016_55, © Springer International Publishing Switzerland
Published Online: 13 Aug 2016

1 Introduction: Errors, Margins and Compensation Strategies in Radiotherapy

1.1 Rationale for Advanced Technologies in the Reirradiation Situation

Reirradiation is probably the most challenging treatment in the radiotherapy field. The radiation tolerance of the normal tissue is reduced compared to the first radiotherapy series unless complete repair of the radiation damage has occurred. Partial recovery has been suggested for some organs such as the spinal cord: Experiments on rhesus monkeys with two courses of radiotherapy (doses of >50 Gy in each course with intervals between 1 and 3 years) showed low rates of myelopathy (Ang et al. 2001), and preliminary clinical patient data support the hypothesis of recovery of the spinal cord (Nieder et al. 2006). However, this is unlikely for the majority of normal tissues after a first course of radiotherapy with a curative radiation dose, despite there being very limited data in the literature. Consequently, the need for effective sparing of critical normal tissue is even more important compared to primary radiotherapy.

Because of this reduced radiation tolerance of the normal tissue in the situation of a locoregional recurrence after primary radiotherapy, one could either reduce the maximum dose such that an acceptable risk of toxicity is met or reduce the exposure of the normal tissue best as possible by minimizing the irradiated volume and maximizing the conformity of the dose distributions.

New technologies in radiation oncology have always been utilized early after their clinical introduction for the purpose of reirradiation as a means to deliver clinically effective doses to the recurrent tumor with optimal dose reduction for the preirradiated normal tissue (Mantel et al. 2013; Chao et al. 2000; Loeffler et al. 1990). Although there is little literature available on the use of novel techniques specifically for reirradiation, this book chapter covers general aspects of target volume definition and radiation delivery in the reirradiation situation and demonstrates the potential improvement by advanced technologies.

1.2 Uncertainties in Radiotherapy and Compensation Strategies

The target volume concept in the reirradiation situation is in principle not different to primary radiotherapy and described in the ICRU reports 50 and 62 (ICRU 1993, 1999) (Fig. 1). The macroscopic tumor is defined as the gross tumor volume (GTV), and safety margins depending on histology and cancer site are applied for generation of the clinical target volume (CTV). Variations in shape, volume, and position of the CTV, for example, due to variable filling of hollow organs or due to breathing motion, are compensated via so-called internal margins, resulting in the internal target volume (ITV). Additional margins are then applied to ensure that the CTV is always exposed to the prescribed treatment dose, resulting in the planning target volume (PTV); setup uncertainties of patients contribute most significantly to these margins. If adequate dose coverage of the PTV is intended, all irradiating techniques deliver some dose outside the PTV, resulting in further increased irradiated volumes of normal tissue. Uncertainties are summarized in Table 1.

In recent years, multiple advanced technologies were introduced into radiotherapy treatment planning and delivery all owing the potential to

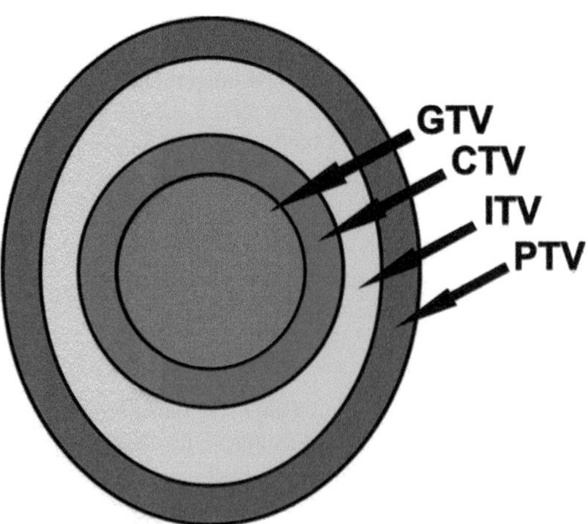

Fig. 1 Target volume concept according to ICRU 62: gross tumor volume (*GTV*); clinical target volume (*CTV*); internal target volume (*ITV*); planning target volume (*PTV*)

Table 1 Uncertainties in radiotherapy treatment planning and delivery

GTV stage	Inter- and intra-observer variability of target volume definition
	Sensitivity and specificity of imaging modality
PTV stage—intra-fractional	Patient motion
	Target motion due to:
	Breathing
	Heartbeat
	Changes of the filling of hollow organs
PTV stage—inter-fractional	Patient setup:
	Rigid setup errors
	Nonrigid setup errors
	Shift of the target position due to:
	Changes of the filling of hollow organs
	Changes of the breathing pattern
	Complex changes of the patients' anatomy (e.g., atelectasis, effusions, etc.)
	GTV regression/progression
	Weight loss of the patient

reduce the margins described above resulting in reduced volumes of normal tissue exposed to mid- and high doses.

GTV Stage Reduction of the GTV is certainly not possible, but modern imaging for target definition using, for example, MRI, SPECT, or PEt allows for more precise and reproducible definition of the recurrent cancer with especially improved differentiation between postirradiation or postsurgical fibrosis and active tumor.

CTV Stage There are no data on the microscopic extension in the situation of loco-regional recurrences after a prior course of radiotherapy. However, it has been suggested, for example, for reirradiation of head-and-neck cancer, that the pattern of treatment failure after confining the target volume to the recurrent GTV with tight safety margins is in-field, which limits the potential benefit of elective nodal irradiation or irradiation of larger volumes where microscopic spread is assumed (Popovtzer et al. 2009). Additionally, the target volume concept needs to be adapted to the individual patient-specific situation: Different target volumes concepts can be considered in patients, where reirradiation intends short-term palliation or where a curative intend is followed.

PTV Stage, Intrafractional Uncertainties Changes of the target position during the treatment fraction may have several reasons: patient motion, breathing motion, cardiac motion, peristaltic motion, and changes of the filling of hollow organs. Depending on the target location and depending on patient individual factors, the above listed uncertainties reach different magnitudes and the contribution of each factor to the total intrafractional uncertainty varies significantly. For example, breathing motion is the dominant uncertainty in the thoracic region but may vary from few millimeters to 3 cm between patients. Management of intrafractional motion is highly challenging because of the short timescale of these uncertainties (e.g., cardiac motion with >1 Hz) as well as the random, unpredictable nature of motion (e.g., patient motion).

PTV Stage, Interfractional Uncertainties Uncertainties of the target position between treatment fractions influence safety margins significantly. The technique of stereotactic radiotherapy has been developed in the 1960s for high-precision radiotherapy of intracranial lesions (Leksell 1951, 1968), and this technique achieved an accuracy of patient setup with residual errors in the range of 1 mm. In the 1990s, the stereotactic principle of patient setup was transferred to the extracranial region, called stereotactic body radiotherapy (SBRT) (Lax et al. 1994). Recently, the need for external coordinates in stereotactic radiotherapy, both cranial and extracranial, has been questioned due to the availability of image guidance (IGRT) (Verellen et al. 2007), which allows verification of the target position prior to each treatment fraction. Besides changes of the target position, systematic changes of tumor volume and shape (regression or progression) and of the normal tissue (e.g., changes of pleural effusion and atelectasis; weight loss of the patient) have been observed during a fractionated course of radiotherapy. Adaptation of the treatment plan to these systematic changes in an adaptive feedback loop is currently a focus of research.

Choice of Irradiation Technique It is important to adjust the irradiation technique to the individual patient case with location of the recurrent tumor, size and volume of the PTV, the type of normal tissue in relationship to the recurrence, and dose distribution of the previous treatment course being the most important factors. Kilovoltage X-rays or electrons may be considered for superficial recurrences and brachytherapy in cases, where implantation of the catheters in a suitable geometry or intraoperatively is reasonable. The standard delivery methods for photon reirradiation are currently intensity-modulated arc techniques such as volumetric modulated arc therapy (VMAT) or RapidArc, which can provide more conformal dose distributions than 3D-conformal techniques (Stieler et al. 2011). Protons and heavy ions offer distinct physical and biological advantages over photons which allow to reduce the dose to normal tissue. Although these properties are of particular interest in the reirradiation situation, there is only limited data on the use of particle therapy for reirradiation published (Plastaras et al. 2014).

1.3 Safety Margins in Radiotherapy

Despite all technological progress, the clinical application of radiotherapy will never be without errors or uncertainties at the planning and delivery stage. Consequently, margins always have to be added to the CTV or GTV if adequate coverage of this target volume is intended. Most important is the differentiation between systematic and random errors (Fig. 2). A systematic error affects all treatment fractions in an identical way and will result in a systematic difference between the intended and delivered dose distribution. An example is target delineation, where a certain part of the tumor is excluded from the target volume because of false-negative imaging for treatment planning. Random errors may affect all treatment fractions as well; however, all errors are centered around the planned position. It is the systematic error component which is most important and which should be minimized with highest effort in the primary and the reirradiation situation. The contribution of the random error component to the overall uncertainty and consequently to the overall safety margin is significantly smaller.

The most commonly used margin concept is a population-based probabilistic concept:

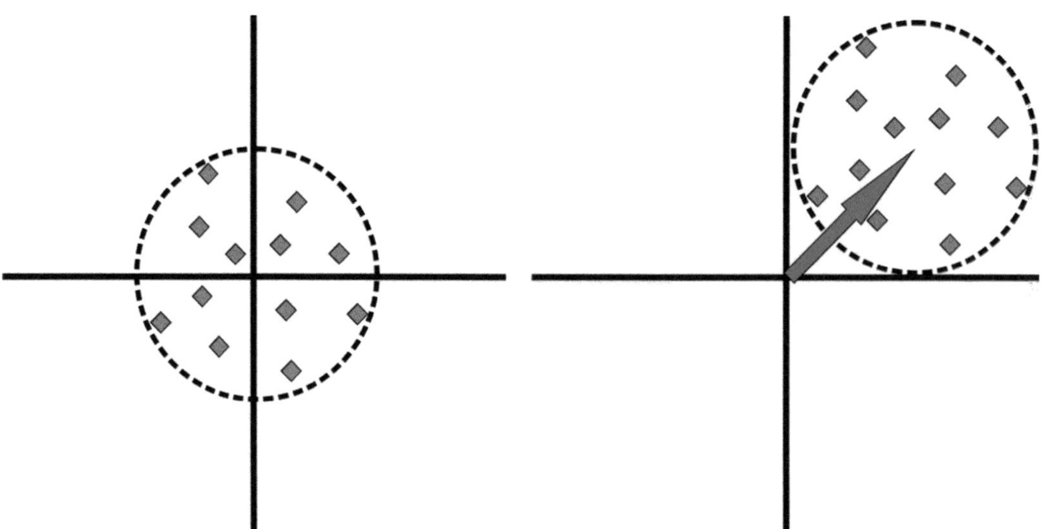

Fig. 2 Random (*left*) and systematic (*right*) uncertainties in radiotherapy treatment

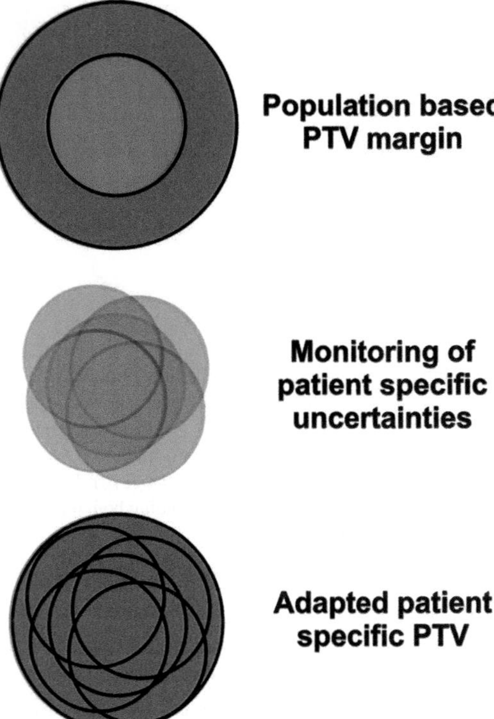

Fig. 3 Work flow of patient individual adaptation of safety margins: (1) Start of treatment with population-based margins; (2) assessment of patient individual uncertainties; and (3) adaptation of safety margins to the patient's individual errors

Application of a certain margin around the target volume ensures that the target volume is treated with at least 95% of the prescribed dose in 90% of the patient population (van Herk 2004). Systematic and random errors of all stages of radiotherapy need to be quantified for a patient population, and these data are used for calculation of population-specific safety margins. A different concept aims at adaptation of the safety margins to the individual, patient-specific uncertainties (Yan et al. 1997): Uncertainties are quantified at the beginning of the treatment course for each patient, and the safety margins and treatment plans are then adapted for the following treatment fractions based on the individual uncertainties (Fig. 3).

In the following of this chapter, we will focus in more detail on the distinct technological advances in external beam radiotherapy and discuss their potential role in the situation of reirradiation.

2 Imaging for Reirradiation

The integration of modern imaging modalities such as CT, MRI, and PET in the treatment planning process has become common practice; however, major advances in more specific imaging technologies have evolved in the last decade, requiring the radiation oncologist to have a detailed understanding of possibilities and limitations of these novel diagnostic modalities. Interdisciplinary discussion with radiologists or nuclear medicine specialists should lead to optimal integration of these modalities into the treatment planning process. Especially the development of image fusion software has significantly advanced in recent years, which was mainly driven by the radiooncological community; we are likely the specialty making greatest clinical use of image fusion, often more so than diagnostic radiologists themselves. Detailed discussion of imaging modalities for the different cancer sites is beyond the scope of this chapter and will be performed in the dedicated chapters of this book. Some important generalized points should be considered:

In the reirradiation situation, the radiation oncologist is frequently confronted with imaging results, which are significantly different to the situation of the primary irradiation (Meerwein et al. 2015): The normal anatomy is substantially altered after repeated surgical interventions and after prior radiotherapy. Especially differentiation between postsurgical/postradiotherapy scarring and recurrent tumor is difficult in many cancer sites: Our morphological imaging techniques of CT and standard MRI sequences are frequently limited in this situation. Additionally, we as radiation oncologists do not only need to differentiate between scarring tissue and recurrent tumor on a diagnostic level (yes or no) but must accurately delineate the recurrence in three dimensions for conformal treatment planning.

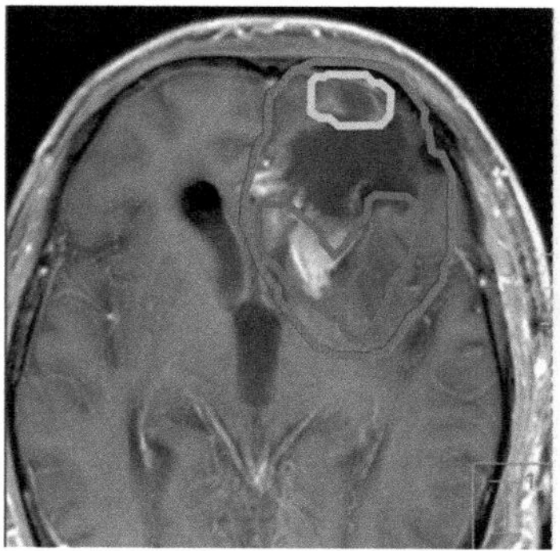
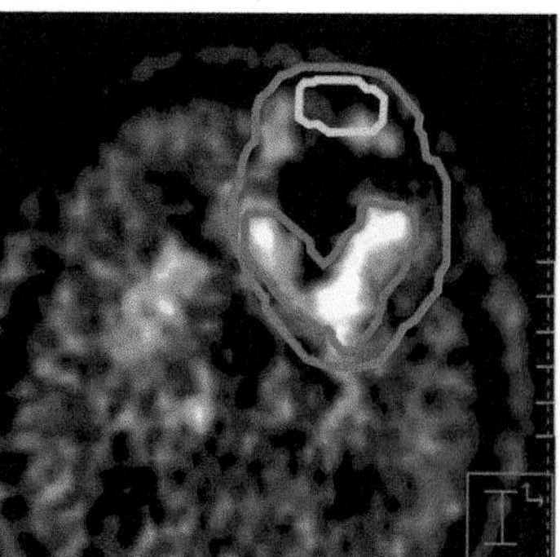
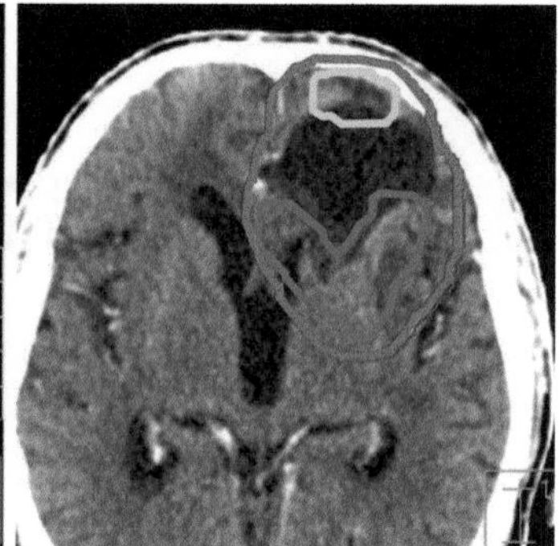

Fig. 4 A 79-year-old patient was treated with standard radiochemotherapy (60 Gy and Temozolomide) to a left frontal glioblastoma. Twelve months later a local recurrence was surgically removed. While the surgeons reported gross total resection, post-OP MRI (within 2 days) showed residual tumor at the very frontal pole (*left image*). The hyperintense region at the posterior of the tumor cavity was attributed to blood. FET-PET however showed marked activity in the dorsal region while the frontal region was inactive (*middle image*). The contrast-enhanced planning CT shows no residual disease (*right image*). *Yellow* GTV MRI, *Blue* GTV PET, *Red* PTV surrounding both regions

The potential advantage of advanced imaging modalities in this situation will be demonstrated exemplarily in two cancer sites.

Malignant gliomas most frequently recur locally within a distance of about 2 cm to the primary lesion, which makes differentiation of recurrent cancer and posttherapeutic changes, especially radiation necrosis, difficult. Amino acid PET imaging in addition to standard MRI imaging was shown to increase sensitivity and especially specificity in diagnosis, grading, and determination of tumor extension of malignant gliomas (Pauleit et al. 2005; Hatakeyama et al. 2008). In the situation of recurrent malignant gliomas, amino acid PET imaging improved the accuracy for differentiation between radiation necrosis and recurrent tumor (Terakawa et al. 2008). Early clinical results suggest that integration of this biological information into target definition in primary radiotherapy and reirradiation of malignant gliomas alters the target volume in a significant proportion of the patients (Rieken et al. 2013; Munck Af Rosenschold et al. 2015; Lee et al. 2009). Additionally, amino acid PET uptake kinetics before reirradiation have shown to be of prognostic value (Niyazi et al. 2012), and the use of PET-based "biological" target volumes may even improve clinical outcome (Grosu et al. 2005) (Fig. 4).

After anterior resection or abdominoperineal resection for rectal cancer, the differentiation between fibrotic masses in the presacral operative bed and a local tumor recurrence is extremely challenging with conventional CT imaging (Lee et al. 1981). This requires the use of further imaging modalities for accurate target volume delineation for reirradiation: Magnetic resonance imaging of recurrent rectal cancer may help to determine infiltration into pelvic structures (Dresen et al. 2010), and dynamic contrast-enhanced imaging may predict R0 resection (Gollub et al. 2013). FDG-PET imaging was reported to allow differentiation between benign scarring tissue and a locally recurrent rectal cancer with high sensitivity and specificity (Ito et al. 1992), and combined PET/CT imaging was shown to further improve the accuracy by avoiding the misinterpretation of displaced pelvic organs as recurrent tumor (Even-Sapir et al. 2004). Integration of this functional imaging into radiotherapy treatment planning with a focal dose escalation in volumes of increased FDG-PET activity has been reported recently (Jingu et al. 2010).

In principle, the requirements for imaging in preparation for reirradiation are comparable to those necessary for high-precision radiotherapy in the primary setting. Here also, there should be no compromise in utilizing possibilities of treatment volume definition as both marginal misses and sequelae due to unnecessarily large treatment volumes are of special issue in the reirradiation situation.

3 Photon External Beam Radiotherapy

3.1 Conventional Two-Dimensional Radiotherapy

Conventional two-dimensional (2D) radiotherapy planning was the standard for decades in photon radiotherapy. Few radiation beams were selected, frequently directly opposing fields, three- or four-field arrangements. Size and shape of the fields were adjusted in 2D simulation X-ray images, and unless the tumor was visible in these planar images, filed shaping was mainly based on bony surrogates instead of the patient individual position, shape, and size of the tumor. Also visualization of normal structures was limited. This makes conventional 2D planning inappropriate for the majority of patients, where reirradiation is intended.

3.2 Three-Dimensional Conformal Radiotherapy

Three-dimensional conformal radiation therapy (3DCRT) has been the standard for most indications in photon radiation therapy in the last years, although it is increasingly replaced by intensity-modulated techniques.

It offers distinct advantages compared to conventional 2D radiotherapy, which are especially important in the reirradiation situation. Target volume definition is based on CT images, and coregistration of further imaging modalities like MRI or PET images is supported by all current treatment planning systems. This allows for more precise definition of both the target and critical organs-at-risk (OAR). These structures are visualized in the beam's eye view for selection of the optimal beam directions and for field shaping aiming at best possible sparing of critical OARs. The benefit of 3D-CRT compared to 2D planning has been demonstrated in a randomized trial: In primary radiotherapy for prostate cancer conformal radiotherapy significantly reduced the incidence of proctitis and rectal bleeding compared to conventional radiotherapy; simultaneously local tumor control was not different between the two techniques (Dearnaley et al. 1999). This potential to reduced doses to the normal tissue with the consequence of reduced side effects is certainly of high clinical value in the reirradiation situation, where such large randomized trials are not possible (Fig. 5).

3.3 Intensity-Modulated Radiotherapy

The technique of intensity-modulated radiotherapy (IMRT) is an advancement of 3D-CRT. In 3D-CRT, homogeneous fluence profiles are delivered from each beam-angle. In contrast, IMRT is characterized by customized nonuniform fluence distributions to achieve certain dosimetric objectives (Fig. 6). 3D-CRT uses forward planning meaning that beams are specified, doses are calculated, and dose distributions in the relevant target volumes and OARs are evaluated at the end of the planning process. This is different to the inverse planning process in IMRT. Patient-specific dosimetric goals (objectives) are defined for all target volumes and OARs at the beginning of the treatment planning; the objectives are most frequently DVH parameters or since more recently biological parameters. These objectives are transferred into an IMRT optimization software, where the best possible beam parameters to achieve the desired dose distribution are calculated in an iterative fashion.

Several techniques are commercially available for delivery of intensity-modulated radiation therapy. For conventional linear accelerators equipped with multileaf collimators, the static (step-and-shoot), the dynamic (sliding window), and rotational (volumetric/intensity-modulated arc therapy) techniques can be distinguished. The static step-and-shoot approach segments each IMRT field into a number of shaped subfields, and the sliding window technique modulates the fluence by moving the multileaf collimators (MLCs) while the radiation is being delivered to the patient. Both approaches achieve the energy fluence modulation by the MLCs, and the radiation is given from different static gantry angles.

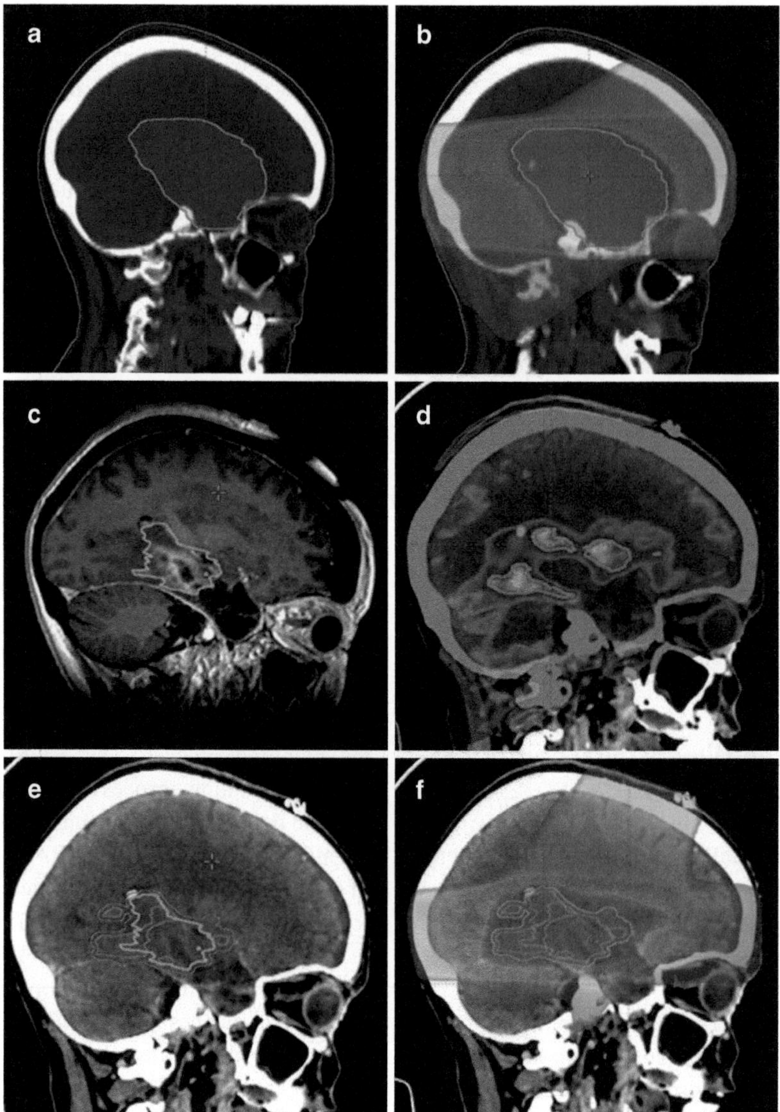

Fig. 5 Case example of reirradiation for a 58-year-old female patient with locally recurrent glioblastoma: Medical history: May 2013: primary diagnosis of glioblastoma; Macroscopically complete resection and adjuvant radiochemotherapy with 60 Gy and concurrent Temozolomide; No adjuvant chemotherapy due to grade III thrombopenia during radiochemotherapy November 2014: new contrast-enhancing nodule in the left temporal lobe; systemic therapy with bevacizumab May 2015: progressive recurrence in the left temporal lobe June 2015: repeat surgery, incomplete resection July 2015: stereotactic re-irradiation with 10 x 3.5 Gy using a PET/MRI-based target volume (**a**) Sagittal reconstruction of the primary volume definition; (**b**) Sagittal reconstruction of the primary irradition; (**c**) Target definition of the local recurrence in the MRI; (**d**)Target definition of the local recurrance in the FET-PET; (**e**) PET based GTV, MRI based GTV and PTV on the CT of the local recurrence; (**f**) Dose distribution for the local recurrent tumor

In contrast, volumetric/intensity-modulated arc therapy (IMAT/VMAT) rotates the linear accelerator around the patient while continuously delivering radiation, thereby applying hundreds of fields, by changing the position of the MLCs and the amount of radiation. A new promising approach still under investigation and not yet clinically available is the 4π- or dynamic-couch

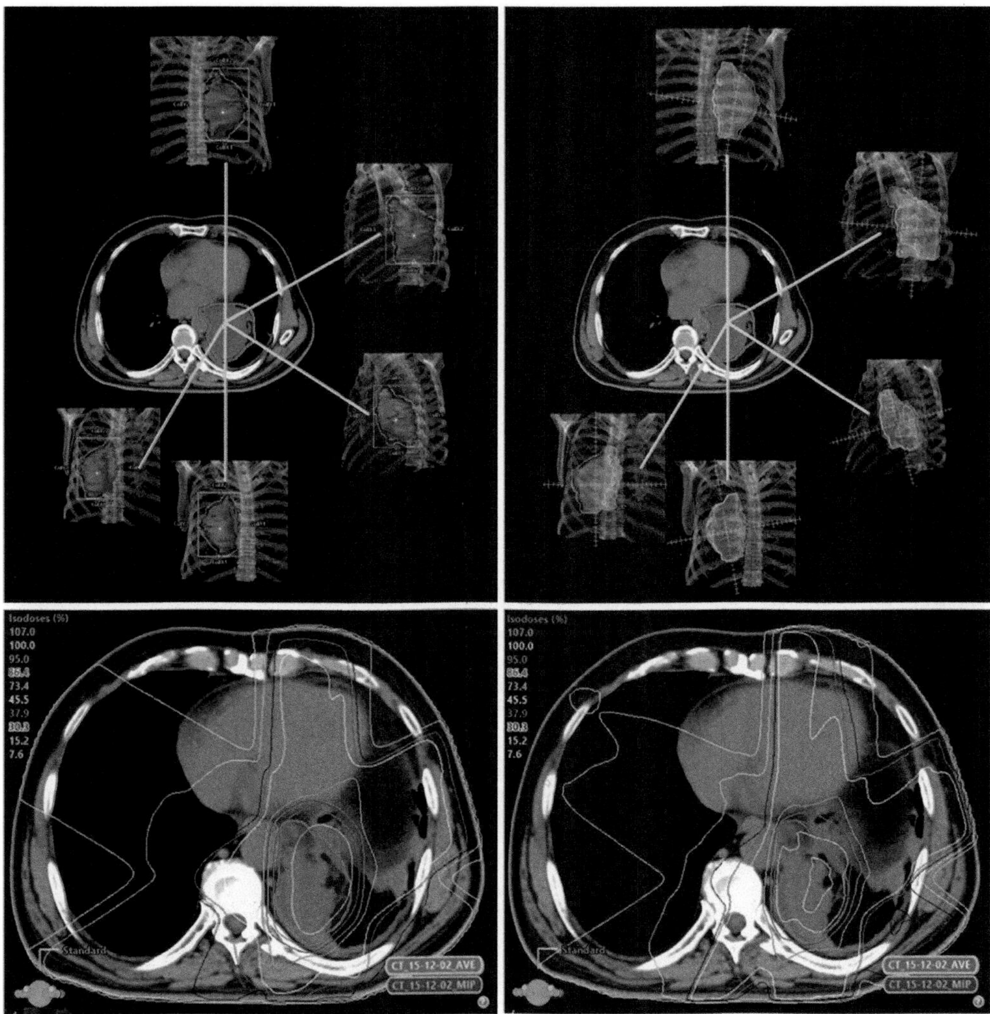

Fig. 6 3D-Conformal radiation therapy (*left*) and intensity-modulated radiotherapy (*right*) for a re-treatment of a lung metastasis. Non-uniform fluence distribution of the IMRT technique allows to more conformally irradiate the tumor and to better spare the organs at risk

rotation technique, which combines the VMAT techniques with continuous rotation of the treatment couch (Smyth et al. 2013; Liang et al. 2015). Major advantages of these rotational techniques are significantly reduced delivery times as well as increased monitor units efficiency. A different IMRT solution is the tomotherapy approach, where the linear accelerator constantly rotates around the patient. The fluence modulation is achieved with a binary collimator, and fan beams are delivered in a CT-like "sliced" fashion, either in spiral or more recently in helical mode (Mackie et al. 1993).

Numerous planning studies have shown the potential of IMRT to generate highly conformal dose distributions, especially for complex, concave-shaped target volumes in close distance to organs-at-risk. In such cases, the sparing of normal tissue is significantly improved compared to 3D-CRT (Nakamura et al. 2014). The superiority or inferiority of one of the above described IMRT delivery techniques has been the issue of countless planning studies and is still highly controversial (Fig. 7). An analytical model was used by Bortfeld and Webb for comparison of TomoTherapy, single-arc VMAT, and static

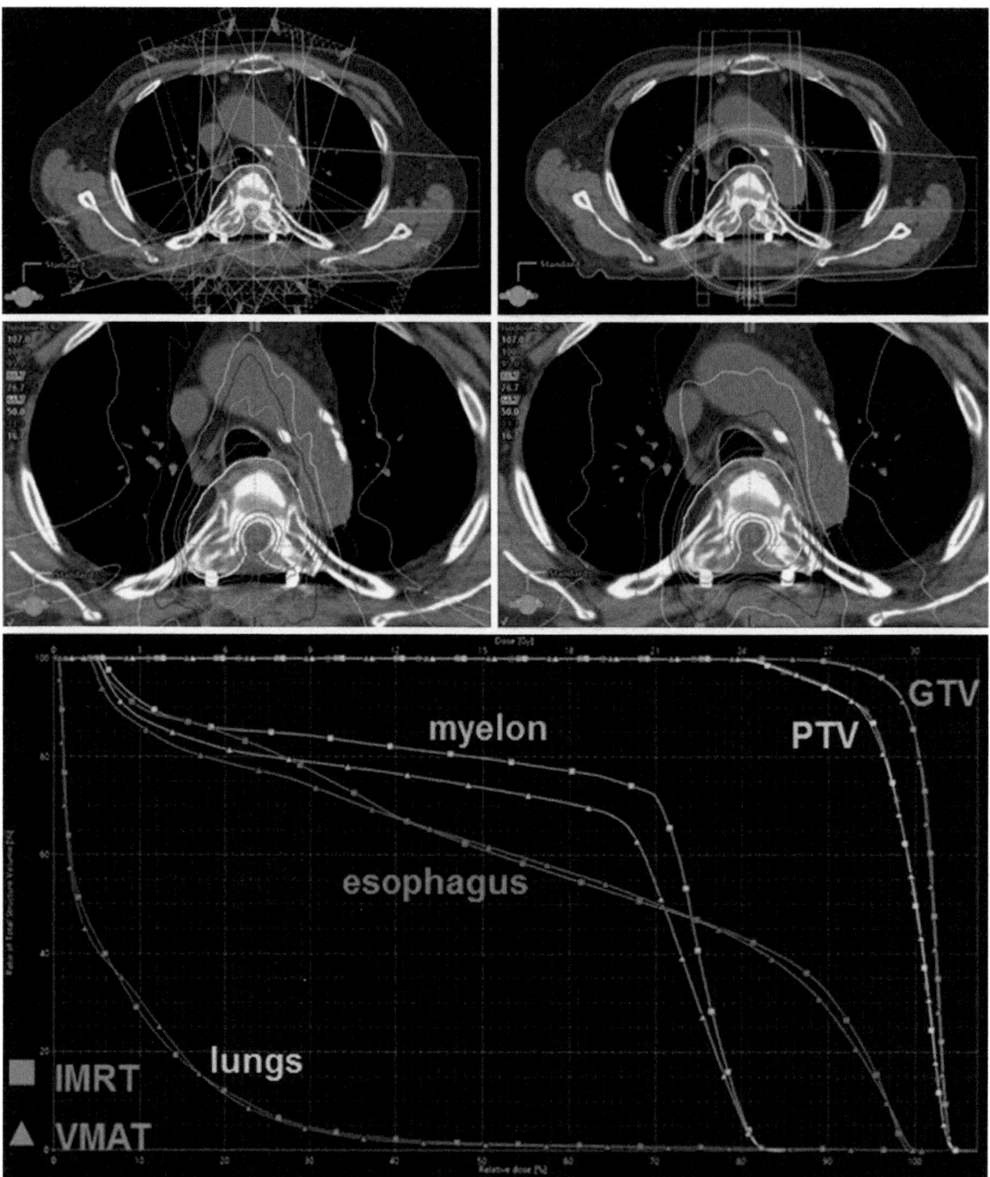

Fig. 7 Sliding window (*left*) and volumetric modulated arc therapy (*right*) treatment planning for re-treatment of a spinal metastasis. On the top the beam setups are shown, in the middle the dose distributions of the two techniques and on the bottom the dose volume histrograms

IMRT (step-and-shoot and sliding window IMRT), and they concluded that the TomoTherapy system has the greatest dose shaping flexibility at cost of decreased efficiency of the treatment delivery (Bortfeld and Webb 2009). However, it needs to be considered that despite these theoretical calculations and other planning studies comparing different IMRT hard- and software, the results of IMRT planning are dependent on the experience of the IMRT team (both physician and physicist) in terms of selection of optimization objectives for the inverse planning (Marnitz et al. 2015).

IMRT treatment planning, delivery, and quality assurance are in principle not different between a primary course of radiotherapy and the reirradiation course. However, some issues need to be considered more in detail in the reirradiation situation.

Unlike in 3D-CRT, IMRT planning distributes low doses over a larger volume of the patient. Additionally, volumes exposed to mid-doses or sometimes even high doses are frequently observed distant to the target volume. This may be of limited relevance in the primary course of treatment but could be deleterious in the reirradiation scenario, if these "hot spots" are located in volumes of normal tissue, where these additional doses exceed the radiation tolerance. Consequently, the physician should not only delineate the standard OARs as done in the primary treatment course; all volumes, where a significant prior irradiation dose had been delivered, should be defined as OARs and separate dose objectives should be defined for these volumes. Such normal structures could be the skin to avoid skin necrosis, joints and muscles to avoid contractures, and bones to avoid osteoradionecrosis.

In the reirradiation case, the radiation tolerance of normal structures is frequently significantly reduced. This is an extremely challenging situation for treatment planning, especially if this normal structure is located immediately next to recurrent cancer. A typical example is a spinal metastasis in the thoracic spine after primary radiotherapy for lung or esophageal cancer. In the situation of the OAR touching the PTV, the maximum dose of the OAR is the minimum dose to the PTV. The physician has now to decide where the dose gradient should be positioned: in the OAR aiming at a homogeneous dose in the PTV or in the PTV aiming at best possible sparing of the OAR at cost of an inhomogeneous dose in the target volume. The latter is certainly the most frequent situation in clinical practice. It is important that the IMRT planning objectives need to be adjusted to this desired dose distribution: Lower doses in the PTV immediately next to the OAR need to be allowed explicitly to the planning algorithm. The magnitude of this "underdosed" PTV depends on the steepness of the dose gradient between the target and the OAR. Mahan et al. reported a dose gradient of 10 %/mm using tomotherapy for retreatment of a spinal metastasis (Mahan et al. 2005). However, multiple variables influence the maximum achievable dose gradient: invariable factor like IMRT hard- and software and variable factors like geometry of target and OAR. For individual optimization of each plan, a ring-shaped help-volume around the OAR could be generated, where the dose gradient between OAR and PTV is to be located. Desired maximum and minimum doses of the OAR and the PTV excluding this help-volume are defined as hard constrains, and the size of the help-volume is step-wise decreased until these constrains can no longer be met by the planning system.

Clinical results of IMRT for reirradiation are promising. Loco-regional recurrent head-and-neck cancer is an example, where IMRT seems to improve outcome compared to conventional radiotherapy or 3D-CRT. Lee et al. reported about reirradiation in 105 patients with loco-regional recurrent head-and-neck cancer, and IMRT was used in 70 % of the patients (Lee et al. 2007). The median prior dose was 62 Gy and the median reirradiation dose was 59.4 Gy. Two-year loco-regional progression-free survival was 50 % and 20 % for patients treated with IMRT and non-IMRT, respectively. This benefit of IMRT remained statistically significant in multivariate analysis with a HR of 0.37. Other groups confirmed these favorable rates of ~50 % 2-year loco-regional control using IMRT (Biagioli et al. 2007; Duprez et al. 2009). Nevertheless, severe late toxicity was still considerable in these series.

Spinal metastases in previously irradiated areas are ideal IMRT indications for pain reduction or because of neurological symptoms (Fig. 8). Here, IMRT allows effective sparing of the spinal cord while treating the vertebral tumor, which is not possible with conventional radiotherapy or 3D-CRT. Milker-Zabel et al. reported the outcome in 19 patients with symptomatic spinal metastases, where a previous irradiation delivered a median dose of 28 Gy (Milker-Zabel et al. 2003). The median reirradiation dose was 39.6 Gy, while the dose to the spinal cord was limited to 20 Gy. With a median follow-up of about 1 year, only one patient developed a local recurrence. Pain relief and improvement of neurological deficits was

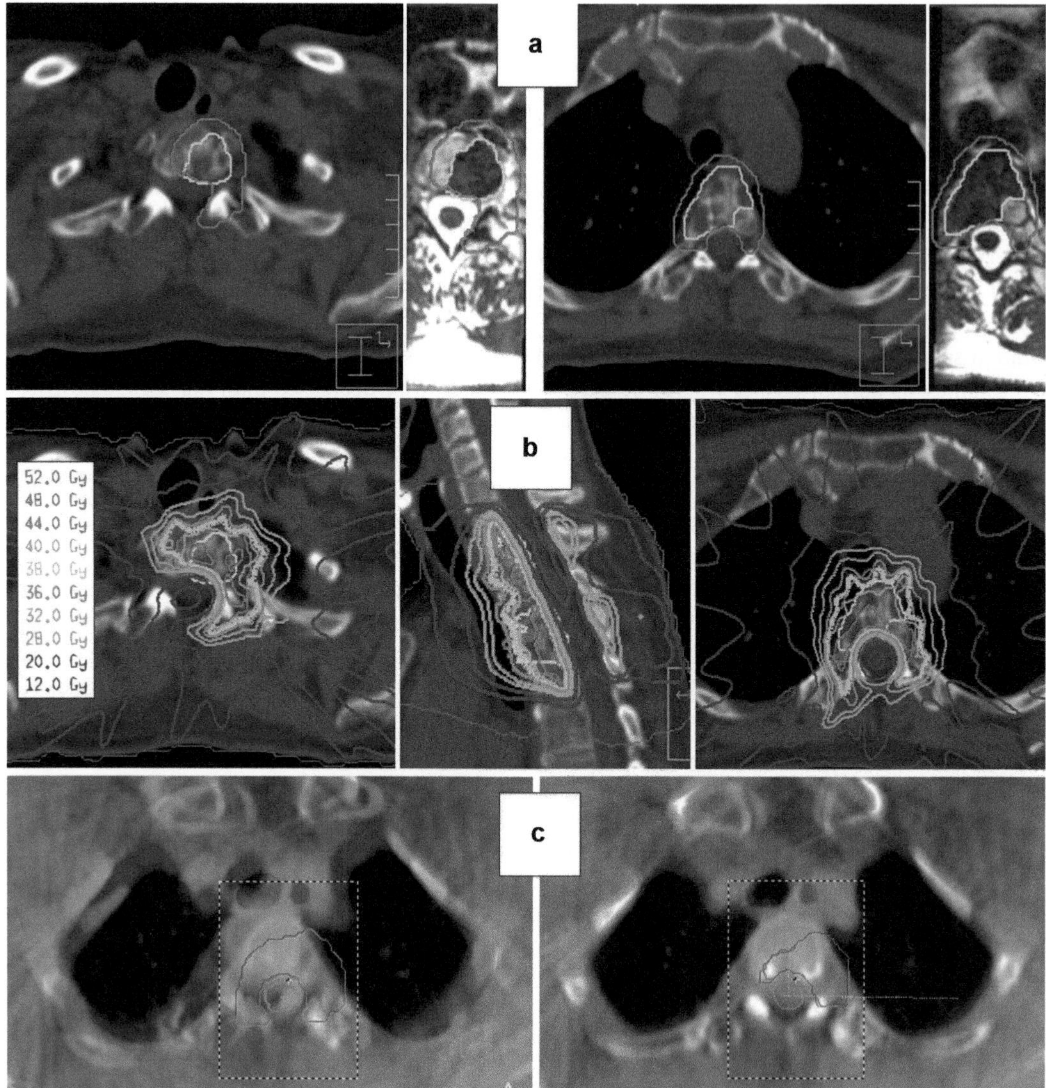

Fig. 8 Case example of a reirradiation for a spinal metastasis in a 62-year-old male patient with metastatic prostate cancer. Medical history: 2010: primary diagnosis of localized prostate cancer; antihormonal therapy, rejection of local therapy. January 2015: locally invasive prostate cancer, several bone metastases including the thoracic spine; laminectomy Th3-6 and tumor debulking; and dorsal instrumentation Th1-Th8. March 2015: postoperative radiotherapy to residual tumor with 5×4 Gy. January 2016: local progression with epidural growth Th4-5; reirradiation with 10×3 Gy. (**a**) Spinal metastases with GTV (*yellow*) based on the MRI and PTV (*red*); (**b**) IMRT dose distributions with a total dose of 40 Gy to the PTV and a maximum dose of 15 Gy to the spinal cord; (**c**) image-guidance using cone-beam CT with superposition of planning CT and verification cone-beam CT before (*left*) and after (*right*) image registration

achieved in 13/16 patients and 5/12 patients, respectively. No acute or late toxicity grade >II was observed. Further data are needed for confirmation of these promising results. Sterzing et al. reported on reirradiation of spinal metastases in 36 patients: The initial irradiation dose was 36.3 Gy on average, and after an interval of 17.5 months a dose of 34.8 Gy was delivered using TomoTherapy IMRT (Sterzing et al. 2010). Promising rates of pain reduction and local control were reported and no severe toxicity was observed.

4 Three and Four Dimensional Treatment Plan Evaluation

If possible, the dose distribution of the first radiotherapy series should be available for treatment planning and plan evaluation. Information on maximum doses or DVH data of the first radiotherapy series is insufficient because of the missing spatial relationship to the current treatment. If this information about the previous dose distribution is not available, for example, because the patient had been treated with 2D conventional planning, this radiotherapy series should be resimulated in the current planning CT. However, one needs to be aware that the resimulation may not reflect the situation at the first irradiation course, because the patient's anatomy could have changed, for example, due to the recurrent tumor or weight changes.

Three-dimensional dose distributions need to be evaluated carefully in terms of target coverage and especially in terms of normal tissue doses. DVHs are helpful tools for evaluation of the dose distributions, but one needs to be aware of the limitations of DVHs, where all spatial information is lost.

If the first treatment series was a 3D-CRT or IMRT irradiation and the treatment plan is digitally available, one could accumulate the dose distributions of the first and the current treatment series for a better risk assessment of the reirradiation. Accumulation of two dose distributions delivered at different times is called 4D dose calculation or 4D planning. Three important issues need to be considered for this 4D dose accumulation.

1. Data about recovery of normal tissue and their modeling in treatment planning and evaluation are rare. Accumulation consequently simulates a worst case scenario without any recovery.
2. Accumulation of physical doses would require conventional fractionation throughout the target and OARs, which is infrequently the case. Single-fraction doses different from 2 Gy should be weighted according to their biological effectiveness using the linear-quadratic model prior to dose accumulation. Calculation of 2 Gy-equivalent total doses (Lebesque and Keus 1991; Maciejewski et al. 1986) is an elegant method, resulting in numbers, which can be compared to tolerance doses for a single course of radiotherapy (Marks et al. 2010).
3. The patient's anatomy of the previous and the current treatment plan is certainly different, which makes 1:1 dose accumulation in the current CT data set misleading. A critical organ could have been displaced by the recurrent tumor, and this displacement of the critical organ in the current CT image relative to the situation of the first treatment course has to be considered in the process of dose accumulation (Fig. 9). Deformable registration between both image data may need to be performed and the

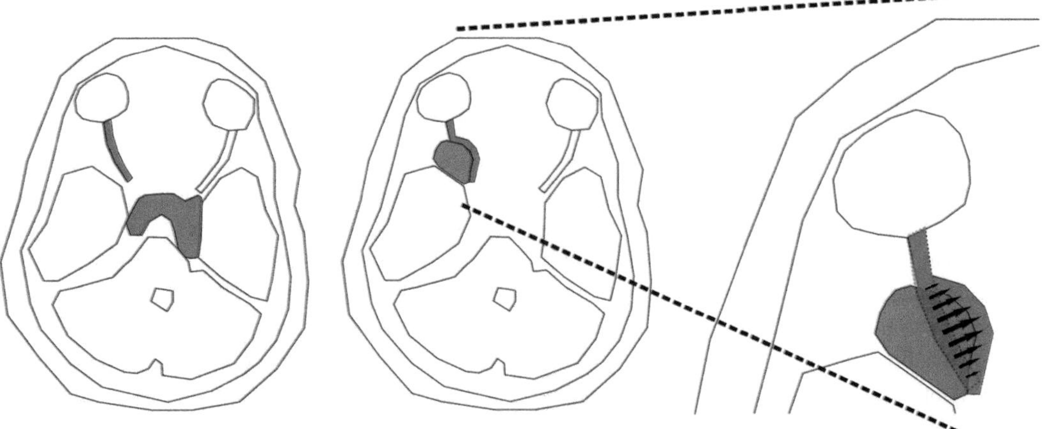

Fig. 9 Illustration of a recurrent skull base tumor (*red*), which causes a displacement of the right optical nerve (*blue*). Accumulation of the dose to this optical nerve from both irradiation series needs to account for this displacement by means of deformable image registration (indicated by vectors)

resulting deformation map applied to the previous dose distribution: The deformed previous dose distribution and the current dose distribution are then accumulated and displayed in the current CT data set with the recurrent tumor and preset location of the relevant OARs (Jumeau et al. 2015). Several commercial solutions are nowadays available to perform such dose accumulations; however, methods to allow the user to evaluate the uncertainty of the deformable registration and subsequent accumulation are missing. Therefore, residual dose distributions, especially in situations with large anatomical change, have to be evaluated carefully (van Rijssel et al. 2014).

5 Stereotactic Radiotherapy and Image Guidance

In the reirradiation situation, the target volume is usually limited to the recurrent macroscopic tumor without extensive elective CTV margins in order to reduce normal tissue exposure (Mantel et al. 2013). Stereotactic intracranial radiotherapy and stereotactic body radiotherapy (SBRT) in combination with image guidance (IGRT) provide an accurate means of highly conformal treatment delivery and patient positioning which can further spare organs-at-risk during reirradiation (Guckenberger et al. 2014).

Patient setup for daily radiotherapy has traditionally been performed by alignment of the room lasers with patient skin marks. This procedure assumes that there is a fixed, rigid relationship between the skin marks and the actual target volume. However, this method of patient setup is one of the major uncertainties in the radiotherapy delivery process contributing significantly to the safety margins (Hurkmans et al. 2001). Patient-specific uncertainties are imperfect alignment of the patient to the laser, mobility of the skin relative to the bony anatomy, and mobility of the tumor relative to the bony anatomy. These setup errors are especially important for treatment plans with steep dose gradients between the target and the organ-at-risk: For IMRT treatment of spinal metastases, it has been shown that patient setup errors as small as 1 mm can increase the dose to the spinal cord by a clinically relevant amount (Guckenberger et al. 2007a) (Fig. 10). Consequently, highly conformal treatment plans using IMRT or Protons pose a significant risk of target underdosage and/or OAR overdosage unless precise patient setup is ensured.

The stereotactic technique has been proven as highly effective for accurate patient setup. Stereotactic radiotherapy has traditionally been defined by a system of external coordinates. This stereotactic system is rigidly fixated to the patient and forms the basis for treatment planning with definition of the isocenter position and patient setup before treatment. In the cranial region, this has been traditionally practiced in an invasive fashion, where the stereotactic frame is fixated to the patient's skull. This offers best accuracy of patient setup; however, the invasiveness of the procedure requires planning and treatment finished within 1 day by means of radiosurgery. Noninvasive techniques for fractionated regimes were developed using thermoplastic mask or bite-block systems; the tradeoff to perform a fractionated treatment courses was a slightly reduced accuracy of patient setup. Initially developed for intracranial treatments, the stereotactic technique has been successfully adopted for extracranial stereotactic radiotherapy (Fig. 11).

Recently, image-guidance techniques have been developed, which are located in the treatment room and allow for daily verification of the patient setup with online correction of setup errors before the start of treatment. It has been shown that these IGRT techniques are at least equivalent in terms of patient setup accuracy compared to invasive frame-based stereotactic radiosurgery in the cranial region (Ramakrishna et al. 2010). The accuracy of patient setup for fractionated stereotactic radiotherapy in the cranial (Guckenberger et al. 2007b) and extracranial region (Guckenberger et al. 2006) is improved with IGRT compared to frame-based stereotactic patient positioning. Additionally, sufficient soft-tissue contrast in these verification images or implantation of radio-opaque markers make verification of the actual tumor position possible, which is important for targets, where mobility

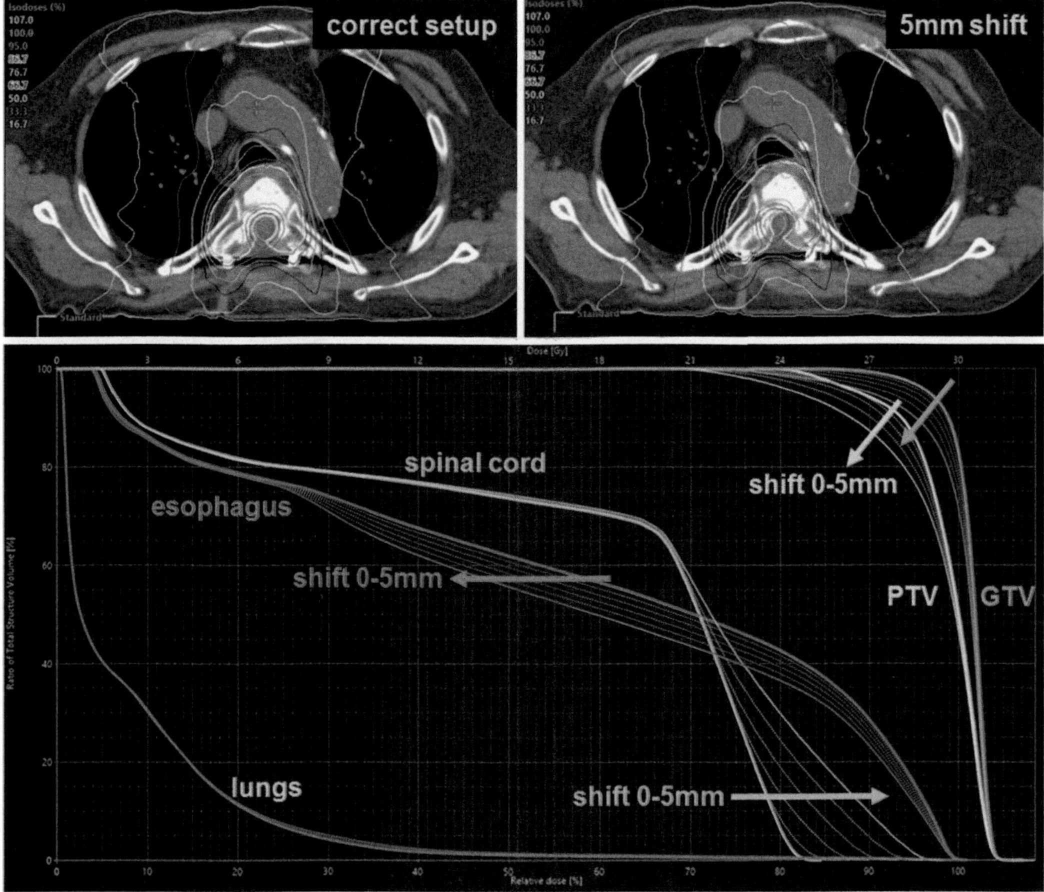

Fig. 10 Effect of set-up errors on dose to organ-at-risk: *Upper left image*: Dose distribution in the axial plane in VMAT plan for a spinal metastasis. *Upper right image*: Simulation of patient set-up error with a lateral shift of 5 mm to the left *Lower image*: Dose to the spinal cord: The *yellow* DVH curve displays the prescribed PTV dose according to the treatment plan. The *turquoise* DVH curves are dose distributions to the spinal cord resulting from simulated set-up errors. DVH curves for the esophagus and GTV are shown in *lilac* and *pink*, respectively

independent from bony anatomy has been described (Fig. 12). A treatment using daily image guidance with online correction of setup errors for high-precision radiotherapy is considered as "frame-less stereotactic radiotherapy": The stereotactic frame is replaced by image guidance with the patient's image as the "system of coordinates" for isocenter localization (Haertl et al. 2013). The available technologies of IGRT are summarized in Table 2.

Some issues, which are considered as especially important in the reirradiation situation, should be discussed.

In the primary course of radiotherapy, IGRT mainly aims at precise as possible delivery of the planned dose to the target volume. This may be different in the reirradiation situation, where precise as possible sparing of the OAR is the primary goal of IGRT. Precise targeting the tumor versus precise avoidance of the OAR could result in different displacement vectors for IGRT in cases where the spatial relationship between target and OAR changed in comparison to the planning situation. Possible causes are shrinkage/progression of the recurrent tumor during radiotherapy or a shift of the tumor position towards the OAR. Such non-rigid patient deformations cannot be corrected with a single couch displacement. Firstly, registration of the whole planning image with the

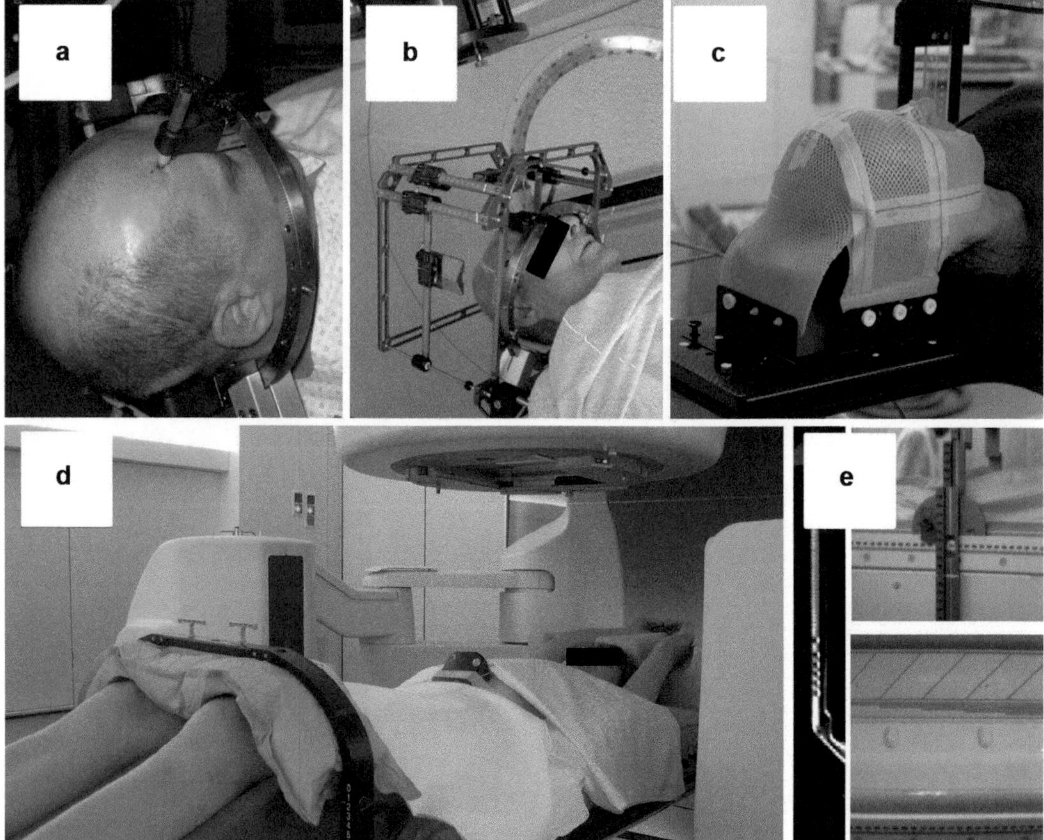

Fig. 11 Stereotactic patient setup: Cranial stereotactic radiotherapy with invasive fixation of the stereotactic ring (**a**) and the attached stereotactic frame with the system of external coordinates (**b**). Thermoplastic mask used in image-guided stereotactic radiotherapy (**c**). Stereotactic body radiotherapy using the Stereotactic bodyframe with a customized vacuum cushion (**d**) and a system of external coordinates (**e**)

whole verification image will result in a single registration vector, which will neither correctly display the situation for the target nor the OAR. Consequently, one should limit the region of interest (ROI) for image registration in IGRT to the volume, which is intended to be treated most precisely: This can be the target or the OAR. Larger uncertainties for volumes outside this ROI then need to be considered. Two separate registrations with the ROI for image registration around the target and around the OAR allow the evaluation of relative motion between these two structures. A compromise could be made to achieve an acceptable level degree of accuracy on the target and OAR level; in cases of changes beyond a certain threshold, replanning should be considered.

Additional irradiation dose due to IGRT could also be an issue of concern in the reirradiation situation. However, similar to the primary course of radiotherapy, the rationale for using IGRT should be evaluated on an individual patient basis before the treatment with consideration of the planned dose distribution and expected setup uncertainties. Additionally, most IGRT systems allow adaptation of imaging parameters to the clinical situation: for example, for cone-beam CT imaging, collimation, and the number of projection images, voltage and mAs influence the imaging dose significantly: If no soft-tissue contrast is needed, the dose for a single cone-beam CT can be reduced to less than 1 mSv (Sykes et al. 2005), which is certainly of limited clinical relevance, even if reirradiation is performed.

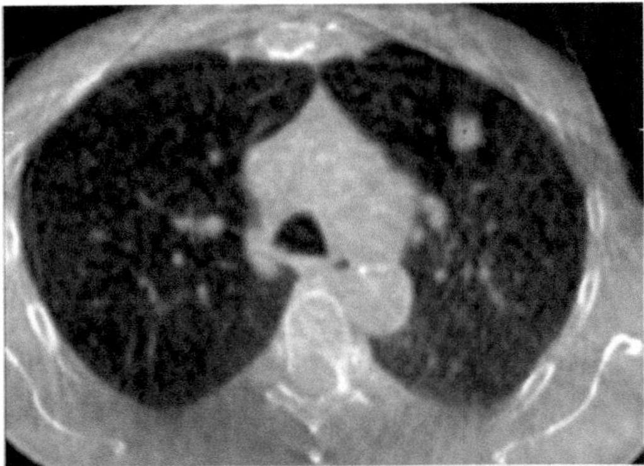

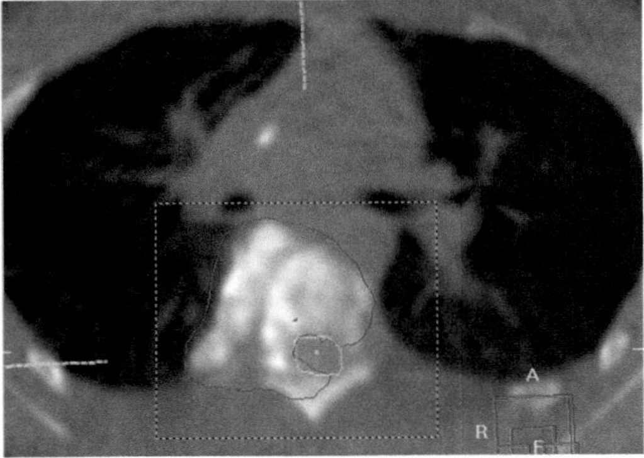

Fig. 12 Image quality of kilo-voltage cone-beam CT for image guidance: *upper image*: targeting of a lung nodule; *lower image*: targeting of a (GTV in *red*) spinal metastasis

Before the IGRT era, frame-based stereotactic radiosurgery with invasive fixation of the frame to the patient's skull offered significantly increased accuracy compared to the noninvasive fractionated approaches. One had to choose between highest accuracy and a fractionated treatment. This is not the case anymore when IGRT is used: Today, the same accuracy can be achieved with IGRT during a fractionated course of treatment. This could be beneficial especially in the reirradiation scenario: Fractionated irradiation may reduce late complications compared to hypo-fractionated regimes or radiosurgery taking advantage of the well-known difference in repair capability between tumors and late responding tissues.

Clinical results using stereotactic patient setup or image guidance in the reirradiation situation are promising, although they can currently not yet be considered standard of practice. Cranial reirradiation frequently used stereotactic patient setup for maximum (re-)positioning accuracy. Detailed clinical results are described in the respective chapter of this book. For example, fractionated stereotactic reirradiation of recurrent high grade gliomas has resulted in acceptable rates of toxicity and promising overall survival compared to historical controls after application of hypo-fractionated doses up to 40 Gy (Shepherd et al. 1997) or stereotactic radiosurgery (Kong et al. 2008). The addition of modern targeted drugs or chemotherapy like temozolomide (Combs et al. 2008), gfitinib (Schwer et al. 2008), or bevacizumab (Gutin et al. 2009; Cuneo et al. 2012) to stereotactic reirradiation may further improve outcome. Similarly, repeated stereotactic radiosurgery has been proven to be feasible for patients with progressive brain metastases with 1-year local control rates of up to 78 % depending on tumor histology (Minniti et al. 2016).

A small number of studies reported clinical results using SBRT in the reirradiation situation. For instance, initial results have been published for recurrent head-and-neck cancer (Rwigema et al. 2010; Heron et al. 2009), lung cancer after previous thoracic radiotherapy (Fig. 13) (Kelly et al. 2010; Poltinnikov et al. 2005; Kilburn et al. 2014), or recurrent gynecological cancer (Guckenberger et al. 2010; Deodato et al. 2009). For lung cancer, small field SBRT for thoracic reirradiation seems to be safe with promising rates of local control exceeding conventional techniques, although overall survival appears to be highly dependent on systemic progression. In contrast, SBRT reirradiation for head-and-neck cancer is limited by the risk of severe late adverse events, which are however less frequent than in patient series with conventional techniques. In summary, SBRT for recurrent extracranial tumors is still in an early stage of establishment, where no recommendations regarding total dose, fractionation, and radiation tolerance of normal tissue are possible.

6 Intrafractional Motion Management

Intrafractional changes of the tumor position could result in decreased target dose coverage with the consequence of reduced local control;

Table 2 Image-guided technologies

	Technique	Radiation dose	3D information	Soft tissue contrast	Real-time imaging	Imaging in treatment position	Pros	Cons
Electronic portal imaging device (EPID)	Use of therapeutic MV beam	None to high	Limited	Very low	Possible	Yes	No doses for imaging of treatment fields; in-beam imaging; real-time imaging	High doses unless imaging of treatment fields; very limited soft tissue contrast; implanted markers required for soft tissue tumors
Stereoscopic kV X-ray	Two stereoscopic X-ray sources and panels	Low	Limited	Low	Possible	Yes	Real-time imaging	Limited soft tissue contrast; implanted markers required for soft tissue tumors
In-room CT scanner	CT on rail; mobile CT scanner	Medium	Full	Excellent	No	No	Volume imaging; best image quality; respiration-correlated imaging	Movement of patient and treatment couch necessary
kV cone-beam CT	Installed orthogonal to treatment beam	Medium	Full	Good	No	Yes	Volume imaging; respiration-correlated imaging	Worse image quality compared with in-room CT imaging
MV cone-beam CT and helical MV CT	MV CBCT: use of treatment beam and EPID; TomoTherapy™	High	Full	Acceptable	No	Yes	Volume imaging; minimized metal artifacts	Suboptimal soft tissue contrast; high imaging doses
Ultrasound	B-mode acquisition and targeting	None	Good	Acceptable	No	Yes	No additional irradiation dose	User dependency; risk of target displacement due to pressure
Active electromagnetic markers	Implanted active electromagnetic markers (Calypso)	None	Limited	None	Yes	Yes	Real-time online information with high frequency	No anatomical information; implanted markers required
Surface scanner	Laser- or video-based surface scanner	None	Surface only	None	Yes	Yes	Real-time imaging; complete surface imaged	Suboptimal correlation between surface and target position for many tumor sites

No absolute values of radiation doses are stated because imaging parameters can be adjusted in most of the systems with large differences in imaging doses; it is distinguished between no additional irradiation dose, low, medium, and high additional irradiation dose

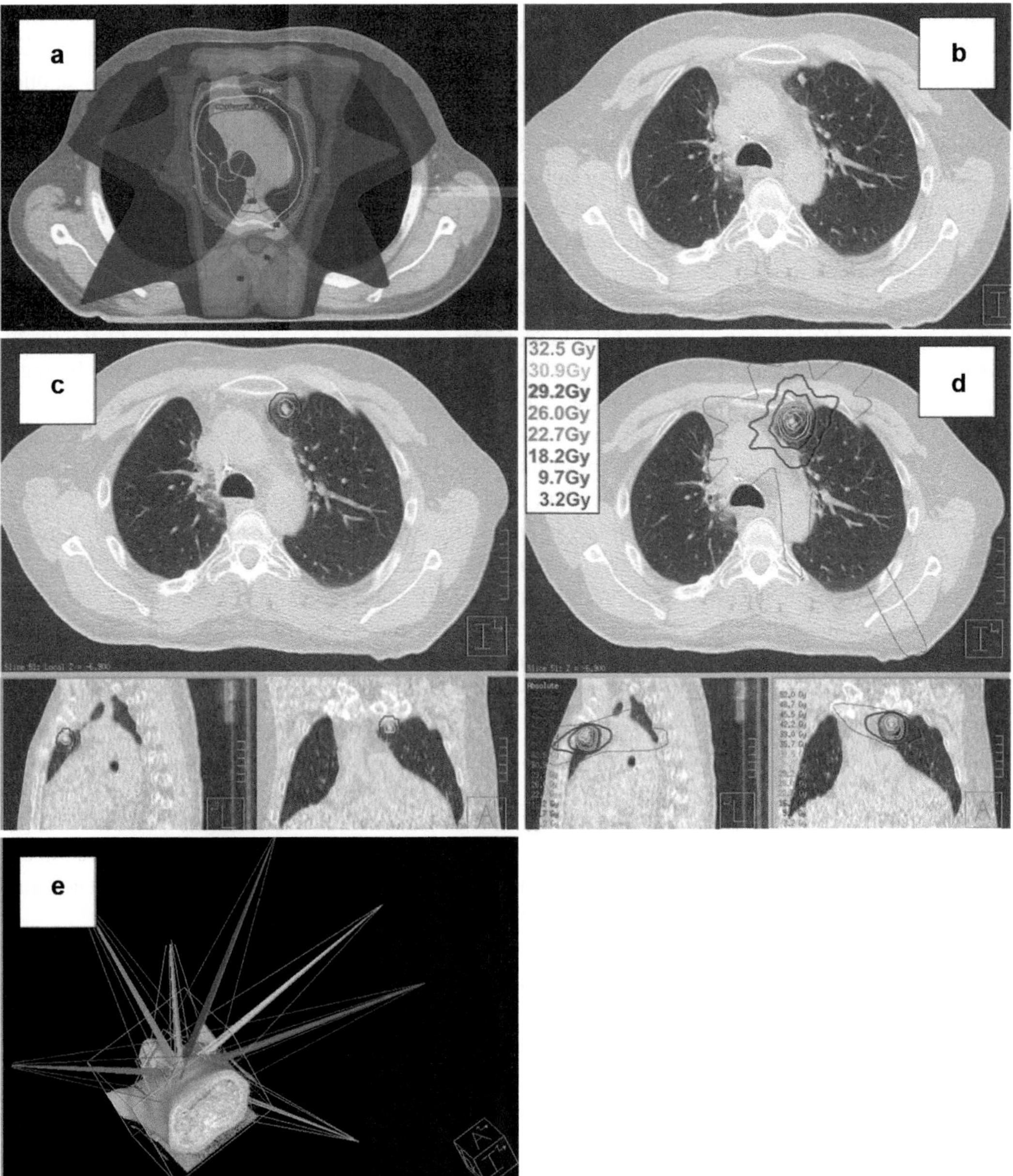

Fig. 13 Case example of retreatment for a solitary lung metastasis with SBRT. Medical history**:** 2007: Primary NSCLC (adeno carcinoma) right lower lobe; three cycles of neo-adjuvant chemotherapy; surgery with lobectomy and mediastinal lymph node dissection; tumor stage: ypT2 ypN2 M0; postoperative adjuvant chemotherapy; postoperative radiotherapy to the mediastinum (55.8 Gy); 2008: Solitary brain metastasis treated with radiosurgery; 2009: Solitary lung metastasis treated with radiosurgery of 26 Gy; (**a**) adjuvant radiotherapy after surgical treatment of N2 disease, (**b**) solitary lung metastasis, (**c**) target volume for SBRT GTV (*yellow*) and PTV (*red*), (**d**) dose distribution of SBRT with delivery of a single fraction of 26 Gy to the 80 % isodose, and (**e**) beam arrangement for SBRT

similarly, intrafractional motion of the OAR could result in increased risk of toxicity. Four sources of intrafractional uncertainties need to be considered: (1) Regarding *motion of the patient* him- or herself, one can distinguish between voluntary motion due to poor compliance and involuntary motion, for example, due to pain, cough, or uncomfortable positioning. (2) *Breathing motion* is a major source of uncertainty in the thoracic and upper abdominal region: Motion amplitudes up to 3 cm for targets located in the chest (Seppenwoolde et al. 2002) or upper abdomen (Brandner et al. 2006) have been described. The predominant direction of breathing-induced tumor motion is the cranio-caudal direction with increased motion amplitudes in the caudal compared to the cranial parts of the lung. Analogously, the influence of breathing motion in the abdominal region decreases from the diaphragm towards caudal. (3) The influence of *cardiac motion* on tumor and OAR position variability is in order of magnitude between 1 and 4 mm. (4) It has been shown that *changes in the filling of hollow organs*, especially rectum and bladder, may influence doses to the target and OAR significantly (Polat et al. 2008). Additionally, peristaltic motion might lead to an additional uncertainty in the dose to the organs-at-risk.

6.1 Patient Motion Management

As described above, we distinguished between voluntary motion and involuntary intrafractional patient motion. The most effective way to reduce involuntary patient motion due to pain is to ensure a comfortable patient setup by using support devices for head, arms, knees, and feet and adjust these to the individual patient. Additionally, appropriate pain medication is essential, which is especially important in the reirradiation situation, where the local tumor is frequently associated with significant pain to the patient. Patient motion due to cough or dyspnea could be reduced by medication or oxygen supply during treatment, respectively.

Passive immobilization is standard practice in primary radiotherapy for many cancer sites, and identical devices should be used in the reirradiation situation: for example, head-shoulder masks or bite-blocks for irradiation in the head-and-neck region and thermoplastic vacuum cushions for immobilization of arms, leg, and the whole body. For total body immobilization in a vacuum cushion, a double-vacuum technique has been developed, where a second vacuum is applied underneath a foil, which is wrapped around the patient: A low pressure underneath the foil presses the patient into the vacuum cushions for effective and comfortable immobilization (Fuss et al. 2004). There is sometimes a tradeoff between immobilization and comfort of the patient: A patient in an uncomfortable positioning device will not be immobilized effectively, whatever device is used. It should also be mentioned that the previously discussed techniques of frame-less image-guided stereotactic radiotherapy still require effective immobilization: Image-guidance aims at minimization of interfractional setup errors, whereas immobilization aims at minimization of intrafractional uncertainties.

Different systems are available for intrafractional monitoring of the patient stability: for example, surface scanners or infrared markers positioned on the surface of the patient. If predefined thresholds of patient motion are violated, interruption of the irradiation should be performed. The patient's surface is then only a surrogate for the actual target position: Target motion independently from patient motion needs to be considered. It is consequently most accurate to repeat image guidance.

6.2 Breathing Motion Compensation

The first step in compensation of breathing motion is quantification of this uncertainty in a patient individual fashion at treatment planning. Fluoroscopic planar imaging is a frequently used technique for measurement of breathing-induced motion of pulmonary tumors; for targets in the upper abdomen, mobility of the diaphragm is used as a surrogate for the actual tumor motion. The advantage of fluoroscopic imaging is the possibility to monitor range and pattern of motion for a longer period of time. Disadvantages are the limitations of 2D planar imaging, where a proportion of pulmonary tumors are not visible and evaluation of the 3D motion trajectory is difficult.

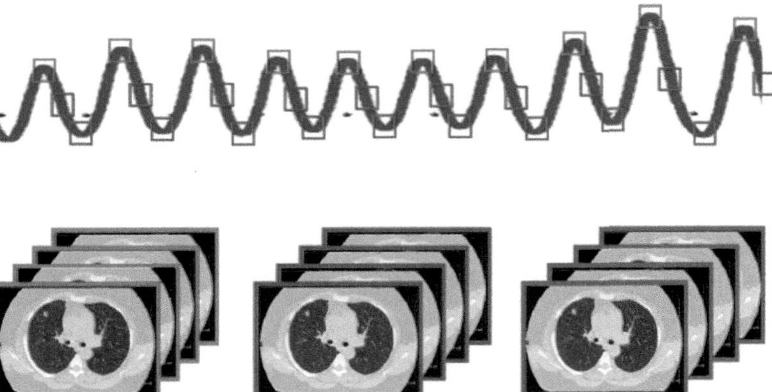

Fig. 14 Respiration correlated 4D-CT: In contrast to conventional CT imaging, each axial patient position is imaged for the duration of at least one breathing cycle by using small table pitches (highly redundant data acquisition). Images or projection data acquired at corresponding phases of the breathing cycle are then sorted/binned such that multiple CT phases at different phases of the breathing cycle are reconstructed

Implantation of radiopaque markers into the target for fluoroscopic 4D imaging is frequently practiced in the lung and liver region; however, the risk of a pneumothorax needs to be considered. The current gold standard for treatment planning is the respiration correlated CT (4D-CT), which allows with a single image acquisition the reconstruction of multiple CT series at different phases of the breathing cycle (Fig. 14). Besides evaluation of the patient individual motion pattern and range, another advantage of respiration correlated CT imaging for treatment planning is the reduction of motion artifacts in the CT images, which could result in incorrect size and shape of the target volume (Fig. 15).

In general, three techniques for breathing motion compensation can be distinguished. (1) Treatment in free breathing, (2) treatment in free breathing with dynamic beams chasing the target or with a dynamic couch performing compensatory motion to keep the target fixed relative to linac coordinates (tracking), and (3) gated beam delivery in only a specific phase of the breathing cycle or in a breath-hold technique. A summary of available motion management strategies is presented in Table 3.

The most frequently used technique treats the patients while they are breathing freely and continuous delivery of static beams is performed.

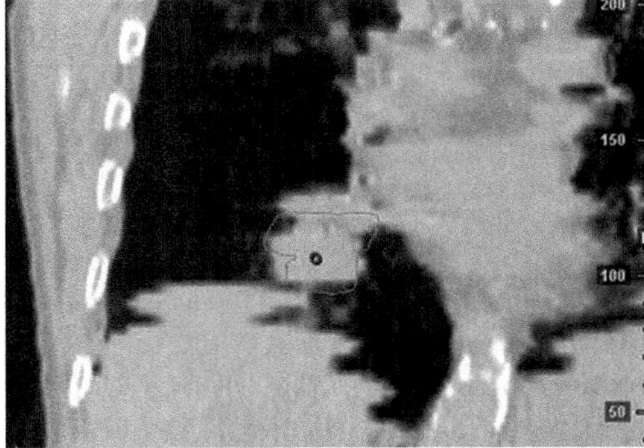

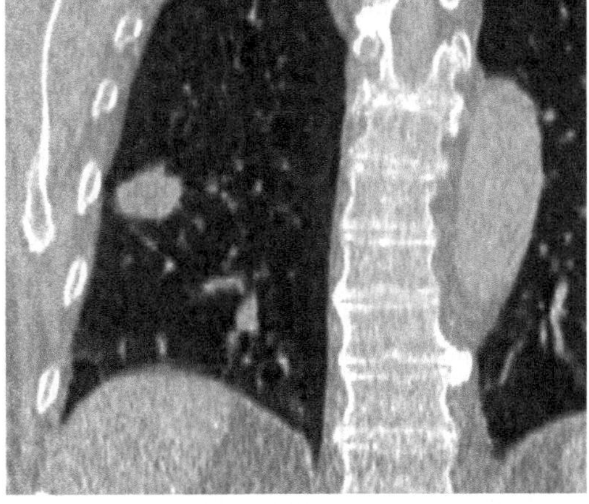

Fig. 15 Two pulmonary tumors, which were highly mobile in fluoroscopy. (*Upper image*) Significant motion artifacts in conventional 3D-CT imaging of the pulmonary target and the dome of the diaphragm; (*Lower image*) absence of motion artifacts in respiration correlated 4D-CT imaging

Table 3 Breathing motion management strategies

Breathing motion management technology	Safety margins	Complexity of treatment planning and delivery	Proportion of beam on time of total treatment time	Comments
Free breathing (ITV)	Large based on internal target volume concept	Low	Optimal	Unnecessary large safety margins
Free breathing (stochastical)	Reduced with mid-ventilation concept	High	Optimal	Preferable for motion amplitudes up to 15–20 mm
Mechanical abdominal compression	Reduced compared to free breathing	Low	Optimal	Only for patients with predominant tumor motion in craniocaudal direction; dependent on patient tolerance
Breath–hold technique	Small	Medium	Patient dependent (pulmonary function and compliance)	Adequate pulmonary function and patient compliance required; reduction of irradiated lung tissue when practiced in inhalation breath-hold technique
Gated beam delivery	Small	High	Low	Significant prolongation of the total treatment time
Tumor tracking	Small	Very high	Optimal	Highly complex

With patients breathing freely, the target volume needs to be adjusted such that it encompasses the tumor completely in all phases of the breathing cycle according to ICRU 62. However, it has been shown that this geometrical target volume concept uses unnecessary large safety margins with the consequence of large volumes of normal tissue within the PTV; smaller safety margins are possible if a stochastic target volume concept is applied (Engelsman et al. 2005). The so-called mid-ventilation concept has been proposed for irradiation in free breathing, where treatment planning and image guidance are based on the average tumor position; this was shown to reduce safety margins significantly compared to the traditional ITV target volume concept (Wolthaus et al. 2008). Recently, intensity-modulated, inverse treatment planning is more frequently used for tumors that move due to respiration. Several studies have evaluated the interplay effect between the motion of the tumor and the motion of the MLC with the conclusion that over a large number of beams and fractions or a high dose per fraction, the interplay effect averages out and is in the order of magnitude of 1–3 % (Ehrbar et al. 2016; Chan et al. 2014).

Tumor tracking is defined as a technique, where the treatment delivery adjusts dynamically to changes of the target position during the breathing cycle. Up to now tracking has been performed clinically using three different techniques: the CyberKnife, the Vero system, and MLC tracking. Most studies have been performed using the CyberKnife, a linear accelerator mounted on an industrial robot, which moves synchronously with breathing motion of the target (Seppenwoolde et al. 2007). The Vero system is a gimbaled linac system, which tracks the tumor using the treatment beam (Depuydt et al. 2014). Another technique, where the irradiation beam chases the moving tumor, makes use of a dynamic multileaf collimator (MLC) (Keall et al. 2006, 2014): The MLC shape is adjusted in real-time to changes of the target position. The third approach is different: A static beam delivery technique is combined with a dynamic couch, where compensatory couch motion opposite to the target motion aims at keeping the target fixed in the beam aperture (Wilbert et al. 2008; Lang et al. 2014).

Gated beam delivery differs significantly, as the irradiation is only performed in a specific phase of the breathing cycle or in breath-hold technique; the irradiation is then paused at the other phases of the breathing cycle. This gated beam delivery results in a significant reduction of the "effective" target motion at cost of prolonged total treatment time (Underberg et al. 2005).

The choice of the appropriate motion management strategy should be dependent on the motion range of the pulmonary target. For motion amplitudes less than 15–20 mm, which is the majority of the patients, there is only a small benefit of gating and tracking in terms of margin reduction (Sonke et al. 2009; Guckenberger et al. 2009b) and treatment with the patient breathing freely is preferable. The benefit of gating and tracking increases for larger motion amplitudes. However, the availability of tracking is currently still limited and gating prolongs the treatment delivery time substantially. Keeping the total treatment time as short as possible is essential as longer treatment times were shown to result in increased intrafractional patient motion and drifts of the target (Purdie et al. 2007).

Similar to treatment planning, 4D target motion needs to be integrated into pretreatment patient setup using image guidance and intrafractional target position monitoring. Different technologies for pretreatment and intratreatment 4D imaging are available. Evaluation of the patient's surface and establishment of a correlation model between the surface motion and the target motion is frequently performed; however, interfractional and intrafractional changes of this correlation model are well known. Pretreatment respiration correlated 4D cone-beam CT is clinically available allowing for precise patient setup with full consideration of breathing motion in the IGRT process (Sonke et al. 2005); however, continuous intrafractional 4D imaging is not possible with this technology. Intrafractional 4D target monitoring has been described using stereoscopic X-ray imaging or using the electronic portal imaging device; however, implantation of markers is necessary for visualization of the targets as described previously.

Regardless which motion management strategy and which technology is chosen, it is important to have a consistent 4D work flow for treatment planning and treatment delivery: A systematic integration of breathing motion into all steps of imaging for treatment planning, target volume definition, image guidance, and treatment delivery is essential (Korreman et al. 2008).

6.3 Management of Cardiac Motion

Only limited research has been performed on the magnitude of cardiac motion and the influence of it on the dose distribution. For lung tumors, a displacement of 1–4 mm, depending on the distance between the tumor and the cardiac or aortic wall, was reported (Seppenwoolde et al. 2002). This might lead to an increase in target volume of about 10% and in some cases to a reduction in target coverage (Chen et al. 2014). For esophageal tumors, the displacement can be up to 10 mm depending on the location of the tumor (Palmer et al. 2014).

Cardiac motion can be compensated with the motion management techniques described above. However, one needs to take into consideration that cardiac motion has a higher frequency compared to respiratory motion, and therefore, it is important that the applied motion management technique has a short delay between the detection of the motion and the compensation of the motion.

6.4 Management of Motion Due Variable Filling of Hollow Organs

Variability of the target position due to changes of the filling of hollow organs is well known in primary radiotherapy, for example, of prostate cancer. Whereas intrafractional variability of the bladder filling is clearly dependent on the total treatment time, changes of the rectal filling could occur on a much shorter timescale and are not predictable.

Several noninvasive and nontechnological techniques have been shown to reduce interfractional and intrafractional target position variability. A diet protocol was shown to reduce moving fecal gas during acquisition of cone-beam CT images (intrafractional motion) and reduce interfractional prostate position variability (Smitsmans et al. 2008). Daily emptying the rectum before treatment by patient-applied rectal enemas has also been shown to reduce interfractional prostate position variability (Fiorino et al. 2008). Similar positive effects are expected for locally recurrent tumors with close relationship to the rectum. Rectal balloons have been shown to fixate the prostate (Wachter et al. 2002); however, the effect of the balloon on different tumor locations or local recurrences is probably small. Daily catheterization of the urinary bladder and refilling with a defined volume of normal saline reduce interfractional bladder volume variability, and a drinking protocol might reduce intrafractional bladder volume variability.

If real-time intrafractional monitoring of the target position is intended, identical technologies as described in the breathing motion management part can be applied. Additionally, electromagnetic transponders may be implanted into or in the vicinity of the tumor and their position can be monitored with a high frequency of 10 Hz.

Two issues may be different between primary radiotherapy and reirradiation regarding intrafractional motion management. Firstly, many patients are in considerable pain because of the locally recurrent tumor, and effective pain medication is difficult in a number of patients; consequently, comfortable patient positioning and a fast treatment delivery work flow are highly important. Techniques, which minimize the total treatment time (e.g., VMAT), may reduce intrafractional uncertainties more efficiently and simultaneously improve patient comfort compared to highly sophisticated techniques, which prolong the treatment time (e.g., gated beam delivery or repeated cone-beam CT scanning during treatment).

Though the implantation of markers into or around the macroscopic tumor is considered a safe procedure in the primary course of radiotherapy, literature data about the safety in the reirradiation situation are missing. The patient's anatomy may be altered due to previous surgery, and radiation-induced fibrosis may increase complication rates. Consequently, the use of imaging systems which do not require invasive implantation of markers may be preferable for retreatments.

7 Adaptive Radiotherapy

Besides changes of the target position, more complex changes have been described during the course of fractionated radiotherapy: for example weight loss of the patients, progression and regression of the macroscopic tumor, changes of oedema, effusion, and pulmonary atelectasis. Such systematic changes of the patient's anatomy compared to the planning situation could influence the delivered dose distributions, and an adaptation of the treatment plan should consequently be considered (Fig. 16).

Adaptive radiation therapy has been defined as a closed-loop, iterative process where the treatment plan is modified based on feedback measurements performed during treatment (Yan et al. 1997). Adaptive radiotherapy is a technique to deal with all uncertainties during a course of radiotherapy; however, this chapter will concentrate on systematic shape and volume changes of the macroscopic tumor and changes of the patient's weight and shape.

The process of adaptive radiotherapy can be divided into several steps. The first step is evaluation of the patient individual random and especially systematic changes compared to the planning stage. If these changes exceed a certain threshold, an adaptation of the treatment plan is performed: This could be an adjustment of the isocenter position as well as replanning to deal with more complex changes. Ideally, this is not only an adaptation of the treatment plan to the current situation but takes changes, which occurred during the treatment course so far, into account (e.g., planning of a compensatory higher

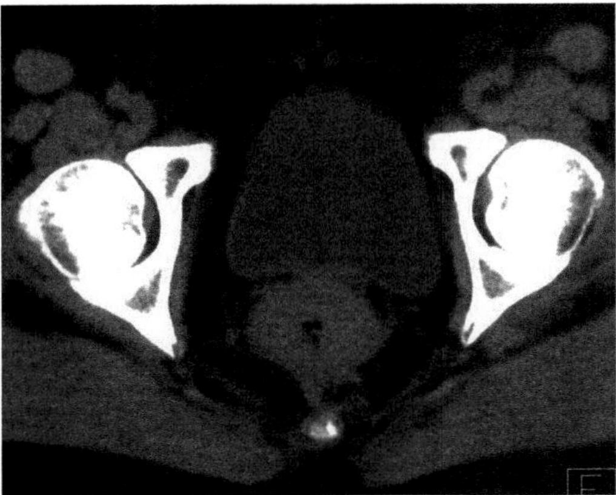

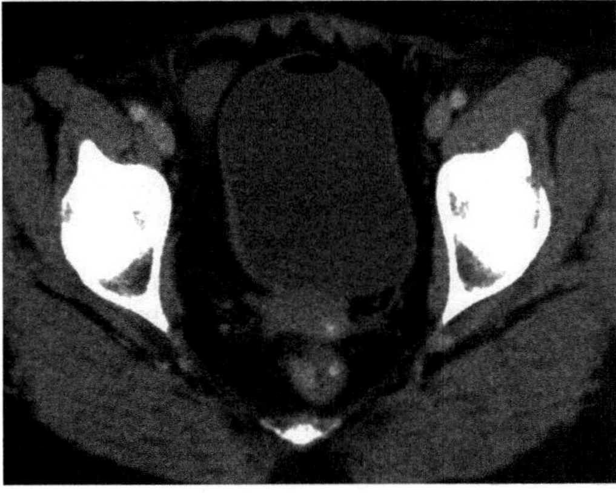

Fig. 16 Locally recurrent cervical cancer: size of the macroscopic tumor at the time prior to treatment planning (*upper image*) and after delivery of a conventionally fractionated dose of 46 Gy (*lower image*); this CT image with significant tumor regression was used for adaptive planning of an SBRT boost

dose to a cold-spot volume). After the adaptation is performed, the feedback loop is re-entered (Fig. 17).

Systematic volume changes of the macroscopic tumor have been described in primary radiotherapy for advanced stage NSCLC, where a continuous decrease of the GTV by 1.2 % per day has been reported (Kupelian et al. 2005). This continuous tumor shrinkage has been confirmed by other groups, whereas progressive disease during radio (chemo) therapy seems to be rare. Similar findings of continuous GTV shrinkage were made during primary radiotherapy for other cancer sites, for example, head-and-neck cancer (Barker et al. 2004) and cervical cancer (Mayr et al. 2006). Shrinkage of the tumor could release pressure from the surrounding tissue with the consequence of critical structures moving into the high dose regions. Additionally, adaptive replanning depending on daily bladder filling has shown to reduce dose to normal tissue considerably (Vestergaard et al. 2013).

Weight loss is a frequently observed phenomenon in cancer patients and is an established prognostic factor for overall survival in a number of cancer sites (Fearon et al. 2011). Weight loss during a course of radiotherapy may have multiple causes, for example, oral, pharyngeal, or esophageal mucositis, diarrhea, simultaneous chemotherapy, or loss of appetite. All means of

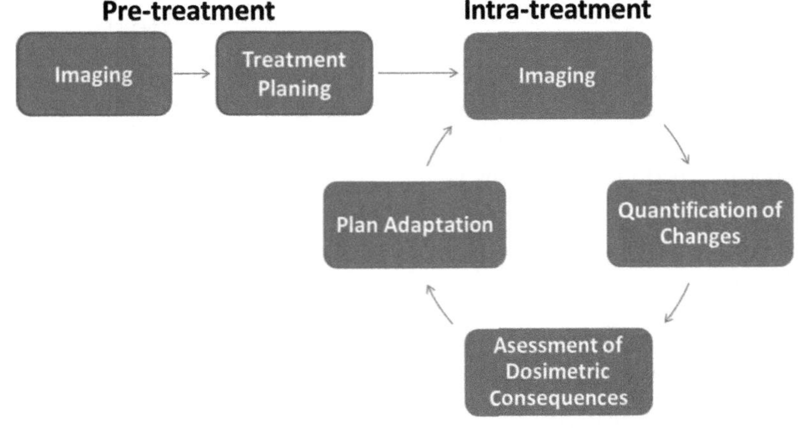

Fig. 17 Schematic illustration of an adaptive feedback loop

prevention and treatment of weight loss should be undertaken. However, if significant weight loss occurs during treatment, it could influence radiotherapy in a clinically relevant way. Weight loss could make immobilization devices like thermoplastic head masks less effective, resulting in increased setup uncertainties or alter dose distributions due to changes of the patient's geometry.

Several issues remain to be solved until adaptation of the treatment beams to a shrinking tumor will find its way into routine clinical practice of primary radiotherapy. The additional work load of replanning needs to be considered. Reliable and fast nonrigid image registration tools are required for dose accumulation of treatment plans, which were planned on different CT data sets. There are no valid data about thresholds and optimal time during the radiotherapy course, when and how frequently adaptation should be performed. There may also be a certain risk of shrinking the treatment fields: Microscopic disease could be excluded from the PTV with the consequence of underdosage and decreased local control.

There are no data in the literature about this type of adaptive radiotherapy specifically in the reirradiation situation. However, one could argue that the risk of normal tissue damage is significantly increased for reirradiation, justifying adaptive radiotherapy despite the increased work load and accepting a potential miss of microscopic disease. Additionally, it is not only the tumor, which might change during the course of radiotherapy: As described above, pulmonary atelectasis, effusions, and edemas could change and alter doses to critical OARs or the target volume. Adaptation of the treatment plans to such changes of the normal tissue could be considered as a safe approach of adaptive radiotherapy and should be performed when observed.

Literature

Ang KK et al (2001) Extent and kinetics of recovery of occult spinal cord injury. Int J Radiat Oncol Biol Phys 50(4):1013–1020

Barker JL Jr et al (2004) Quantification of volumetric and geometric changes occurring during fractionated radiotherapy for head-and-neck cancer using an integrated CT/linear accelerator system. Int J Radiat Oncol Biol Phys 59(4):960–970

Biagioli MC et al (2007) Intensity-modulated radiotherapy with concurrent chemotherapy for previously irradiated, recurrent head and neck cancer. Int J Radiat Oncol Biol Phys 69(4):1067–1073

Bortfeld T, Webb S (2009) Single-arc IMRT? Phys Med Biol 54(1):N9–N20

Brandner ED et al (2006) Abdominal organ motion measured using 4D CT. Int J Radiat Oncol Biol Phys 65(2):554–560

Bzdusek K et al (2009) Development and evaluation of an efficient approach to volumetric arc therapy planning. Med Phys 36(6):2328–2339

Chan C et al (2014) Intensity-modulated radiotherapy for lung cancer: current status and future developments. J Thorac Oncol 9(11):1598–1608

Chao KS et al (2000) Intensity-modulated radiation therapy in head and neck cancers: the Mallinckrodt experience. Int J Cancer 90(2):92–103

Chen T et al (2014) Frequency filtering based analysis on the cardiac induced lung tumor motion and its impact on the radiotherapy management. Radiother Oncol 112(3):365–370

Combs SE et al (2008) Radiochemotherapy with temozolomide as re-irradiation using high precision fractionated stereotactic radiotherapy (FSRT) in patients with recurrent gliomas. J Neurooncol 89(2):205–210

Cuneo KC et al (2012) Safety and efficacy of stereotactic radiosurgery and adjuvant bevacizumab in patients with recurrent malignant gliomas. Int J Radiat Oncol Biol Phys 82(5):2018–2024

Dearnaley DP et al (1999) Comparison of radiation side-effects of conformal and conventional radiotherapy in prostate cancer: a randomised trial. Lancet 353(9149):267–272

Deodato F et al (2009) Stereotactic radiotherapy in recurrent gynecological cancer: a case series. Oncol Rep 22(2):415–419

Depuydt T et al (2014) Treating patients with real-time tumor tracking using the Vero gimbaled linac system: implementation and first review. Radiother Oncol 112(3):343–351

Dresen RC et al (2010) Absence of tumor invasion into pelvic structures in locally recurrent rectal cancer: prediction with preoperative MR imaging. Radiology 256(1):143–150

Duprez F et al (2009) Intensity-modulated radiotherapy for recurrent and second primary head and neck cancer in previously irradiated territory. Radiother Oncol 93(3):563–569

Ehrbar S et al (2016) Three-dimensional versus four-dimensional dose calculation for volumetric modulated arc therapy of hypofractionated treatments. Z Med Phys 26(1):45–53

Engelsman M et al (2005) How much margin reduction is possible through gating or breath hold? Phys Med Biol 50(3):477–490

Even-Sapir E et al (2004) Detection of recurrence in patients with rectal cancer: PET/CT after abdominoperineal or anterior resection. Radiology 232(3):815–822

Fearon K et al (2011) Definition and classification of cancer cachexia: an international consensus. Lancet Oncol 12(5):489–495

Fiorino C et al (2008) Evidence of limited motion of the prostate by carefully emptying the rectum as assessed by daily MVCT image guidance with helical tomotherapy. Int J Radiat Oncol Biol Phys 71(2):611–617

Fuss M et al (2004) Repositioning accuracy of a commercially available double-vacuum whole body immobilization system for stereotactic body radiation therapy. Technol Cancer Res Treat 3(1):59–67

Goitein M (2010) Trials and tribulations in charged particle radiotherapy. Radiother Oncol 95(1):23–31

Gollub MJ et al (2013) Prognostic aspects of DCE-MRI in recurrent rectal cancer. Eur Radiol 23(12):3336–3344

Grosu AL et al (2005) Reirradiation of recurrent high-grade gliomas using amino acid PET (SPECT)/CT/MRI image fusion to determine gross tumor volume for stereotactic fractionated radiotherapy. Int J Radiat Oncol Biol Phys 63(2):511–519

Guckenberger M et al (2006) Cone-beam CT based image-guidance for extracranial stereotactic radiotherapy of intrapulmonary tumors. Acta Oncol 45(7):897–906

Guckenberger M et al (2007a) Precision required for dose-escalated treatment of spinal metastases and implications for image-guided radiation therapy (IGRT). Radiother Oncol 84(1):56–63

Guckenberger M et al (2007b) Reliability of the bony anatomy in image-guided stereotactic radiotherapy of brain metastases. Int J Radiat Oncol Biol Phys 69(1):294–301

Guckenberger M et al (2009a) Is a single arc sufficient in volumetric-modulated arc therapy (VMAT) for complex-shaped target volumes? Radiother Oncol 93(2):259–265

Guckenberger M et al (2009b) Potential of image-guidance, gating and real-time tracking to improve accuracy in pulmonary stereotactic body radiotherapy. Radiother Oncol 91(3):288–295

Guckenberger M et al (2010) Stereotactic body radiotherapy for local boost irradiation in unfavourable locally recurrent gynaecological cancer. Radiother Oncol 94(1):53–59

Guckenberger M et al (2014) Definition of stereotactic body radiotherapy: principles and practice for the treatment of stage I non-small cell lung cancer. Strahlenther Onkol 190(1):26–33

Gutin PH et al (2009) Safety and efficacy of bevacizumab with hypofractionated stereotactic irradiation for recurrent malignant gliomas. Int J Radiat Oncol Biol Phys 75(1):156–163

Haertl PM et al (2013) Frameless fractionated stereotactic radiation therapy of intracranial lesions: impact of cone beam CT based setup correction on dose distribution. Radiat Oncol 8:153

Hashimoto T et al (2006) Repeated proton beam therapy for hepatocellular carcinoma. Int J Radiat Oncol Biol Phys 65(1):196–202

Hatakeyama T et al (2008) 11C-methionine (MET) and 18F-fluorothymidine (FLT) PET in patients with newly diagnosed glioma. Eur J Nucl Med Mol Imaging 35(11):2009–2017

Heron DE et al (2009) Stereotactic body radiotherapy for recurrent squamous cell carcinoma of the head and neck: results of a phase I dose-escalation trial. Int J Radiat Oncol Biol Phys 75(5):1493–1500

Hurkmans CW et al (2001) Set-up verification using portal imaging; review of current clinical practice. Radiother Oncol 58(2):105–120

ICRU (1993) International commission on radiation units and measurements: prescribing, recording and reporting photon beam therapy, report 50. ICRU, Bethesda

ICRU (1999) International commission on radiation units and measurements: prescribing, recording and reporting photon beam therapy, report 62. ICRU, Bethesda

Ito K et al (1992) Recurrent rectal cancer and scar: differentiation with PET and MR imaging. Radiology 182(2):549–552

Jingu K et al (2010) Focal dose escalation using FDG-PET-guided intensity-modulated radiation therapy boost for postoperative local recurrent rectal cancer: a planning study with comparison of DVH and NTCP. BMC Cancer 10:127

Jumeau R et al (2015) Optimization of reirradiation using deformable registration. Int J Radiat Oncol Biol Phys 93(3):E599

Keall PJ et al (2006) Geometric accuracy of a real-time target tracking system with dynamic multileaf collimator tracking system. Int J Radiat Oncol Biol Phys 65(5):1579–1584

Keall PJ et al (2014) The first clinical implementation of electromagnetic transponder-guided MLC tracking. Med Phys 41(2):020702

Kelly P et al (2010) Stereotactic body radiation therapy for patients with lung cancer previously treated with thoracic radiation. Int J Radiat Oncol Biol Phys 78(5):1387–1393

Kilburn JM et al (2014) Thoracic re-irradiation using stereotactic body radiotherapy (SBRT) techniques as first or second course of treatment. Radiother Oncol 110(3):505–510

Kong DS et al (2008) Efficacy of stereotactic radiosurgery as a salvage treatment for recurrent malignant gliomas. Cancer 112(9):2046–2051

Korreman SS, Juhler-Nottrup T, Boyer AL (2008) Respiratory gated beam delivery cannot facilitate margin reduction, unless combined with respiratory correlated image guidance. Radiother Oncol 86(1):61–68

Kupelian PA et al (2005) Serial megavoltage CT imaging during external beam radiotherapy for non-small-cell lung cancer: observations on tumor regression during treatment. Int J Radiat Oncol Biol Phys 63(4):1024–1028

Lang S et al (2014) Development and evaluation of a prototype tracking system using the treatment couch. Med Phys 41(2):021720

Lax I et al (1994) Stereotactic radiotherapy of malignancies in the abdomen. Methodological aspects. Acta Oncol 33(6):677–683

Lebesque JV, Keus RB (1991) The simultaneous boost technique: the concept of relative normalized total dose. Radiother Oncol 22(1):45–55

Lee JK et al (1981) CT appearance of the pelvis after abdomino-perineal resection for rectal carcinoma. Radiology 141(3):737–741

Lee N et al (2007) Salvage re-irradiation for recurrent head and neck cancer. Int J Radiat Oncol Biol Phys 68(3):731–740

Lee IH et al (2009) Association of 11C-methionine PET uptake with site of failure after concurrent temozolomide and radiation for primary glioblastoma multiforme. Int J Radiat Oncol Biol Phys 73(2):479–485

Leksell L (1951) The stereotaxic method and radiosurgery of the brain. Acta Chir Scand 102(4):316–319

Leksell L (1968) Cerebral radiosurgery. I. Gammathalanotomy in two cases of intractable pain. Acta Chir Scand 134(8):585–595

Liang J et al (2015) Trajectory modulated arc therapy: a fully dynamic delivery with synchronized couch and gantry motion significantly improves dosimetric indices correlated with poor cosmesis in accelerated partial breast irradiation. Int J Radiat Oncol Biol Phys 92(5):1148–1156

Lin R et al (1999) Nasopharyngeal carcinoma: repeat treatment with conformal proton therapy – dose-volume histogram analysis. Radiology 213(2): 489–494

Loeffler JS et al (1990) The treatment of recurrent brain metastases with stereotactic radiosurgery. J Clin Oncol 8(4):576–582

Maciejewski B, Taylor JM, Withers HR (1986) Alpha/beta value and the importance of size of dose per fraction for late complications in the supraglottic larynx. Radiother Oncol 7(4):323–326

Mackie TR et al (1993) Tomotherapy: a new concept for the delivery of dynamic conformal radiotherapy. Med Phys 20(6):1709–1719

Mahan SL et al (2005) Evaluation of image-guided helical tomotherapy for the retreatment of spinal metastasis. Int J Radiat Oncol Biol Phys 63(5):1576–1583

Mantel F, Flentje M, Guckenberger M (2013) Stereotactic body radiation therapy in the re-irradiation situation – a review. Radiat Oncol 8:7

Marks LB, Ten Haken RK, Martel MK (2010) Guest editor's introduction to QUANTEC: a users guide. Int J Radiat Oncol Biol Phys 76(3 Suppl):S1–S2

Marnitz S et al (2015) Which technique for radiation is most beneficial for patients with locally advanced cervical cancer? Intensity modulated proton therapy versus intensity modulated photon treatment, helical tomotherapy and volumetric arc therapy for primary radiation – an intraindividual comparison. Radiat Oncol 10:91

Marucci L et al (2006) Conservation treatment of the eye: conformal proton reirradiation for recurrent uveal melanoma. Int J Radiat Oncol Biol Phys 64(4):1018–1022

Mayr NA et al (2006) Serial therapy-induced changes in tumor shape in cervical cancer and their impact on assessing tumor volume and treatment response. AJR Am J Roentgenol 187(1):65–72

Meerwein CM et al (2015) Post-treatment surveillance of head and neck cancer: pitfalls in the interpretation of FDG PET-CT/MRI. Swiss Med Wkly 145:w14116

Milker-Zabel S et al (2003) Clinical results of retreatment of vertebral bone metastases by stereotactic conformal radiotherapy and intensity-modulated radiotherapy. Int J Radiat Oncol Biol Phys 55(1):162–167

Minniti G et al (2016) Repeated stereotactic radiosurgery for patients with progressive brain metastases. J Neurooncol 126(1):91–97

Munck Af Rosenschold P et al (2015) Impact of [18F]-fluoro-ethyl-tyrosine PET imaging on target definition for radiation therapy of high-grade glioma. Neuro Oncol 17(5):757–763

Nakamura K et al (2014) Recent advances in radiation oncology: intensity-modulated radiotherapy, a clinical perspective. Int J Clin Oncol 19(4):564–569

Nieder C et al (2006) Update of human spinal cord reirradiation tolerance based on additional data from 38 patients. Int J Radiat Oncol Biol Phys 66(5): 1446–1449

Niyazi M et al (2012) Re-irradiation in recurrent malignant glioma: prognostic value of [18F]FET-PET. J Neurooncol 110(3):389–395

Otto K (2008) Volumetric modulated arc therapy: IMRT in a single gantry arc. Med Phys 35(1):310–317

Palmer J et al (2014) Motion of the esophagus due to cardiac motion. PLoS One 9(2):e89126

Pauleit D et al (2005) O-(2-[18F]fluoroethyl)-L-tyrosine PET combined with MRI improves the diagnostic assessment of cerebral gliomas. Brain 128(Pt 3):678–687

Plastaras JP, Berman AT, Freedman GM (2014) Special cases for proton beam radiotherapy: re-irradiation, lymphoma, and breast cancer. Semin Oncol 41(6): 807–819

Polat B et al (2008) Intra-fractional uncertainties in image-guided intensity-modulated radiotherapy (IMRT) of prostate cancer. Strahlenther Onkol 184(12):668–673

Poltinnikov IM et al (2005) Combination of longitudinal and circumferential three-dimensional esophageal dose distribution predicts acute esophagitis in hypofractionated reirradiation of patients with non-small-cell lung cancer treated in stereotactic body frame. Int J Radiat Oncol Biol Phys 62(3):652–658

Popovtzer A et al (2009) The pattern of failure after reirradiation of recurrent squamous cell head and neck cancer: implications for defining the targets. Int J Radiat Oncol Biol Phys 74(5):1342–1347

Purdie TG et al (2007) Cone-beam computed tomography for on-line image guidance of lung stereotactic radiotherapy: localization, verification, and intrafraction tumor position. Int J Radiat Oncol Biol Phys 68(1):243–252

Ramakrishna N et al (2010) A clinical comparison of patient setup and intra-fraction motion using frame-based radiosurgery versus a frameless image-guided radiosurgery system for intracranial lesions. Radiother Oncol 95(1):109–115

Rieken S et al (2013) Analysis of FET-PET imaging for target volume definition in patients with gliomas treated with conformal radiotherapy. Radiother Oncol 109(3):487–492

Rwigema JC et al (2010) Fractionated stereotactic body radiation therapy in the treatment of previously-irradiated recurrent head and neck carcinoma: updated report of the University of Pittsburgh experience. Am J Clin Oncol 33(3):286–93

Schwer AL et al (2008) A phase I dose-escalation study of fractionated stereotactic radiosurgery in combination with gefitinib in patients with recurrent malignant gliomas. Int J Radiat Oncol Biol Phys 70(4):993–1001

Seppenwoolde Y et al (2002) Precise and real-time measurement of 3D tumor motion in lung due to breathing and heartbeat, measured during radiotherapy. Int J Radiat Oncol Biol Phys 53(4):822–834

Seppenwoolde Y et al (2007) Accuracy of tumor motion compensation algorithm from a robotic respiratory tracking system: a simulation study. Med Phys 34(7): 2774–2784

Shepherd SF et al (1997) Hypofractionated stereotactic radiotherapy in the management of recurrent glioma. Int J Radiat Oncol Biol Phys 37(2):393–398

Smitsmans MH et al (2008) The influence of a dietary protocol on cone beam CT-guided radiotherapy for prostate cancer patients. Int J Radiat Oncol Biol Phys 71(4):1279–1286

Smyth G et al (2013) Trajectory optimization for dynamic couch rotation during volumetric modulated arc radiotherapy. Phys Med Biol 58(22):8163–8177

Sohn M, Weinmann M, Alber M (2009) Intensity-modulated radiotherapy optimization in a quasi-periodically deforming patient model. Int J Radiat Oncol Biol Phys 75(3):906–914

Sonke JJ et al (2005) Respiratory correlated cone beam CT. Med Phys 32(4):1176–1186

Sonke JJ et al (2009) Frameless stereotactic body radiotherapy for lung cancer using four-dimensional cone beam CT guidance. Int J Radiat Oncol Biol Phys 74(2):567–574

Sterzing F et al (2010) Spinal cord sparing reirradiation with helical tomotherapy. Cancer 116(16):3961–3968

Stieler F et al (2011) Reirradiation of spinal column metastases: comparison of several treatment techniques and dosimetric validation for the use of VMAT. Strahlenther Onkol 187(7):406–415

Sykes JR et al (2005) A feasibility study for image guided radiotherapy using low dose, high speed, cone beam X-ray volumetric imaging. Radiother Oncol 77(1): 45–52

Teoh M et al (2011) Volumetric modulated arc therapy: a review of current literature and clinical use in practice. Br J Radiol 84(1007):967–996

Terakawa Y et al (2008) Diagnostic accuracy of 11C-methionine PET for differentiation of recurrent brain tumors from radiation necrosis after radiotherapy. J Nucl Med 49(5):694–699

Underberg RW et al (2005) Benefit of respiration-gated stereotactic radiotherapy for stage I lung cancer: an analysis of 4DCT datasets. Int J Radiat Oncol Biol Phys 62(2):554–560

van Herk M (2004) Errors and margins in radiotherapy. Semin Radiat Oncol 14(1):52–64

van Rijssel MJ et al (2014) A critical approach to the clinical use of deformable image registration software. In response to Meijneke et al. Radiother Oncol 112(3):447–448

Verellen D et al (2007) Innovations in image-guided radiotherapy. Nat Rev Cancer 7(12):949–960

Vestergaard A et al (2013) Adaptive plan selection vs. re-optimisation in radiotherapy for bladder cancer: a dose accumulation comparison. Radiother Oncol 109(3): 457–462

Wachter S et al (2002) The influence of a rectal balloon tube as internal immobilization device on variations of volumes and dose-volume histograms during treatment course of conformal radiotherapy for prostate cancer. Int J Radiat Oncol Biol Phys 52(1):91–100

Wilbert J et al (2008) Tumor tracking and motion compensation with an adaptive tumor tracking system (ATTS): system description and prototype testing. Med Phys 35(19):3911–9921

Wolthaus JW et al (2008) Comparison of different strategies to use four-dimensional computed tomography in treatment planning for lung cancer patients. Int J Radiat Oncol Biol Phys 70(4):1229–1238

Yan D et al (1997) Adaptive radiation therapy. Phys Med Biol 42(1):123–132

Proton Beam Reirradiation

Mark W. McDonald and Kevin P. McMullen

Contents

The original version of this chapter was revised. An erratum to this chapter can be found at 10.1007/978-3-319-41825-4_78.

M.W. McDonald, MD (✉)
Department of Radiation Oncology, Winship Cancer Institute of Emory University, 1365 Clifton Road NE, Suite A1300, Atlanta, GA 30322, USA
e-mail: mark.mcdonald@emory.edu

K.P. McMullen, MD
Department of Radiation Oncology, The Cancer Center at Columbus Regional Health, 2400 E 17th Street, Columbus, IN 47201, USA
e-mail: kmcmullen@crh.org

Abstract

Proton therapy is a modality of radiation therapy with unique physical properties relative to photon (X-ray) therapy. Each proton beam is modulated to deposit the maximum radiation dose in the target, with essentially no radiation to tissues beyond the target. Compared to photon treatments, highly conformal treatment plans can typically be developed with fewer proton beams, significantly reducing the overall exposure of nontarget tissues to radiation. Given the narrow therapeutic window of reirradiation, proton therapy is of great interest as a mechanism to potentially avoid or reduce toxicities of reirradiation by limiting the volume of nontarget tissues receiving additional radiation dose. In some diseases, proton reirradiation may improve outcomes by facilitating safer radiation dose escalation to recurrent and potentially radioresistant tumors or providing better target coverage while respecting constraints to critical normal structures. In uncommon cases, proton therapy may permit reirradiation when the dosimetry achieved with other modalities is felt to preclude safe reirradiation. Clinical experience with proton reirradiation is currently limited to relatively small patient series and is highly heterogeneous. To better understand the value of proton therapy in reirradiation relative to other radiation modalities, prospective evaluation with more homogenous patient populations is needed to evaluate predefined end points

Med Radiol Radiat Oncol (2016)
DOI 10.1007/174_2016_71, © Springer International Publishing Switzerland
Published Online: 20 Jul 2016

based on rational clinical hypotheses. In this chapter, the rationale and published clinical results of proton therapy for reirradiation are reviewed for a variety of disease sites, with case examples provided.

1 Background

Proton therapy is a modality of radiation therapy distinguished from photon (X-ray)-based treatments by the unique physical properties of protons. Protons have an energy-dependent finite range in tissue. The rate of energy deposition increases as the protons slow down, yielding a peak in ionization (dose deposition) in the terminal range of the beam, followed by an abrupt falloff to essentially no radiation dose as the protons come to rest. This is known as the Bragg peak of proton therapy (Paganetti 2012; Lomax 2009). Compared to a single photon beam, a single proton beam has a lower entrance dose to normal tissues, puts its maximal energy in the target (rather than near the surface of the patient), and has no meaningful exit dose beyond the target. As a result, highly conformal plans can typically be developed with fewer treatment beams, reducing the overall exposure of nontarget tissues to radiation (Lomax et al. 2004). In addition, compared to photons, proton therapy provides a sharper lateral beam penumbra (dose buildup region) at depths up to about 17 cm in water (Suit et al. 2003).

These physical properties of proton therapy provide unique and heightened opportunities in treatment planning to reduce overall radiation exposure, achieve areas of significant radiation reduction or complete avoidance adjacent to the target, create steep dose gradients adjacent to critical normal structures, and more safely escalate radiation dose to targets adjacent to critical structures. In clinical use since the 1950s, proton therapy has had a rising profile due to technological advancements, continued interest in reducing potential toxicities of radiation therapy, and increased accessibility with a growing number of proton treatment facilities opening globally.

2 Patient Selection for Proton Reirradiation

Reirradiation often has a narrow therapeutic window, and in each case the clinician must balance the clinical benefit of additional radiation for local tumor control against what may be significant risks of toxicity to previously irradiated normal tissues. Anticipated acute toxicities of reirradiation may be deemed excessive or unbearable in heavily pretreated patients. Often of greater concern than acute toxicities are the potential significant late toxicities to normal structures, which may be life altering or even fatal. These concerns must be carefully weighed against the potential benefit of obtaining local control or local palliation. Proton therapy may be selected to reduce radiation exposure to nontarget tissues or achieve regions of complete radiation avoidance in an effort to mitigate the potential toxicities of treatment. In cases where the proximity of critical structures or other constraints would result in significantly compromised target coverage or require significant dose reduction with photon techniques, the dosimetric advantages of proton therapy may facilitate improved target coverage and/or delivery of a higher radiation dose with the intent of improving the likelihood of curative therapy or more durable local control. Proton therapy may therefore be a useful tool to improve the therapeutic ratio of reirradiation and potentially to extend the option of reirradiation to patients otherwise unsuitable for reirradiation with other modalities.

Data-driven patient selection criteria for reirradiation are sparse. Many applications of reirradiation are given with clear palliative intent, and the goals of palliative reirradiation can be met in the great majority of cases with photon techniques. However, practitioners may confront special clinical circumstances where the utilization of more costly palliative proton therapy appears justified. For example, the authors have used palliative proton therapy in a patient with an undefined presumed genetic predisposition that resulted in heightened radiosensitivity. Two prior attempted courses of palliative photon therapy for metastatic osseous spine disease resulted in extraordinary gastrointestinal toxicity requiring hospitalization on both occasions.

Proton therapy was subsequently used to palliate the spine and avoid dose to the viscera anterior to the spine. Outside these uncommon clinical scenarios, there are no substantive clinical data to support the increased economic costs of palliative reirradiation with proton therapy. This application is likely to remain based on the clinical judgment of practitioners facing uncommon scenarios and constrained by restrictions from healthcare payers.

Patients considered for definitive or curative intent reirradiation generally have nonmetastatic disease (or controlled or controllable systemic disease), a good performance status, and a disease process which suggests that successful locoregional therapy could achieve either a long-term disease control or cure (McDonald et al. 2011). As a modality of external beam irradiation, proton therapy may be considered an alternative to photon-based reirradiation with three-dimensional conformal radiation therapy, intensity-modulated radiation therapy (IMRT), volumetric-modulated arc therapy (VMAT), or stereotactic body radiation therapy (SBRT). Other reirradiation options such as intraoperative radiotherapy (IORT) and brachytherapy have profoundly different dosimetry with unique applications and indications. Practitioners benefit from having access to the broadest array of potential treatment options to tailor therapy to the clinical circumstances. There is no single modality that would be appropriate for every clinical reirradiation scenario.

3 Treatment Planning Considerations in Proton Reirradiation

The distinct physical properties of protons entail special treatment planning considerations and uncertainties (ICRU 2007). These uncertainties and considerations have increased importance in reirradiation, as there are often more organs or structures deemed at risk with more stringent dose constraints and the potential for more significant toxicity should those dose constraints be exceeded.

Although not a unique consideration to proton therapy, patient weight loss (or weight gain), changes in tumor size or morphology, and other potential alterations in tissues within the beam path(s) during retreatment can lead to significant changes in proton dosimetry which could result in unanticipated variations in dose to organs at risk (Mannina et al. 2014). Compared to photon therapy, proton therapy is significantly more sensitive to differences in tissue heterogeneities within the beam path (Paganetti 2012). In situations of anticipated dynamic tissue heterogeneity – such as treatment of the sinuses, where obstructive secretions and inflammatory sinusitis can vary over a treatment course – patients should be frequently reimaged to monitor for dynamic changes that may require adaptive planning. Proton beam arrangements should be selected in a fashion that limit the effect of potential changes in tissue heterogeneity that would risk overdosing critical organs by assessing "worst case" scenarios for plan robustness (Li 2012).

Patients with metal hardware, such as spinal fixation, can pose a tremendous challenge in proton therapy due to the loss of critical CT information needed to accurately calculate proton range, mixed alloy hardware or implants which include materials of varying density, and issues of dose perturbations at the tissue/hardware interface including dose shadowing distal to the hardware. The clinical impact of these uncertainties can be mitigated through the use of metal artifact reduction algorithms for CT simulation (Andersson et al. 2014), incorporating multiple beams with varied angles of incidence relative to the hardware, the use of passive scattered protons rather than pencil beam scanning (Verburg and Seco 2013), and integration of photon therapy for some portion of the total treatment.

Organ motion is an important treatment planning consideration for all radiation modalities and poses special challenges in proton therapy, which are elsewhere reviewed in depth (De Ruysscher et al. 2015). Rigorous patient immobilization and positioning accuracy with pretreatment image verification are essential in proton therapy, both for protection of critical normal structures and also to minimize changes in beam path heterogeneities which can markedly affect dose distributions.

While the majority of clinical experience with proton therapy has been with 3D conformal proton therapy using passive beam scattering techniques, or more recently, uniform scanning, pencil beam scanning (PBS) is the most recent technological advance in the delivery of proton therapy. Older proton techniques provide a uniform dose with a uniform spread-out Bragg peak (SOBP) across the entire treatment field and often require a manual, iterative approach to treatment plan optimization. In contrast, PBS utilizes magnetic steering of a narrow proton beam and can vary the dose distribution across the field and adjust the width of the SOBP across the field so that the dose deposition more closely matches the target geometry. PBS planning techniques include single field uniform dose, in which each treatment field is optimized to deliver a uniform dose to the target, and multifield optimization, in which, similar to photon-based IMRT, inverse optimization is used to create a composite target dose distribution from constituent treatment fields that individually may deliver a highly heterogeneous dose distribution. These newer proton therapy techniques, utilizing a treatment planning objective-based clinical workflow more similar to photon-based IMRT, generally offer improved dose distributions compared to 3D conformal proton plans using passive scattering. They are the focus of significant ongoing work in proton treatment planning optimization, validation, assessments of treatment plan robustness, and adaptive proton therapy in response to dynamic changes through the treatment course.

4 Proton Reirradiation of Radiation-Associated Neoplasms

Benign and malignant neoplasms in patients with prior radiation are uncommon but often devastating complications of prior radiotherapy. Population data from the US Surveillance, Epidemiology, and End Results (SEER) cancer registries suggest the excess risk of a second solid tumor in adult patients is 0.005 % at 15 years after radiotherapy (Berrington de Gonzalez et al. 2011). The incidence of second malignancies in children is much higher (Bassal et al. 2006), presumably related to heightened radiosensitivity, more frequent underlying genetic syndromes, and a longer available latency period to develop second neoplasms in children compared to patients treated as adults.

In a report with long-term follow-up of 963 patients with hereditary retinoblastoma, patients treated with radiotherapy had almost twice the absolute excess risk of cancer compared to those managed without radiation (Kleinerman et al. 2005). Of interest, the cumulative incidence of second malignancy at 40 years was 32.9 % in patients treated with orthovoltage radiation, but for those treated with megavoltage techniques (in which radiation scatter to nontarget tissues was reduced), the cumulative incidence was reduced to 26.3 %. These data support the clinical goal of minimizing radiation dose to nontarget tissues, particularly in patients at heightened risk of secondary malignancy.

Radiobiologic modeling predicts a reduced incidence of secondary malignancy in adult and pediatric patients treated with proton therapy compared to photon techniques (Simone et al. 2012; Zhang et al. 2013). Although the risk of second malignant neoplasms is greatest in children and young adults receiving radiation therapy, they are not insignificant in adult patients. For example, meta-analysis of patients receiving radiotherapy for prostate cancer highlights an increased risk of bladder and colorectal cancers following radiation (Wallis et al. 2016). Compared to photon therapy, proton therapy was associated with a reduced risk of second malignant neoplasms in adult patients in a retrospective matched cohort analysis (Chung et al. 2013). We are unaware of any published clinical data on proton therapy in patients with radiation-induced malignancies or second cancers. Due to its reduced radiation exposure to nontarget tissues, proton therapy is an appealing option when radiotherapy is indicated in management of these patients who have a demonstrated heightened sensitivity to radiotherapy.

Figure 1 shows an example of proton therapy in treatment of a patient with a recurrent, clival meningioma in a previously irradiated adult survivor of childhood glioma.

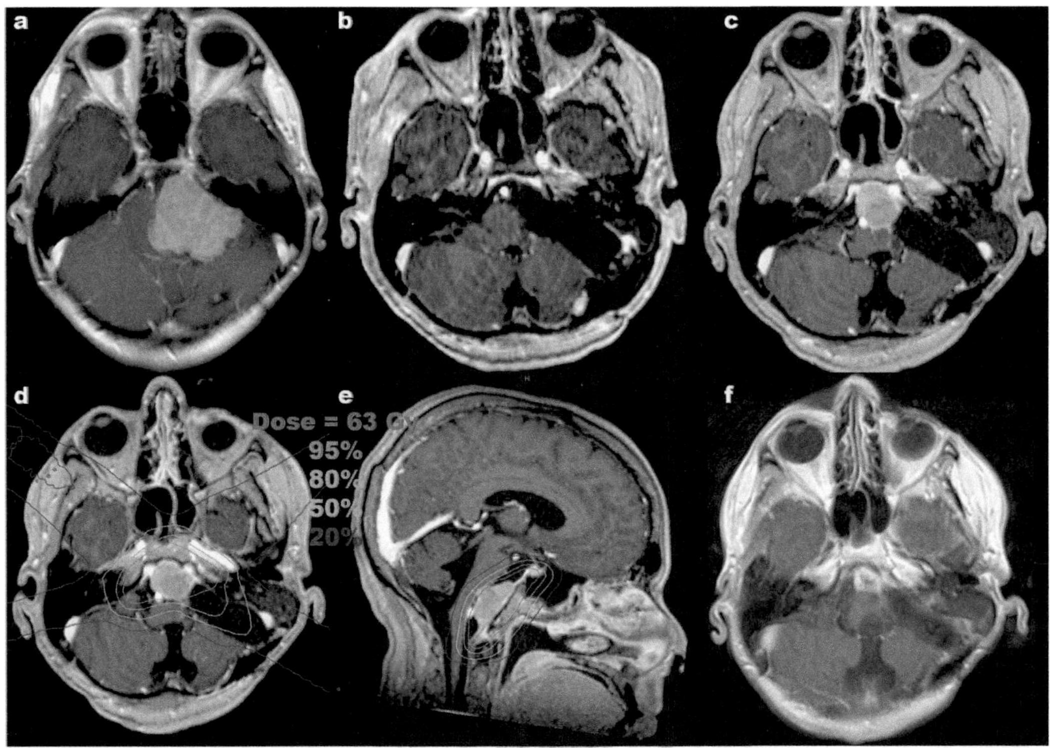

Fig. 1 A 40-year-old male was treated for a radiation-induced atypical clival meningioma. He had a history of a pediatric posterior fossa tumor, reported as a glioblastoma, and had received radiation therapy 30 years prior: 30 Gy to the whole brain and a 55 Gy boost to the posterior fossa with 6 MV photons. Pathology slides from his original tumor had been destroyed. He presented with left-sided hearing loss, dysphagia, and balance disturbance and was found to have a large left cerebellar-pontine angle/posterior clival meningioma with brainstem compression (**a**). Surgical debulking was undertaken via a two-stage approach including lateral suboccipital craniotomy with pathology showing a WHO grade 2 meningioma. A near-total resection of tumor was obtained (**b**). Unfortunately he suffered left cranial nerve VI and VII palsies with neurotrophic keratopathy eventually requiring left eye enucleation and multiple lower cranial nerve palsies with dysarthria and dysphagia requiring permanent tracheostomy and gastrostomy tube feeding. Within 6 months from surgery, his tumor had regrown and was again approximating the brainstem (**c**). No further surgery was advised. He was referred for proton therapy due to concern about brainstem tolerance to additional radiation considering his prior radiation and surgical trauma. A treatment plan was generated using a combination of through and patch fields (keeping the brainstem at the aperture edge) and anterior oblique fields with distal blocking of the brainstem to avoid delivery of any radiation through the brainstem. Two schemas were used of four fields each. The prescription dose was 63 Gy (RBE) in 35 fractions, allowing the surface of the brainstem to receive an additional 50 Gy (RBE) (**d**, **e**). Because of his debilitated condition, daily anesthesia was required to comply with immobilization. The first posttreatment MRI at 6 weeks showed central tumor necrosis and transient enlargement of the tumor without clinical worsening. At 12 months postradiation, his MRI showed significant regression of tumor, volumetrically reduced from 6 to 2.2 cm^3 (**f**). At 37 months from radiation, the patient had continued radiographic regression of tumor

5 Proton Reirradiation of Chordoma

Chordomas are rare primary bone tumors with a high propensity for local recurrence even after aggressive surgery and radiotherapy. For clival chordomas, maximizing tumor debulking and optimizing residual tumor coverage by high-dose radiotherapy are associated with superior outcomes (McDonald et al. 2016a). For patients with recurrent disease after prior radiation, treatment options are limited. While effective targeted drug therapies are desperately needed in chordoma, local control measures remain the mainstay of treatment.

Salvage surgery alone rarely achieves a durable period of disease stability and has a reported 2-year overall survival of 63 % (Fagundes et al. 1995). Reirradiation options are typically constrained by the prior dose delivered to closely adjacent critical normal structures, particularly the spinal cord for extracranial chordomas and the brainstem and optic apparatus for clival chordomas. Small intracranial recurrences are often amenable to stereotactic radiosurgery (SRS) with satisfactory local control, although there is a not insignificant risk of marginal failure of about 15 % (Kano et al. 2011).

Researchers at the now-closed Indiana University Health Proton Therapy Center reported on 16 previously irradiated patients with recurrent or progressive chordoma (McDonald et al. 2013a). Half the patients underwent salvage surgery in management of their recurrent or progressive disease. At a median of 37 months after a median prior dose of 75.2 Gy, patients were retreated to an additional median dose of 75.6 Gy (RBE). At a median follow-up of 23 months, the 2-year estimate of local control was 85 % and overall survival 80 %. The 2-year estimate of late grade 3+ toxicity was 19 %. The disease control in this experience with aggressive proton reirradiation compares very favorably to other interventions in a population with a historically poor prognosis.

Figure 2 is an example of proton therapy in reirradiation of a recurrent cervical spine chordoma.

6 Proton Reirradiation of Gliomas

Recurrent or progressive infiltrative glioma develops in almost all patients after initial therapy. In the absence of high-quality data on optimal management, patients with recurrent glioma are typically evaluated for further resection, chemotherapy, reirradiation, and other interventions based on tumor histology, genetic factors, size, location, and patient performance status, among other factors (Stupp et al. 2014). For glioblastoma, the most common malignant primary brain tumor in adults, the standard of care for initial management is maximal safe surgical

Fig. 2 A 67-year-old man was reirradiated for a cervical spine chordoma. He presented with dysphagia and imaging showed a destructive mass at C2 extending into the prevertebral space (**a**; tumor outlined in *red*). He underwent transoral partial resection with pathology showing chordoma and was observed. Imaging one year later showed a bulky recurrence (**b**; tumor outlined in *red*). After neurosurgical evaluation, the morbidity of re-resection was felt to be too great and he was referred for proton therapy. He was treated to 75.6 Gy (RBE) in 42 fractions by another physician (**c**, gross tumor volume outlined in *red*). Due to concern for potential surgical seeding, a large treatment volume was defined which covered the soft palate, resulting in permanent xerostomia and dental caries. Three years after proton therapy, the tumor remained stable in size but he developed a solitary supraclavicular nodal metastasis, which was completely excised. At 38 months from radiation, imaging showed progression of the primary tumor. A 6-month trial of imatinib was undertaken with repeat imaging showing further tumor progression now encroaching upon the cervical spinal cord (**d**; tumor outlined in *magenta*). He was referred for neurosurgical decompression and posterior spine stabilization, which achieved clearance around the spinal cord, although complete surgical resection was not possible. He was then retreated with proton therapy to 78 Gy (RBE) in 38 fractions, 4 years after his prior radiation therapy (**e**, **f**; gross tumor volume outlined in *red*). A CT myelogram was performed in the immobilization devices to define the cervical spinal cord. CT simulation was performed with an orthopedic metal artifact reduction algorithm in light of his spine stabilization hardware and dental amalgam artifacts. He was treated with two complex alternating schemas of through and patch fields, the first schema involving six fields and the second involving five fields. The spinal cord was blocked by all beams to keep the spinal cord surface dose at the 50 % isodose line. His lifetime dose distribution is shown (**g**, **h**). The maximum spinal cord point dose was 54.9 Gy from his initial course, 46.5 Gy from his reirradiation and cumulative lifetime maximum point dose 97.5 Gy (75.4 Gy to 0.5 cm^3). He did not develop any oral mucositis during reirradiation and had only grade 1 odynophagia and grade 1 dermatitis. Three months after reirradiation, he started planned adjuvant therapy with erlotinib which was stopped after 1 month due to skin toxicity. At 6 months after reirradiation, he had a focus of posterior oropharyngeal wall soft tissue necrosis treated with hyperbaric oxygen. Unfortunately, the soft tissue necrosis progressed, leading to exposure of bone and required tracheostomy and gastrostomy tube feeding. He survived for two years after reirradiation without evidence of tumor progression or spinal cord myelopathy but died from a sudden carotid artery rupture, highlighting the significant risks of high dose retreatment

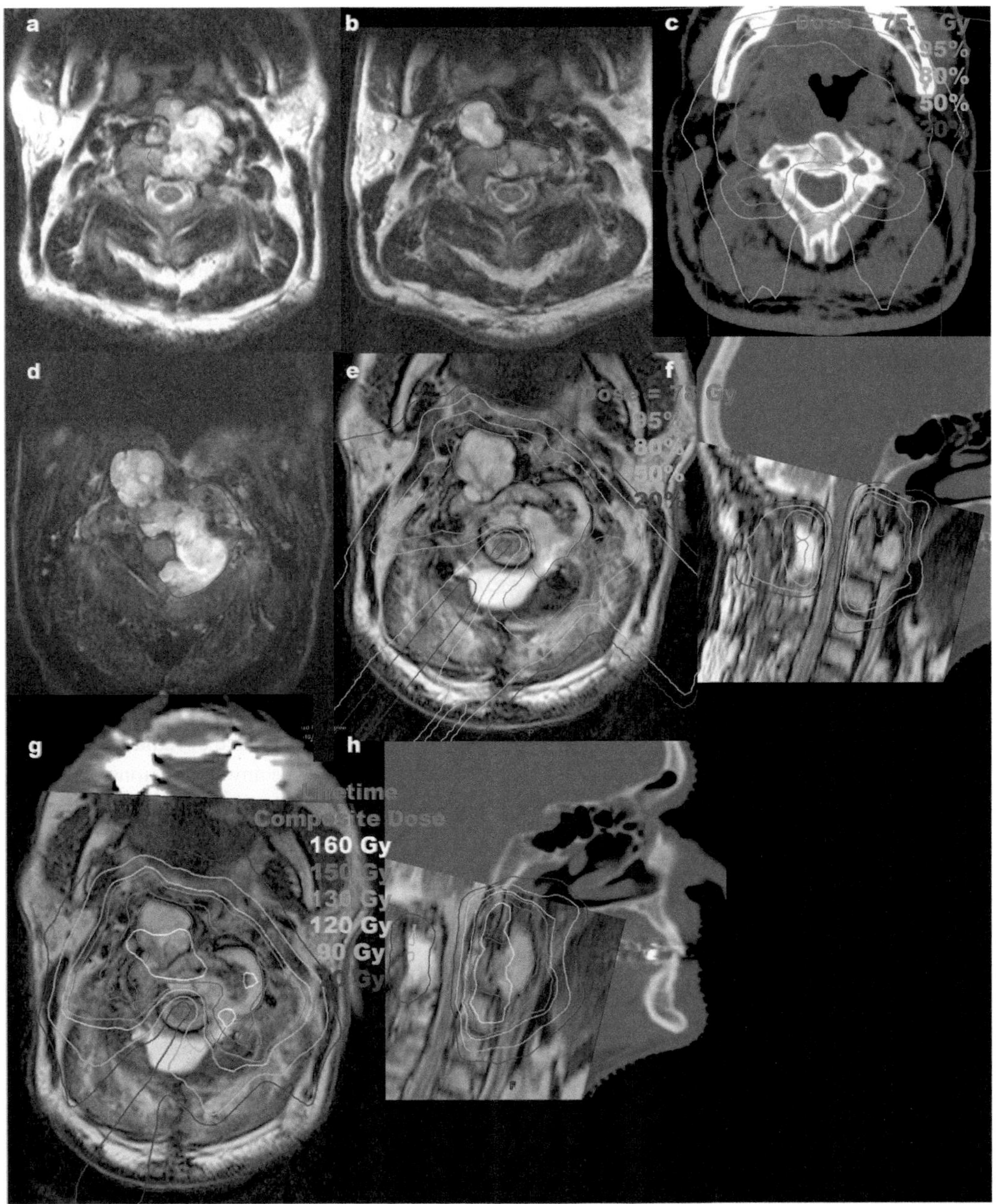
a
b
c
95%
80%
50%
d
e
f
g
h
160 Gy
120 Gy

resection followed by radiotherapy with concurrent and adjuvant temozolomide (Stupp et al. 2009). The median progression-free survival is approximately 7 months. The Radiation Therapy Oncology Group is currently enrolling patients in a randomized phase II trial for patients with recurrent or progressive glioblastoma in which patients are randomized to bevacizumab alone or bevacizumab plus hypofractionated reirradiation to 35 Gy in 10 fractions. This trial should provide valuable prospective evidence to evaluate the potential benefit of early incorporation of reirradiation.

One of the most significant clinical concerns with reirradiation of gliomas is the risk of brain radiation necrosis. Proton therapy is theoretically appealing because highly conformal reirradiation can be delivered with lower dose to adjacent nontarget brain tissue. However, this would not reduce the risk of central radiation necrosis occurring within the reirradiation target. Furthermore, modern photon techniques of hypofractionated reirradiation for high-grade gliomas have been associated with no discernable or very low risk of radiation necrosis (Fogh et al. 2010). This is presumably due at least in part to the limited survival time of patients. For these reasons, the routine application of proton therapy in reirradiation of high-grade gliomas may not translate into measurable clinical improvements in toxicity.

If prognostic tools improve to accurately identify better prognosis patients (whose longer survival time would presumably place them at greater risk of radiation necrosis and neurocognitive effects of reirradiation), proton reirradiation may be of benefit in these select patients. Proton therapy may be a useful tool in prospective dose-escalation trials of reirradiation. A similar strategy is being employed in an open phase I/II trial at the University of Heidelberg evaluating the role of carbon ion therapy in recurrent gliomas (grades 2–4). The phase I component is designed to establish a recommended carbon ion dose via dose escalation from 30 to 48 Gy equivalent (GyE) in 3 GyE fractions, while the phase II component will compare 12-month survival against photon reirradiation to 36 Gy in 2 Gy fractions (Combs et al. 2010).

Researchers at the now-closed Indiana University Health Proton Therapy Center reported on 20 patients with recurrent gliomas who were treated with proton reirradiation (Galle et al. 2015). Three had grade I or II gliomas, 4 grade III, and 13 grade IV. The patient population was heterogeneous in terms of prior therapy and utilization of concurrent chemotherapy. Additionally, the dose of reirradiation varied from hypofractionated regimens to full dose reirradiation in conventional fractionation. Protracted fractionation was generally used in patients with a long time interval from prior radiation therapy (up to 12 years) based on a belief that such patients may be longer-term survivors. The median dose of reirradiation was 59.4 Gy (RBE) (range 37.5–60) for grade III tumors and 54 Gy (RBE) (range 30–60) for grade IV tumors. The median survival after reirradiation was 10.2 months for grade III tumors and 8.2 months for grade IV tumors. With reference to prior radiation dosimetry, efforts were made to direct proton reirradiation beams to minimize the volume of reirradiated brain. There was a 10 % crude incidence of radiation necrosis. It is difficult to derive any conclusions from such heterogeneous data, but it is quite uncommon to deliver full course reirradiation, and the apparent reasonably low risk of radiation necrosis is provocative even if the benefit of full dose reirradiation is unknown.

Figure 3 illustrates an example of proton therapy in reirradiation of a patient with a recurrent WHO grade III anaplastic astrocytoma.

7 Proton Salvage Craniospinal Irradiation

Salvage craniospinal irradiation has been reported, primarily in children, in treatment of recurrent and disseminated ependymoma (Merchant et al. 2008), recurrent medulloblastoma after prior CSI (Massimino et al. 2009), and for other histologies with neuroaxis dissemination after prior focal radiation (Wei et al. 2012). Researchers at St. Jude Children's Research Hospital reported on varied techniques of salvage reirradiation for recurrent ependymoma. For those treated with

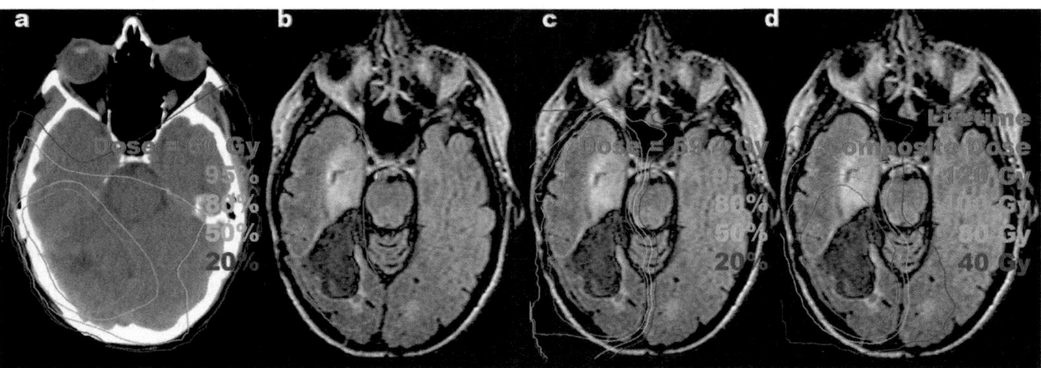

Fig. 3 A 48-year-old woman was reirradiated for a recurrent glioma. She had a history of a complete resection of right posterior temporal anaplastic astrocytoma (grade III) and received adjuvant radiation therapy to 60 Gy in 30 fractions (**a**) without chemotherapy. Seven years later she developed episodes of confusion prompting MRI scan that revealed local recurrence of non-enhancing tumor with progression of FLAIR abnormality into the anterior ipsilateral temporal lobe highly suspicious for tumor. She underwent radical subtotal resection guided by functional MRI, confirming recurrent grade III astrocytoma, IDH-1 intact, with residual inoperable tumor. She was offered reirradiation with proton therapy to 59.4 Gy (RBE) in 33 fractions with concurrent temozolomide. The residual tumor and the target volume for reirradiation are shown in *orange* (**b**). Proton therapy was used to avoid radiation to the contralateral hemisphere and to minimize dose to the brainstem (**c**). The previous tumor region received a cumulative dose of 120 Gy between the two courses separated by 7 years (**d**). She developed bone marrow suppression requiring dose de-escalation of temozolomide in the later course of therapy. Within 1 year, the patient developed brain parenchymal radiation necrosis that was treated with bevacizumab and hyperbaric oxygen treatment. She developed a sustained contralateral hemiparesis with dysarthria. Eighteen months after reirradiation, the patient was alive with no radiographic evidence of tumor progression

salvage CSI, standard photon technique with opposed lateral brain fields was used, with custom blocking designed to limit the brainstem and spinal cord to a maximum cumulative radiation dose of 55.8 Gy. While effective at shielding critical structures and limiting cumulative radiation dose, lateral blocks also shield a volume of cerebrospinal fluid and leptomeningeal space potentially harboring microscopic disease. This could theoretically reduce the effectiveness of salvage CSI and allow for reseeding. Others have used IMRT to attenuate dose to previously irradiated critical structures while maintaining coverage of the surrounding target volume (Wei et al. 2012), but this cannot achieve complete sparing in the same way as lateral blocks.

Using the finite distal range of proton therapy, researchers at the now-closed Indiana University Health Proton Therapy Center reported a novel technique to block a critical structure on lateral fields and then fill in or "plug" dose to cover the target volume lateral to the structure. The resulting plan created a "donut" hole of complete dose avoidance surrounding the critical structure. Two example cases were highlighted in which critical structures were felt to require complete sparing from additional radiation dose: one child receiving salvage CSI for recurrent and disseminated medulloblastoma in which the optic chiasm was spared, and one adult with recurrent and disseminated anaplastic meningioma in which the previously irradiated portion of the lateral brainstem was spared. Compared to lateral photon fields with blocks and with IMRT, this proton technique improved coverage of the planning target volume while reducing the mean and maximum dose to the critical organs at risk (McDonald et al. 2013b).

Similarly, a case report from researchers at the University of Pennsylvania reported on the use of pencil beam scanning proton therapy to deliver salvage craniospinal irradiation with brainstem sparing (Hill-Kayser and Kirk 2015). The case involved a child with a posterior fossa ependymoma whose prior radiation delivered a maximum brainstem dose of 60 Gy (RBE). Ten months later, spinal dissemination was detected and salvage CSI to 36 Gy (RBE) followed by focal tumor boosts was offered, using pencil beam scanning to limit the surface of the brainstem to an additional 5 Gy (RBE).

In addition to the ability to create regions of complete dose avoidance if necessary around previously irradiated critical structures, proton therapy offers the advantage of no exit dose to viscera anterior to the spine during CSI, which is expected to reduce both acute and late toxicity by complete radiation avoidance. Retrospective cohort analysis supports reduced acute gastrointestinal and hematologic toxicities with proton CSI compared to photon CSI in adult patients treated for medulloblastoma (Brown et al. 2013). Additionally, retrospective cohort analysis found that, compared to photon CSI, proton CSI was associated with fewer late endocrine abnormalities in children treated for standard risk medulloblastoma (Eaton et al. 2015). Radiobiologic modeling predicts that proton CSI is associated with a reduced risk of secondary malignancies compared to photon techniques (Zhang et al. 2013). These data support the role of proton therapy in craniospinal irradiation for patients of all ages.

8 Proton Reirradiation of Ocular Melanomas

Proton therapy is an established modality of treatment for ocular melanomas with a very high rate of local control and favorable toxicity profile (Dendale et al. 2006; Desjardins et al. 2012). In addition to close collaboration with a specialized ophthalmologist, the treatment requires a dedicated patient setup, planning software, and expertise which may not be available at every proton treatment center. However, the shallow beam range and therefore low proton energy required for treatment means that proton therapy for ocular melanomas is also available at a number of centers with low-energy cyclotrons unsuitable for treatment of broader indications. A systematic review and meta-analysis suggested charged particle therapy for uveal melanoma was associated with lower rates of local recurrence, retinopathy, and cataract formation than plaque brachytherapy (Wang et al. 2013).

Choroidal melanomas arising in proximity to the optic disk (juxtapapillary) may be inappropriate for plaque brachytherapy due to inability to properly position the plaque for adequate tumor coverage. Stereotactic radiosurgery (SRS), hypofractionated stereotactic radiation therapy (SRT), and proton beam therapy have been used for posterior choroidal melanomas with success. A comparative treatment planning study of SRT and proton beam therapy for choroidal melanomas arising near the optic disk or fovea centralis found superior dosimetry with proton therapy in the majority of cases (Hocht et al. 2005). Clinical data from the Clatterbridge Cancer Centre and Sheffield Ocular Oncology Service compared outcomes for patients treated with SRS compared to proton therapy for choroidal melanomas (Sikuade et al. 2015). SRS and proton therapy were selected for patients with tumors considered either too large for plaque brachytherapy or for those located too close (<2.5 mm) to the optic disk for plaque placement. While tumor control was very high with both treatments, their analysis found a statistically significant lower rate of severe vision loss with proton therapy compared to SRS for patients whose tumors touched the optic nerve and for those >3 mm from the fovea. It may be that the fractionation used for proton therapy in this series (53.1 Gy (RBE) in 4 fractions) conferred fewer late effects compared to SRS (35 Gy at the 50% isodose line in 1 fraction) or that other confounding factors were related to the difference in visual preservation.

Researchers at the Massachusetts General Hospital (MGH) reported on 31 patients with recurrent uveal melanoma who received a second course of proton therapy (Marucci et al. 2006). Nearly all the patients had received 70 Gy (RBE) in 5 fractions for both the initial course and the salvage course of proton therapy. At a mean follow-up of 50 months, the 5-year estimate of local control after salvage proton therapy was 69%. The 5-year eye retention rate was 55%, with 27% of those who retained their eye having useful vision of 20/200 or better. Of the nine patients undergoing enucleation, five were due to local recurrence and four due to intractable pain.

Researchers at the Helmholtz-Zentrum Berlin reported on 48 patients with recurrent uveal melanoma after a variety of prior treatments (54 % previously irradiated) who received salvage proton beam radiation, with most receiving 60 Gy (RBE) in 4 fractions. At a mean follow-up time of 81 months, the 10-year estimate of local tumor control after proton reirradiation was 92.1 %. One patient required enucleation for local recurrence. At 5 years after salvage proton therapy, 24 % had useful vision of 20/200 or better. Compared to the MGH experience, the improved tumor control and lower rate of enucleation may be related to fewer patients having had prior radiation treatment or differences in other confounding variables such as tumor size. Together these data suggest that salvage proton reirradiation yields eye preservation in the majority of patients and preservation of useful vision in about a quarter of patients.

While overall survival is not compromised by local therapy with plaque brachytherapy compared to enucleation for choroidal melanomas (Diener-West et al. 2001), it is unclear whether further local therapy provides comparable survival to enucleation for recurrent disease. The MGH group compared survival outcomes for their 31 patients receiving salvage proton therapy to a cohort of 42 patients undergoing enucleation. Patients selected for enucleation had, on average, larger tumors than those selected for reirradiation. The 5-year survival estimate for those treated with reirradiation was 63 % compared to 36 % for those enucleated ($p=0.040$) suggesting that survival is not compromised by salvage proton therapy compared to enucleation (Marucci et al. 2011).

9 Proton Reirradiation of Head and Neck Cancers

Despite aggressive therapy, locoregional disease failure remains common in many head and neck cancers. Reirradiation is a potentially curative treatment option for appropriately selected patients, although only a small percentage of patients achieve long-term survival (McDonald et al. 2011). The toxicities of head and neck reirradiation can be significant. A prospective multi-institutional trial using an accelerated hyperfractionated reirradiation regimen interdigitated with chemotherapy reported early grade 3 or higher toxicities in 77 % of patients. While many were hematologic, radiation mucositis occurred in 16 % and gastrointestinal toxicity in 48 %. Grade 3 or higher late radiation toxicities were reported in 37 %. In total, treatment-related deaths occurred in 8 % (Langer et al. 2007). These results drive the desire to improve the therapeutic ratio of reirradiation. Proton therapy may be advantageous in reducing the volume of previously irradiated tissues receiving additional radiation dose, potentially reducing toxicities of retreatment. Proton therapy may also enable the option of retreatment for patients whose prior radiation dose distribution is felt to preclude the safe delivery of additional radiation using other modalities.

Researchers from the now-closed Indiana University Health Proton Therapy Center reported on 61 adult patients with recurrent, progressive, or second primary head and neck malignancies after prior radiotherapy (McDonald et al. 2016b). The most frequent histologies were squamous cell (54.2 %), adenoid cystic (11.0 %), and undifferentiated (8.2 %) carcinoma. The great majority of cases (90.2 %) involved skull base tumor sites, and 45 % had macroscopic intracranial perineural spread or direct intracranial tumor extension. These patients had been referred from over 30 separate institutions and practices, most often because there were felt to be no appropriate photon-based reirradiation treatment options. The patients were heavily pretreated; 18 % had received two to four prior courses of radiotherapy, 52.5 % had undergone two or more prior surgeries, and 59 % had received prior chemotherapy.

Patients were treated to a median dose of 66 Gy (RBE) for microscopic residual disease and 70 Gy (RBE) for gross residual disease. Concurrent chemotherapy was used in a minority of patients (29.5 %). With a median follow-up time of 15.2 months (28.7 months in those alive), the 2-year estimate of overall survival was 32.7 % and median survival 16.8 months. In a competing risk analysis with death as a competing risk, the

2-year cumulative incidence estimate for local failure was 19.7 % and distant metastasis 38.3 %. Acute toxicity of maximum grade 2 occurred in 47.5 %, grade 3 in 13.1 %, and grade 5 in 1.6 %. Late toxicity of maximum grade 2 occurred in 22.6 %, grade 3 in 15.1 %, grade 4 in 5.7 %, and grade 5 in 3.8 %. There were a total of three treatment-related deaths.

Given the heterogeneity and complexity of this patient population, it is difficult to assess the relative merits of proton reirradiation. Outcomes appear comparable to series of patients treated with photon-based reirradiation, despite a patient population with more adverse risk factors and largely felt ineligible for additional photon therapy. For many of these patients, proton therapy was used to extend a reirradiation option to those who would otherwise likely have received supportive care alone or palliative chemotherapy in a minority. Compared to historical expectations of survival outcomes with supportive care and palliative chemotherapy, the patient survival outcomes appear favorable.

Investigators at the Northwestern Medicine Chicago Proton Center and the ProCure Proton Therapy Center in Somerset, New Jersey, reported a pooled analysis of 92 patients who received proton therapy as reirradiation for recurrent or metachronous head and neck cancers (Romesser et al. 2016). The most frequent histologies were squamous cell carcinoma (56.5 %), adenocarcinoma (9.8 %), and sarcomas (5.4 %). The most common tumor site was the oropharynx (85.5 %), followed by the nasal cavity and paranasal sinuses (13 %), with 8.7 % being skull base tumors. Patients were heavily pretreated: 17.4 % had two or more prior course of radiotherapy and 48.9 % had prior chemotherapy.

The median dose of reirradiation was 60.6 Gy (RBE) and 47.8 % of patients received concurrent chemotherapy. With a median follow-up time of 10.4 months (13.3 months in those alive), the 1-year estimate of overall survival was 65.2 %. In a competing risk analysis with death as a competing risk, the 1-year cumulative incidence estimate for local failure was 25.1 %. The Kaplan-Meier estimate of distant metastasis at 1 year was 16 %. There were no reported acute grade 4 or 5 toxicities. Late toxicities of grade 4 occurred in 7.2 % and grade 5 in 2.9 % with two treatment-related deaths.

Figures 4 and 5 illustrate the use of proton therapy in patients with recurrent head and neck cancer.

10 Proton Reirradiation of Lung Cancer

Researchers from MD Anderson Cancer Center (MDACC) reported on 33 patients treated with proton therapy for intrathoracic recurrence of non-small cell lung cancer (McAvoy et al. 2013). After a median prior dose of 63 Gy, patients received a median reirradiation dose of 66 Gy (RBE) at a median time of 36 months from prior radiation. Relative to the initial tumor, the retreatment was infield in 57.5 %, marginal in 6 %, and out of field for 36 %. For the majority (85 %), reirradiation was given for a centrally located tumor. Roughly half had received chemotherapy prior to reirradiation and 24 % received concurrent chemotherapy with reirradiation. After a median follow-up time of 11 months (21 months in those alive), the 1-year Kaplan-Meier estimate of overall survival was 47 %, locoregional control 54 %, and freedom from distant metastases 39 %. Grade ≥3 esophageal toxicity occurred in 9 %, grade ≥3 pulmonary toxicity in 21.2 %, and there was 1 grade 3 cardiac toxicity. Toxicity was similar to other experiences with retreatment of NSCLC. Locoregional control remained problematic and the risk of distant metastasis was high. While these data cannot provide insight into the relative merit of proton therapy compared to other modalities for reirradiation of NSCLC, they do provide clinical experience with the feasibility and tolerance of proton reirradiation.

Subsequently, the MDACC researchers reported their combined experience of reirradiation with proton therapy and IMRT (McAvoy et al. 2014). They found no association between treatment technique and pulmonary or esophageal toxicity but did note a correlation between grade ≥2 pulmonary toxicity and increasing volume of lung receiving 10 Gy (V10) during

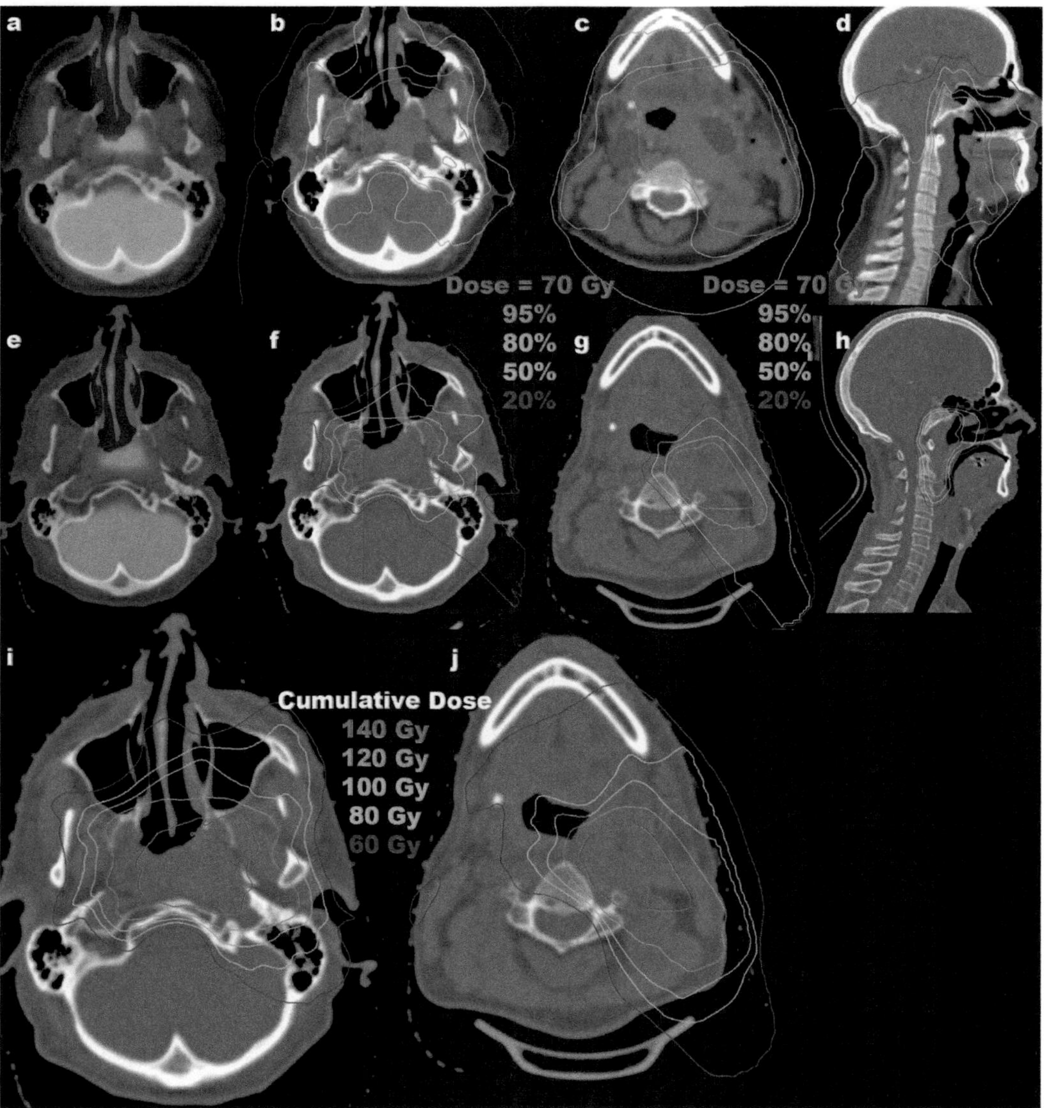

Fig. 4 A 48-year-old man was reirradiated for recurrent nasopharyngeal squamous cell carcinoma. He presented with headaches, left-sided otalgia, and a serous otitis media and was found to have a nasopharyngeal mass (**a**) extending down the oropharyngeal wall to the level of the larynx with associated ipsilateral necrotic neck adenopathy. His pathology was negative for p16. He was treated with tomotherapy to 70 Gy in 35 fractions (**b–d**) with three cycles of 100 mg/m^2 cisplatin chemotherapy (third cycle dose reduced). He had profound xerostomia and dysphagia with over 70 lb of weight loss and remained gastrostomy tube dependent 9 months after radiation. Follow-up PET/CT showed resolution of hypermetabolic uptake but with residual centrally necrotic nodal adenopathy. Six months after radiation, an FNA of the nodal mass confirmed residual viable neck disease and a repeat PET/CT 7 months after radiation showed recurrent disease in the nasopharynx (**e**), biopsy proven. Given the short time interval from prior radiation and persistent disease in the neck, further radiation was not offered. Palliative chemotherapy was recommended. After seeking a second opinion, he was referred for an opinion on salvage proton reirradiation. At the time of our evaluation, he has a KPS of 80 %, his weight had been stable over the past 3 months, and a PET/CT scan showed no evidence of distant metastatic disease. He was offered reirradiation to 70 Gy in 35 fractions (**f–h**) and received concurrent weekly cetuximab, carboplatin, and paclitaxel. He developed no oral mucositis during treatment and gained 12 lb during the course of reirradiation with improved oral intake. He continued to gain weight after reirradiation although he still required a gastrostomy tube. Cumulative lifetime dose distribution is shown (**i, j**). A PET/CT scan 3 months after reirradiation showed a complete response. Unfortunately, he later developed intracranial tumor progression and died at 8 months from reirradiation

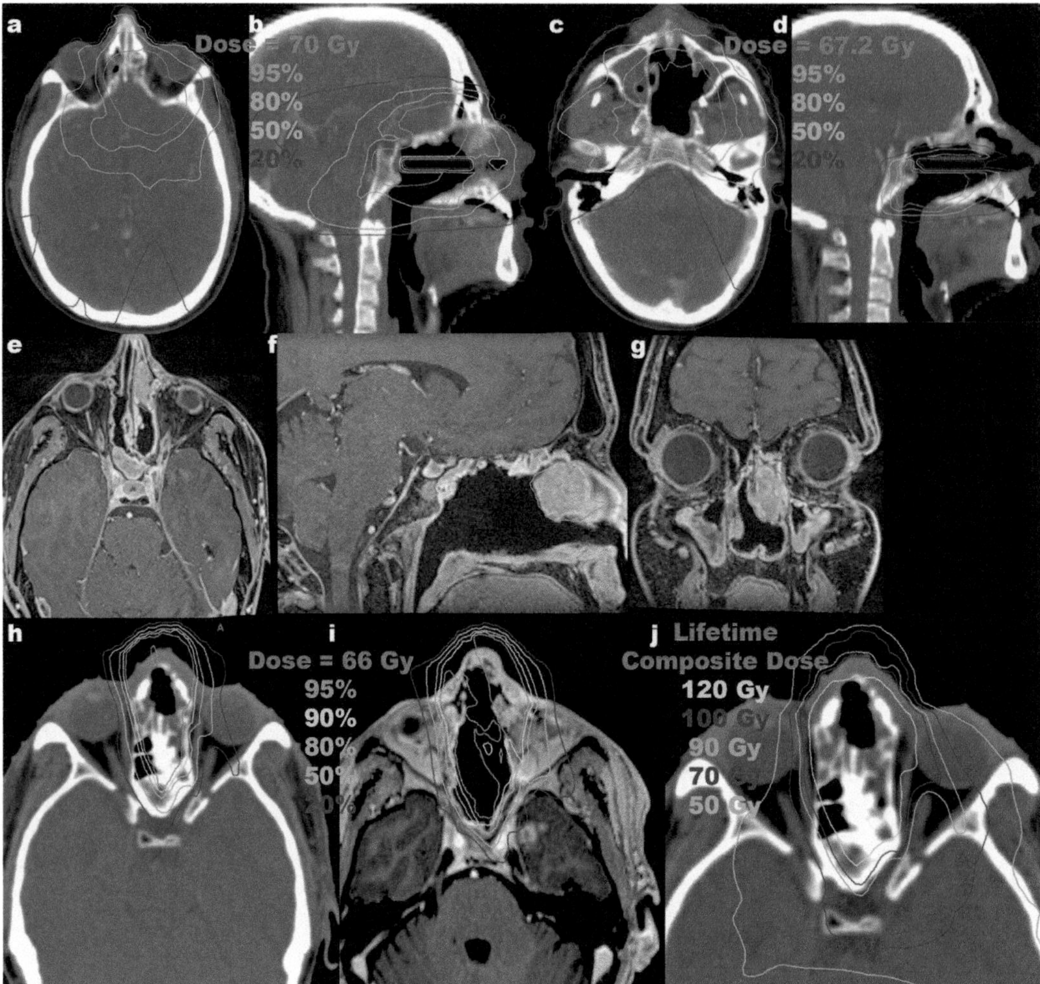

Fig. 5 A 34-year-old man was treated for a recurrent sinonasal poorly differentiated adenocarcinoma. He originally presented with a sphenoid sinus primary with left orbital extension. The pathology was felt consistent with sinonasal undifferentiated carcinoma. He underwent induction chemotherapy followed by concurrent chemoradiation therapy to 70 Gy using IMRT (**a**, **b**). Imaging suggested a complete response and endoscopic exploration and resection identified no residual tumor. He developed radiation retinopathy of the left eye with loss of useful vision. Three years later, he developed recurrent disease versus a second primary in the left nasal cavity (within the prior radiation volume) involving the sphenopalatine foramen and pterygoid canal and abutting the infraorbital nerve. It was biopsied as an intermediate grade adenocarcinoma. He was then reirradiated with concurrent cisplatin, receiving 67.2 Gy in 1.4 Gy fractions given twice daily with IMRT (**c**, **d**). He had another complete response to therapy and went on to develop moderate trismus as well as a focus of grade 1 (asymptomatic) radiation necrosis in the left temporal lobe. Ten months after reirradiation, there was concern for recurrent disease in the anterior nasal cavity on PET/CT scan, and an MRI 14 months after reirradiation showed enhancing tumor in the anterior left nasal cavity (**e–g**), biopsy confirmed as a poorly differentiated adenocarcinoma. This was largely outside of his reirradiation volume but within the 80 % isodose line of his original radiation volume. He underwent an endoscopic endonasal craniofacial resection with involved surgical margins and both perineural and angiolymphatic space invasion. Tumor involved the crista galli and the lamina papyracea, which was removed, but did not grossly invade the periorbita. He sought evaluation at two major academic centers for further reirradiation, but in light of his two prior courses of treatment, the risk: benefit ratio of further radiation was deemed unfavorable. He was then referred for consideration of reirradiation with proton therapy. A recent postoperative PET/CT scan and a repeat MRI showed no evidence of recurrence or distant metastatic disease, and proton therapy was offered. He declined concurrent chemotherapy with repeat reirradiation. Proton therapy was used to maximize sparing of his right eye (**h**), which had his only useful vision, and to minimize additional dose to the area of his preexisting left temporal lobe radiation necrosis (**i**). The lifetime cumulative dose is shown (**j**). Unfortunately, he developed distant metastatic disease to the liver and lung at 4 months and succumbed to metastatic disease

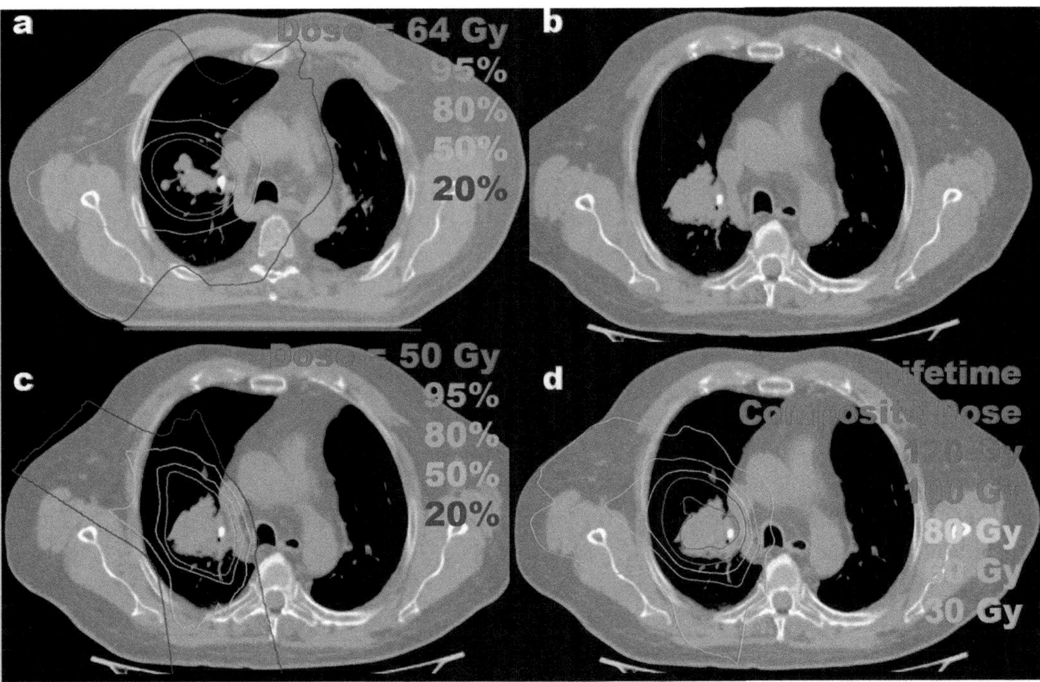

Fig. 6 An 80-year-old man was treated for recurrent solitary lung metastasis from colon adenocarcinoma. Five years after surgery for a pathologic T3 N0 colon adenocarcinoma, he developed hemoptysis and was found to have a solitary right perihilar metastasis, biopsied as adenocarcinoma consistent with his colon primary. Given his advanced age and medical comorbidities including hypertensive cardiomyopathy, and obstructive pulmonary disease from asbestosis with poor pulmonary function tests, he was not a candidate for surgical metastasectomy. He then received thoracic radiotherapy with IMRT to 64 Gy (**a**) with concurrent capecitabine. Eighteen months later he developed recurrent hemoptysis, and a CT (**b**) showed recurrence of the previously treated right perihilar metastasis, now measuring just over 5 cm in size, without evidence of other distant disease on PET/CT. He was not felt to be a candidate for additional external beam radiation or stereotactic body radiotherapy in light of his prior radiation and tumor size. He was then referred for salvage proton therapy. He was treated with a field-in-field technique, delivering 30 Gy (RBE) in 10 fractions to a larger volume and 50 Gy (RBE) in 10 fractions at the 80% isodose line to the gross tumor volume with more limited margin (**c**). In the absence of 4D CT capability and gated delivery, a respiratory compression belt was used to minimize respiratory excursion, and a slow CT was acquired to create an average image over several respiratory cycles. Beam angles were selected to treat through lung which had previously been irradiated to significant dose and avoid increasing the lifetime lung V20. Three beam angles were used: a right anterior oblique, left posterior oblique, and a PA. His lifetime dose distribution is shown (**d**). His hemoptysis resolved with reirradiation and he had no acute toxicities of treatment. In follow-up imaging, he had a persistent right hilar mass that could represent fibrosis or residual tumor but without clear progression. He did later develop intrabronchial progressive disease outside of the reirradiation field. At 45 months after reirradiation, he was alive off therapy

reirradiation, as well as V20, mean lung dose, and composite (lifetime) mean lung dose. These findings support a planning objective of minimizing nontarget lung exposure to additional radiation using the most conformal modality available.

Figure 6 shows an example of a patient treated with proton therapy for reirradiation of a solitary lung metastasis.

11 Proton Reirradiation of Esophageal Cancer

Putative advantages of proton therapy in reirradiation of esophageal cancer include reduced cardiac and lung dose, potentially reducing the risk of cardiopulmonary complications. Esophageal mucosal toxicity would not be anticipated to be different from other external beam modalities but likely lower than with brachytherapy, which has been associated with a fairly high risk of stricture, ulceration, and perforation (Sharma et al. 2002).

Researchers at the University of Pennsylvania reported on 14 patients receiving proton reirradiation for esophageal cancer who had been treated on a prospective study of proton reirradiation (Fernandes et al. 2015). Patients were retreated to a median dose of 54 Gy at a median interval of 32 months from their initial radiation treatment course, which had delivered a median prior dose of 54 Gy. One patient was deemed infeasible due to development of a pleural effusion which necessitated that 30 % of the reirradiation dose be delivered with IMRT due to the increased proton range uncertainties in the setting of the pleural effusion. One grade 5 and one grade 3 esophageal ulceration occurred, both thought to be related to persistent tumor rather than radiation. Of the ten patients presenting with dysphagia, 70 % had partial or complete improvement. The median survival after reirradiation was 14 months. Nine patients developed further infield tumor progression and six developed distant metastatic disease.

12 Proton Reirradiation of Rectal Cancer

Prior to total mesorectal excision (TME), locally recurrent rectal cancer was estimated to occur in up to one-third of patients, and approximately one-half of these recurrences arose without evidence of distant metastatic disease (Moriya 2006). Following preoperative short-course radiotherapy and TME, long-term data from a randomized controlled trial reported a 10-year local recurrence risk of 5 % (van Gijn et al. 2011), which still yields a large number of cases given the high incidence of colorectal cancer.

A common approach in previously irradiated patients selected for curative intent salvage therapy is preoperative reduced dose reirradiation with concurrent chemotherapy followed by reassessment for radical resection and IORT (Konski et al. 2012). Compared to more favorable locations such as anastomotic recurrences, presacral and posterolateral recurrences are associated with a low likelihood of radical surgical resectability, significant rates of morbidity and mortality, and poorer outcomes (Kusters et al. 2009). The dose of reirradiation has typically been limited, with 30 Gy in conventional fractionation being a common prescription, because of the risk of toxicity to previously irradiated bowel and neurovascular tissues. Because these low doses are extremely unlikely to eradicate gross disease, reirradiation is generally a palliative treatment when surgery is not a component of treatment.

Proton therapy may be considered for preoperative reirradiation in an effort to reduce the dose to previously irradiated bowel and bladder. Through improved avoidance of pelvic viscera, proton therapy may be hypothesized to reduce the risk of urinary toxicity, small bowel obstruction, or fistula compared to less conformal treatments. Improved target conformality and normal tissue avoidance may allow for dose-escalated preoperative proton reirradiation, which may be hypothesized to improve the likelihood of tumor response and subsequent R0 resection.

For patients managed without surgery, proton therapy also offers the possibility of dose escalation and treatment with radical intent. Other modalities which may be considered for radical reirradiation include SBRT (Defoe et al. 2011) and interstitial brachytherapy (Bishop et al. 2015). Potential advantages of proton therapy in radical reirradiation include the ability to target recurrences that are not anatomically accessible or otherwise unsuitable for interstitial therapy (e.g., encasement of neurovascular structures) or are too large or poorly defined to be suitable targets for SBRT. Clinical outcomes data of proton reirradiation are too sparse to judge the merits of any of these hypotheses.

Figures 7 and 8 are examples of the application of radical proton therapy with concurrent chemotherapy in patients with recurrent rectal cancer.

Researchers from the University of Pennsylvania reported outcomes for seven patients with locally recurrent rectal cancer treated on a prospective study of proton reirradiation (Berman et al. 2014). At a median of 39 months after a median prior dose of 50.4 Gy, patients received an additional 45–64.8 Gy

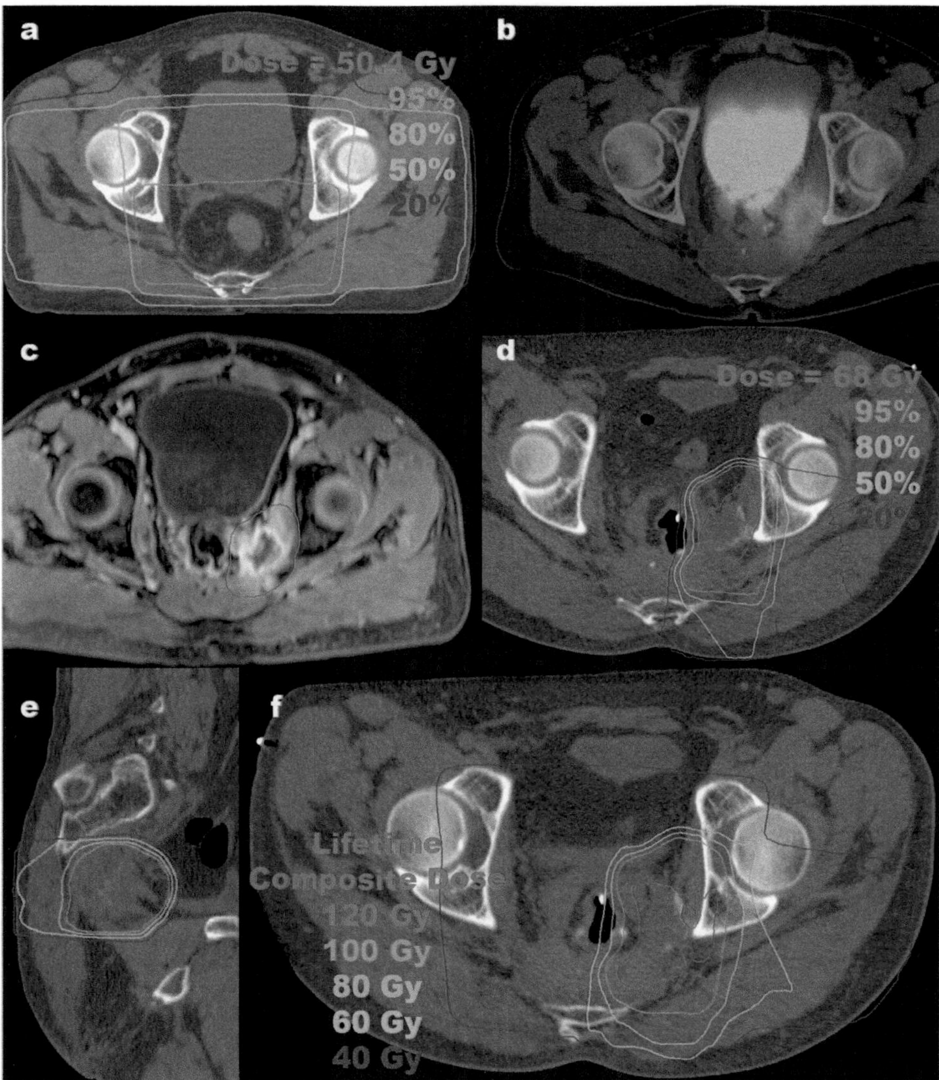

Fig. 7 A 63-year-old man was reirradiated for a posterolateral pelvic side wall recurrence of rectal adenocarcinoma. He originally presented with a T2 N2 rectal adenocarcinoma, KRAS wild type, and was treated with preoperative radiation therapy to 50.4 Gy with continuous infusion 5-fluorouracil (**a**). He then underwent a low anterior resection with a pathologic complete response, with 0/3 lymph nodes being involved. He had poor tolerance of planned adjuvant capecitabine and so received no adjuvant therapy. Four and a half years after surgery, he developed a rising CEA with a PET/CT showing a hypermetabolic (SUV 4.2) mass at the left pelvic sidewall (**b**), with a CT-guided FNA showing recurrent adenocarcinoma consistent with his rectal primary. He was not felt to be a candidate for radical surgical resection due to tumor location. He was referred for salvage proton therapy, which was initially denied by insurance. He received FOLFOX4 plus bevacizumab for 4 months while awaiting insurance approval, with stabilization of disease. Oxaliplatin was stopped early due to acute reaction. Pelvic MRI was obtained to assess the extent of disease (**c**). He was then treated with salvage proton therapy, planned to 70 Gy (RBE) in 38 fractions (he elected to stop at 68 Gy (RBE) due to travel arrangements) with continuous infusion fluorouracil (**d**, **e**). It was decided to allow the lateral rectal wall to receive an additional 50 Gy (RBE), assuming some interval normal tissue recovery in the intervening years since prior radiotherapy. The lifetime cumulative dose distribution is also shown (**f**). A PET/CT scan at 3 months after reirradiation showed a complete response and his CEA had normalized. Three years after reirradiation, he had a rising CEA again, and a PET/CT scan showed a solitary focus of osseous metastatic disease in the left ischium, biopsy proven, at which point he elected observation. He remains alive 4 and a half years after reirradiation without rectal bleeding, ulceration, or colostomy

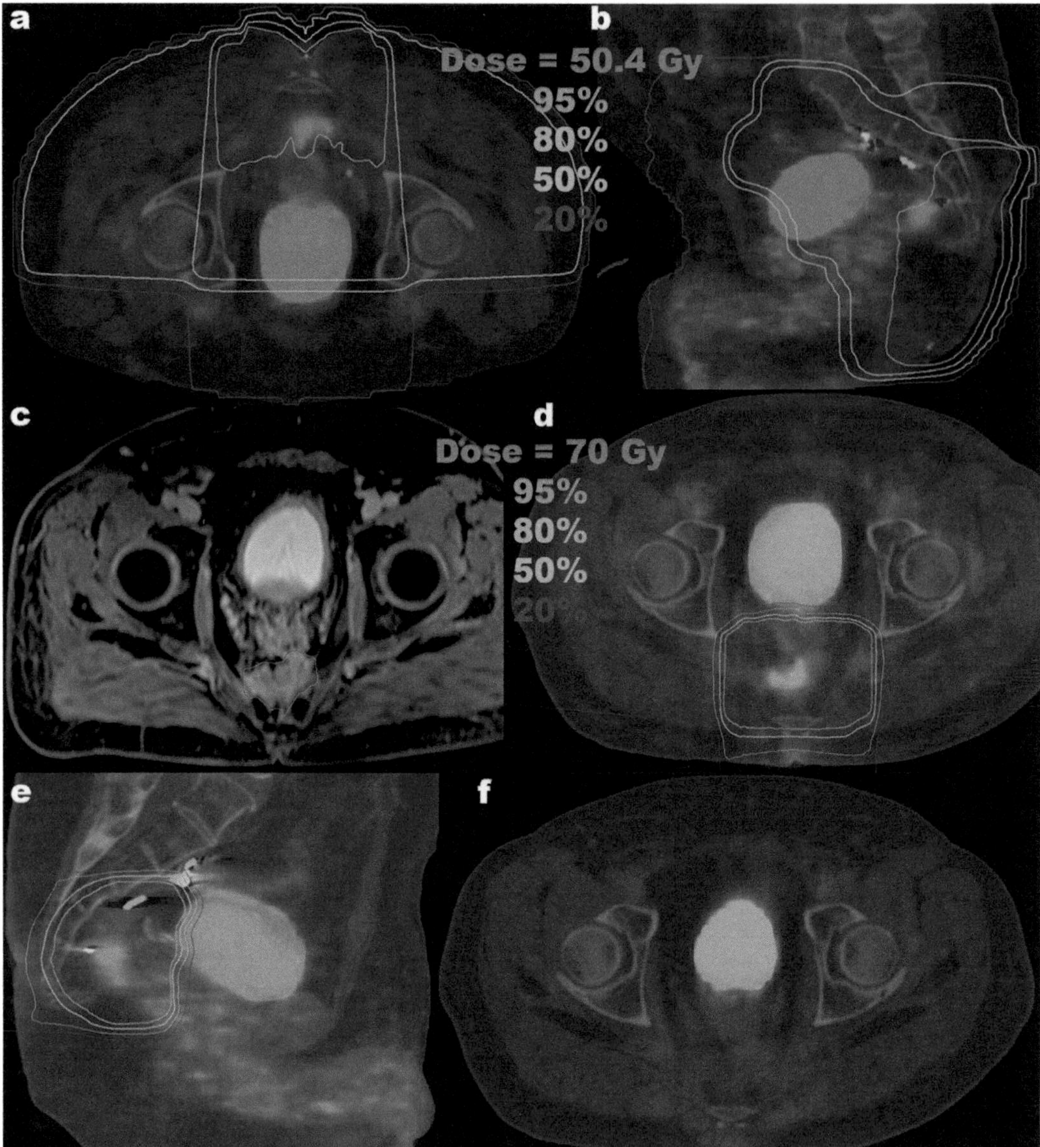

Fig. 8 A 63-year-old man was treated for a presacral recurrence of rectal adenocarcinoma. His original treatment was an abdominal perineal resection (APR) for a pathologic T2 N0 rectal adenocarcinoma with uninvolved surgical margins and no lymphovascular space invasion. No adjuvant therapy was indicated. Two years later, a rising CEA prompted a PET/CT scan which showed a hypermetabolic focus in the presacral space, biopsied by fine needle aspiration which confirmed locally recurrent adenocarcinoma, without evidence of regional or distant metastatic disease. It was not felt to be surgically resectable without significant morbidity. He was treated with 3DCRT to 50.4 Gy (**a**, **b**: dose shown on PET/CT scan) with concurrent capecitabine with a complete response on subsequent PET/CT scan. One year later, his CEA was rising again and PET/CT and MRI (**c**) showed recurrence of the previously treated lesion without evidence of regional or distant metastatic disease. He was then referred for salvage therapy with protons and again received concurrent capecitabine. On exam he had fairly pronounced radiation fibrosis of the sacral skin (bolus had been applied over the buttocks during prior radiation). He was reirradiated with proton therapy to 70 Gy (RBE) with three fields: a PA and steeply angled left and right oblique fields to improve skin sparing during reirradiation (**d**, **e**). Proton therapy was readily able to avoid the bladder and a small amount of bowel in the cranial portion of the field which was not in close proximity to the target. At 3 months postradiation, his CEA had normalized and a CT scan showed stability of the presacral thickening. At 5 months postradiation, a repeat PET/CT scan showed a complete response (**f**). At 32 months from completion of reirradiation, he remains without evidence of recurrent disease

(mean 61.2 Gy) with proton therapy. Most (6/7) received concurrent 5-FU-based chemotherapy and two patients had R2 (macroscopically incomplete) surgical resections as part of management. At a median follow-up of 14 months, there had been one complete response, one patient with progressive disease, and five partial responses, two of whom later developed another local recurrence. In dosimetric comparison to alternate prospectively developed treatment plans using IMRT, proton therapy was associated with reduced dose to bowel. There were three acute (and transient) grade 3 toxicities and three late grade 4 toxicities (two bowel obstructions and one enterovaginal fistula thought due to progressive tumor).

Researchers from the Hyogo Ion Beam Medical Center have also reported on three cases of particle reirradiation of recurrent rectal cancer (two proton, one carbon ion) (Mokutani et al. 2015). Treatment was given with radical intent (proton dose 74 Gy in 34 fractions) without concurrent chemotherapy and achieved durable control of the treated tumor in two of the cases with the third developing another local re-recurrence approximately 30 months after reirradiation.

Conclusions

Clinical experience with reirradiation using proton beam therapy is increasing. The rationale for proton reirradiation is often to avoid or reduce toxicities of reirradiation by limiting the volume of nontarget tissues receiving additional radiation dose. In some diseases, proton reirradiation may improve outcomes by facilitating safe dose escalation or providing better target coverage while respecting constraints to critical normal structures. In uncommon cases, proton therapy may permit reirradiation when the dosimetry achieved with other modalities is felt to preclude safe reirradiation. The existing data on proton reirradiation is limited to small series and is highly heterogeneous. To better understand the value of proton therapy in reirradiation relative to other radiation modalities, prospective evaluation with more homogenous patient populations is needed to evaluate predefined end points based on rational clinical hypotheses.

References

Andersson KM, Ahnesjo A, Vallhagen Dahlgren C (2014) Evaluation of a metal artifact reduction algorithm in CT studies used for proton radiotherapy treatment planning. J Appl Clin Med Phys 15(5):4857

Bassal M, Mertens AC, Taylor L, Neglia JP, Greffe BS, Hammond S, Ronckers CM, Friedman DL, Stovall M, Yasui YY, Robison LL, Meadows AT, Kadan-Lottick NS (2006) Risk of selected subsequent carcinomas in survivors of childhood cancer: a report from the Childhood Cancer Survivor Study. J Clin Oncol 24(3):476–483

Berman AT, Both S, Sharkoski T, Goldrath K, Tochner Z, Apisarnthanarax S, Metz JM, Plastaras JP (2014) Proton reirradiation of recurrent rectal cancer: dosimetric comparison, toxicities, and preliminary outcomes. Int J Particle Ther 1(1):2–13

Berrington de Gonzalez A, Curtis RE, Kry SF, Gilbert E, Lamart S, Berg CD, Stovall M, Ron E (2011) Proportion of second cancers attributable to radiotherapy treatment in adults: a cohort study in the US SEER cancer registries. Lancet Oncol 12(4):353–360

Bishop AJ, Gupta S, Cunningham MG, Tao R, Berner PA, Korpela SG, Ibbott GS, Lawyer AA, Crane CH (2015) Interstitial brachytherapy for the treatment of locally recurrent anorectal cancer. Ann Surg Oncol 22(S3):596–602

Brown AP, Barney CL, Grosshans DR, McAleer MF, de Groot JF, Puduvalli VK, Tucker SL, Crawford CN, Khan M, Khatua S, Gilbert MR, Brown PD, Mahajan A (2013) Proton beam craniospinal irradiation reduces acute toxicity for adults with medulloblastoma. Int J Radiat Oncol Biol Phys 86(2):277–284

Chung CS, Yock TI, Nelson K, Xu Y, Keating NL, Tarbell NJ (2013) Incidence of second malignancies among patients treated with proton versus photon radiation. Int J Radiat Oncol Biol Phys 87(1):46–52

Combs SE, Burkholder I, Edler L, Rieken S, Habermehl D, Jakel O, Haberer T, Haselmann R, Unterberg A, Wick W, Debus J (2010) Randomised phase I/II study to evaluate carbon ion radiotherapy versus fractionated stereotactic radiotherapy in patients with recurrent or progressive gliomas: the CINDERELLA trial. BMC Cancer 10:533

De Ruysscher D, Sterpin E, Haustermans K, Depuydt T (2015) Tumour movement in proton therapy: solutions and remaining questions: a review. Cancers (Basel) 7(3):1143–1153

Defoe SG, Bernard ME, Rwigema JC, Heron DE, Ozhasoglu C, Burton S (2011) Stereotactic body radiotherapy for the treatment of presacral recurrences from rectal cancers. J Cancer Res Ther 7(4):408–411

Dendale R, Lumbroso-Le Rouic L, Noel G, Feuvret L, Levy C, Delacroix S, Meyer A, Nauraye C, Mazal A, Mammar H, Garcia P, D'Hermies F, Frau E, Plancher C, Asselain B, Schlienger P, Mazeron JJ, Desjardins L (2006) Proton beam radiotherapy for uveal melanoma: results of Curie Institut-Orsay proton therapy center (ICPO). Int J Radiat Oncol Biol Phys 65(3):780–787

Desjardins L, Lumbroso-Le Rouic L, Levy-Gabriel C, Cassoux N, Dendale R, Mazal A, Delacroix S, Sastre X, Plancher C, Asselain B (2012) Treatment of uveal melanoma by accelerated proton beam. Dev Ophthalmol 49:41–57

Diener-West M, Earle JD, Fine SL, Hawkins BS, Moy CS, Reynolds SM, Schachat AP, Straatsma BR, Collaborative Ocular Melanoma Study G (2001) The COMS randomized trial of iodine 125 brachytherapy for choroidal melanoma, III: initial mortality findings. COMS Report No. 18. Arch Ophthalmol 119(7): 969–982

Eaton BR, Esiashvili N, Kim S, Patterson B, Weyman EA, Thornton LT, Mazewski C, MacDonald TJ, Ebb D, MacDonald SM, Tarbell NJ, Yock TI (2015) Endocrine outcomes with proton and photon radiotherapy for standard risk medulloblastoma. Neuro Oncol, available online ahead of print

Fagundes MA, Hug EB, Liebsch NJ, Daly W, Efird J, Munzenrider JE (1995) Radiation therapy for chordomas of the base of skull and cervical spine: patterns of failure and outcome after relapse. Int J Radiat Oncol Biol Phys 33(3):579–584

Fernandes A, Berman AT, Mick R, Both S, Lelionis K, Lukens JN, Ben-Josef E, Metz JM, Plastaras JP (2016) A prospective study of proton beam reirradiation for esophageal cancer. Int J Radiat Oncol Biol Phys 95(1):483–487

Fogh SE, Andrews DW, Glass J, Curran W, Glass C, Champ C, Evans JJ, Hyslop T, Pequignot E, Downes B, Comber E, Maltenfort M, Dicker AP, Werner-Wasik M (2010) Hypofractionated stereotactic radiation therapy: an effective therapy for recurrent high-grade gliomas. J Clin Oncol 28(18):3048–3053

Galle JO, McDonald MW, Simoneaux V, Buchsbaum JC (2015) Reirradiation with proton therapy for recurrent gliomas. Int J Particle Ther 2(1):11–18

Hill-Kayser C, Kirk M (2015) Brainstem-sparing craniospinal irradiation delivered with pencil beam scanning proton therapy. Pediatr Blood Cancer 62(4):718–720

Hocht S, Stark R, Seiler F, Heufelder J, Bechrakis NE, Cordini D, Marnitz S, Kluge H, Foerster MH, Hinkelbein W (2005) Proton or stereotactic photon irradiation for posterior uveal melanoma? A planning intercomparison. Strahlenther Onkol 181(12): 783–788

ICRU (2007) Prescribing, recording, and reporting proton-beam therapy: treatment planning. J ICRU 7(2):95–122

Kano H, Iqbal FO, Sheehan J, Mathieu D, Seymour ZA, Niranjan A, Flickinger JC, Kondziolka D, Pollock BE, Rosseau G, Sneed PK, McDermott MW, Lunsford LD (2011) Stereotactic radiosurgery for chordoma: a report from the North American Gamma Knife Consortium. Neurosurgery 68(2):379–389

Kleinerman RA, Tucker MA, Tarone RE, Abramson DH, Seddon JM, Stovall M, Li FP, Fraumeni JF Jr (2005) Risk of new cancers after radiotherapy in long-term survivors of retinoblastoma: an extended follow-up. J Clin Oncol 23(10):2272–2279

Konski AA, Suh WW, Herman JM, Blackstock AW Jr, Hong TS, Poggi MM, Rodriguez-Bigas M, Small W Jr, Thomas CR Jr, Zook J (2012) ACR appropriateness criteria(R)-recurrent rectal cancer. Gastrointest Cancer Res 5(1):3–12

Kusters M, Dresen RC, Martijn H, Nieuwenhuijzen GA, van de Velde CJ, van den Berg HA, Beets-Tan RG, Rutten HJ (2009) Radicality of resection and survival after multimodality treatment is influenced by subsite of locally recurrent rectal cancer. Int J Radiat Oncol Biol Phys 75(5):1444–1449

Langer CJ, Harris J, Horwitz EM, Nicolaou N, Kies M, Curran W, Wong S, Ang K (2007) Phase II study of low-dose paclitaxel and cisplatin in combination with split-course concomitant twice-daily reirradiation in recurrent squamous cell carcinoma of the head and neck: results of Radiation Therapy Oncology Group Protocol 9911. J Clin Oncol 25(30):4800–4805

Li Z (2012) Toward robust proton therapy planning and delivery. Transl Cancer Res 1(3):217–226

Lomax AJ (2009) Charged particle therapy: the physics of interaction. Cancer J 15(4):285–291

Lomax AJ, Bohringer T, Bolsi A, Coray D, Emert F, Goitein G, Jermann M, Lin S, Pedroni E, Rutz H, Stadelmann O, Timmermann B, Verwey J, Weber DC (2004) Treatment planning and verification of proton therapy using spot scanning: initial experiences. Med Phys 31(11):3150–3157

Mannina E Jr, Bartlett G, Wallace D, McMullen K (2014) Steroid-induced adaptive proton planning in a pediatric patient with low grade glioma: a case report and literature review. Pract Radiat Oncol 4(1):50–54

Marucci L, Lane AM, Li W, Egan KM, Gragoudas ES, Adams JA, Collier JM, Munzenrider JE (2006) Conservation treatment of the eye: conformal proton reirradiation for recurrent uveal melanoma. Int J Radiat Oncol Biol Phys 64(4):1018–1022

Marucci L, Ancukiewicz M, Lane AM, Collier JM, Gragoudas ES, Munzenrider JE (2011) Uveal melanoma recurrence after fractionated proton beam therapy: comparison of survival in patients treated with reirradiation or with enucleation. Int J Radiat Oncol Biol Phys 79(3):842–846

Massimino M, Gandola L, Spreafico F, Biassoni V, Luksch R, Collini P, Solero CN, Simonetti F, Pignoli E, Cefalo G, Poggi G, Modena P, Mariani L, Potepan P, Podda M, Casanova M, Pecori E, Acerno S, Ferrari A, Terenziani M, Meazza C, Polastri D, Ravagnani F, Fossati-Bellani F (2009) No salvage using high-dose chemotherapy plus/minus reirradiation for relapsing previously irradiated medulloblastoma. Int J Radiat Oncol Biol Phys 73(5):1358–1363

McAvoy SA, Ciura KT, Rineer JM, Allen PK, Liao Z, Chang JY, Palmer MB, Cox JD, Komaki R, Gomez DR (2013) Feasibility of proton beam therapy for reirradiation of locoregionally recurrent non-small cell lung cancer. Radiother Oncol 109(1):38–44

McAvoy S, Ciura K, Wei C, Rineer J, Liao Z, Chang JY, Palmer MB, Cox JD, Komaki R, Gomez DR (2014) Definitive reirradiation for locoregionally recurrent non-small cell lung cancer with proton beam therapy or intensity modulated radiation therapy: predictors of high-grade toxicity and survival outcomes. Int J Radiat Oncol Biol Phys 90(4):819–827

McDonald MW, Lawson J, Garg MK, Quon H, Ridge JA, Saba N, Salama JK, Smith RV, Yeung AR, Yom SS, Beitler JJ, Expert Panel on Radiation O-H, Neck C (2011) ACR appropriateness criteria retreatment of recurrent head and neck cancer after prior definitive radiation expert panel on radiation oncology-head and neck cancer. Int J Radiat Oncol Biol Phys 80(5):1292–1298

McDonald MW, Linton OR, Shah MV (2013a) Proton therapy for reirradiation of progressive or recurrent chordoma. Int J Radiat Oncol Biol Phys 87(5):1107–1114

McDonald MW, Wolanski MR, Simmons JW, Buchsbaum JC (2013b) Technique for sparing previously irradiated critical normal structures in salvage proton craniospinal irradiation. Radiat Oncol 8:14

McDonald MW, Linton OR, Moore MG, Ting JY, Cohen-Gadol AA, Shah MV (2016a) Influence of residual tumor volume and radiation dose coverage in outcomes for clival chordoma. Int J Radiat Oncol Biol Phys 95(1):304–311

McDonald MW, Zolali-Meybodi O, Lehnert SJ, Cohen-Gadol AA, Moore MG (2016b) Reirradiation of recurrent and second primary head and neck cancer with proton therapy. Int J Radiat Oncol Biol Phys 94(4):930–931

Merchant TE, Boop FA, Kun LE, Sanford RA (2008) A retrospective study of surgery and reirradiation for recurrent ependymoma. Int J Radiat Oncol Biol Phys 71(1):87–97

Mokutani Y, Yamamoto H, Uemura M, Haraguchi N, Takahashi H, Nishimura J, Hata T, Takemasa I, Mizushima T, Doki Y, Mori M (2015) Effect of particle beam radiotherapy on locally recurrent rectal cancer: three case reports. Mol Clin Oncol 3(4):765–769

Moriya Y (2006) Treatment strategy for locally recurrent rectal cancer. Jpn J Clin Oncol 36(3):127–131

Paganetti H (2012) Proton therapy physics, Series in medical physics and biomedical engineering. CRC Press, Boca Raton

Romesser PB, Cahlon O, Scher ED, Hug EB, Sine K, DeSelm C, Fox JL, Mah D, Garg MK, Chang JH, Lee NY (2016) Proton beam re-irradiation for recurrent head and neck cancer: multi-institutional report on feasibility and early outcomes. Int J Radiat Oncol Biol Phys 95(1):386–395

Sharma V, Mahantshetty U, Dinshaw KA, Deshpande R, Sharma S (2002) Palliation of advanced/recurrent esophageal carcinoma with high-dose-rate brachytherapy. Int J Radiat Oncol Biol Phys 52(2):310–315

Sikuade MJ, Salvi S, Rundle PA, Errington DG, Kacperek A, Rennie IG (2015) Outcomes of treatment with stereotactic radiosurgery or proton beam therapy for choroidal melanoma. Eye (Lond) 29(9):1194–1198

Simone CB 2nd, Kramer K, O'Meara WP, Bekelman JE, Belard A, McDonough J, O'Connell J (2012) Predicted rates of secondary malignancies from proton versus photon radiation therapy for stage I seminoma. Int J Radiat Oncol Biol Phys 82(1):242–249

Stupp R, Hegi ME, Mason WP, van den Bent MJ, Taphoorn MJ, Janzer RC, Ludwin SK, Allgeier A, Fisher B, Belanger K, Hau P, Brandes AA, Gijtenbeek J, Marosi C, Vecht CJ, Mokhtari K, Wesseling P, Villa S, Eisenhauer E, Gorlia T, Weller M, Lacombe D, Cairncross JG, Mirimanoff RO (2009) Effects of radiotherapy with concomitant and adjuvant temozolomide versus radiotherapy alone on survival in glioblastoma in a randomised phase III study: 5-year analysis of the EORTC-NCIC trial. Lancet Oncol 10(5):459–466

Stupp R, Brada M, van den Bent MJ, Tonn JC, Pentheroudakis G, Group EGW (2014) High-grade glioma: ESMO Clinical Practice Guidelines for diagnosis, treatment and follow-up. Ann Oncol 25(Suppl 3):iii93–101

Suit H, Goldberg S, Niemierko A, Trofimov A, Adams J, Paganetti H, Chen GT, Bortfeld T, Rosenthal S, Loeffler J, Delaney T (2003) Proton beams to replace photon beams in radical dose treatments. Acta Oncol 42(8):800–808

van Gijn W, Marijnen CA, Nagtegaal ID, Kranenbarg EM, Putter H, Wiggers T, Rutten HJ, Pahlman L, Glimelius B, van de Velde CJ (2011) Preoperative radiotherapy combined with total mesorectal excision for resectable rectal cancer: 12-year follow-up of the multicentre, randomised controlled TME trial. Lancet Oncol 12(6):575–582

Verburg JM, Seco J (2013) Dosimetric accuracy of proton therapy for chordoma patients with titanium implants. Med Phys 40(7):071727

Wallis CJ, Mahar AL, Choo R, Herschorn S, Kodama RT, Shah PS, Danjoux C, Narod SA, Nam RK (2016) Second malignancies after radiotherapy for prostate cancer: systematic review and meta-analysis. BMJ 352:i851

Wang Z, Nabhan M, Schild SE, Stafford SL, Petersen IA, Foote RL, Murad MH (2013) Charged particle radiation therapy for uveal melanoma: a systematic review and meta-analysis. Int J Radiat Oncol Biol Phys 86(1):18–26

Wei RL, Nguyen ST, Yang JN, Wolff J, Mahajan A (2012) Salvage craniospinal irradiation with an intensity modulated radiotherapy technique for patients with disseminated neuraxis disease. Pract Radiat Oncol 2(4):e69–e75

Zhang R, Howell RM, Giebeler A, Taddei PJ, Mahajan A, Newhauser WD (2013) Comparison of risk of radiogenic second cancer following photon and proton craniospinal irradiation for a pediatric medulloblastoma patient. Phys Med Biol 58(4):807–823

Brain Tumours

Joshua D. Palmer, Colin Champ, Susan C. Short, and Shannon E. Fogh

Contents

The original version of this chapter was revised. An erratum to this chapter can be found at 10.1007/978-3-319-41825-4_78.

J.D. Palmer
Department of Radiation Oncology, James Comprehensive Cancer Center, The Ohio State University Columbus, Ohio, USA

C. Champ
Department of Radiation Oncology, University of Pittsburgh Medical Center, Pittsburgh, PA, USA

S.C. Short (✉)
UCL Cancer Institute, London, UK
e-mail: S.C.Short@leeds.ac.uk

S.E. Fogh, MD
Department of Radiation Oncology, University of California, San Francisco, CA, USA
e-mail: Shannon.Fogh@ucsf.edu

Abstract

Historically, radiation oncologists have approached re-irradiating brain tumours with caution due to the potential risks of central nervous system late toxicity, especially radionecrosis, which may occur months or years following treatment. There is, however, a paucity of prospective data addressing this approach. Re-irradiation of brain tumours is attracting more interest as our understanding of the tolerance of the brain to radiation evolves. Furthermore, developments in radiation treatment approaches, technology and imaging enable highly accurate targeting of biologically relevant tumour volumes. Thanks to recent advancements in molecular-targeted therapy, further exploration of the role of re-irradiation – primary or in combination with novel agents – is needed.

Med Radiol Radiat Oncol (2016)
DOI 10.1007/174_2016_66, © Springer International Publishing Switzerland
Published Online: 16 Aug 2016

1 Introduction

The current standard of care for glioblastoma multiforme (GBM) is radiotherapy with concurrent and adjuvant temozolomide. Recent data suggest that the addition of the device NovoTTF (tumour-treating fields) to adjuvant temozolomide improves progression-free and overall survival for GBM patients (Stupp et al. 2015). Temozolomide is associated with a 5-year overall survival of 9.8 % versus 1.9 % with radiotherapy alone (Stupp et al. 2009). Because of the infiltrating nature of gliomas, they frequently recur and despite an increase in survival rates, the majority of patients progress within 1–2 years. With regard to anaplastic astrocytomas and low-grade gliomas, radiotherapy remains the standard first-line treatment, although other approaches are under investigation. Time to local recurrence is longer in lower-grade tumours; however, the majority ultimately also recur. Salvage therapy is indicated in the majority of recurrent gliomas and most patients receive chemotherapy or surgery at relapse. Further neurosurgical intervention is frequently limited because of the high risk of operative morbidity in these infiltrative tumours and systemic options can be impacted by resistance to therapy. A local agent without systemic toxicity would be ideal, as a significant proportion of patients experience a reduced bone marrow reserve at progression, complicating further systemic treatment.

Historically, radiation oncologists have been cautious about re-irradiating brain tumours because of concerns of late toxicity when exceeding normal tissue constraints, especially radionecrosis, which can occur several months to many years following treatment. There is, however, a lack of prospective data addressing this approach, and most information is from relatively small reported clinical series. Re-irradiation for brain tumours is now attracting more interest as our understanding of the tolerance of normal brain tissue evolves. Developments in radiation technology and imaging also enable highly accurate targeting of biologically relevant tumour volumes.

In this chapter, we discuss the radiobiological principles behind re-irradiation of central nervous system (CNS) tumours and look at the current evidence and future directions for development.

2 Overview of Treatment Options for Recurrent Gliomas

External beam radiotherapy is an integral part of therapy for the treatment of low- and high-grade gliomas. The exact timing of radiotherapy for low-grade gliomas is controversial, but most patients will receive radiotherapy at some point during the course of their disease. The vast majority of gliomas recur within 2 cm of the original surgical site (Hess et al. 1994; Wong et al. 1999).

At relapse, treatment options have included further surgical resection, systemic chemotherapy and more recently re-irradiation. Currently, there is no agreed standard of care.

The extent of surgical resection at relapse is frequently limited by the infiltrative nature of these tumours and the need to avoid severe neurological deficit from further surgical intervention. For those patients able to undergo further surgical resection, the use of impregnated carmustine wafers in the surgical cavity improved median survival by 8 weeks in a placebo-controlled study (Brem et al. 1995). There are attempts at improving the rate of complete resections for first-line and repeat resection in glioblastoma using a fluorescent compound named protoporphyrin IX (PpIX) which is derived from 5-aminolevulinic acid (5-ALA). Studies have shown that PpIX accumulates preferentially in malignant glioma cells and is highly fluorescent with a maximum absorption of 440 nm. This property can be exploited intraoperatively to demarcate malignant cells for resection during a fluorescence-guided surgery (Ngyuen and Tsien 2013). Clinical studies have shown this compound can improve the rate of complete resections (Quick-Weller et al. 2016). Both surgical resection and re-irradiation are considered local therapies which independently have demonstrated acceptable median survival times of 8–11 months. The combination of both modalities in the setting of recurrent high-grade glioma is less well studied, but Palmer et al. (2015) demonstrated that the addition of re-resection to re-irradiation added no additional survival benefit. Typically, the use of repeat surgical resection appears most efficacious in the setting of a small recurrence in an operable location in which resection is expected to alleviate symptomatic requirement of steroids.

There are few randomised controlled clinical trials in the treatment of recurrent glioma. Wong et al. (1999) published a review on outcomes and prognostic factors for recurrent gliomas treated within phase II clinical trials. From the eight studies reviewed, the progression-free survival at 6 months was 21 %, median progression-free survival was 10 weeks and median overall survival was 30 weeks. GBM patients had significantly poorer outcomes than anaplastic astrocytoma patients. Results were also worse for those with more than two prior operations or two prior chemotherapy regimens.

Huncharek and Muscat (1998) published a systematic review of outcomes from treatment of high-grade gliomas at relapse. This included 40 trials (36 non-randomised controlled trials and 4 randomised controlled trials). Thirty-two of the trials addressed the outcome post chemotherapy; 7 were radiation therapy trials. The nitrosoureas were associated with significantly extended time to tumour progression compared to all other drugs (26.9 weeks). The nitrosoureas and platinums were the most active drugs with regard to overall survival (32 weeks). Average median survival for patients treated with radiation was 44.7 weeks but selection bias prevented comparison with chemotherapy studies.

The use of temozolomide at recurrence has been investigated in several phase II studies with varying dose regimes and seems to be associated with improved progression-free and overall survival (Yung et al. 1999; Wick et al. 2004, 2007). New information on biomarker selection for patients who are likely to be sensitive to temozolomide may alter the proportion of patients who are deemed suitable for this treatment (Weller et al. 2015).

One of the main limitations of systemic therapy is that a significant proportion of patients have grade III/IV haematological toxicity from first-line chemotherapy. Therefore, a significant proportion has reduced bone marrow reserve at progression. Current standard treatment is to offer chemotherapy or a novel agent along with chemotherapy, but a local agent without systemic toxicity would be advantageous in these circumstances.

Re-irradiation for gliomas has attracted controversy in the past but is receiving more attention due to advances in radiotherapy techniques and imaging modalities, which may reduce concerns related to the risk of late neurological toxicity.

3 The Biology of Late Central Nervous System Toxicity

Historically, CNS toxicity following irradiation has been divided into three phases – early (days-weeks after), early delayed (1–6 months after and including somnolence syndrome and Lhermitte's phenomenon due to transient demyelination) and late (greater than 6 months following irradiation). Early and early-delayed toxicity are normally reversible and spontaneously resolve whereas late toxicity is normally progressive and irreversible.

Late injury is characterised pathologically by demyelination, vascular changes and ultimately necrosis. Therefore, much focus has been on the radioresponse of the vasculature and the oligodendrocyte population. Radiation induces damage to endothelial cells and the loss of 02A progenitor cells, which results in failure to replace oligodendrocytes and subsequent demyelination. There is an additional role involving astrocytes, microglia, neurons and neural stem cells. The biology of late CNS toxicity is therefore thought to be a complex dynamic process involving many cell types and interactions with no known effective means of prevention or treatment (Tofilon and Fike 2000; Wong and van der Kogel 2004; Wong et al. 2015).

Available animal data come mainly from studies investigating spinal cord tolerance to irradiation. The pathogenesis of radiation toxicity and recovery potential in the brain is assumed to be similar to the spinal cord, and the structures of the central nervous system are assumed to have a low α/β ratio (Hall and Giaccia 2005; Withers 1985). Preclinical data suggest that there is significant recovery following irradiation. Therefore, the toxicity resulting from retreatment depends on dose, volume and time between exposures. A conservative estimate is that up to 50% recovery may occur within 1–2 years post initial treatment if doses that fall below full tolerance were given at first exposure. In preclinical models within the spinal cord, no microscopic lesions were seen with a cumulative dose less than 110 Gy (Ang et al. 2001).

4 Factors for Predicting Better Survival

Carson et al. (2007) published an evaluation on prognostic factors for patients with recurrent high-grade gliomas based on ten prospective phase I and II trials and using a recursive partitioning analysis (RPA) to define seven prognostic groups. Relevant prognostic factors included performance status, initial histology, age and corticosteroid use. They concluded that patients with recurrent gliomas entering clinical trials have widely variable outcomes, many of which depend on initial clinical characteristics and demographics. In addition, time from initial radiation to re-irradiation (12 months) has been shown to be strongly prognostic (Combs et al. 2013b). These may be applicable in selecting patients for re-irradiation, patient counselling and treatment avoidance or design for future clinical trials.

5 Evidence for Re-irradiation

There are over 50 clinical studies in the literature on the re-irradiation of gliomas. The majority of these studies are retrospective and use a variety of techniques including brachytherapy, fractionated stereotactic radiotherapy, radiosurgery and conformal radiotherapy with or without new systemic agents (see Table 1). As well as using differing techniques, the available data uses a wide range of doses and volumes highlighting the fact that no standard approach exists in this context

Table 1 Summary of the largest re-irradiation studies for patients with recurrent gliomas

Author	Case number	Technique/dose	Median survival
Brachytherapy			
Scharfen et al. (1992)	66 GBM	Brachytherapy I-125 64.4 Gy	11.3 months
Sneed et al. (1997)	66 GBM 45 WHO III	Brachytherapy I-125 64.4 Gy	11.7 months 12.3 months
Gabayan et al. (2006)	81 GBM 14 WHO III	Gliasite brachytherapy 60 Gy at 10 mm	35.9 weeks 43.6 weeks
Tselis et al. (2007)	84 GBM	Brachytherapy Ir-192 40 Gy	37 weeks
Fabrini et al. (2009)	18 GBM 3 WHO III	HDR brachytherapy 18 Gy	8.0 months
Stereotactic radiosurgery			
Shrieve et al. (1995)	86 GBM	Stereotactic radiosurgery 13 Gy	10.5 months
Cho et al. (1999)	46 GBM	Stereotactic radiosurgery 17 Gy	11.0 months
Combs et al. (2005a)	32 GBM	Stereotactic radiosurgery Median 15 Gy (10–20 Gy)	10.0 months
Combs et al. (2005b)	54 GBM 39 WHO III	Stereotactic radiotherapy 36 Gy (15–62 Gy) 5 × 2 Gy conventional fractionation	8.0 months 16.0 months
Kong et al. (2008)	65 GBM 49 WHO III	Stereotactic radiosurgery 16 Gy	13.0 months 26.0 months
Patel et al. (2009)	36 GBM	Stereotactic radiosurgery 18 Gy Fractionated stereotactic radiotherapy 36 Gy in 6 fractions	8.5 months 7.4 months
Cuneo et al. (2012)	49 GBM	Stereotactic radiosurgery 15 Gy	10 months

(continued)

Table 1 (continued)

Author	Case number	Technique/dose	Median survival
Hypofractionated stereotactic radiotherapy			
Shepherd et al. (1997)	33 GBM	Hypofractionated conformal radiotherapy Escalation 20–50 Gy	11.0 months
Hudes et al. (1999)	19 GBM 1 WHO III	Stereotactic hypofractionated radiotherapy Escalation 24 Gy (3 Gy/F) – 35 Gy (3.5 Gy/F)	10.5 months
Lederman et al. (2000)	88 GBM	Stereotactic hypofractionated radiotherapy Median 24 Gy in 4 fractions	7.0 months
Grosu et al. (2005)	44 GBM	Stereotactic hypofractionated radiotherapy 36 PET/SPECT 30 Gy 8 CT/MRI (6 × 5 Gy)	9.0 months 5.0 months
Fokas et al. (2009)	53 GBM	Stereotactic hypofractionated radiotherapy 30 Gy in 10 fractions	9.0 months
Fogh et al. (2010)	105 GBM 42 WHO III	Stereotactic hypofractionated radiotherapy Median 35 Gy in 10 fractions	11.0 months 10.0 months
Palmer et al. (2015)	161 GBM 59 WHO III	Stereotactic hypofractionated radiotherapy Median 35 Gy in 10 fractions	10.8 months
Conventionally fractionated stereotactic radiotherapy			
Arcicasa et al. (1999)	31 GBM	Fractionated conventional 2D radiotherapy 34.5 Gy in 23 fractions (1.5 Gy/F)	13.7 months
Cho et al. (1999)	25 GBM	Conventional fractionated radiotherapy 37.5 Gy in 15 fractions	12.0 months
Koshi et al. (2007)	11 GBM 14 WHO III	Stereotactic radiotherapy 22 Gy in 8 fractions/8 F (+ hyperbaric oxygen)	11.0 months 19.0 months
Combs et al. (2008)	8 GBM 10 WHO III 7 WHO II	Stereotactic radiotherapy 36 Gy in 2 Gy per fraction (+ temozolomide 50 mg/m^2)	9.0 months

(Nieder et al. 2006). There are, therefore, severe limitations when comparing these studies that are compounded by a lack of standardised recording of radiotherapy variables and toxicity outcomes.

5.1 Conformal Radiotherapy

Over the past decade, there have been improvements in radiotherapy and imaging techniques to improve target definition. 3D conventional radiotherapy using co-registered magnetic resonance imaging (MRI) has improved target definition and allows the dose to normal structures to be reduced. Further developments such as IMRT (intensity-modulated radiotherapy) can improve this further by improving conformality at the target using multiple modulated beams. With re-irradiation planning and treatment, the intention is generally to treat the area of recurrence with an adequate margin while avoiding the total dose to critical organs at risk within the CNS, such as the optic nerves or the brainstem, making highly conformal approaches very appealing in this context (Figs. 1 and 2).

5.2 Stereotactic Radiosurgery/ Fractionated Stereotactic Radiotherapy

In brain radiotherapy, stereotactic methods offer optimal precision of target definition while minimising dose to the surrounding tissues. This treatment technique usually utilises exact positioning of the patient using a frame-based structure for three-dimensional localisation.

Stereotactic radiosurgery (delivered using the Leksell Gamma Knife, adapted linear accelerators, CyberKnife and other devices) is a non-invasive, highly conformal radiotherapy technique. It allows very accurate dose delivery

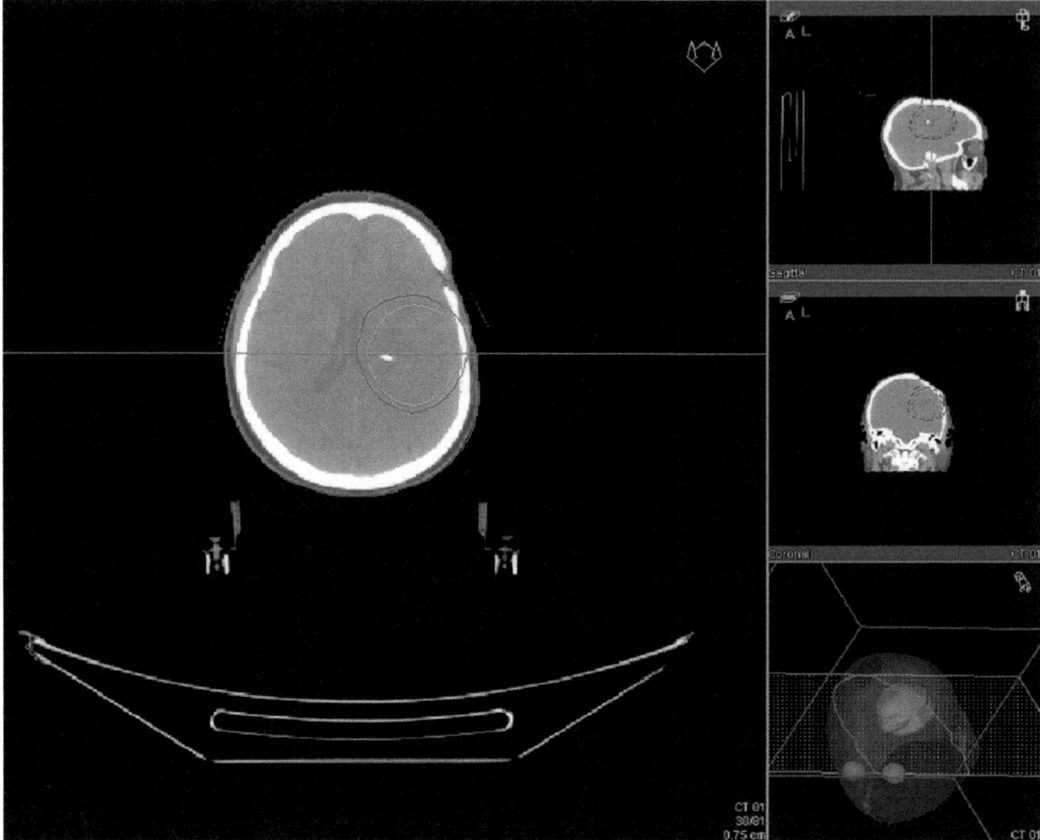

Fig. 1 CT and MRI-fused planning images for a patient treated for a recurrent glioma. Ten years previously treated with 55 Gy in 30 fractions over 6 weeks. Re-irradiated with 30 Gy in 6 fractions over 2 weeks. *CTV* (*Blue contour*) contrast-enhancing volume on T1-weighted MRI, *PTV* (*Red contour*) CTV + 0.5 cm margin

with the patient in a fixed head frame, and multiple beam sources produce a steep dose gradient at the edge of the target, therefore allowing a highly precise dose to be delivered to tumour while sparing the surrounding normal tissues and organs at risk. The treatment is limited to smaller volumes as the risk of radiotherapy-related side effects increases with both volume treated and dose. The treatment is usually given in a single fraction (Figs. 3 and 4).

In fractionated stereotactic radiotherapy, the dose is divided over several fractions, which is made possible by using relocatable head frames or image-guided frameless systems. This has the radiobiological advantage of sparing toxicity to normal tissues due to fractionation and the allowance of normal tissue repair during treatment. This technique can therefore be used to treat larger volumes compared to stereotactic radiosurgery (Fig. 5).

Shepherd et al. (1997) reported on 29 recurrent high-grade glioma patients treated with a variety of doses of stereotactic hypofractionated re-irradiation who had a median survival of 11 months. This compared favourably to a matched cohort of patients treated with nitrosourea chemotherapy with a median survival of 7 months. In this study, a stereotactic radiotherapy dose of >40 Gy was found to be a significant predictor of radiation damage. There was also a trend towards higher risk of complications for larger volumes irradiated.

More recent data on response to radiosurgery or fractionated stereotactic radiotherapy in the retreatment of high-grade glioma reported a median survival of 8 months with radiologi-

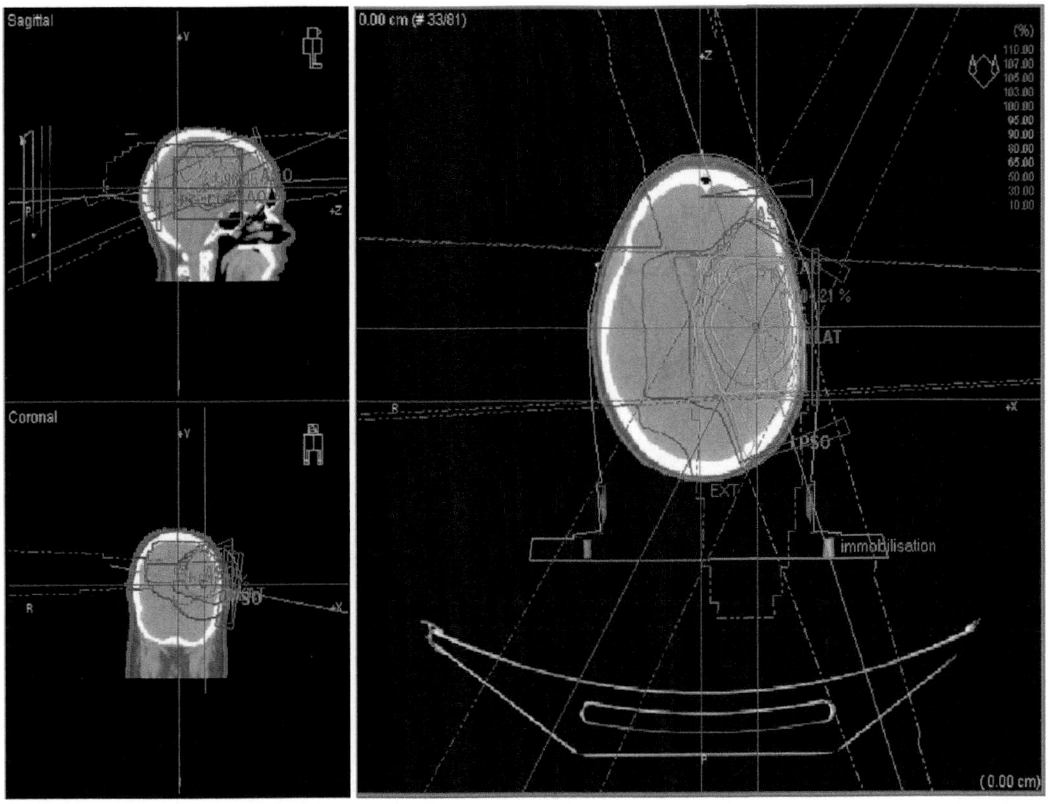

Fig. 2 Image showing four-field conformal radiotherapy axial plan for the same patient

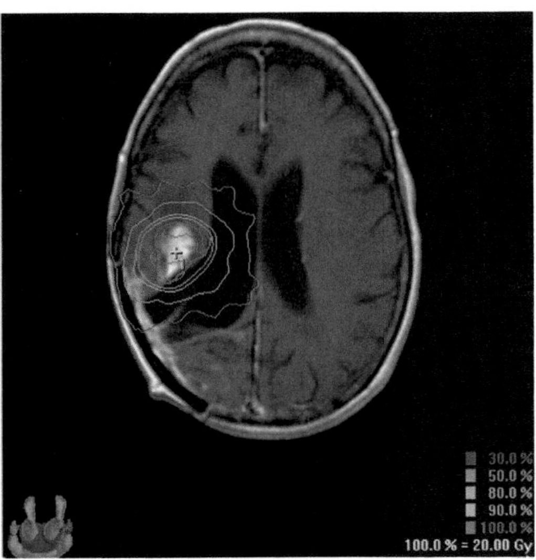

Fig. 3 A 57-year-old patient with recurrent glioblastoma of the right temporal lobe anterior to the surgical resection cavity. The targeted volume was 12.3 ml. The patient was treated with SRS to a dose of 18 Gy prescribed to the 90 % isodose line

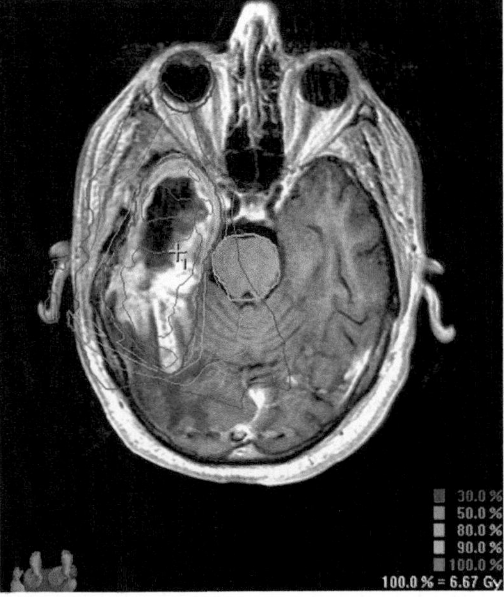

Fig. 4 A 44-year-old patient with recurrent glioblastoma of the right temporal lobe. The targeted volume was 123.3 ml. The patient was treated with FSRT to a dose of 36 Gy in 6 fractions prescribed to the 90 % isodose line due to the large tumour volume and close proximity of critical structures

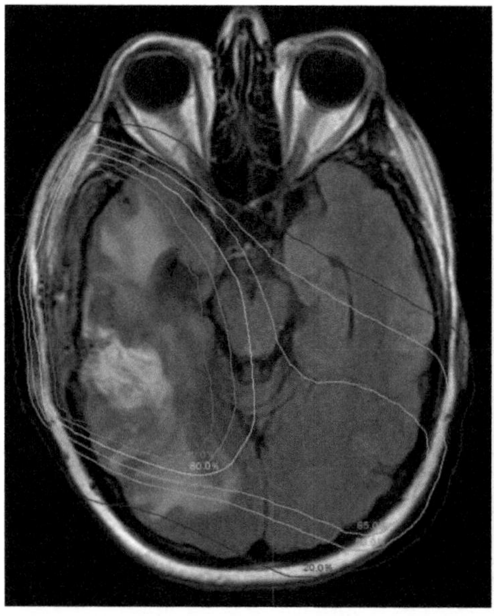

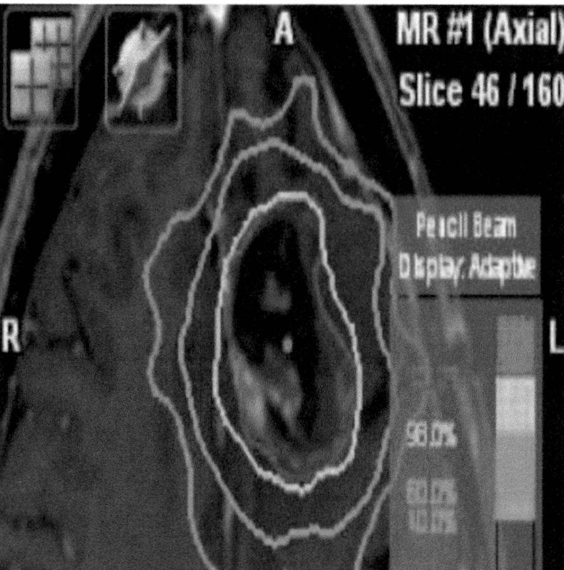

Fig. 5 MRI images used for radiation treatment planning. The *left panel* depicts a conformal radiation treatment plan with large portions of the brain receiving at least 50 % of the prescription dose (*blue isodose line*). The *right panel* depicts a fractionated stereotactic radiation treatment plan with a much steeper dose gradient with less brain receiving at least 40 % of the prescription dose (*blue isodose line*)

cal response rate of 40 % based on MRI criteria (Patel et al. 2009).

There is an ongoing clinical trial at the National Cancer Institute addressing hypofractionated stereotactic radiation therapy dose escalation (NCT02709226). The study is a phase I 3+3 design trial with three pre-planned dose levels: 3.5 Gy × 10 fractions, 3.5 Gy × 12 fractions and 3.5 Gy × 14 fractions.

5.3 Brachytherapy

Brachytherapy delivers radiation over a short distance therefore requiring the radiation source to be placed in close contact with the volume being treated. Most studies in the brain have used ^{125}I or ^{192}I. Placement of multiple sources of radiation around the surgical cavity is technically challenging to ensure an adequate and even dose distribution. A recent review by Combs et al. (2007) reports on the available but limited data on brachytherapy for recurrent gliomas (see Table 1). It should be noted that patients who are selected for brachytherapy are normally those with resectable tumours, good performance status and small volume of disease. High reoperation rates and radionecrosis incidence have been reported using these techniques.

5.4 Radiobiology of Re-irradiation of Gliomas

Although the biology of re-irradiation responses in the CNS remains to be fully understood, there is now a significant body of clinical and pre-clinical data which allow broad conclusions to be drawn and recommendations made. Mayer and Sminia (2008) identified and analysed 21 re-irradiation studies and reviewed the available clinical data on re-irradiation of gliomas with respect to tolerance of the normal brain tissue. They found that the incidence of toxicity, including radionecrosis, may be significantly under-reported since only symptomatic necrosis is likely to be recorded. According to their analysis, the major factor contributing to necrosis was the total dose received. There was no correlation between time to re-irradiation and the development of necrosis, although the minimum time interval between treatments in this data set was 3 months. Importantly, they concluded that the incidence of necrosis did not increase significantly until the total cumulative dose reached 100 Gy.

5.5 Conclusions Based on Clinical Evidence

Despite a large body of clinical work, there remains no standard protocol for re-irradiation of brain tumours. The clinical data are limited by the variety of techniques that have been used, which may be associated with different risks of toxicity. Specific toxicity is also often poorly reported in these studies and important variables are often not recorded.

Further limitations of the clinical evidence include problems distinguishing necrosis from recurrence on imaging. It is well established that standard, T1-weighted MRI sequences distinguish poorly between recurrent tumour and necrosis, which can often appear as a new enhancing lesion. The poor dose definitions also make comparisons between studies difficult. Some studies have used concomitant chemotherapy, which may have been a confounding factor. There are very few data on the quality of life following re-irradiation – an important consideration in a poor prognostic group (Nieder et al. 2008).

Overall, though, available data suggest that there may be a select group of patients with recurrent glioma in whom re-irradiation may be a safe and effective approach.

Ideally, radiotherapy should be highly conformal to keep the treated volume as small as possible and reduce late side effects to organs at risk and normal brain tissue. Many series suggest that limiting the target volume to approximately 4–5 cm minimises the risk of toxicity and suggests that if larger volumes are being targeted then consideration should be made for reducing the dose.

Most recurrent glioma patients will have received the equivalent of 55–60 Gy in 1.8–2 Gy per fraction when they were initially treated, and therefore not more than 40 Gy equivalent in a hypofractionated regime should be delivered when re-irradiating, aiming to keep the total dose less than 100 Gy (Mayer and Sminia 2008).

Available data do not suggest that there is an obvious limitation on the time between treatment courses, although most clinicians would not treat within a year, as these patients are likely to have primary treatment resistance.

Performance status of the patient and the potential impact on their quality of life should be taken into account. Consideration should be given to the impact of prolonged treatment courses in the context of poor prognosis disease.

6 Imaging

6.1 Target Definition

Contrast-enhanced thin-sliced MRI imaging using gadolinium remains the gold standard imaging modality for target delineation for gliomas. The problems are that following surgery or radiotherapy, the signal change based on gadolinium enhancement can be non-specific making accurate target definition a challenge. Most gliomas recur within 4 cm from the margin of the original lesion, and this is often where non-specific signal change due to surgery and prior treatment are also apparent (Gaspar et al. 1992; Chan et al. 2002).

To optimise the outcome of radiotherapy treatment, improved target definition is of paramount importance. In this context, alternative biological imaging may improve the definition of the relevant target, for example, amino acid PET (SPECT)/CT/MRI image fusion to determine the gross tumour volume is currently under investigation (GLIAA-NCT01252459).

Typically, the gross tumour volume is delineated as the new or progressive contrast-enhancing lesion. For stereotactic radiosurgery or fractionated stereotactic techniques, typically no margin is added; however, based on physician preference or other treatment parameters, a small 1–2 mm margin may be added. Recently, several studies have assessed the value of adding a lower dose to the surrounding T2/FLAIR volume due to the possibility that this may encompass low-grade or transforming tumour (Clark et al. 2014).

6.2 Diagnosing Radionecrosis

There is no gold standard imaging modality that can distinguish true tissue necrosis from tumour recurrence associated with recurrence (Ullrich et al. 2008). Conventional MRI techniques have limitations when discriminating tumour recurrence and treatment-induced injury. This may become possible with advances in imaging technology such as perfusion-weighted, diffusion-weighted and magnetic resonance spectroscopy (Bobek-Billewicz et al. 2010). Early studies using ^{18}F-FDG PET reported sensitivities of 81–86 % and specificities of 40–94 % when distinguishing between radiation necrosis and recurrent tumour (Langleben and Segall 2000). Further studies are awaited but co-registration of MRI and amino acid tracers may improve the diagnostic accuracy (Chen 2007; Götz and Grosu 2013).

6.3 Diagnosing Progression

For many years, the Macdonald criteria developed in 1990 was the gold standard in assessing response to treatment in high-grade gliomas. These criteria were based on two-dimensional tumour measurements and clinical assessments (Macdonald et al. 1990). These criteria focused on the contrast-enhancing lesions only and have limited use to differentiate pseudoprogression from true progression. The new standardised response criteria for glioma clinical trials are the updated Response Assessment Criteria in Neuro-Oncology (RANO) criteria developed in 2010 (Wen et al. 2010). These updated criteria differentiate between measurable and non-measurable lesions on contrast-enhanced CT, MRI T1 post-contrast and T2 imaging. A measurable lesion is defined as a contrast-enhancing lesion with clearly demarcated margins, seen on two or more axial slices with a maximum diameter of at least 10 mm excluding a cystic cavity. Non-measurable lesions are those with cystic or necrotic components or a surgical cavity. For these lesions, the peripheral nodular component is considered measurable. Criteria for progression of disease based on RANO criteria include a 25 % or more increase in enhancing lesions despite increasing steroid dose; a significant increase in non-enhancing T2/FLAIR, not attributable to other causes; any new lesions; and clinical deterioration.

The diagnosis of true tumour progression can be difficult as approximately 20–30 % of patients may develop pseudoprogression after concurrent chemoradiotherapy (Brandsma et al. 2008). Pseudoprogression is a manifestation of treatment-related effects and is more likely in MGMT-methylated glioblastoma patients. Newer imaging techniques have been developed which may also aid in the differentiation between early tumour progression and pseudoprogression. Perfusion MRI imaging measuring cerebral blood volume changes may predict early tumour progression as true tumour progression manifests as an increase in relative cerebral blood volume (rCBV), and radionecrosis more likely manifests with a relative decrease in rCBV (Surapaneni et al. 2015). Additionally, diffusion-weighted MRI imaging and apparent diffusion coefficient maps may also predict early tumour progression as true progression is more likely correlated with low ADC values (Chu et al. 2013).

7 Combination Treatment

Few studies have addressed the addition of conventional cytotoxics when re-irradiating brain tumours. Some of the studies combining new agents with radiotherapy are described below. The combination of temozolomide and re-irradiation has been found to be safe and effective. In a study combining fractionated stereotactic radiotherapy and concomitant temozolomide in 25 patients with recurrent gliomas, median survival from re-irradiation was 8 months. Treatment was completed in all patients as scheduled without interruptions greater than 3 days, and no severe treatment-related side effects were observed (Combs et al. 2008). In a phase II trial, concurrent temozolomide delivered with conventional radiotherapy achieved an overall response rate of 20.6 % with a median progression-free survival of 10.1 months. The combined therapy was well tolerated and HR-QOL was improved (Osman 2014).

Darakchiev et al. (2008) reported on 34 patients with recurrent GBM and following re-resection who were treated by implantation with ^{125}I seeds and Gliadel wafers to the resection bed. They documented that patients with a Karnofsky performance status less than 70 were more likely to have a worse outcome. One-year survival was 66 % but this was a small, non-randomised study, and brain necrosis was observed in 24 % of cases associated with a tumour volume of >30 cm^3.

Gefitinib (an inhibitor of epidermal growth factor receptor's (EGFR) tyrosine kinase domain) has also been given with fractionated stereotactic radiotherapy with dose escalation up to 36 Gy in 3 fractions in a small phase I study in the re-irradiation setting of GBM and WHO grade III gliomas. Treatment was well tolerated and median OS was reported at 10 months (Schwer et al. 2008).

Gutin et al. (2009) combined hypofractionated stereotactic radiotherapy (30 Gy in 5 fractions) with bevacizumab (a humanised monoclonal antibody to vascular endothelial growth factor (VEGF)). They documented a 50 % response rate in the GBM population and a median overall survival of 12.5 months. It has also been reported in an individual case report that bevacizumab may reverse radiation-induced necrosis. In a patient with temporal lobe necrosis following radiotherapy for nasopharyngeal cancer, radiologically defined necrosis was reversed using this drug (Wong et al. 2008). Torcuator et al. (2009) reported on a further group of six patients with biopsy-proven radionecrosis. These six received bevacizumab; all had a radiological response and three also improved clinically. A small randomised double-blind placebo-controlled trial with 14 patients confirmed that bevacizumab might be a treatment option for patients with radiation necrosis (Levin et al. 2011). There is an ongoing cooperative group phase II trial, NRG 1205, which randomises patients between bevacizumab alone and hypofractionated radiation to 35 Gy in 10 fractions with bevacizumab (NCT02671981).

Panobinostat (an oral pan-histone deacetylase (HDAC) inhibitor) has been administered with fractionated stereotactic radiotherapy to 35 Gy in 10 fractions. Panobinostat was given in escalating doses in this phase I trial using a 3+3 design. Panobinostat was well tolerated and a maximum tolerated dose was not found. The median overall survival for patients receiving the maximum dose of 30 mg was 16.1 months (Shi et al. 2016).

Immune checkpoint inhibitors have shown antitumour activity in both solid tumours and preclinical glioma models. CHECKMATE-143 is a phase I trial for recurrent glioblastoma patients evaluating the safety and tolerability of combination immunotherapy nivolumab and ipilimumab. Nivolumab is a PD-1 inhibitor and ipilimumab targets CTLA-4. Results were presented at the American Society of Clinical Oncology 2015 annual meeting, demonstrating the combination is safe with no drug-related deaths and five patients experienced grade 3 or 4 adverse events with the combination immunotherapy, including colitis, cholecystitis, diabetic ketoacidosis, confusion and increased lipase. The 6-month survival rate was 75 % (Sampson et al. 2015). There is an ongoing cooperative group trial NRG-BN002 assessing the safety of the immune checkpoint inhibitors ipilimumab and nivolumab in the maintenance temozolomide phase of treatment (NCT02311920). Additionally, there is a phase I trial combining pembrolizumab (anti PD-1), bevacizumab and hypofractionated radiation in recurrent glioblastoma (NCT02313272).

Dietary manipulation in preclinical models has demonstrated the ability to inhibit the growth of glioma cells and synergize with radiation therapy to improve overall survival (http://www.ncbi.nlm.nih.gov/pubmed/22563484). Several forms of dietary manipulation are typically recommended including the ketogenic and calorie restriction diets. Retrospective studies in GBM patients appeared promising demonstrating that the dietary manipulation was feasible during concurrent chemoradiotherapy (Champ et al. 2014). In addition, a pilot study (ERGO) conducted in recurrent glioblastoma demonstrated a ketogenic diet is safe and feasible with a median survival of 32 weeks (Rieger et al. 2014). One major issue using dietary manipulation is the lack of palatability of the restrictive ketogenic diet and potential side effects associated with long-term carbohydrate restriction. A recent preclinical study demonstrated that a less stringent, supplemented high-fat, low-carbohydrate diet is a viable treatment alternative to the ketogenic diet and may be more easily tolerated (Martuscello et al. 2015). There are two ongoing clinical trials combining a low-carbohydrate (ketogenic) diet with re-irradiation in recurrent GBM patients (NCT02149459, ERGO2-NCT01754350).

Data such as these may broaden the applicability of re-irradiation even further since co-treatment with new agents may improve response rates and/or improve the therapeutic ratio by reducing the risk of major side effects.

8 Clinical Impact of Late Central Nervous System Toxicity

The suitability for re-irradiation must be considered on an individual patient basis and when the potential for benefit outweighs the risks. The impact on an individual's quality of life from late toxicity must not be underestimated. Patients may experience worsening of their presenting symptoms due to the original tumour, including focal neurological deficits. Any high-dose brain irradiation is also associated with a risk of memory problems, cognitive impairment and personality change. Focal normal tissue damage as a result of re-irradiation may also be associated with higher seizure risk, and an expanding mass related to radionecrosis may require surgical intervention to relieve pressure symptoms.

There are few prospective studies addressing quality of life prospectively in recurrent glioblastoma. However, there is prospective data that correlates patient's symptom burden, neurocognitive function and quality of life with overall survival in newly diagnosed GBM patients. Analysis of the RTOG 0525 study net clinical benefit (NCB) as measured by a collection of neurocognitive tests, quality of life assessments and symptom burden demonstrated that baseline and early change in the NCB measures were associated with decreased rates of survival (Armstrong et al. 2013). Similar associations have been noted in the Avaglio trial (Taphoorn et al. 2015). It is important that future prospective recurrent GBM studies include quality of life, symptom burden and/or neurocognitive function assessments as these are important measures that correlate with patient survival.

9 Future Directions

There have been a number of attempts in newly diagnosed and recurrent GBM clinical trials to combine standard therapy with novel targeted therapy. Largely these trials have failed (cilengitide, bevacizumab) to demonstrate a survival benefit (Stupp et al. 2014; Gilbert et al. 2014). This is not surprising given the TCGA analysis of glioblastoma patients demonstrated marked mutational heterogeneity with patients categorised within four main groups (Brennan et al. 2013). In the era of personalised or tailored therapy, it is becoming clear that targeted therapies must be administered to patients most likely to benefit. The best example of this is the excellent results of rindopepimut, a unique epidermal growth factor receptor (EGFR) vIII peptide sequence conjugated to keyhole limpet hemocyanin, which is an immunotherapy targeting patients with EGFRvIII deletion mutations and has demonstrated immune responses as well as a median survival of 21.8 months (Schuster et al. 2015). The ongoing ACT IV phase III trial will build on this paradigm of targeting specific patient populations within glioblastoma. Thus trials administering targeted therapies to patients based on validated biomarkers are most likely to demonstrate efficacy. In addition, there are many patients who are unable to have adequate tumour tissue to undergo mutational analysis and genome sequencing in order to tailor therapy. New research suggests that circulating exosomes (ctDNA, miRNA) may aid in the diagnosis and treatment of patients with glioblastoma. Especially in light of the marked inter- and intra-tumour heterogeneity, these very promising biomarkers have the capability of profiling the whole tumour genome (Westphal and

Lamszus 2015). An alternative is to administer a modality whose mechanism does not rely on specific mutations or pathways such as NovoTTF or high LET radiation (carbon ions). There is retrospective data comparing carbon ion with photon radiotherapy which favours carbon ions (Combs et al. 2013a). Based on these results, a randomised trial is underway CLEOPATRA (NCT01165671). NovoTTF (Optune), a device worn on the patient's scalp that disrupts mitosis by transmitting low intensity, alternating electric fields across the tumour, has demonstrated improved progression-free and overall survival in newly diagnosed glioblastoma patients (Stupp et al. 2015). NovoTTF is currently under study in combination with bevacizumab and radiotherapy in recurrent glioblastoma (NCT01925573).

Conclusions

Recurrent glioblastoma is a difficult disease to treat as these patients have a limited survival and few studies adequately demonstrate a clear benefit. It is important that these patients are seen at centres with multidisciplinary teams to address the risks and benefits of surgery, systemic therapy and re-irradiation.

There is a patient group with recurrent gliomas for whom re-irradiation may be appropriate. The available literature suggests that re-irradiation is safe in well-selected patients, but as we have discussed, there are limitations with the available evidence. With advances in functional imaging technology, new approaches to target definition deserve investigation. The additional benefit of conventional cytotoxics is unknown but the new agent combinations look promising for further studies.

Prospective trials are needed to compare re-irradiation to newer systemic agents or re-irradiation in combination with newer agents. The impact on quality of life of re-irradiation with or without systemic therapies is an important component that has not been adequately addressed to date.

Acknowledgement Susan C. Short and Jennifer E. Gains authored the brain tumours chapter for the first edition of this textbook. The present chapter is based on their updated manuscript.

References

Ang K, Jiang GL, Feng Y (2001) Extent and kinetics of recovery of occult spinal cord injury. Int J Radiat Oncol Biol Phys 50:1013–1020

Arcicasa M, Roncadin M, Bidoli E et al (1999) Re-irradiation and lomustine in patients with relapsed high grade gliomas. Int J Radiat Oncol Biol Phys 43:789–793

Armstrong TS, Wefel JS, Wang M et al (2013) Net clinical benefit analysis of radiation therapy oncology group 0525: a phase III trial comparing conventional adjuvant temozolomide with dose-intensive temozolomide in patients with newly diagnosed glioblastoma. J Clin Oncol 31:4076–4084

Bobek-Billewicz B, Stasik-Pres G, Majchrzak H (2010) Differentiation between brain tumour recurrence and radiation injury using perfusion, diffusion-weighted imaging and MR spectroscopy. Folia Neuropathol 48:81–92

Brandsma D, Stalpers L, Taal W et al (2008) Clinical features, mechanisms, and management of pseudoprogression in malignant gliomas. Lancet Oncol 9:453–461

Brem H, Piantadosi S, Burger PC et al (1995) Placebo controlled trial of safety and efficacy of intraoperative controlled delivery by biodegradable polymers of chemotherapy for recurrent gliomas. Lancet 345:1008–1012

Brennan CW, Verhaak RG, McKenna A et al (2013) The somatic genomic landscape of glioblastoma. Cell 155:462–477

Carson K, Grossman S, Fisher J (2007) Prognostic factors for survival in adult patients with recurrent glioma enrolled onto the new approaches to brain tumour therapy CNS consortium phase I and phase II clinical trials. J Clin Oncol 25:2601–2606

Champ CE, Palmer JD, Volek JS et al (2014) Targeting metabolism with a ketogenic diet during the treatment of glioblastoma multiforme. J Neurooncol 117:125–131

Chan JL, Lee SW, Fraass BA (2002) Survival and failure patterns of high grade gliomas after three-dimensional conformal radiotherapy. J Clin Oncol 20:1635–1642

Chen W (2007) Clinical applications of PET in brain tumours. J Nucl Med 48:1468–1481

Cho KH, Hall WA, Gerbi BJ et al (1999) Single dose versus fractionated stereotactic radiotherapy for recurrent gliomas. Int J Radiat Oncol Biol Phys 45:1133–1141

Chu HH, Choi SH, Ryoo I et al (2013) Differentiation of true progression from pseudoprogression in glioblastoma treated with radiation therapy and concomitant temozolomide: comparison study of standard and high-b-value diffusion-weighted imaging. Radiology 269:831–840

Clark GM, McDonald AM, Nabors LB et al (2014) Hypofractionated stereotactic radiosurgery with concurrent bevacizumab for recurrent malignant gliomas: the University of Alabama at Birmingham experience. Neuro Oncol Pract 1:172–177

Combs SE, Widmer V, Thilman C et al (2005a) Stereotactic radiosurgery (SRS): treatment option for recurrent glioblastoma multiforme. Cancer 104:2168–2173

Combs SE, Thilmann C, Edler L et al (2005b) Efficacy of fractionated stereotactic re-irradiation in recurrent gliomas: long term results in 172 patients treated in a single institution. J Clin Oncol 23:8863–8869

Combs S, Debus J, Schulz-Ertner D (2007) Radiotherapeutic alternatives for previously irradiated recurrent gliomas. BMC Cancer 7:167

Combs S, Bischof M, Welzel T (2008) Radiochemotherapy with temozolomide as re-irradiation using high precision fractionated stereotactic radiotherapy (FSRT) in patients with recurrent gliomas. J Neurooncol 89:205–210

Combs SE, Bruckner T, Mizoe JE et al (2013a) Comparison of carbon ion radiotherapy to photon radiation alone or in combination with temozolomide in patients with high-grade gliomas: explorative hypothesis-generating retrospective analysis. Radiother Oncol 108:132–135

Combs SE, Edler L, Rausch R et al (2013b) Generation and validation of a prognostic score to predict outcome after re-irradiation of recurrent glioma. Acta Oncol 52:147–152

Cuneo KC, Vredenburgh JJ, Sampson JH et al (2012) Safety and efficacy of stereotactic radiosurgery and adjuvant bevacizumab in patients with recurrent malignant gliomas. Int J Radiat Oncol Biol Phys 82:2018–2024

Darakchiev B, Albright R, Breneman J (2008) Safety and efficacy of permanent iodine-125 seed implants and carmustine wafers in patients with recurrent glioblastoma multiforme. J Neurosurg 108:236–242

Fabrini MG, Perrone F, De Franco L et al (2009) Perioperative high-dose-rate brachytherapy in the treatment of recurrent malignant gliomas. Strahlenther Onkol 185:524–529 (erratum:703)

Fogh SE, Andrews DW, Glass J et al (2010) Hypofractionated stereotactic radiation therapy: an effective therapy for recurrent high-grade gliomas. J Clin Oncol 28:3048–3053

Fokas E, Wacker U, Gross MW et al (2009) Hypofractionated stereotactic re-irradiation of recurrent glioblastomas: a beneficial treatment option after high dose radiotherapy. Strahlenther Onkol 185:235–240

Gabayan AJ, Green SB, Sanan A et al (2006) Gliasite brachytherapy for treatment of recurrent malignant gliomas: a retrospective multi-institutional analysis. Neurosurgery 58:701–709

Gaspar LE, Fisher BJ, Macdonald DR et al (1992) Supratentorial malignant glioma: patterns of recurrence and implications for external beam local treatment. Int J Radiat Oncol Biol Phys 24:55–57

Gilbert MR, Dignam JJ, Armstrong TS et al (2014) A randomized trial of bevacizumab for newly diagnosed glioblastoma. N Engl J Med 370:699–708

Götz I, Grosu AL (2013) [(18)F]FET-PET imaging for treatment and response monitoring of radiation therapy in malignant glioma patients – a review. Front Oncol 3:104

Grosu A, Weber W, Franz M et al (2005) Re-irradiation of recurrent high grade gliomas using amino acid PET (SPECT)/CT/MRI fusion to determine gross tumour volume for stereotactic fractionated radiotherapy. Int J Radiat Oncol Biol Phys 63:511–519

Gutin P, Iwamoto F, Beal K et al (2009) Safety and efficacy of bevacizumab with hypofractionated stereotactic irradiation for recurrent malignant gliomas. Int J Radiat Oncol Biol Phys 75:156–163

Hall EJ, Giaccia AJ (2005) Radiobiology for the radiologist, 6th edn. Lippincott Williams and Wilkins, Philadelphia

Hess CF, Schaaf JC, Kortmann RD et al (1994) Malignant glioma: patterns of failure following individually tailored limited volume irradiation. Radiother Oncol 30:146–149

Hudes RS, Corn BW, Werner-Wasik M et al (1999) A phase I dose escalation study of hypofractionated stereotactic radiotherapy as salvage therapy for persistent or recurrent malignant glioma. Int J Radiat Oncol Biol Phys 43:293–298

Huncharek M, Muscat J (1998) Treatment of recurrent high grade astrocytoma; results of a systematic review of 1,415 patients. Anticancer Res 18:1303–1311

Kong DS, Lee JI, Park K et al (2008) Efficacy of stereotactic radiosurgery as a salvage treatment for recurrent malignant gliomas. Cancer 112:2046–2051

Koshi K, Yamamoto H, Nakahara A et al (2007) Fractionated stereotactic radiotherapy using gamma unit after hyperbaric oxygenation on recurrent high-grade gliomas. J Neurooncol 82:297–303

Langleben DD, Segall GM (2000) PET in differentiation of recurrent brain tumour from radiation injury. J Nucl Med 41:1861–1867

Lederman G, Wronski M, Arbit E (2000) Treatment of recurrent glioblastoma multiforme using fractionated stereotactic radiosurgery and concurrent paclitaxel. Am J Clin Oncol 23:155–159

Levin VA, Bidaut L, Hou P et al (2011) Randomized double-blind placebo-controlled trial of bevacizumab therapy for radiation necrosis of the central nervous system. Int J Radiat Oncol Biol Phys 79:1487–1495

Macdonald D, Cascino T, Schold SJ et al (1990) Response criteria for phase II studies of supratentorial malignant glioma. J Clin Oncol 8:1277–1280

Martuscello RT, Vedam-Mai V, McCarthy DJ et al. (2015) A supplemented high-fat low-carbohydrate diet for the treatment of glioblastoma. Clin Cancer Res 22:2482–2495

Mayer R, Sminia P (2008) Reirradiation tolerance of the human brain. Int J Radiat Oncol Biol Phys 70:1350–1360

Ngyuen QT, Tsien RY (2013) Fluorescence-guided surgery with live molecular navigation — a new cutting edge. Nat Rev Cancer 13:653–662

Nieder C, Adam M, Molls M et al (2006) Therapeutic options for recurrent high-grade glioma in adult patients: recent advances. Crit Rev Oncol Hematol 60:181–193

Nieder C, Astner ST, Mehta MP et al (2008) Improvement, clinical course, and quality of life after palliative radiotherapy for recurrent glioblastoma. Am J Clin Oncol 31:300–305

Osman MA (2014) Phase II trial of temozolomide and reirradiation using conformal 3D-radiotherapy in recurrent brain gliomas. Ann Transl Med 2:44

Palmer JD, Siglin J, Yamoah K et al (2015) Re-resection for recurrent high-grade glioma in the setting of re-irradiation: more is not always better. J Neurooncol 124:215–221

Patel M, Siddiqui F, Jin J-Y et al (2009) Salvage re-irradiation for recurrent glioblastoma with radiosurgery: radiographic response and improved survival. J Neurooncol 92:185–191

Quick-Weller J, Lescher S, Forster MT et al (2016) Combination of 5-ALA and iMRI in re-resection of recurrent glioblastoma. Br J Neurosurg 8:1–5

Rieger J, Bahr O, Maurer GD et al (2014) ERGO: a pilot study of ketogenic diet in recurrent glioblastoma. Int J Oncol 44:1843–1852

Sampson JH, Vlahovic G, Sahebjam S et al. (2015) Preliminary safety and activity of nivolumab and its combination with ipilimumab in recurrent glioblastoma (GBM): CHECKMATE-143. J Clin Oncol ASCO Ann Meet Proc 33(3010S)

Scharfen CO, Sneed PK, Wara WM et al (1992) High activity iodine-125 interstitial implant for gliomas. Int J Radiat Oncol Biol Phys 24:583–591

Schuster J, Lai RK, Recht LD et al (2015) A phase II, multicenter trial of rindopepimut (CDX-110) in newly diagnosed glioblastoma: the ACT III study. Neuro Oncol 17:854–861

Schwer A, Damek D, Kavanagh B et al (2008) A phase I dose escalation study of fractionated stereotactic radiosurgery in combination with gefitinib in patients with recurrent malignant gliomas. Int J Radiat Oncol Biol Phys 70:993–1001

Shepherd S, Laing R, Cosgrove V et al (1997) Hypofractionated stereotactic radiotherapy in the management of recurrent glioma. Int J Radiat Oncol Biol Phys 37:393–398

Shi W, Palmer JD, Werner-Wasik M et al. (2016) Phase I trial of panobinostat and fractionated stereotactic re-irradiation therapy for recurrent high grade gliomas. J Neurooncol 127:535–539

Shrieve DC, Alexander E 3rd, Wen PY et al (1995) Comparison of stereotactic radiosurgery and brachytherapy in the treatment of recurrent glioblastoma multiforme. Neurosurgery 36:275–282

Sneed PK, McDermott MW, Gutin PH (1997) Interstitial brachytherapy procedures for brain tumours. Semin Surg Oncol 13:157–166

Stupp R, Hegi ME, Mason WP et al (2009) Effects of radiotherapy with concomitant and adjuvant temozolomide versus radiotherapy alone on survival in glioblastoma in a randomised phase II study: 5-year analysis of the EORTC-NCIC trial. Lancet Oncol 10:459–466

Stupp R, Hegi ME, Gorlia T et al (2014) Cilengitide combined with standard treatment for patients with newly diagnosed glioblastoma with methylated MGMT promoter (CENTRIC EORTC 26071-22072 study): a multicentre, randomised, open-label, phase 3 trial. Lancet Oncol 15:1199–1208

Stupp R, Taillibert S, Kanner AA et al (2015) Maintenance therapy with tumor-treating fields plus temozolomide vs temozolomide alone for glioblastoma. JAMA 314:2535–2543

Surapaneni K, Kennedy BC, Yanagihara TK et al (2015) Early cerebral blood volume changes predict progression after convection-enhanced delivery of topotecan for recurrent malignant glioma. World Neurosurg 84:163–172

Taphoorn MJ, Henriksson R, Bottomley A et al (2015) Health-related quality of life in a randomized phase III study of bevacizumab, temozolomide, and radiotherapy in newly diagnosed glioblastoma. J Clin Oncol 33:2166–2175

Tofilon P, Fike J (2000) The radioresponse of the central nervous system: a dynamic process. Radiat Res 153:357–370

Torcuator R, Zuniga R, Mohan YS (2009) Initial experience with bevacizumab treatment for biopsy confirmed cerebral radiation necrosis. J Neurooncol 94:63–68

Tselis N, Kolotas C, Birn G et al (2007) CT guided interstitial HDR brachytherapy for recurrent glioblastoma multiforme. Long term results. Strahlenther Onkol 183:563–570

Ullrich RT, Kracht LW, Jacobs AH (2008) Neuroimaging in patients with gliomas. Semin Neurol 28:484–494

Weller M, Tabatabai G, Kästner B et al (2015) MGMT promoter methylation is a strong prognostic biomarker for benefit from dose-intensified temozolomide rechallenge in progressive glioblastoma: the DIRECTOR trial. Clin Cancer Res 21:2057–2064

Wen PY, Macdonald DR, Reardon DA et al (2010) Updated response assessment criteria for high-grade gliomas: response assessment in neuro-oncology working group. J Clin Oncol 28:1963–1972

Westphal M, Lamszus K (2015) Circulating biomarkers for gliomas. Nat Rev Neurol 11:556–566

Wick W, Steinbach JP, Kuker WM et al (2004) One week on/one week off: a novel active regime of temozolomide for recurrent glioblastoma. Neurology 62:2113–2115

Wick A, Felsberg J, Steinbach JP et al (2007) Efficacy and tolerability of temozolomide in an alternating weekly regimen in patients with recurrent glioma. J Clin Oncol 25:3357–3361

Withers HR (1985) Biological basis for altered fractionation schemes. Cancer 55:2086–2095

Wong CS, van der Kogel AJ (2004) Mechanisms of radiation injury to the central nervous system: implications for neuroprotection. Mol Interv 4:273–284

Wong ET, Hess KR, Gleason MJ et al (1999) Outcomes and prognostic factors in recurrent glioma patients enrolled into phase II clinical trials. J Clin Oncol 17:2572–2579

Wong E, Huberman M, Lu X-Q (2008) Bevacizumab reverses cerebral radiation necrosis. J Clin Oncol 26:5049

Wong CS, Fehlings MG, Sahgal A (2015) Pathobiology of radiation myelopathy and strategies to mitigate injury. Spinal Cord 53:574–580

Yung WK, Prados MD, Yaya-Tur R et al (1999) Multicentre phase II trial of temozolomide in patients with anaplastic astrocytoma or anaplastic oligoastrocytoma at first relapse. Temodal Brain Tumour Group. J Clin Oncol 17:2762–2771

Eye Tumors

Helen A. Shih, Alexei V. Trofimov, and John E. Munzenrider

Contents

The original version of this chapter was revised. An erratum to this chapter can be found at 10.1007/978-3-319-41825-4_78.

H.A. Shih, MD (✉)
Central Nervous System and Eye Services, Department of Radiation Oncology, Massachusetts General Hospital, 30 Fruit Street, Boston, MA 02114, USA
e-mail: hshih@mgh.harvard.edu

A.V. Trofimov, PhD
Physics Division, Department of Radiation Oncology, Massachusetts General Hospital, 30 Fruit Street, Boston, MA 02114, USA
e-mail: atrofimov@mgh.harvard.edu

J.E. Munzenrider, MD
Department of Radiation Oncology, Massachusetts General Hospital, 30 Fruit Street, Boston, MA 02114, USA

Abstract

Reirradiating the eye after ocular irradiation is a relatively rare occurrence since the eye is irradiated infrequently as a primary target. Because of the intrinsic sensitivity of the structures in the eye to radiation, significant efforts are made to minimize the dose received incidentally by the eye during treatment of tumors of the orbit or periorbital areas or of other head and neck or central nervous system sites. Capitalizing upon technological advances that enable increased radiation dose conformality to the primary disease with minimization of excess radiation dose to the nontargeted parts of the eye permits for safer radiation treatment, both at primary indication and at reirradiation. This chapter will discuss the need for radiation oncologists to be aware of the differing threshold doses for complications involving various parts of the eye, specifically the lens, optic nerve, macula, and retina, as well as the tolerance of the lacrimal gland and the tear-producing cells in the eyelids. Recommendations are provided for determining the advisability of attempting reirradiation of the eye after primary treatment with low, intermediate, or high doses. Advantages of focused radiation therapy techniques, specifically external beam proton therapy and episcleral radionuclide plaque brachytherapy for primary treatment or for reirradiation of discrete ocular tumors, are discussed. Finally, the existing literature on proton therapy used in reirradiation of ocular melanomas is described.

Med Radiol Radiat Oncol (2016)
DOI 10.1007/174_2016_33, © Springer International Publishing Switzerland
Published Online: 13 Apr 2016

1 Background

Radiation oncologists should be knowledgeable regarding tolerance doses for the cornea, lens, retina, macula, and optic nerve (Emami et al. 1991; Parsons et al. 1983). They must also know that radiation damage to the lacrimal gland and tear-producing cells in the eyelids will decrease tear production and may result in a "dry eye" syndrome. Mild cases can be effectively managed with artificial tear preparations, but more severe cases may require tarsorrhaphy or plugging of the lacrimal duct. In extreme cases, corneal scarring may lead to significant visual loss and eye loss due to intractable eye pain.

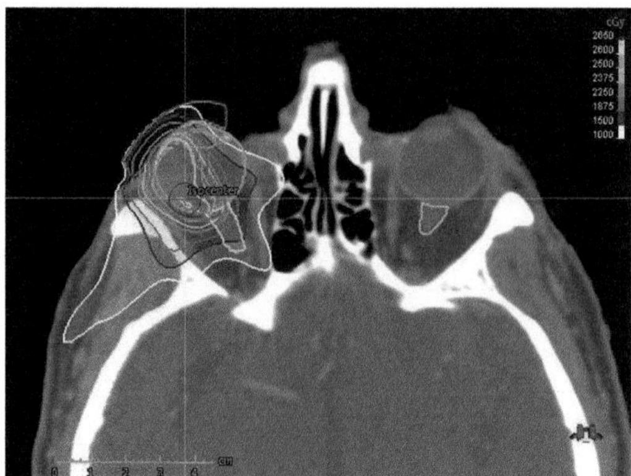

Fig. 1 Intensity-modulated radiation therapy for an eye metastasis. Dose delivered was 25 Gy in five fractions

2 Primary Ocular Treatment

2.1 Metastatic Lesions

Primary treatment to the eye itself is most commonly given for metastatic lesions (Rudoler et al. 1997; Tsina et al. 2005; Kamran et al. 2014). Such lesions commonly spread to the eye from breast or lung cancers, although metastases from other primary sites may also be seen (Ferry and Font 1974). The eye can be considered as part of the central nervous system (CNS), since it develops as an evagination of the diencephalon. Metastatic spread to both the eye and the brain occurs solely via hematogenous spread, since both organs lack lymphatics. Because of their common routes of metastatic spread, patients with ocular metastases frequently also have brain metastases diagnosed prior to, simultaneous with, or following the appearance of the ocular lesion. If either the eye or the brain has already been irradiated prior to the appearance of metastasis in the other organ, treatment of the site currently involved must consider what, if any, dose the eye or the brain has received from prior irradiation given to the other organ for metastatic lesions there. Highly conformal radiation treatment techniques such as intensity-modulated radiation therapy can be employed to achieve minimization of unwanted dose to surrounding nontarget cranial tissues (Fig. 1).

2.2 Primary Ocular Tumors and Benign Ocular and Orbital Conditions

Primary tumors, specifically melanomas, lymphomas, vascular lesions, and retinoblastomas, present for treatment less frequently than do metastatic ocular lesions. Doses for primary ocular tumors vary widely. Ocular melanomas receive very high uniform doses (50–70 Gy in four or five fractions) most commonly with proton radiation, and similar or even higher nonhomogeneous doses are delivered with episcleral radionuclide plaque therapy (Courdi et al. 2010; Dendale et al. 2006; Gragoudas et al. 2002; Egger et al. 2001; The American Brachytherapy Society – Ophthalmic Oncology Task Force 2014; Badiyan et al. 2014; Barker et al. 2014; Sagoo et al. 2011; Semenova and Finger 2013). Intermediate doses (36–46 Gy) are given for retinoblastoma (Mouw et al. 2014; Merchant et al. 2002; Pradhan et al. 1997) and sometimes even lower doses for ocular lymphomas (Harada et al. 2014; Munch-Petersen et al. 2015; Fasola et al. 2013). Benign ocular conditions, such as macular degeneration; vascular tumors, such as choroidal hemangiomas; and benign orbital conditions, such as Graves' ophthalmopathy and orbital pseudotumor, may also be treated with radiation (Jackson et al. 2015; Chan et al. 2010; Petersen et al. 1990; Lanciano et al. 1990). In the former condition, only the immediate macular area is targeted, while in the latter two conditions, the entire globe posterior to the ora is irradiated despite the fact that the pathological condition being targeted is in the extraocular muscles or the orbit, rather than within the globe itself. Relatively low doses (10–20 Gy) are given to patients with benign conditions (Barak et al. 2005; Chen et al. 2014; Chan et al. 2010; Petersen et al. 1990; Mourits et al. 2000; Cardosa et al. 2012). More recent investigation with stereotactic radiotherapy doses of 16 or 24 Gy for age-related macular degeneration find early efficacy in data reported at 2 years, but long-term data will be required to assess late toxicity and may impact on eligibility of potential future reirradiation (Jackson et al. 2015). Similar efficacy has been reported with the use of proton therapy of 16 or 24 Gy(RBE) divided in two fractions (Chen et al. 2014).

3 Reirradiation

3.1 Reirradiation After Low Doses Given for Benign Diseases

The low doses given for macular degeneration can be repeated with relatively little risk, although the efficacy of intraocular anti-angiogenic drugs has largely supplanted the use of radiotherapy for macular degeneration. A recent update of indications for treatment of benign disease concluded that macular degeneration is no longer an indication for radiotherapy (Van Houtte et al. 2005). Relatively low doses (20 Gy in 10 fractions) are given to the eye with fractionated external beam photon therapy for Graves' ophthalmopathy and orbital pseudotumor. That dose can typically be repeated with a low risk of significant morbidity, other than possibly cataract formation if the lens was not adequately shielded during either the first or the second course of treatment. However, there is little if any data available in the literature regarding indications for and either the efficacy or the risk of retreating patients previously irradiated for these conditions.

3.2 Reirradiation After Intermediate Doses Given for Retinoblastomas, Lymphomas, and Metastatic Carcinomas

Patients with these tumors usually are treated with fractionated external beam supervoltage photon therapy to doses of 30–46 Gy ranging at 1.8–3.0 Gy per fraction. The target may include the posterior globe only in patients with posterior retinoblastomas or metastatic lesions. The entire globe posterior to the ora serrata is treated in retinoblastoma patients with more anteriorly located tumors and in patients with diffuse lymphomatous or carcinomatous involvement of the retina or the vitreous. When the aim is to treat only the retina posterior to the equator, appropriate planning and treatment techniques can limit the lens dose to ≤4 Gy, a subthreshold level for cataractogenesis (Parsons et al. 1983). When the target volume extends anteriorly to the ora serrata, the probability of radiation-induced cataract is increased. The threshold dose for radiation retinopathy or optic neuritis is >20 Gy. However, symptomatic retinopathy or optic neuropathy is seen relatively infrequently after doses of the order of 40–46 Gy. Reirradiation after an initial course would likely result in cataract formation, unless the dose to the lens could be kept to a very low level, perhaps by using focused treatment techniques such as proton therapy, episcleral radionuclide plaque therapy, or stereotactic radiotherapy. The use of such focused techniques could also limit the volume of retina and possibly the dose to the macula or the optic nerve. However, systemic treatment, with chemotherapy in patients with ocular lymphomas, retinoblastomas, or metastatic carcinomas may preclude the need to consider reirradiation. Local treatments, using cryotherapy, laser photocoagulation, or radionuclide episcleral plaque therapy, are effective for focally recurrent disease in retinoblastoma patients, and the indication for external beam reirradiation of such patients arises rarely, if at all.

3.3 Reirradiation After High Doses Given for Ocular Melanomas

Ocular melanomas receive very high uniform doses (50–70 Gy in 4 or 5 fractions) with proton beam radiation. Similar or even higher nonhomogeneous doses are also delivered to such tumors with episcleral radionuclide plaque therapy, delivered over 4–8 days, depending upon the intensity of the radiation sources in the plaque at the time of placement. These focused techniques deliver the prescribed dose of radiation to only that portion of the eye containing the tumor. An example of a patient treated twice with proton therapy for a uveal melanoma that subsequently failed marginally is demonstrated in Fig. 2. Non-involved eye structures located away from the tumor receive little or no dose, although small portions of the eye immediately adjacent to the tumor and eye structures through which the beam passes en route to the tumor may also receive the prescribed dose.

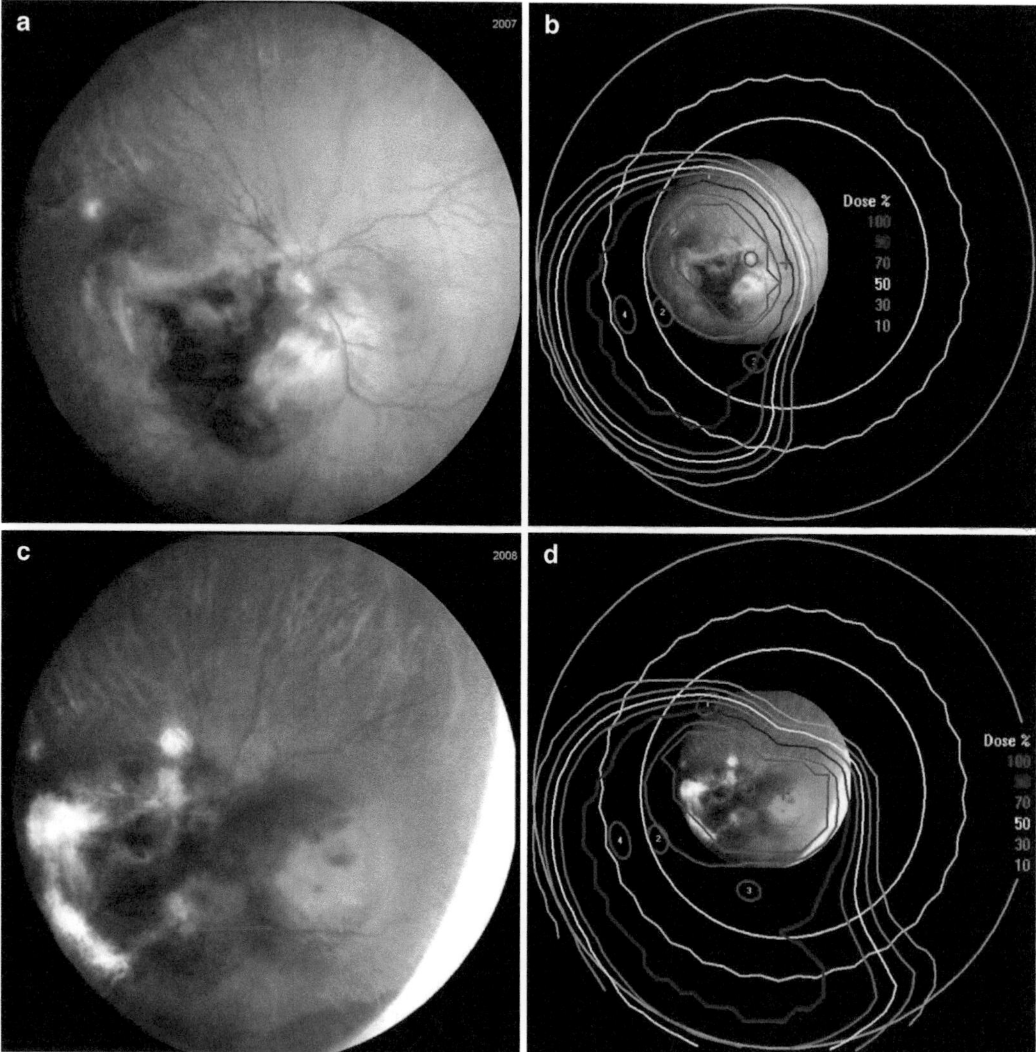

Fig. 2 Uveal melanoma recurrence. An 81-year-old man with a primary left uveal melanoma (**a**) who was treated with proton therapy to 50 Gy(RBE) in five fractions (**b**). He recurred along the lateral margin to the primary tumor 14 months later (**c**) at which time he was reirradiated to 70 Gy(RBE) in five fractions (**d**)

Reirradiation of new tumors arising away from the initially treated volume and, in certain cases, regrowing immediately adjacent to or even within the previously irradiated volume can be carried out with proper patient selection. Marucci et al. (2006) evaluated the outcomes of a second course of proton beam radiation therapy (PBRT) in 31 patients with recurrent uveal melanoma. Mean interval between the first and the second PBRT course was 50.2 months (range, 8–165 months). Most patients (87 %) received 70 Gy(RBE) (gray-relative biological effectiveness; biological correction to be equivalent to photon doses) for both the initial and the second treatment course. Visual acuity was 20/200 or better in 30 patients initially and in 22 patients at the time of the second treatment. The mean follow-up time after the second treatment was 50 months (range, 6–164 months). When last seen, 20 tumors had either regressed or showed no evident tumor progression. Nine eyes (29 %) were enucleated, five for local recurrence and four because of intractable pain. The 5-year eye retention rate was 55 % (95 % confidence interval, 25.2–77.4). Six of the 22 patients who retained their eye (27 %) had useful vision (20/200 or better). This small retrospective study demonstrated that a second course of PBRT for recurrent uveal melanoma to total doses between 118 and 140 Gy(RBE) was associated with a moderately good probability of local control and a relatively low enucleation rate. Although most patients lost their vision, the majority were able to retain the reirradiated eye.

In a subsequent study, survival in patients with recurrent melanomas was retrospectively compared between those treated by enucleation and those who were reirradiated (Marucci et al. 2011). Patients selected for reirradiation were slightly older than those treated with enucleation (56 vs. 61 years, respectively). Both initial and recurrent tumors were larger in patients treated with enucleation than in those who were reirradiated. Tumor location and the presence or absence of ciliary body involvement did not differ significantly between the groups. The median follow-up after enucleation and after retreatment was longer in the enucleated patients (79 and 59 months, respectively). Median survival duration in the enucleated and reirradiated groups was 42 and 90 months, respectively. The median time free of metastases was 38 months in enucleated patients and 97 months in reirradiated patients. At 5 years after surgery or reirradiation, the probability of overall survival was 36 % and 63 %, respectively ($p=0.040$, log-rank test). The probability of freedom from metastases was 31 % and 66 %, respectively ($p=0.028$, log-rank test). These differences persisted after adjustment for largest tumor diameter and volume at the time of reirradiation or enucleation. Results of this analysis suggested that survival in reirradiated patients was not compromised by their receiving a second course of proton beam therapy, relative to that of those treated with enucleation.

Most recently, Riechardt et al. (2014) reported on their experience of salvage irradiation with proton therapy. Unlike the prior report of patients receiving only proton therapy with both courses of treatment, this study of 48 patients received a variety of types of initial therapy, including 26 with radiotherapy, 21 with ruthenium-106 plaque brachytherapy, 1 with CyberKnife radiation, and 4 with proton therapy. Overall the local tumor control among the 48 patients was 92 % at a median of 10-year follow-up. Two of the three second recurrences were in patients who had previously been irradiated with proton therapy and CyberKnife. Late effects are reported with all patients together such that the attributable toxicity from two courses of radiation is more difficult to assess but overall visual acuity remained stable for the first year after proton reirradiation but then declined thereafter. Other late effects included cataracts (corrective surgery in 25 % of patients) and vitreous hemorrhage (vitrectomy performed in 12.5 % of patients).

3.4 Reirradiation of Pterygia

These benign irregular fleshy-colored fibrovascular growths can obscure vision when they progress into the visual axis of the cornea. Recurrence occurs in 20–30 % of primarily excised lesions and in 30–60 % of re-excised lesions. Treatment with a strontium-90 beta-ray applicator to doses ranging from 18 Gy in a single fraction to 60 Gy in six fractions has been employed, with recurrence rates ranging from 2 to 12 % (Paryani et al. 1994; Van den Brenk 1968). Recurrence and complication rates are both higher following reirradiation (Wilder et al. 1992; Dusenbery et al. 1992).

4 Summary

Reirradiation of the eye can be successfully accomplished in carefully selected patients with recurrent ocular tumors, specifically uveal melanomas and retinoblastomas. Conformal treatment planning techniques combined with focused treatment techniques can target primarily the tumor and exclude to the extent possible critical ocular structures, thus providing patients with recurrent tumors an option of effective treatment with retention of their eye and a smaller but nonzero possibility of visual preservation.

References

Badiyan SN, Rao RC, Apicelli AJ et al (2014) Outcomes of iodine-125 plaque brachytherapy for uveal melanoma with intraoperative ultrasonography and supplemental transpupillary thermotherapy. Int J Radiat Oncol Biol Phys 88:801–805

Barak A, Hauser D, Yipp P et al (2005) A phase I trial of stereotactic external beam radiation for subfoveal choroidal neovascular membranes in age-related macular degeneration. Br J Radiol 78:827–831

Barker CA, Francis JH, Cohen GN et al (2014) 106Ru plaque brachytherapy for uveal melanoma: factors associated with local tumor recurrence. Brachytherapy 13:584–590

Cardosa CC, Giordani AJ, Wolosker AM et al (2012) Protracted hypofractionated radiotherapy for Graves' ophthalmopathy: a pilot study of clinical and radiologic response. Int J Radiat Oncol Biol Phys 82:1285–1291

Chan RV, Yonekawa Y, Lane AM et al (2010) Proton beam irradiation using a light-field technique for the treatment of choroidal hemangiomas. Ophthalmologica 224:209–216

Chen L, Kim IK, Lane AM et al (2014) Proton beam irradiation for non-AMD CNV: 2-year results of a randomised clinical trial. Br J Ophthalmol 98:1212–1217

Courdi A, Caujolle JP, Grange JD et al (2010) Results of proton therapy of uveal melanomas treated in Nice. Int J Radiat Oncol Biol Phys 45:5–11

Dendale R, Lumbroso-Le Rouic L, Noel G et al (2006) Proton beam radiotherapy for uveal melanoma: results of Curie Institut-Orsay proton therapy center (ICPO). Int J Radiat Oncol Biol Phys 65:780–787

Dusenbery KE, Alul IH, Holland EJ et al (1992) Beta-irradiation of recurrent pterygia: results and complications. Int J Radiat Oncol Biol Phys 24:315–320

Egger E, Schalenbourg A, Zografos L et al (2001) Maximizing local tumor control and survival after proton beam radiotherapy of uveal melanoma. Int J Radiat Oncol Biol Phys 151:138–147

Emami B, Lyman J, Brown A et al (1991) Tolerance of normal tissue to therapeutic irradiation. Int J Radiat Oncol Biol Phys 21:109–122

Fasola CE, Jones CE, Huang DD et al (2013) Low-dose radiation therapy (2 Gy x 2) in the treatment of orbital lymphoma. Int J Radiat Oncol Biol Phys 86:930–935

Ferry AP, Font R (1974) Carcinoma metastatic to the eye and orbit: a clinicopathological study of 227 eyes. Arch Ophthalmol 92:276–286

Gragoudas E, Li W, Lane AM et al (2002) Evidence-based estimates of outcome in patients irradiated for intraocular melanoma. Arch Ophthalmol 120:1665–1671

Harada K, Murakami N, Kitaguchi M et al (2014) Localized ocular adnexal mucosa-associated lymphoid tissue lymphoma treated with radiation therapy: a long-term outcome in 86 patients with 104 treated eyes. Int J Radiat Oncol Biol Phys 88:650–654

Jackson TL, Chakravarthy U, Slakter JS et al (2015) Stereotactic radiotherapy for neovascular age-related macular degeneration: year 2 results of the INTREPID study. Ophthalmology 122:138–145

Kamran SC, Collier JM, Lane AM et al (2014) Outcomes of proton therapy for the treatment of uveal metastases. Int J Radiat Oncol Biol Phys 90:1044–1050

Lanciano R, Fowble B, Sergott RC et al (1990) The results of radiotherapy for orbital pseudotumor. Int J Radiat Oncol Biol Phys 18:407–411

Marucci L, Lane AM, Li W et al (2006) Conservation treatment of the eye: conformal proton reirradiation for recurrent uveal melanoma. Int J Radiat Oncol Biol Phys 64:1018–1022

Marucci L, Ancukiewicz M, Lane AM et al (2011) Uveal melanoma recurrence after fractionated proton beam therapy: comparison of survival in patients treated with reirradiation or with enucleation. Int J Radiat Oncol Biol Phys 79:842–846

Merchant T, Gould CJ, Hilton NE et al (2002) Ocular preservation after 36 Gy external beam radiation therapy for retinoblastoma. J Pediatr Hematol Oncol 224:246–249

Mourits MP, van Kempen-Harteveld ML, Garcia MBG et al (2000) Radiotherapy for Graves' orbitopathy: randomised placebo-controlled study. Lancet 355:1505–1509

Mouw KW, Sethi RV, Yeap BY et al (2014) Proton radiation therapy for the treatment of retinoblastoma. Int J Radiat Oncol Biol Phys 90:863–869

Munch-Petersen HD, Rasmussen PK, Coupland SE et al (2015) Ocular adnexal diffuse large B-cell lymphoma: a multicenter international study. JAMA Ophthalmol 133:165–173

Parsons JT, Fitzpatrick CJ, Hood CL et al (1983) The effects of irradiation on the eye and optic nerve. Int J Radiat Oncol Biol Phys 9:609–622

Paryani SB, Scotta WP, Wells JW et al (1994) Management of pterygium with surgery and radiation therapy. Int J Radiat Oncol Biol Phys 28:101–103

Petersen IA, Kriss JP, McDougall IR et al (1990) Prognostic factors in radiotherapy of Graves' ophthalmopathy. Int J Radiat Oncol Biol Phys 19:259–264

Pradhan DG, Sandridge AL, Mullaney P et al (1997) Radiation therapy for retinoblastoma: a retrospective study of 120 patients. Int J Radiat Oncol Biol Phys 39:3–13

Riechardt AI, Cordini D, Dobnet B et al (2014) Salvage proton beam therapy in local recurrent uveal melanoma. Am J Ophthalmol 158:948–956

Rudoler SB, Shields CL, Corn BW et al (1997) Functional vision is improved in the majority of patients treated with external-beam radiotherapy for choroid metastases: a multivariate analysis of 188 patients. J Clin Oncol 15:1244–1251

Sagoo MS, Shields CL, Mashayekhi A et al (2011) Plaque radiotherapy for juxtapapillary choroidal melanoma. Tumor control in 650 consecutive cases. Ophthalmology 118:402–407

Semenova E, Finger PT (2013) Palladium-103 radiation therapy for small choroidal melanoma. Ophthalmology 120:2353–2357

The American Brachytherapy Society – Ophthalmic Oncology Task Force (2014) The American Brachytherapy Society consensus guidelines for plaque brachytherapy of uveal melanoma and retinoblastoma. Brachytherapy 13:1–14

Tsina EK, Lane AM, Zacks DN et al (2005) Treatment of metastatic tumors of the choroid with proton beam irradiation. Ophthalmology 112:337–343

Van den Brenk HA (1968) Results of prophylactic postoperative irradiation in 1300 cases of pterygium. Am J Roentgenol 103:723–727

Van Houtte P, Roelandts M, Devriendt D et al (2005) Radiation therapy of benign diseases. What's new eight years after? Cancer Radiother 9:427–434

Wilder RB, Buatti JM, Kittleson JM et al (1992) Pterygium treated with excision and postoperative beta irradiation. Int J Radiat Oncol Biol Phys 23:533–537

Re-irradiation in Head and Neck Cancer

Johannes A. Langendijk

Contents

The original version of this chapter was revised. An erratum to this chapter can be found at 10.1007/978-3-319-41825-4_78.

J.A. Langendijk, MD, PhD
Department of Radiation Oncology, University Medical Center Groningen, University of Groningen, Groningen, The Netherlands
e-mail: j.a.langendijk@umcg.nl

Abstract

Re-irradiation for loco-regional failure of head and neck cancer or second primary tumours in previously irradiated areas after a full course of (chemo-)radiation poses a challenging problem for radiation oncologists. Salvage surgery remains the standard of care, which however, is the case in only 20 % of the cases. Chemotherapy alone is not considered a curative treatment option.

Curatively intended (chemo-)radiation should be considered in well-selected cases and can be administered safely with a reasonable chance of long-term survival (approximately 15–20 %) but at the cost of severe increased acute and late toxicity. The results of taxane-based chemo-re-irradiation protocols are most promising.

In case of adverse prognostic factors, immediate postoperative (chemo-)re-irradiation after salvage surgery can be administered safely and significantly improves loco-regional control. Severe treatment-related morbidity remains of major concern. However, most series on re-irradiation published so far did not use fractionation schedules and techniques considered most optimal. Improvement of the therapeutic ratio can be expected from altered fractionation schedules, by limiting the target volume to the high-risk areas and by using more advanced radiation technologies.

Future studies should focus on new developments that proved to be effective in the

Med Radiol Radiat Oncol (2016)
DOI 10.1007/174_2016_76, © Springer International Publishing Switzerland
Published Online: 13 Aug 2016

primary treatment of head and neck squamous cell cancer (HNSCC). In this respect, new induction chemotherapy regimens using TPF and the addition of cetuximab to radiation are of great interest as these approaches might improve loco-regional control and overall survival without increasing treatment-related morbidity.

1 Introduction

Radiotherapy plays a pivotal role in the curative treatment of head and neck squamous cell carcinoma (HNSCC). Currently, the majority of patients with HNSCC have locally advanced disease and are treated with radiotherapy either alone or in combination with other modalities, such as surgery, chemotherapy and/or biological targeting agents. Despite the advances made in the primary treatment of HNSCC, still 30–50% of all curatively treated patients will develop a loco-regional recurrence (Blanchard et al. 2013, 2015). In addition, for those who survive, there is a constant threat of the development of a new head and neck tumour. In a meta-analysis, the incidence of second primary tumours (SPTs) was 14.2% (Haughey et al. 1992). Given that most patients received radiation treatment to the primary site as well as to the regional lymph node areas, the vast majority of these recurrences and SPTs will occur in previously irradiated areas.

In most cases the previous radiation dose administered is just below the generally accepted tolerance dose of the normal tissues, and although some recovery is likely to occur over time, the exact additional dose that can be administered safely to these normal structures remains to be determined. Therefore, in the re-irradiation setting, most radiation oncologists are much more reluctant with regard to the radiation dose to the normal tissues in general and in particular to the most critical structures, such as the spinal cord, the larynx and the optic nerves and chiasm. On the other hand, in order to achieve satisfactory rates of loco-regional tumour control, the total dose administered to the high-risk areas should at least be in the range of what is normally considered curative. Therefore, recurrent and second primary HNSCC after curative (chemo-)radiation in previously irradiated areas poses an important and difficult therapeutic challenge for radiation oncologists. In this chapter, a number of issues related to curatively intended re-irradiation either or not in combination with other modalities will be discussed.

2 A Changing Population

In the last decades, a major progress has been made in the treatment of patients with HNSCC. In particular, the addition of concomitant chemotherapy (Langendijk et al. 2004; Pignon et al. 2009; Blanchard et al. 2013, 2015) and cetuximab (Bonner et al. 2006, 2010) to radiation and the introduction of altered fractionation schedules (Baujat et al. 2010; Blanchard et al. 2011) have resulted in a significant improvement of loco-regional tumour control and overall survival. These new treatment regimens have gained conceptual acceptance and are now considered standard among patients with HNSCC in the organ preservation as well as in the unresectable setting. In most studies reporting on the results of (chemo-)re-irradiation in HNSCC, patients included received their initial treatment before the 1990s most likely with conventional fractionation schedules and without the addition of chemotherapy (Weppelmann et al. 1992; Spencer et al. 1999; Schaefer et al. 2000; De Crevoisier et al. 1998, 2001). Moreover, in that period, planning CT scans and 3D dose calculations were not routinely used, and most patients were treated after direct simulation. The same accounts for patients treated with primary surgery and postoperative radiotherapy. Since the publication of the results of two prospective randomised studies, an increasing number of patients are now treated with postoperative concomitant chemo-radiation instead of postoperative radiotherapy alone (Bernier et al. 2004; Cooper et al. 2004), in particular in case of high-risk factors for loco-regional failure, such as positive surgical margins and lymph node metastases with extranodal spread (Bernier et al. 2005). As a consequence of these changes in what is currently considered standard treatment, there are two major concerns. First, it should be noted that loco-regional failures among patients currently treated with CT-guided 3D conformal radiotherapy or intensity-modulated radiotherapy (IMRT) with altered fractionation schedules and/or in combination with concomitant chemotherapy are less frequent than after conventional RT alone, suggesting the selection of more radioresistant cases compared to those described in earlier studies. Therefore, it should be questioned as to whether translation of the results obtained from these earlier studies on re-irradiation to patients that underwent more effective initial treatment regimens is justified. Tumours recurring in previously irradiated areas after more effective chemoradiation regimens will originate from perhaps more radioresistant clonogens, and we cannot rule out that (chemo-)re-irradiation could be less effective in these patients than after conventionally fractionated radiotherapy alone. Indeed Nagar et al. found that both disease-free survival and overall survival after chemo-re-irradiation were markedly and significantly worse among those that were initially treated with chemo-radiation as compared to those who initially received radiotherapy alone (Nagar et al. 2004). In that study, none of the patients that received chemoradiation as initial treatment were disease-free at 1 year and all patients died within 2 years after chemo-re-irradiation. Moreover, in a retrospective study including re-irradiated HNC patients from nine consecutive phases I–II trials, initial treatment with chemo-radiation was an adverse prognostic factor for overall survival (Choe et al. 2011). These results support the hypothesis that the current population of patients with recurrent HNC in previously irradiated areas considered for re-irradiation have less favourable outcome when initially treated with chemo-radiation than those included in earlier reports that mainly included patients initially treated with radiotherapy alone.

3 Patient Selection

As re-irradiation, either or not in combination with other modalities, is associated with a considerable risk on severe acute and late treatment-related side effects, proper selection of patients is essential to further improve the therapeutic ratio. From this point of view, identification of reliable and validated prognostic factors is essential. Moreover, the possibility of alternative treatment approaches should be taken into consideration, and the previous radiation treatment should be analysed thoroughly.

3.1 Prognostic Factors

There are a number of methodological problems with regard to the identification and validation of prognostic factors in the re-irradiation setting, including (1) differences in eligibility criteria and subsequent heterogeneity of the study populations among the different studies, (2) the retrospective design of most studies, (3) the relatively limited number of patients included with insufficient power to detect clinically relevant prognostic factors and (4) the large variety of treatment regimens used. Nevertheless, despite these methodological shortcomings, there are a limited number of prognostic factors that seem to be important.

Tanvetyanon et al. reported on a retrospective analysis on prognostic factors for survival among patients treated with curatively intended salvage re-irradiation for head and neck cancer (Tanvetyanon et al. 2009). The study population was composed of patients with recurrent tumours as well as SPTs, and 46 out of 103 patients underwent salvage surgery and postoperative re-irradiation. With this nomogram, the probability of death at 24 months after initiation of re-irradiation can be predicted with a combination of prognostic factors, including comorbidity (based on the Charlson index), organ dysfunction prior to re-irradiation, isolated neck recurrence, tumour bulk and time interval between completion of previous therapy and initiation of re-irradiation. The performance of this nomogram showed good agreement between predicted and observed outcomes, with a C-index of 0.75. The factors included in this nomogram generally reflect the most frequently reported prognostic factors in the re-irradiation setting (Stell 1989; Spencer et al. 2001, 2008). However, the number of patients in this analysis was relatively small, and other potential prognostic factors such as recurrent versus SPT, total dose of radiation, previous chemo-radiation (Spencer et al. 2001, 2008) and radiation technique were not identified as significant prognostic factors. Nevertheless, the nomogram could be a useful tool to select patients with favourable outcome for the more intensified (chemo-)re-irradiation strategies.

Choe et al. reported on a retrospective multivariable analysis of 166 previously irradiated patients with locally advanced non-metastatic HNC that were either treated with salvage surgery followed by adjuvant concurrent chemo-re-irradiation or definitive chemo-re-irradiation (Choe et al. 2011). They identified four independent prognostic factors for overall survival, including salvage surgery before chemo-re-irradiation (yes/no), previous chemo-radiation (yes/no), total dose of re-irradiation (<60/≥60 Gy) and interval between end of first treatment to initiation of chemo-re-irradiation (<36/≥36 months). The 5-year overall survival of patients with 0–1 adverse prognostics factors was around 30 %, compared to 10 % and 0 % for those with 2 and 3–4 adverse prognostic factors, respectively. This latter model is a rather simple and therefore very practical tool to stratify patients into distinct risk groups and to support decision-making for the most suitable salvage strategy.

More recently, Riaz et al. reported on the development of a nomogram that predicts 2-year loco-regional control after re-irradiation either as single modality or combined with surgery or concurrent chemotherapy. This nomogram included five prognostic factors, including stage, tumour site, organ dysfunction, salvage surgery and total dose of re-irradiation (Riaz et al. 2014).

An important finding in two of the aforementioned studies was that comorbidity and preexisting organ dysfunction were important prognostic factors (Tanvetyanon et al. 2009; Riaz et al. 2014). More specifically, the median overall survival among patients with neither significant comorbidity nor pretreatment organ dysfunction was 59.6 months which was markedly better compared to those with both comorbidity and organ dysfunction, in whom the median survival was only 5.5 months with no survivors beyond 2 years of follow-up ($p<0.001$) (Tanvetyanon et al. 2009). These two factors are probably important because they may increase the risk of cancer-related death due to poor treatment tolerance and compliance and/or increase the risk of non-cancer-related death. Moreover, organ dysfunction, which is mainly due to radiation-induced toxicity from the previous treatment, may also be a surrogate marker of a more aggressive biological behaviour of the tumour. Hence, given the large impact on overall survival, both factors may interact negatively with (chemo-)re-irradiation, but may also be a competing risk of death.

3.2 Alternative Treatment Options

Before deciding for (chemo)re-irradiation, other treatment options should be taken into account as well. In particular in case of resectable loco-regional recurrences and/or SPTs, surgery should be considered and is traditionally regarded as the standard of care (Gilbert and Kagan 1974; Pradhan et al. 1980; Goodwin 2000), while chemotherapy and (chemo-)re-irradiation have been reserved for unresectable cases or as adjuvant modality after salvage surgery (De Crevoisier et al. 1998, 2001). However, only approximately 20 % of the patients are candidates for curative resections (Ridge 1993; Mabanta et al. 1999). In addition, the results of salvage surgery are relatively poor. The results of a meta-analysis on salvage surgery in HNSCC, based on 1,633 patients from 32 studies, revealed a 5-year overall survival rate of approximately 40 % (Goodwin 2000). The 5-year survival tended to be better among patients with recurrent cancer of the larynx (48 %) and oral cavity (43 %) than among those with recurrent disease in the oropharynx (26 %). Better outcome of salvage surgery in patients with laryngeal and hypopharyngeal cancer with loco-regional recurrences after concurrent chemo-radiation has been confirmed in a recent retrospective study (Putten et al. 2015). Of the 66 patients that developed loco-regional recurrence after concurrent chemo-radiation, 22 underwent salvage surgery (33 %). Independent favourable predictive factors for salvage surgery were younger age and laryngeal cancer. The 5-year overall survival rate was 27 % as compared to 0 % in patients that were not salvaged by surgery. However, this higher survival rate came at the cost of 14 % major complications.

It should be noted that survival data were not available stratified by stage or interval between primary and recurrence, demonstrating one of the limitations of the aforementioned meta-analysis (Goodwin 2000). In this regard, Zafareo et al., who reported on the results of a retrospective study on the role of salvage surgery in patients with recurrent squamous cell carcinoma of the oropharynx (Zafereo et al. 2009), showed that the outcome after salvage surgery may depend on a number of other prognostics factors. These authors identified 199 patients with locally recurrent oropharyngeal cancers, after excluding patients with regional metastases only or distant metastases, who had been treated with definitive radiotherapy in the past. Out of these 199 patients, only 41 (21 %) were selected for salvage surgery and the 3-year overall survival was 42 %. The results of that study indicated that favourable surgical salvage candidates are younger, have smaller recurrent tumours for which it is possible to obtain free surgical margins and have no recurrent neck disease. Other studies showed that the interval between the previous treatment (Stell 1991; Llewelyn and Mitchell 1997; Agra et al. 2006) and recurrence and disease stage (Lacy et al. 1999; Goodwin 2000; Agra et al. 2003, 2008) are important adverse prognostic factors for salvage surgery as well. Nevertheless, the risk of developing a second recurrence after salvage surgery remains high, with approximately two-thirds of the patients developing such an event within the first year of salvage surgery (Kim et al. 2007; Zafereo et al. 2009), emphasising the potential importance of postoperative (chemo)re-irradiation, which will be discussed later.

The results after salvage surgery alone and the fact that postoperative (chemo-)re-irradiation may be indicated after salvage surgery should be taken into account when deciding for either primary (chemo-)re-irradiation or salvage surgery. From this point of view, it is worthwhile to notice that the outcome after salvage surgery followed by postoperative (chemo-)re-irradiation appears to be superior to that after (chemo-)re-irradiation alone. Salama et al. reported a 5-year progression-free survival of 51 % after postoperative (chemo-)re-irradiation, which was significantly better as compared to (chemo-)re-irradiation in which the progression-free survival was only 19 % (Salama et al. 2006). In addition, Kasperts et al. reported on the results of a retrospective study that included 39 patients that underwent surgery for SPTs or loco-regional recurrences followed by postoperative re-irradiation without chemotherapy (Kasperts et al. 2006). All patients had positive surgical margins and/or lymph node metastases with extra-nodal spread and were therefore considered to have a high or very high risk for loco-regional failure. In this study, the 3-year loco-regional control and overall survival rates were 74 % and 44 %, respectively. These results did not significantly differ from the results obtained among patients that underwent surgery and postoperative radiotherapy as initial treatment.

It should also be noted that, as in the case of intensified (chemo-)re-irradiation, complications after salvage surgery in a previously irradiated area are an important problem as well, reported in approximately 20–40 % of the cases (Goodwin 2000). As expected, the frequency of complications is larger following more extensive surgery required for stage III and IV disease. Wound complications seem to be a manageable problem, although occurring in a considerable proportion of patients (approximately 50 %) (Langendijk et al. 2005; Agra et al. 2008; Putten et al. 2015). However, perioperative deaths are relatively rare. Nowadays, the availability of myocutaneous flaps, as well as free flaps with microvascular anastomosis, provides the surgeon with a wide array of opportunities to bring non-irradiated tissue into the surgical field for reconstruction.

Chemotherapy alone for recurrent HNSCC is generally not considered a curative treatment option, although progress has been made in the treatment of metastatic and recurrent disease among patients not suitable for more aggressive local treatments such as salvage surgery or re-irradiation. In case of systemic treatment alone, platinum-based chemotherapy is considered the current standard (Hong et al. 1983; Forastiere et al. 1992; Arnold et al. 2004; Gibson et al. 2005; Sacco and Cohen 2015). The only regimen that showed significant outcome improvement as compared to platinum-based chemotherapy alone in approximately 30 % is the combination of platinum, fluorouracil and cetuximab (Sacco and Cohen 2015). The addition of cetuximab to platinum-based chemotherapy with fluorouracil revealed an overall survival improvement from 7.4 months with chemotherapy alone group to 10.1 months after chemotherapy plus cetuximab (Vermorken et al. 2008). Although these results are encouraging, systemic treatment alone cannot be regarded as curative treatment option in the long term and should be reserved for patients with recurrent disease that are not eligible for intensified loco-regional treatment anymore and/or for those with distant metastases. Indeed, in a retrospective analysis, Datta et al. found that patients with residual or recurrent disease after curative radiotherapy showed better outcome after chemo-radiation compared to chemotherapy alone with a 5-year overall survival rate of 19 % after chemo-radiation versus no survivors at 5 years after chemotherapy alone (Datta et al. 2003). However, randomised controlled trials comparing these two strategies are still lacking, and we can therefore not rule out that selection bias may account for at least part of the beneficial effect of chemo-radiation compared to chemotherapy alone.

3.3 Recurrence Analysis

Given that patients developing loco-regional recurrences and/or SPTs in previously irradiated areas have been treated with more aggressive regimens and the fact that more advanced radiation delivery techniques, such as IMRT, are being used, allowing for better dose conformation to the target volume reference to the tissues outside the target volume, it becomes increasingly important to analyse the exact location of the loco-regional recurrence reference to the initial radiation dose distributions. If the radiation dose at the site of recurrence is significantly lower than the prescribed dose at the gross tumour volume (GTV), e.g. in the case of a recurrence in an electively treated neck, or in case of geographical miss, that loco-regional failure is less likely to be due to intrinsic radioresistance, and (chemo-)re-irradiation will probably be more effective than in case of loco-regional failures occurring in a high-dose area. For this reason, all cases considered for (chemo-)re-irradiation should be subjected to a thorough 3D reconstruction and analysis of the initial treatment portals and dose distributions. This so-called 'recurrence analysis', using both planning CT of the initial treatment co-registered with the CT scan of the recurrence preferably combined with other advanced imaging modalities such as positron emission tomography (PET) and/or MRI, is an essential step in the decision process for curative (chemo-)re-irradiation.

4 Primary (Chemo-) re-irradiation

As most patients initially underwent a full course of radiotherapy, it is reasonable to assume that radiation-resistant tumour clonogens exist and that a second course of radiation alone to the same or lower dose would not likely sterilise these resistant clones. There are a number of potential options to overcome the problem of radioresistance, including dose escalation and by radiation-sensitising strategies, e.g. the addition of chemotherapy and/or molecular-targeting therapies.

4.1 Re-irradiation Alone

A number of authors reported on the results of re-irradiation with external beam radiotherapy alone. In the older studies, patients were generally treated with standard fractionation and conventional radiation techniques (Stevens et al. 1994), sometimes combined with brachytherapy. In these older studies, the local control rates varied from 27 % in case of recurrent tumours to 60 % in case of SPTs, while the 5-year overall survival rate varied from 17 % among patients with recurrent tumours to 37 % among those with SPTs (Skolyszewski et al. 1980). For some subsets, the outcome was markedly better, e.g. in the series of Wang et al. who only included early-stage second primary laryngeal tumours, the 5-year overall survival was 93 % (Wang and McIntyre 1993). The problem with the reports on re-irradiation alone is that they are all retrospective, based on single centre experiences, including highly selected patient and heterogeneous patient groups, treated with rather outdated radiation technologies.

More recently, some authors reported on re-irradiation alone with more modern techniques, such as 3D-CRT and IMRT (Dawson et al. 2001). A total of 34 patients with a SPT ($n=26$) or loco-regional recurrence ($n=8$) were treated with a second course of high-dose radiotherapy. Patients were selected for re-irradiation in case of inoperable and/or unresectable tumours to a total dose of 60 Gy with conventional fractionation. The loco-regional control rate after 2 years was 27 % and the 3-year overall survival was 22 %.

4.2 Is There a Dose-Effect Relationship?

In the primary treatment of HNSCC, dose escalation by hyperfractionated regimens provides higher loco-regional control rates without a significant increase in late radiation-induced morbidity. Although there are no phase III studies on dose escalation in the re-irradiation setting, the results of retrospective analyses suggest that higher radiation doses are associated with better loco-regional tumour control.

A significant association between total re-irradiation dose and outcome was found by Datta et al. (2003). The population of this study was composed of 124 patients with residual or recurrent lesions treated with either re-irradiation alone or in combination with induction or concomitant chemotherapy. The total response rate was significantly higher when the total dose of re-irradiation was ≥40 Gy (91 versus 33 %, $p<0.001$), which also translated in a significant difference in overall survival (multivariate analysis).

Schaefer et al. treated 32 patients with external beam split-course radiation therapy with concomitant hydroxyurea and 5-fluorouracil for 5 days followed by 9 days of rest (Schaefer et al. 2000). This cycle was repeated every 2 weeks until a cumulative soft tissue radiation dose of 110 Gy (including prior radiation therapy) was reached. In this study, the median overall survival and progression-free survival among patients treated with ≤50 Gy were 9.0 and 14.2 months compared to 0.0 and 5.0 months, respectively, among patients that received a total dose of 40–49 Gy.

In another study, patients that received a dose of >50 Gy had a significantly better overall survival rate compared to those that received ≤50 Gy, which remained significant in the multivariate analysis (HR 0.45; 95 % CI 0.26–0.76; $p=0.002$) (Choe et al. 2011). Similar results were shown by Riaz et al. who found that radiation dose was an independent prognostic factor for loco-regional control in a multivariable analysis, with a hazard ratio of 0.57 (95 % ci, 0.38–0.85) for patients treated with 50 Gy or higher as compared to patients treated with a dose of less than 50 Gy (Riaz et al. 2014).

Salama et al. (2006) reported on the results achieved in 115 patients with loco-regionally recurrent non-metastatic or second primary HNSCC treated in seven consecutive phases I–II protocols at the University of Chicago with high-dose chemo-re-irradiation. In patients treated with a total dose ≥58 Gy, the 3-year loco-regional control rate, progression-free survival and overall survival was 56 %, 38 % and 30 %, respectively, which was significantly better compared to those treated with a total dose of <58 Gy, in which the 3-year loco-regional control rate, progression-free survival and overall survival was 33 %, 21 % and 6 %, respectively. The total dose turned out to be an independent prognostic factor in the multivariate analysis. This dose-effect relationship was most pronounced in the subset of patients with unresectable disease. More recently, Choe et al. found that the total dose of re-irradiation was an independent prognostic factor for overall survival, with a hazard ratio of 0.35 (95 % ci, 0.23–0.53; $p<0.001$) for patients that received <60 Gy versus patients that received 60 Gy or more (Choe et al. 2011).

However, in other studies no significant dose-effect relationships were found, which may also be due to the low number of patients included in these studies resulting in too low statistical power to detect clinically relevant differences between the various dose levels.

These results at least suggest that higher dose levels of re-irradiation result in better loco-regional control and/or overall survival rates. However, it remains difficult to determine the most appropriate dose level in this setting, as it remains unclear if the better survival rates after higher dose levels may be contributed to better patient selection. Given that most patients with recurrent tumours already failed after a curative dose of 66–70 Gy of the previous treatment, it is very unlikely that sufficient loco-regional control rate can be achieved when a much lower dose will be used in the re-irradiation setting. The same line of reasoning is applicable for SPTs in previously irradiated areas. There is no reason to believe that a lower dose of radiation than usually applied in the primary setting will result in satisfactory loco-regional control rates.

Therefore, in case of curatively intended (chemo-)re-irradiation, a total dose of at least 60 Gy with standard fractionation or a biologically equivalent dose using hyperfractionation is required. Preferably, hyperfractionation with a moderate reduction of the overall treatment time of radiation (Fu et al. 2000) will be most optimal in this setting.

4.3 Chemo-re-irradiation

In a previous report, an overview regarding the results achieved with chemo-re-irradiation was provided (Kasperts et al. 2005). In summary, in most of these series, chemotherapy mainly consisted of 5-FU and hydroxyurea, as originally described by Vokes et al. (1989) using alternating chemo-re-irradiation protocols. In these series, 2-year overall survival rates varying between 5 and 45 % have been reported (Weppelmann et al. 1992; Spencer et al. 1999; Schaefer et al. 2000).

The first prospective multi-institutional trial testing a re-irradiation plus chemotherapy regimen was conducted by the RTOG (RTOG protocol 9610) (Spencer et al. 2008). In this study, 79 patients with unresectable recurrent and second primary tumours were enrolled and analysed. The 2- and 5-year survival rates were 15 % and 3.8 %, respectively. The 5-year overall survival rate in this study was somewhat disappointing, but is similar to that reported by others (De Crevoisier et al. 1998). These results were obtained at the cost of considerable acute and late toxicity. In total, 17.7 % and 7.6 % of the patients experienced grade 4 and grade 5 mainly haematological acute toxicity. Late toxicity was mainly related to radiotherapy with 19.4 % grade 3 and 30 % grade 4 toxicities. Approximately 70 % of the patients were tube-feeding dependent at the last follow-up.

The trials that reported higher survival rates generally used more effective chemotherapy regimens and higher total doses of re-irradiation and/or included patients treated with postoperative chemo-re-irradiation (Langendijk et al. 2006; Milano et al. 2005).

In the primary setting, the results of a number of prospective studies showed that induction chemotherapy with taxanes, cisplatin and 5-FU (TPF) followed by radiotherapy or concomitant chemo-radiation is more effective than induction chemotherapy with cisplatin and 5-FU alone. The addition of taxanes in the chemo-re-irradiation setting is of interest as the results of preclinical data suggest that taxanes are particularly effective in radiotherapy-resistant squamous cell carcinoma cell lines (Britten et al. 1998).

During the last 5 years, a number of authors reported on (chemo-)re-irradiation protocols containing taxanes (Hehr et al. 2005; Kramer et al. 2005; Langer et al. 2007).

Kramer et al. (2005) reported on the results obtained in 38 patients with recurrent unresectable HNSCC that were treated in two prospective phases I–II trials at the Fox Chase Cancer Center. Patients were treated with split-course re-irradiation and concomitant cisplatin and paclitaxel. In this study, the 2-year overall survival was 35 %, with a progression-free survival at 1 year of 33 %, with increased but acceptable treatment-related morbidity.

Of note is the phase II study conducted by the RTOG (RTOG protocol 9911) (Langer et al. 2007). The study population of this study was composed of 105 patients with loco-regional recurrences or SPTs in previously irradiated areas. The protocol consisted of twice-daily radiation (1.5 Gy per fraction bid) for 5 days every 2 weeks up to a total dose of 60 Gy combined with cisplatin 15 mg/m^2 daily and paclitaxel 20 mg/m^2 daily for 5 days every other week. The protocol showed reasonable compliance with 74 % of the patients completing the planned chemotherapy and 76 % of the patients receiving at least 52.5 Gy of radiation. However, the toxicity of this protocol was substantial, with a relatively high incidence of treatment-related deaths and late grade 4 or worse toxicities. Grade 4 or worse acute radiation-induced and haematologic toxicity presented in 28 % and 21 % of the cases, respectively. There were 8 % treatment-related deaths of which 5 % in the acute phase. In addition, there were three fatal late complications, including two carotid haemorrhages and one death attributable to oral-cutaneous fistula and soft tissue necrosis. The median overall survival was 12.1 months and the 1- and 2-year overall survival rates were 50.2 % and 25.9 %, respectively, which was significantly better than observed in RTOG 9601 in which the 1- and 2-year survival rates were 47.1 and 16.9 % ($p=0.044$).

It should be stressed that definitive conclusions from these relatively small phase II studies are difficult to draw, but the results of taxane-based chemo-re-irradiation regimens are certainly promising with relatively impressive tumour control and survival rates but at the cost of increased and significant acute and late morbidity. As compared to the previously reported RTOG protocol (RTOG 9601), the results of taxane-based chemo-re-irradiation protocols appear to be better.

Based on these results, the question arises as to whether concurrent chemo-re-irradiation yields better results than chemotherapy alone containing cisplatin either or not in combination with taxanes, which was investigated in a prospective randomised study (RTOG 0421) (Wong et al. 2006). Unfortunately, this study was terminated due to poor patient accrual.

4.4 Re-irradiation Combined with Cetuximab

The results of a phase III randomised study in the primary setting demonstrated that the epidermal growth factor receptor (EGFR) inhibitor cetuximab given concomitantly with radiotherapy significantly improved LRC and OS compared to radiotherapy alone without any increase in radiation-induced toxicity (Bonner et al. 2010). Therefore, the use of agents directed against specific molecular targets in general and the EGFR receptor in particular might be a more promising approach. This is supported by the fact that the use of anti-EGFR targeting alone (cetuximab) has been shown to be effective in refractory HNSCC patients, progressing under salvage chemotherapy (Baselga et al. 2005). The number of reports on the combination of re-irradiation and cetuximab is increasing (Balermpas et al. 2009; Jensen et al. 2010; Lartigau et al. 2013; Dornoff et al. 2015).

Worth mentioning is the multicentre phase II study on the efficacy and safety of hypofractionated stereotactic body radiotherapy (SBRT) in combination with 5 weekly injections of cetuximab among 60 patients with inoperable recurrent HNC patients or patients with SPTs (Lartigau et al. 2013). All patients had previous radiotherapy, 85 % had previous surgery and 48 % had previous chemotherapy. At 3 months, the response rate was 58 % and the 1-year overall survival rate was 48 %, while acute toxicity was limited, mainly skin toxicity. One patient died from toxic death. The authors concluded that this approach seems to be effective and tolerable with regard to acute and late toxicity.

Although promising, it remains difficult to draw definitive conclusions from this study as the total dose of re-irradiation was relatively low and lacks direct comparison with other approaches.

Given the mild toxicity, this approach warrants further evaluation in well-designed future re-irradiation studies in which the radiation protocol should be further optimised.

5 Postoperative Re-irradiation

As mentioned in one of the previous paragraphs, salvage surgery is considered the treatment of choice for recurrent and second primary HNSCC in previously irradiated areas. Patients eligible for surgery should have non-metastatic disease, with limited tumours that can be surgically resected with sufficient margins, without unacceptable morbidity, and be considered medically fit to undergo surgery.

Although salvage surgery alone can be relatively successful in a well-selected subset of patients (McLaughlin et al. 1996; Ganly et al. 2005), results become worse in more advanced recurrent stages (Agra et al. 2006). Moreover, in case of risk factors for loco-regional recurrence, such as positive surgical margins and lymph node metastases with extranodal spread (Langendijk et al. 2005; Jonkman et al. 2007), the risk on loco-regional failure will increase and postoperative (chemo-)re-irradiation could be considered (Kasperts et al. 2006).

The GORTEC/GETTEC reported on a prospective phase III study in which 130 patients that underwent salvage surgery were randomly assigned to receive full-dose re-irradiation (60 Gy) combined with concomitant chemotherapy (5-FU and hydroxyurea) versus no adjuvant treatment (Janot et al. 2008). All patients had recurrent tumours or SPTs in previously irradiated areas and underwent a macroscopic complete resection. In the majority of patients, the surgical margins were sufficient. A significant improvement with regard to loco-regional tumour control (HR, 2.73; 95% CI, 1.66–4.51; $p<0.0010$) and disease-free survival (HR, 1.68; 95% CI, 1.13–2.50; $p=0.01$) was observed in those patients that were assigned to receive postoperative chemo-re-irradiation compared to those that underwent surgery alone. However, this benefit in disease-free survival did not translate into a significant improvement of the overall survival, which may be due to the higher incidence of distant metastases in the chemo-re-irradiation arm. The most serious acute side effect was grade 3–4 mucositis, which occurred in 28% of the patients. The gain in loco-regional tumour control and disease-free survival was achieved at the cost of significantly higher rates of grade 3–4 late side effects (39 versus 10% at 2 years, respectively). It should be noted that patients allocated to the wait-and-see arm received salvage chemo-re-irradiation at the time of loco-regional recurrence after salvage surgery, which was the case in 25% of the cases. In this regard, this study could be considered as a comparison between immediate versus delayed postoperative chemo-re-irradiation.

If the chemo-re-irradiation regimen as described in the GETTEC/GORTEC trial is the most optimal approach remains to be determined. As mentioned earlier, Kasperts et al. achieved a loco-regional control rate of 70% after 3 years among high-risk patients with either positive surgical margins or extra-nodal spread, with similar rates of late toxicity (Kasperts et al. 2006).

In conclusion, high-dose postoperative chemo-re-irradiation can be administered with a moderate but acceptable increase in late radiation-induced toxicity. More importantly, the results indicate that postoperative chemo-re-irradiation significantly improves loco-regional tumour control among patients at risk for a second failure. Therefore, postoperative (chemo-)re-irradiation should be considered in these cases, in particular given the very low loco-regional control rate after salvage surgery alone that was only 20% at 2 years. However, in the light of the high rate of late toxicity, the exact postoperative regimen in the re-irradiation setting requires further optimisation, e.g. by optimising the fractionation schedule and radiation technique and/or the addition of biological targets such as EGFR inhibitors, which do not interfere with radiation-induced side effects.

6 How to Reduce Treatment-Related Morbidity?

Treatment-related morbidity can be reduced by a number of measures, including reduction of the target volume for radiation and the use of selective radioprotectors. In the primary treatment, radiation-induced side effects mainly depend on total dose and are volume irradiated, illustrated by numerous reports on normal tissue complication probability (NTCP) models for different late side effects such as xerostomia and swallowing dysfunction. In the re-irradiation setting, no NTCP models are available. There are only some retrospective data that suggests a relationship of dose and volume of re-irradiated tissues as the most important prognostic factor for radiation-induced late side effects (Pomp et al. 1988; Stevens et al. 1994). To achieve a reduction of the irradiated volume of normal tissues, two main strategies have been applied, including attempts to redefine the clinical target volume and the use of advanced and emerging radiation delivery techniques.

6.1 Target Volume Definition Reduction

Elective nodal treatment, either by surgery or radiotherapy, is commonly applied in the primary treatment of HNSCC in case the probability of occult nodal metastases is 20 % or higher (Weiss et al. 1994; Gregoire et al. 2000). This threshold of 20 % is more or less arbitrarily determined taking into account the expected treatment-related morbidity reference to the expected improvement of regional control that can be achieved with elective treatment of the regional lymph node areas. As the probability of late radiation-induced morbidity will be higher in the case of (chemo-) re-irradiation and will increase with larger volumes irradiated (Langlois et al. 1985), it should be questioned whether elective nodal areas should be included in the target volume in case of (chemo-)re-irradiation as well.

In the majority of recently published series, the clinical target volume (CTV) was confined to the GTV with limited margins around the GTV in case of primary (chemo-)re-irradiation or limited to the high-risk areas in case of postoperative re-irradiation (Nagar et al. 2004; Hehr et al. 2005; Kasperts et al. 2006; Langendijk et al. 2006; Langer et al. 2007; Sulman et al. 2009; Heron et al. 2009, 2010; Berger et al. 2010; Chen et al. 2011).

Popovtzer et al. (2009) performed a retrospective analysis on patterns of failure in 66 patients treated with curatively intended re-irradiation in whom the targets in all patients only encompassed the recurrent GTV with limited margins. Out of the 47 loco-regional recurrences, 45 (96 %) occurred within the recurrent GTV area, except for two patients, who developed a true out-of-field recurrence (4 %). Similar results were found by other investigators (Nagar et al. 2004; Hehr et al. 2005; Kasperts et al. 2006; Langendijk et al. 2006; Langer et al. 2007; Sulman et al. 2009; Heron et al. 2009, 2010; Berger et al. 2010; Chen et al. 2011).

These results indicate that in primary or postoperative (chemo-)re-irradiation, limitation of the CTV to the high-risk area or GTV with some margin is safe and should be considered particularly in case the elective nodal areas encompass heavily treated structures.

6.2 New Radiation Techniques

In many patients referred for re-irradiation, it is difficult to achieve an adequate dose distribution with conventional 3D conformal techniques, particularly in case of concave and U-shaped target volumes near organs at risk (OARs) such as the spinal cord that has reached radiation tolerance. In these cases, it is not unusual to compromise the dose to the target in favour of limiting the dose to OARs, which may be associated with higher loco-regional failure rates (Nutting et al. 2011). Given the described dose-effect relationships for tumour control, both dose escalation in the target volume and maximal reduction of the dose distribution in OARs are even more important in the re-irradiation than in the primary setting. In this respect, the use of advanced radiation delivery techniques becomes increasingly important.

6.3 Intensity-Modulated Radiotherapy

Intensity-modulated radiotherapy (IMRT) is a radiation technique in which the intensity of multiple beams can be optimised in order to conform the radiation dose to the target volumes, while reducing the dose to adjacent critical structures. The initial experiences with IMRT in the primary setting have provided encouraging results regarding loco-regional tumour control, overall survival and in particular reduction of side effects (Lee et al. 2006; McMillan et al. 2006; Pow et al. 2006; Vergeer et al. 2009; Christianen et al. 2016), such as xerostomia and dysphagia. As IMRT permits increased possibilities to conform the dose to the target volume, it promises to both reduce toxicity and improve loco-regional tumour control. A limited number of authors reported on the results achieved with IMRT in the re-irradiation setting (Sulman et al. 2009; Chen et al. 2011; Sher et al. 2010).

Sulman et al. (2009) reported on the results of a retrospective analysis including 78 consecutive patients treated with curatively intended re-irradiation (median total dose, 60 Gy) either following salvage surgery or in combination with chemotherapy. The results with regard to loco-regional tumour control and overall survival were promising with 2-year actuarial rates of 64 % and 58 %, respectively. Severe late radiation-induced side effects occurred in 20 % of the cases. The authors mentioned that this incidence of late radiation-induced toxicity appears to be less common than reported by others using conventional radiation techniques, suggesting a benefit in therapeutic ratio.

In another retrospective study from the Dana-Farber Cancer Institute, 35 patients received concomitant chemo-re-irradiation using IMRT to a median total dose of 60 Gy (Sher et al. 2010). The loco-regional control and overall survival rates at 2 years were 67 % and 48 %, respectively, and thus comparable to those reported by Sulman et al. (2009).

Chen et al. reported on the first prospective study on high-dose re-irradiation using daily image guidance with IMRT (Chen et al. 2011). They included 21 patients who were treated with IMRT confined to the GTV with limited margins without chemotherapy together with daily helical megavoltage CT scans before each fraction. The 2-year loco-regional control rate was 65 % and there were no treatment-related toxic deaths. Fibrosis of the neck was the most frequently reported late side effect. Of note is that 57 % of the patients were gastrostomy tube dependent at last follow-up.

More recently, Duprez et al. reported on the long-term results of a retrospective study that included 67 patients with recurrent HNC treated with IMRT to a total dose of 70 Gy (conventional fractionation) (Duprez et al. 2009). In this study, the 5-year loco-regional control rate was 32 % with an overall survival rate of 22 % after 5 years. The cumulative incidence of grade III and IV late toxicity was 66 % after 5 years.

The results from these studies indicate that high rates of loco-regional control can be achieved with high-dose re-IMRT with or without chemotherapy, but that the development of severe late radiation-induced side effects remains of major concern, although the incidence of these side effects appears to be somewhat lower than observed after conventional radiation techniques. Long-term survival is possible but at the costs of high rates of grade 3 and 4 toxicities (Duprez et al. 2009).

6.4 Stereotactic Radiotherapy

Further reduction of the dose to OARs can be achieved by improving delivery accuracy using, e.g. stereotactic radiation techniques. Recently, Heron et al. presented the results of a phase I study testing the safety and efficacy of stereotactic body radiotherapy (SBRT) among patients with HNSCC in previously irradiated areas (Heron et al. 2010). In this study, the target volume was confined to the radiographic and clinical areas of gross tumour, augmented by PET-CT when available. The 80 % isodose was intended to cover at least 90 % of the target volume. Then, the dose was escalated from 5 fractions of 5 Gy to 5 fractions of 8.8 Gy. A total number of 25 patients were included of which 65 % also received chemotherapy. The treatment was well tolerated, no dose limiting toxicities were encountered and the maximum tolerated dose was not reached. However, the response rates were relatively low with only four objective responses with a maximum duration of 4 months. No significant association was found between total dose of radiation and objective response. This approach will be further investigated in a phase II study combining SBRT with the highest dose level with cetuximab.

In another study, 36 patients with local recurrences from various tumours sites in the head and neck region were treated with fractionated stereotactic radiotherapy (Roh et al. 2009). In this study, the PTV encompassed the radiographic GTV with a 2–3 mm margin. A complete response was achieved in 43 % of the patients, while in 37 % of the cases, a partial response was achieved. However, the exact efficacy of this approach remains difficult to assess as one of the major limitations of this study was that tumour dose and fractionation was determined on an individual basis according to a number of factors, such as previous radiation dose, interval, performance status and estimated remaining tolerance of adjacent normal tissues. In 13 patients (30 %), grade III acute complications were noted, while late complications were noted in three patients (one bone necrosis and two soft tissue necrosis).

More recently, Kress et al. (2015) found a 2-year overall survival and loco-regional recurrence rates of 24 % and 28 %, respectively, in 85 HNC patients after re-irradiation with hypofractionated stereotactic radiotherapy, with very low grade 3 late toxicity rates (5.9 %). In this study different fractionation schedules were used.

Given the small size of these studies and the heterogeneity regarding the study populations as well as the different fractionation schedules used, it remains difficult to draw definitive conclusion from these two studies. One of the advantages of using stereotactic radiation techniques could be the use of image-guided high precision repositioning in order to be able to safely reduce the margins from CTV to PTV. However, using higher dose per fraction, as was the case in both studies, could counterbalance this advantage of volume reduction. Using higher doses per fraction to the GTV only assumes that the radiographic GTV only contains the tumour tissue rather than the normal tissue, which is very unlikely. The three major complications in the latter study could be contributed to the use of these higher doses per fraction.

It is clear that the most optimal fractionation when using stereotactic radiation techniques remains to be determined, in particular when combined with systemic agents.

Conclusions

Loco-regional failure of HNSCC or second primary tumours in previously irradiated areas after a full course of (chemo)radiation poses a challenging problem for radiation oncologists, but remains a potentially curable disease.

Whenever feasible, salvage surgery remains the standard of care, which is the case in approximately 20 % of the cases. In case of adverse prognostic factors, immediate postoperative (chemo-)re-irradiation after salvage surgery can be administered safely and significantly improves loco-regional control. Despite relatively high rates of late radiation-induced complications, adjuvant (chemo-)re-irradiation should be considered in case there is an increased risk on loco-regional recurrence, such as in case of positive surgical margins and/or lymph node metastases with extranodal spread.

In case of unresectable loco-regional failures or SPTs, curatively intended (chemo-)radiation should be considered in well-selected cases. The results of taxane-based chemo-re-irradiation protocols are promising with a reasonable percentage of long-term survivors.

Severe treatment-related morbidity remains of major concern in case of chemo-re-irradiation. The initial treatment modality (e.g. radiotherapy alone or chemo-radiation) should be taken into account, and 'recurrence analysis' should be part of the diagnostic procedure when (chemo-)re-irradiation is considered. The clinical target volume can be confined to the GTV with limited margins in case of primary (chemo-)re-irradiation or to the high-risk areas in the postoperative setting. Limiting the target volume using the most advanced radiation delivery techniques (IMRT and stereotactic radiotherapy) to the high-risk areas appears to be of outstanding importance to reduce the radiation-induced morbidity and thus the therapeutic ratio, but care must be taken with regard to the use of high-dose per fraction. Moreover, outcomes in terms of loco-regional control and survival after IMRT are very promising.

Future studies should focus on new developments that proved to be effective in the primary treatment of HNSCC. In this respect, new induction chemotherapy regimens such as TPF and the addition of cetuximab to radiation are of great interest as these approaches might improve loco-regional control and overall without increasing treatment-related morbidity.

References

Agra IM, Carvalho AL, Pontes E, Campos OD, Ulbrich FS, Magrin J, Kowalski LP (2003) Postoperative complications after en bloc salvage surgery for head and neck cancer. Arch Otolaryngol Head Neck Surg 129(12):1317–1321

Agra IM, Carvalho AL, Ulbrich FS, de Campos OD, Martins EP, Magrin J, Kowalski LP (2006) Prognostic factors in salvage surgery for recurrent oral and oropharyngeal cancer. Head Neck 28(2):107–113

Agra IM, Carvalho AL, Pinto CA, Martins EP, Filho JG, Soares FA, Kowalski LP (2008) Biological markers and prognosis in recurrent oral cancer after salvage surgery. Arch Otolaryngol Head Neck Surg 134(7):743–749

Arnold DJ, Goodwin WJ, Weed DT, Civantos FJ (2004) Treatment of recurrent and advanced stage squamous cell carcinoma of the head and neck. Semin Radiat Oncol 14(2):190–195

Balermpas P, Hambek M, Seitz O, Rodel C, Weiss C (2009) Combined cetuximab and reirradiation for locoregional recurrent and inoperable squamous cell carcinoma of the head and neck. Strahlenther Onkol 185(12):775–781

Baselga J, Trigo JM, Bourhis J, Tortochaux J, Cortes-Funes H, Hitt R, Gascon P, Amellal N, Harstrick A, Eckardt A (2005) Phase II multicenter study of the antiepidermal growth factor receptor monoclonal antibody cetuximab in combination with platinum-based chemotherapy in patients with platinum-refractory metastatic and/or recurrent squamous cell carcinoma of the head and neck. J Clin Oncol 23(24):5568–5577

Baujat B, Bourhis J, Blanchard P, Overgaard J, Ang KK, Saunders M, Le Maître A, Bernier J, Horiot JC, Maillard E, Pajak TF, Poulsen MG, Bourredjem A, O'Sullivan B, Dobrowsky W, Andrzej H, Skladowski K, Hay JH, Pinto LH, Fu KK, Fallai C, Sylvester R, Pignon JP; MARCH Collaborative Group (2010) Hyperfractionated or accelerated radiotherapy for head and neck cancer. Cochrane Database Syst Rev (12):CD002026

Berger B, Belka C, Weinmann M, Bamberg M, Budach W, Hehr T (2010) Reirradiation with alternating docetaxel-based chemotherapy for recurrent head and neck squamous cell carcinoma: update of a single-center prospective phase II protocol. Strahlenther Onkol 186(5):255–261

Bernier J, Domenge C, Ozsahin M, Matuszewska K, Lefebvre JL, Greiner RH, Giralt J, Maingon P, Rolland F, Bolla M, Cognetti F, Bourhis J et al (2004) Postoperative irradiation with or without concomitant chemotherapy for locally advanced head and neck cancer. N Engl J Med 350(19):1945–1952

Bernier J, Cooper JS, Pajak TF, van Glabbeke M, Bourhis J, Forastiere A, Ozsahin EM, Jacobs JR, Jassem J, Ang KK, Lefèbvre JL (2005) Defining risk levels in locally advanced head and neck cancers: a comparative analysis of concurrent postoperative radiation plus chemotherapy trials of the EORTC (#22931) and RTOG (# 9501). Head Neck 27(10):843–850

Blanchard P, Hill C, Guihenneuc-Jouyaux C, Baey C, Bourhis J, Pignon JP, MACH-NC and MARCH Collaborative Groups (2011) Mixed treatment comparison meta-analysis of altered fractionated radiotherapy and chemotherapy in head and neck cancer. J Clin Epidemiol 64(9):985–992

Blanchard P, Bourhis J, Lacas B, Posner MR, Vermorken JB, Hernandez JJ, Bourredjem A, Calais G, Paccagnella A, Hitt R, Pignon JP, Meta-Analysis of Chemotherapy in Head and Neck Cancer, Induction Project, Collaborative Group (2013) Taxane-cisplatin-fluorouracil as induction chemotherapy in locally advanced head and neck cancers: an individual patient data meta-analysis of the meta-analysis of chemotherapy in head and neck cancer group. J Clin Oncol 31(23):2854–2860

Blanchard P, Lee A, Marguet S, Leclercq J, Ng WT, Ma J, Chan AT, Huang PY, Benhamou E, Zhu G, Chua DT, Chen Y, Mai HQ, Kwong DL, Cheah SL, Moon J, Tung Y, Chi KH, Fountzilas G, Zhang L, Hui EP, Lu TX, Bourhis J, Pignon JP, MAC-NPC Collaborative Group (2015) Chemotherapy and radiotherapy in nasopharyngeal carcinoma: an update of the MAC-NPC meta-analysis. Lancet Oncol 16(6):645–655

Bonner JA, Harari PM, Giralt J, Azarnia N, Shin DM, Cohen RB, Jones CU, Sur R, Raben D, Jassem J, Ove R, Kies MS, Baselga J, Youssoufian H, Amellal N, Rowinsky EK, Ang KK (2006) Radiotherapy plus cetuximab for squamous-cell carcinoma of the head and neck. N Engl J Med 354(6):567–578

Bonner JA, Harari PM, Giralt J, Cohen RB, Jones CU, Sur RK, Raben D, Baselga J, Spencer SA, Zhu J, Youssoufian H, Rowinsky EK, Ang KK (2010) Radiotherapy plus cetuximab for locoregionally advanced head and neck cancer: 5-year survival data from a phase 3 randomised trial, and relation between cetuximab-induced rash and survival. Lancet Oncol 11(1):21–28

Britten RA, Perdue S, Opoku J, Craighead P (1998) Paclitaxel is preferentially cytotoxic to human cervical tumor cells with low Raf-1 kinase activity: implications for paclitaxel-based chemo radiation regimens. Radiother Oncol 48(3):329–334

Chen AM, Farwell DG, Luu Q, Cheng S, Donald PJ, Purdy JA (2011) Prospective trial of high-dose reirradiation using daily image guidance with intensity-modulated radiotherapy for recurrent and second primary head-and-neck cancer. Int J Radiat Oncol Biol Phys 80(3):669–676

Choe KS, Haraf DJ, Solanki A, Cohen EE, Seiwert TY, Stenson KM, Blair EA, Portugal L, Villaflor VM, Witt ME, Vokes EE, Salama JK (2011) Prior chemoradiotherapy adversely impacts outcomes of recurrent and second primary head and neck cancer treated with concurrent chemotherapy and reirradiation. Cancer 117(20):4671–4678

Christianen ME, van der Schaaf A, van der Laan HP, Verdonck-de Leeuw IM, Doornaert P, Chouvalova O, Steenbakkers RJ, Leemans CR, Oosting SF, van der Laan BF, Roodenburg JL, Slotman BJ, Bijl HP, Langendijk JA (2016) Swallowing sparing intensity modulated radiotherapy (SW-IMRT) in head and neck cancer: clinical validation according to the model-based approach. Radiother Oncol 118(2):298–303

Cooper JS, Pajak TF, Forastiere AA, Jacobs J, Campbell BH, Saxman SB, Kish JA, Kim HE, Cmelak AJ, Rotman M, Machtay M, Ensley JF et al (2004) Postoperative concurrent radiotherapy and chemotherapy for high-risk squamous-cell carcinoma of the head and neck. N Engl J Med 350(19):1937–1944

Datta NR, Nagar YS, Singh S, Naryan L (2003) Loco-regional failures in head and neck cancer: can they be effectively salvaged by nonsurgical therapeutic modalities? Int J Clin Oncol 8(1):31–39

Dawson LA, Myers LL, Bradford CR, Chepeha DB, Hogikyan ND, Teknos TN, Terrell JE, Wolf GT, Eisbruch A (2001) Conformal re-irradiation of recurrent and new primary head-and-neck cancer. Int J Radiat Oncol Biol Phys 50(2):377–385

de Crevoisier R, Bourhis J, Domenge C, Wibault P, Koscielny S, Lusinchi A, Mamelle G, Janot F, Julieron M, Leridant AM, Marandas P, Armand JP et al (1998) Full-dose reirradiation for unresectable head and neck carcinoma: experience at the Gustave-Roussy Institute in a series of 169 patients. J Clin Oncol 16(11):3556–3562

de Crevoisier R, Domenge C, Wibault P, Koscielny S, Lusinchi A, Janot F, Bobin S, Luboinski B, Eschwege F, Bourhis J (2001) Full dose reirradiation combined with chemotherapy after salvage surgery in head and neck carcinoma. Cancer 91(11):2071–2076

Dornoff N, Weiß C, Rödel F, Wagenblast J, Ghanaati S, Atefeh N, Rödel C, Balermpas P (2015) Reirradiation with cetuximab or cisplatin-based chemotherapy for recurrent squamous cell carcinoma of the head and neck. Strahlenther Onkol 191(8):656–664

Duprez F, Madani I, Bonte K, Boterberg T, Vakaet L, Derie C, De Gersem W, De De neve W (2009) Intensity-modulated radiotherapy for recurrent and second primary head and neck cancer in previously irradiated territory. Radiother Oncol 93(3):563–569

Forastiere AA, Metch B, Schuller DE, Ensley JF, Hutchins LF, Triozzi P, Kish JA, McClure S, VonFeldt E, Williamson SK (1992) Randomized comparison of cisplatin plus fluorouracil and carboplatin plus fluorouracil versus methotrexate in advanced squamous-cell carcinoma of the head and neck: a Southwest Oncology Group study. J Clin Oncol 10(8):1245–1251

Fu KK, Pajak TF, Trotti A, Jones CU, Spencer SA, Phillips TL, Garden AS, Ridge JA, Cooper JS, Ang KK (2000) A Radiation Therapy Oncology Group (RTOG) phase III randomized study to compare hyperfractionation and two variants of accelerated fractionation to standard fractionation radiotherapy for head and neck squamous cell carcinomas: first report of RTOG 9003. Int J Radiat Oncol Biol Phys 48(1):7–16

Ganly I, Patel S, Matsuo J, Singh B, Kraus D, Boyle J, Wong R, Lee N, Pfister DG, Shaha A, Shah J (2005) Postoperative complications of salvage total laryngectomy. Cancer 103(10):2073–2081

Gibson MK, Li Y, Murphy B, Hussain MH, DeConti RC, Ensley J, Forastiere AA (2005) Randomized phase III evaluation of cisplatin plus fluorouracil versus cisplatin plus paclitaxel in advanced head and neck cancer (E1395): an intergroup trial of the Eastern Cooperative Oncology Group. J Clin Oncol 23(15):3562–3567

Gilbert H, Kagan AR (1974) Recurrence patterns in squamous cell carcinoma of the oral cavity, pharynx, and larynx. J Surg Oncol 6(5):357–380

Goodwin WJ Jr (2000) Salvage surgery for patients with recurrent squamous cell carcinoma of the upper aerodigestive tract: when do the ends justify the means? Laryngoscope 110(3 Pt 2 Suppl 93):1–18

Gregoire V, Coche E, Cosnard G, Hamoir M, Reychler H (2000) Selection and delineation of lymph node target volumes in head and neck conformal radiotherapy. Proposal for standardizing terminology and procedure based on the surgical experience. Radiother Oncol 56(2):135–150

Haughey BH, Gates GA, Arfken CL, Harvey J (1992) Meta-analysis of second malignant tumors in head and neck cancer: the case for an endoscopic screening protocol. Ann Otol Rhinol Laryngol 101(2 Pt 1):105–112

Hehr T, Classen J, Belka C, Welz S, Schafer J, Koitschev A, Bamberg M, Budach W (2005) Reirradiation alternating with docetaxel and cisplatin in inoperable recurrence of head-and-neck cancer: a prospective phase I/II trial. Int J Radiat Oncol Biol Phys 61(5):1423–1431

Heron DE, Ferris RL, Karamouzis M, Andrade RS, Deeb EL, Burton S, Gooding WE, Branstetter BF, Mountz JM, Johnson JT, Argiris A, Grandis JR et al (2009) Stereotactic body radiotherapy for recurrent squamous cell carcinoma of the head and neck: results of a phase I dose-escalation trial. Int J Radiat Oncol Biol Phys 75(5):1493–1500

Heron DE, Rwigema JC, Gibson MK, Burton SA, Quinn AE, Ferris RL (2010) Concurrent cetuximab with stereotactic body radiotherapy for recurrent squamous cell carcinoma of the head and neck: a single institution matched case-control study. Am J Clin Oncol 34(2):165–172

Hong WK, Schaefer S, Issell B, Cummings C, Luedke D, Bromer R, Fofonoff S, D'Aoust J, Shapshay S, Welch J, Levin E, Vincent M et al (1983) A prospective randomized trial of methotrexate versus cisplatin in the treatment of recurrent squamous cell carcinoma of the head and neck. Cancer 52(2):206–210

Janot F, De Raucourt D, Benhamou E, Ferron C, Dolivet G, Bensadoun RJ, Hamoir M, Gery B, Julieron M, Castaing M, Bardet E, Gregoire V et al (2008) Randomized trial of postoperative reirradiation combined with chemotherapy after salvage surgery compared with salvage surgery alone in head and neck carcinoma. J Clin Oncol 26(34):5518–5523

Jensen AD, Bergmann ZP, Garcia-Huttenlocher H, Freier K, Debus J, Münter MW (2010) Cetuximab and radiation for primary and recurrent squamous cell carcinoma of the head and neck (SCCHN) in the elderly and multi-morbid patient. A single center experience. Head Neck Oncol 2:34

Jonkman A, Kaanders JH, Terhaard CH, Hoebers FJ, van den Ende PL, Wijers OB, Verhoef LC, de Jong MA, Leemans CR, Langendijk JA (2007) Multicenter validation of recursive partitioning analysis classification for patients with squamous cell head and neck carcinoma treated with surgery and postoperative radiotherapy. Int J Radiat Oncol Biol Phys 68(1):119–125

Kasperts N, Slotman B, Leemans CR, Langendijk JA (2005) A review on re-irradiation for recurrent and second primary head and neck cancer. Oral Oncol 41(3):225–243

Kasperts N, Slotman BJ, Leemans CR, de Bree R, Doornaert P, Langendijk JA (2006) Results of postoperative reirradiation for recurrent or second primary head and neck carcinoma. Cancer 106(7):1536–1547

Kim AJ, Suh JD, Sercarz JA, Abemayor E, Head C, Funk G, Blackwell KE (2007) Salvage surgery with free flap reconstruction: factors affecting outcome after treatment of recurrent head and neck squamous carcinoma. Laryngoscope 117(6):1019–1023

Kramer NM, Horwitz EM, Cheng J, Ridge JA, Feigenberg SJ, Cohen RB, Nicolaou N, Sherman EJ, Babb JS, Damsker JA, Langer CJ (2005) Toxicity and outcome analysis of patients with recurrent head and neck cancer treated with hyperfractionated split-course reirradiation and concurrent cisplatin and paclitaxel chemotherapy from two prospective phase I and II studies. Head Neck 27(5):406–414

Kress MAS, Sen N, Unger KR, Lominska CE, Deeken JF, Davidson BJ, Newkirk KA, Hwang J, Harter KW (2015) Safety and efficacy of hypofractionated stereotactic body reirradiation in head and neck cancer: long-term follow-up of a large series. Head Neck 37(10):1403–1409

Lacy PD, Spitznagel EL Jr, Piccirillo JF (1999) Development of a new staging system for recurrent oral cavity and oropharyngeal squamous cell carcinoma. Cancer 86(8):1387–1395

Langendijk JA, Leemans CR, Buter J, Berkhof J, Slotman BJ (2004) The additional value of chemotherapy to radiotherapy in locally advanced nasopharyngeal carcinoma: a meta-analysis of the published literature. J Clin Oncol 22(22):4604–4612

Langendijk JA, Slotman BJ, van der Waal I, Doornaert P, Berkof J, Leemans CR (2005) Risk-group definition by recursive partitioning analysis of patients with squamous cell head and neck carcinoma treated with surgery and postoperative radiotherapy. Cancer 104(7):1408–1417

Langendijk JA, Kasperts N, Leemans CR, Doornaert P, Slotman BJ (2006) A phase II study of primary reirradiation in squamous cell carcinoma of head and neck. Radiother Oncol 78(3):306–312

Langer CJ, Harris J, Horwitz EM, Nicolaou N, Kies M, Curran W, Wong S, Ang K (2007) Phase II study of low-dose paclitaxel and cisplatin in combination with split-course concomitant twice-daily reirradiation in recurrent squamous cell carcinoma of the head and neck: results of Radiation Therapy Oncology Group Protocol 9911. J Clin Oncol 25(30):4800–4805

Langlois D, Eschwege F, Kramar A, Richard JM (1985) Reirradiation of head and neck cancers. Presentation of 35 cases treated at the Gustave Roussy Institute. Radiother Oncol 3(1):27–33

Lartigau EF, Tresch E, Thariat J, Graff P, Coche-Dequeant B, Benezery K, Schiappacasse L, Degardin M, Bondiau PY, Peiffert D, Lefebvre JL, Lacornerie T, Kramar A (2013) Multi institutional phase II study of concomitant stereotactic reirradiation and cetuximab for recurrent head and neck cancer. Radiother Oncol 109(2):281–285

Lee NY, de Arruda FF, Puri DR, Wolden SL, Narayana A, Mechalakos J, Venkatraman ES, Kraus D, Shaha A, Shah JP, Pfister DG, Zelefsky MJ (2006) A comparison of intensity-modulated radiation therapy and concomitant boost radiotherapy in the setting of concurrent chemotherapy for locally advanced oropharyngeal carcinoma. Int J Radiat Oncol Biol Phys 66(4): 966–974

Llewelyn J, Mitchell R (1997) Survival of patients who needed salvage surgery for recurrence after radiotherapy for oral carcinoma. Br J Oral Maxillofac Surg 35(6):424–428

Mabanta SR, Mendenhall WM, Stringer SP, Cassisi NJ (1999) Salvage treatment for neck recurrence after irradiation alone for head and neck squamous cell carcinoma with clinically positive neck nodes. Head Neck 21(7):591–594

McLaughlin MP, Parsons JT, Fein DA, Stringer SP, Cassisi NJ, Mendenhall WM, Million RR (1996) Salvage surgery after radiotherapy failure in T1-T2 squamous cell carcinoma of the glottic larynx. Head Neck 18(3):229–235

McMillan AS, Pow EH, Kwong DL, Wong MC, Sham JS, Leung LH, Leung WK (2006) Preservation of quality of life after intensity-modulated radiotherapy for early-stage nasopharyngeal carcinoma: results of a prospective longitudinal study. Head Neck 28(8):712–722

Milano MT, Vokes EE, Salama JK, Stenson KM, Kao J, Witt ME, Mittal BB, Argiris A, Weichselbaum RR, Haraf DJ (2005) Twice-daily reirradiation for recurrent and second primary head-and-neck cancer with gemcitabine, paclitaxel, and 5-fluorouracil chemotherapy. Int J Radiat Oncol Biol Phys 61(4):1096–1106

Nagar YS, Singh S, Datta NR (2004) Chemo-reirradiation in persistent/recurrent head and neck cancers. Jpn J Clin Oncol 34(2):61–68

Nutting CM, Morden JP, Harrington KJ, Urbano TG, Bhide SA, Clark C, Miles EA, Miah AB, Newbold K, Tanay M, Adab F, Jefferies SJ, Scrase C, Yap BK, A'Hern RP, Sydenham MA, Emson M, Hall E, PARSPORT trial management group (2011) Parotid-sparing intensity modulated versus conventional radiotherapy in head and neck cancer (PARSPORT): a phase 3 multicentre randomised controlled trial. Lancet Oncol 12(2):127–136

Pignon JP, le Maître A, Maillard E, Bourhis J, MACH-NC Collaborative Group (2009) Meta-analysis of chemotherapy in head and neck cancer (MACH-NC): an update on 93 randomised trials and 17,346 patients. Radiother Oncol 92(1):4–14

Pomp J, Levendag PC, van Putten WL (1988) Reirradiation of recurrent tumors in the head and neck. Am J Clin Oncol 11(5):543–549

Popovtzer A, Gluck I, Chepeha DB, Teknos TN, Moyer JS, Prince ME, Bradford CR, Eisbruch A (2009) The pattern of failure after reirradiation of recurrent squamous cell head and neck cancer: implications for defining the targets. Int J Radiat Oncol Biol Phys 74(5):1342–1347

Pow EH, Kwong DL, McMillan AS, Wong MC, Sham JS, Leung LH, Leung WK (2006) Xerostomia and quality of life after intensity-modulated radiotherapy vs. conventional radiotherapy for early-stage nasopharyngeal carcinoma: initial report on a randomized controlled clinical trial. Int J Radiat Oncol Biol Phys 66(4): 981–991

Pradhan SA, Rajpal RM, Kothary PM (1980) Surgical management of postradiation residual/recurrent cancer of the base of the tongue. J Surg Oncol 14(3): 201–206

Putten L, Bree R, Doornaert PA, Buter J, Eerenstein SE, Rietveld DH, Kuik DJ, Leemans CR (2015) Salvage surgery in post-chemo radiation laryngeal and hypopharyngeal carcinoma: outcome and review. Acta Otorhinolaryngol Ital 35(3):162–172

Riaz N, Hong JC, Sherman EJ, Morris L, Fury M, Ganly I, Wang TJ, Shi W, Wolden SL, Jackson A, Wong RJ, Zhang Z, Rao SD, Lee NY (2014) A nomogram to predict loco-regional control after re-irradiation for head and neck cancer. Radiother Oncol 111(3):382–387

Ridge JA (1993) Squamous cancer of the head and neck: surgical treatment of local and regional recurrence. Semin Oncol 20(5):419–429

Roh KW, Jang JS, Kim MS, Sun DI, Kim BS, Jung SL, Kang JH, Yoo EJ, Yoon SC, Jang HS, Chung SM, Kim YS (2009) Fractionated stereotactic radiotherapy as reirradiation for locally recurrent head and neck cancer. Int J Radiat Oncol Biol Phys 74(5):1348–1355

Sacco AG, Cohen EE (2015) Current treatment options for recurrent or metastatic head and neck squamous cell carcinoma. J Clin Oncol 33(29):3305–3313

Salama JK, Vokes EE, Chmura SJ, Milano MT, Kao J, Stenson KM, Witt ME, Haraf DJ (2006) Long-term outcome of concurrent chemotherapy and reirradiation for recurrent and second primary head-and-neck squamous cell carcinoma. Int J Radiat Oncol Biol Phys 64(2):382–391

Schaefer U, Micke O, Schueller P, Willich N (2000) Recurrent head and neck cancer: retreatment of previously irradiated areas with combined chemotherapy and radiation therapy-results of a prospective study. Radiology 216(2):371–376

Sher DJ, Haddad RI, Norris CM Jr, Posner MR, Wirth LJ, Goguen LA, Annino D, Balboni T, Allen A, Tishler RB (2010) Efficacy and toxicity of reirradiation using intensity-modulated radiotherapy for recurrent or second primary head and neck cancer. Cancer 116(20):4761–4768

Skolyszewski J, Korzeniowski S, Reinfuss M (1980) The reirradiation of recurrences of head and neck cancer. Br J Radiol 53(629):462–465

Spencer SA, Wheeler RH, Peters GE, Beenken SW, Meredith RF, Smith J, Conner W, Salter MM (1999) Concomitant chemotherapy and reirradiation as management for recurrent cancer of the head and neck. Am J Clin Oncol 22(1):1–5

Spencer SA, Harris J, Wheeler RH, Machtay M, Schultz C, Spanos W, Rotman M, Meredith R (2001) RTOG 96-10: reirradiation with concurrent hydroxyurea and 5-fluorouracil in patients with squamous cell cancer of the head and neck. Int J Radiat Oncol Biol Phys 51(5):1299–1304

Spencer SA, Harris J, Wheeler RH, Machtay M, Schultz C, Spanos W, Rotman M, Meredith R, Ang KK (2008) Final report of RTOG 9610, a multi-institutional trial of reirradiation and chemotherapy for unresectable recurrent squamous cell carcinoma of the head and neck. Head Neck 30(3):281–288

Stell PM (1989) Survival times in end-stage head and neck cancer. Eur J Surg Oncol 15(5):407–410

Stell PM (1991) Time to recurrence of squamous cell carcinoma of the head and neck. Head Neck 13(4): 277–281

Stevens KR Jr, Britsch A, Moss WT (1994) High-dose reirradiation of head and neck cancer with curative intent. Int J Radiat Oncol Biol Phys 29(4):687–698

Sulman EP, Schwartz DL, Le TT, Ang KK, Morrison WH, Rosenthal DI, Ahamad A, Kies M, Glisson B, Weber R, Garden AS (2009) IMRT reirradiation of head and neck cancer-disease control and morbidity outcomes. Int J Radiat Oncol Biol Phys 73(2):399–409

Tanvetyanon T, Qin D, Padhya T, Kapoor R, McCaffrey J, Trotti A (2009) Survival outcomes of squamous cell carcinoma arising from sinonasal inverted papilloma: report of 6 cases with systematic review and pooled analysis. Am J Otolaryngol 30(1):38–43

Vergeer MR, Doornaert PA, Rietveld DH, Leemans CR, Slotman BJ, Langendijk JA (2009) Intensity-modulated radiotherapy reduces radiation-induced morbidity and improves health-related quality of life: results of a nonrandomized prospective study using a standardized follow-up program. Int J Radiat Oncol Biol Phys 74(1):1–8

Vermorken JB, Mesia R, Rivera F, Remenar E, Kawecki A, Rottey S, Erfan J, Zabolotnyy D, Kienzer HR, Cupissol D, Peyrade F, Benasso M et al (2008) Platinum-based chemotherapy plus cetuximab in head and neck cancer. N Engl J Med 359(11):1116–1127

Vokes EE, Panje WR, Schilsky RL, Mick R, Awan AM, Moran WJ, Goldman MD, Tybor AG, Weichselbaum RR (1989) Hydroxyurea, fluorouracil, and concomitant radiotherapy in poor-prognosis head and neck cancer: a phase I-II study. J Clin Oncol 7(6):761–768

Wang CC, McIntyre J (1993) Re-irradiation of laryngeal carcinoma – techniques and results. Int J Radiat Oncol Biol Phys 26(5):783–785

Weiss MH, Harrison LB, Isaacs RS (1994) Use of decision analysis in planning a management strategy for the stage N0 neck. Arch Otolaryngol Head Neck Surg 120(7):699–702

Weppelmann B, Wheeler RH, Peters GE, Kim RY, Spencer SA, Meredith RF, Salter MM (1992) Treatment of recurrent head and neck cancer with 5-fluorouracil, hydroxyurea, and reirradiation. Int J Radiat Oncol Biol Phys 22(5):1051–1056

Wong SJ, Machtay M, Li Y. Locally recurrent, previously irradiated head and neck cancer: concurrent re-irradiation and chemotherapy, or chemotherapy alone? J Clin Oncol 2006; 24(17): 2653–8.

Zafereo ME, Hanasono MM, Rosenthal DI, Sturgis EM, Lewin JS, Roberts DB, Weber RS (2009) The role of salvage surgery in patients with recurrent squamous cell carcinoma of the oropharynx. Cancer 115(24):5723–5733

Nasopharyngeal Carcinoma

Wai Tong Ng, Oscar S.H. Chan, Henry C.K. Sze, and Anne W.M. Lee

Contents

The original version of this chapter was revised. An erratum to this chapter can be found at 10.1007/978-3-319-41825-4_78.

W.T. Ng, MD • O.S.H. Chan, FRCR
H.C.K. Sze, FRCR
Department of Clinical Oncology, Pamela Youde Nethersole Eastern Hospital, Hong Kong, China
e-mail: ngwt1@ha.org.hk; chansh2@ha.org.hk; sck056@ha.org.hk

A.W.M. Lee, MD (✉)
Department of Clinical Oncology, The University of Hong Kong, Hong Kong, China

The University of Hong Kong – Shenzhen Hospital, Hong Kong, China
e-mail: awmlee@hku.hk

Abstract

Despite advances in technology and improved treatment outcome of nasopharyngeal carcinoma (NPC), local recurrence still represents a major mode of failure particularly in patients with locally advanced disease. It can occur years after the primary treatment and is often associated with devastating local symptoms. Salvage nasopharyngectomy is usually reserved for early relapse disease, while majority of the patients have to rely on re-irradiation as the only chance of cure. Due to the close proximity to adjacent critical structures and previous exposure to high-dose irradiation, the therapeutic window is extremely narrow. The increasing use of chemo-irradiation as the primary treatment may also mean local recurrence occurring in modern era is a clone of tumor cells that is more therapy resistant and difficult to eradicate. Nonetheless, there is a stark paucity of prospective studies to guide our current management for this challenging condition. Better under-

DOI 10.1007/174_2016_48, © Springer International Publishing Switzerland
Published Online: 07 May 2016

standing of the radiobiological factors, improvement in radiotherapy techniques, and integration with systemic treatment might enhance the disease control and minimize treatment toxicities. Personalized treatment approach and novel systemic treatment will be the future direction.

1 Introduction

Radiotherapy (RT) is the primary treatment modality for non-metastatic nasopharyngeal carcinoma (NPC). With the development of technology (both in RT technique and diagnostic imaging), together with the addition of chemotherapy for patients with advanced locoregional disease, the treatment outcome has improved substantially. The overall local recurrence rate has decreased to around 5–15 % in contemporary series using intensity-modulated RT (IMRT) (Wang et al. 2013; Lee et al. 2014; Sun et al. 2014; Jiang et al. 2015; Setton et al. 2015). However, T4 disease still often remains problematic, the recurrence rate varied widely from 15 to 45 % despite modern treatment techniques (Cao et al. 2013; Kong et al. 2014; Lee et al. 2014; Sun et al. 2014; Jiang et al. 2015; Setton et al. 2015).

Recurrent NPC is a devastating disease. Patients with local recurrence often suffer from serious symptoms including intractable pain, bleeding, and cranial nerve palsies. Salvage by surgery is feasible mainly for early recurrence in centers with surgical expertise. Unfortunately, majority of patients already had extensive involvement at the time when recurrence was detected and re-irradiation is their only chance of salvage. But this is increasingly difficult because existence of radioresistant clonogens is highly likely in recurrences that develop despite adequate tumor coverage to high dose by the primary course. In addition, recurrent tumors in the fibrotic microenvironment after the primary course RT are likely to be more hypoxic and radioresistant. Furthermore, the therapeutic window is extremely narrow due to the anatomical proximity of critical organs at risk (OAR) and varying degree of residual sublethal damage caused by the primary course of RT. Development of serious treatment toxicities often adds to the suffering.

Moreover, comprehensive prospective data are lacking; our current practice is guided mainly by retrospective studies on small numbers of selected patients. Major uncertainties in optimal radiation dose fractionation and the potential role of chemotherapy remain to be resolved. In this chapter, available data will be summarized to provide as much knowledge as possible on locally recurrent NPC and re-irradiation, in an attempt to derive logical answers for overcoming the challenges.

2 Natural Behavior and Pattern of Failure

The time between primary treatment and local recurrence varies widely. Unlike other head and neck cancers, NPC has a predilection for late recurrence. The median latency reported was 1.9 years (range, 0.6–11.9) in the series of 847 patients by Lee et al. (1999) and 2.2 years (range, 0.3–24.3) in the series by Li et al. (2012). The proportion of local recurrence detected within 2 years was 48–57 % (Lee et al. 1999; Li et al. 2012; Setton et al. 2015), between 2 and 5 years in 35–39 % (Lee et al. 1999; Li et al. 2012) and more than 5 years in 9–17 % (Lee et al. 1999; Li et al. 2012). The importance of early detection cannot be overemphasized as this is the most significant prognostic factor. In addition to vigilant assessment in the first 5 years, long follow-up is indicated.

The clinical presentation of locally recurrent NPC varies; the symptoms may mimic late toxicities induced by RT, making early diagnosis a challenge. In a series by Li et al. (2012) on 351 patients with local relapse, the commonest symptoms include blood-stained nasal discharge (38 %), cranial nerve palsies (36 %), and headache (31 %). Tinnitus, nasal obstruction, and hearing loss tended to be less frequent; 10 % of the patients had no obvious symptoms.

The stage distribution at the time of recurrence varies widely among different series. More than 60 % of patients had rT3–4 disease at the time of detection. Furthermore, patients with local recurrence also showed high incidence of other failures. In the series by Lee et al. (1999), 25 and 8 % had coexisting nodal and distant relapse respectively. Thorough work-up is indicated before decision on salvage method.

3 Local Persistence Versus Local Recurrence

Distinction should be made between persistent lesion (tumor that does not completely regress following primary treatment) and recurrent disease (tumor that reemerges after complete regression) as they reflect different tumor biology and different outcome. The time point to determine genuine disease persistence is not easy because it takes time for tumors to regress after RT. Kwong et al. (1999) showed that the incidence of positive histology decreased from 29 % in the first week after completion of RT to 12 % by the ninth week and then rose again. The 5-year local failure-free rate was 82 % for patients who achieved early histological remission (<5 weeks), 77 % for those with delayed remission (5–12 weeks), but only 54 % for those with persistent tumors after 12 weeks despite subsequent salvage treatment.

Brachytherapy (intracavitary or interstitial) has been widely used for superficial persistent disease yielding excellent results with 5-year local failure-free rate of 90 % or above for patients with initial T1–2 tumors (Leung et al. 2000a; Kwong et al. 2001; Law et al. 2002). For more bulky persistent disease, single-fraction stereotactic radiosurgery (SRS) and fractionated stereotactic radiotherapy (SRT) have been shown to achieve favorable local control (Chua et al. 1999 and 2003; Yau et al. 2004; Zheng et al. 2004). In general, most studies showed that persistent disease had a better prognosis than recurrence. However, it should be cautioned that some of the "persistent tumors," particularly those diagnosed by early biopsy, may spontaneously regress even without further treatment. Genuine persistence due to primary radioresistance or inadequate RT dose coverage as in gross intracranial extension could have a very poor prognosis.

4 Detection of Local Recurrence

Instead of conventional fiberoptic endoscopy, Wang et al. (2012) reported that narrowband imaging endoscopy could improve the detection rate of mucosal recurrent lesions (88 % for both sensitivity and specificity), but postradiation effects may cause false-positive results. Radiological imaging is needed for exclusion of deep-seated or submucosal recurrence. Magnetic resonance imaging (MRI) is preferred over computed tomography (CT) because of its superiority in soft tissue delineation (Liang et al. 2009). However, MRI is not very reliable in differentiating between persistent/recurrent tumor and post-RT fibrosis, and attempts to improve its accuracy have been made using diffusion-weighted imaging (DWI) (Hong et al. 2013) and intravoxel incoherent motion (IVIM) (Lai et al. 2013). Functional imaging with combined positron emission tomography-CT (PET-CT) is increasingly used. Yen et al. (2003) reported that PET-CT was superior to MRI in detecting residual/recurrent NPC with improved sensitivity (100 % vs. 62 %), specificity (93 % vs. 44 %), and accuracy (96 % vs. 49 %). In a recent meta-analysis, both PET-CT and single-photon emission computed tomography (SPECT) were shown to be very accurate for the detection of local residual/recurrent NPC and were superior to MRI in distinguishing recurrent NPC from post-RT changes: the pooled specificity estimates for PET-CT (93 %) and SPECT (81 %) were significantly higher than MRI (76 %) (Wei et al. 2015). Nevertheless, post-RT mucosal inflammatory changes/mucositis or osteonecrosis can lead to false-positive results in PET-CT.

Elevated level of circulating cell-free Epstein-Barr virus (EBV) deoxyribonucleic acid (DNA) in plasma/serum from NPC patients is valuable as a prognostic factor (Lin et al. 2004; Leung et al. 2006) and for monitoring diseases status. Elevated EBV DNA was found in 55–96 % of patients with distant metastases, but varied from 0 to 67 % in patients with local/locoregional recurrence (Leung et al. 2003; Hong et al. 2004; Hou et al. 2011; Chai et al. 2012; Hsu et al. 2013). The accuracy in detecting local recurrence is less certain.

The use of transoral nasopharyngeal brush biopsy for EBV DNA to detect local NPC recurrence has been reported (Lam et al. 2015). In a series by Hao et al. (2004), nasopharyngeal swab with PCR-based latent membrane protein (LMP)-1 gene and Epstein-Barr nuclear antigen (EBNA)-1 gene detection was used to monitor local recurrence in 84 NPC patients. Of the 12 patients who were positive for both LMP-1 and EBNA-1, 11 developed local recurrence (sensitivity 91.7 %, specificity 98.6 %). This method is convenient and simple but may not be reliable in detecting deep-seated lesions.

5 Treatment Consideration

5.1 Rationale of Aggressive Treatment and Treatment Options

For patients with isolated local failure, aggressive treatment is warranted. In a study of 200 patients with isolated local relapse (Yu et al. 2005), it was found that patients who received radical salvage treatment by either surgery or RT had a significantly better overall survival (OS) than those who received chemotherapy only.

It is difficult to compare the efficacy of surgery versus re-irradiation as resectable cases generally have more favorable clinical factors such as low disease volume, early r-T categories, good performance status, and minimal comorbidity. No randomized trial comparing these two modalities has been conducted. Retrospective studies suggested that the local salvage rates by either modality were very similar (Lee et al. 2012). However, in view of the high incidence of serious late toxicities incurred by re-irradiation, surgical salvage should be considered as far as feasible. Depending on the disease extent, various surgical techniques have been developed ranging from endoscopic resection, transoral robotic resection for small tumor without parapharyngeal space involvement (Tsang et al. 2013) to open nasopharyngectomy via different approaches (Chan 2014). Excellent long-term local control rates up to 70 % have been reported with no significant negative impact on patients' quality of life (QOL) (Chan et al. 2012).

However, for patients with more extensive local tumor infiltration or positive resection margin after salvage surgery, re-irradiation as a curative treatment is often unavoidable, and the challenge is to develop novel RT techniques and optimal dose fractionation to improve outcomes and reduce late toxicity.

5.2 Radiobiological Factors

Re-irradiation dose is one of the most important factors affecting the salvage rate; the general consensus is that re-irradiation tumor dose $\geq$ 60 Gy is needed for effective salvage (Pryzant et al. 1992). Lee et al. (1997) also showed that the hazard of failure decreased by 1.7 % per Gy_{10} of re-irradiation biologically effective dose ($\alpha/\beta = 10$ Gy) (C_2-BED). However, the risk of late toxicity is a grave concern. Pryzant et al. (1992) found that the incidence of severe late toxicity increased significantly when total dose by the two courses of RT exceeded 100 Gy (39 % vs. 4 % at 5 years). The striving for optimal balance between successful treatment and significant late complication has long been a great challenge.

The following clinical and laboratory studies have attempted to enhance understanding about damage by the two courses and the maximum tolerable dose. The clinical study by Lee et al. (1997) showed that late toxicity was affected by radiation doses at both courses: the hazard increased by 4.2 and 1.2 % per Gy_3 of primary treatment (C_1-BED) and re-irradiation (C_2-BED) (assuming $\alpha/\beta = 3$ Gy). A subsequent study by Lee et al. (2000) further showed that partial recovery of normal tissues took place following the primary course; the total tolerable BED (Σ-BED) was higher than that expected with a single-course treatment (C_1-BED). The Σ-BED that incurred 20 % toxicity at 5 years was estimated to be 129 % of C_1-BED, and there was a trend of decreasing risk with increasing interval between the courses in patients with a treatment gap ≥ 2 years ($P = 0.07$):

$$C_2\text{-BED} = 129\ \%\ \text{Full-tolerance}\ C_1\text{-BED} - C_1\text{-BED}$$

As their above studies included all symptomatic late complications (except xerostomia), the complication rates of individual OAR were actually much lower than 20 %.

This formula of estimation is very similar to the suggestion by van der Kogel (1993) that the maximum tolerable total dose in two courses amounted to 130 % of the maximum tolerable dose in a single course. In addition, he suggested the 100 % tolerable dose should be higher than the usual maximum dose constraint in the primary course since a higher risk should be accepted for re-irradiation (e.g., 60 Gy instead of 50 Gy for spinal cord):

$$C_2\text{-BED} = 130\ \%\ \text{Full-tolerance}\ C_1\text{-BED} - C_1\text{-BED}$$

Many have since studied the late complication rates from re-irradiation, focusing on the central nervous system (CNS) structures. Nieder et al. (2005 and 2006) analyzed the data from a total of 78 patients receiving $\Sigma - \text{BED}$ ranging from 102 to 205 Gy_2 ($\alpha/\beta = 2$ Gy) to their spinal cords and developed a score system which divided patients into three risk groups according to the $\Sigma - \text{BED}$, time interval before re-treatments, and the BED of any one course. The risk of myelopathy increased from 3 % to 25 % to 90 % from the low-risk to the high-risk groups. They suggested that the risk of radiation-induced myelopathy was small if $\Sigma - \text{BED} \leq 135\ Gy_2$ ($\alpha/\beta = 2$ Gy) for cervical/thoracic cord as long as BED of each course was ≤ 98 Gy_2 and the interval between the courses was at least 6 months. The formula recommended for the second course BED was:

$$C_2\text{-BED} = 135\,Gy_2 - C_1\text{-BED}$$

Mayer and Sminia (2008) studied the incidence of clinically symptomatic necrosis from the re-irradiation of gliomas. In contrast to the spinal cord, they found a large volume effect for normal brain tissues, but no correlation between the incidence of radionecrosis and the time interval before re-treatment (the minimum interval in their series was 3 months). Radiation-induced brain necrosis occurred only when the cumulative equivalent dose in 2 Gy fractions (EQD_2) was > 100 Gy.

The study by Sulman et al. (2009) on severe toxicity (those leading to hospitalization, corrective surgery, or death) from re-irradiation by IMRT for other head and neck cancers suggested that there was 50 % recovery for CNS structures 12 months after the primary course; their recommended formula for planning re-irradiation was:

$$C_2\text{-BED} = \text{Full-tolerance}\ C_1\text{-BED} - 50\ \%\ C_1\text{-BED}$$

Jones and Grant (2014) derived a more detailed formula for estimating the tolerable C_2-BED for CNS structures as a function of the remaining dose tolerance and the treatment gap:

$$\frac{C_2\text{-BED}}{\text{Full tolerance}\ C_1\text{-BED}} = \left(1 - \frac{C_1\text{-BED}}{\text{Full tolerance}\ C_1\text{-BED}}\right)^{\frac{1}{r+1}}$$

where, taking a more cautious approach, $r = 1.5 + e^{[1.2(t-1)]}$ and t = treatment gap in years. The tolerable C_2 dose can be calculated from the C_2-BED taking into account the fractionation scheme and the corresponding α/β ratio.

These observations concurred with findings from animal experiments regarding late damage on CNS by re-irradiation and the estimated tolerance (Ruifrok et al. 1992; Ang et al. 1993; Mason et al. 1993; Wong et al. 1993). Partial recovery ranging from 20 to 55 % has been reported. The amount of recovery depends on the initial dose, the interval between the two courses, their fractionation schedules, the age and the species of

Table 1 Estimation of maximum tolerable re-irradiation dose by different models basing on the assumption that the 100 % tolerance dose for an OAR by a single course is 60 Gy, the dose received at the primary course is 50 Gy, and the numbers of fractions are 35 and 30 for the first and second courses respectively

	Lee et al. (2000)	Nieder et al. (2005, 2006)	Sulman et al. (2009)	Jones and Grant (2014)
Full-tolerance C_1 dose	60 Gy	N/A	60 Gy	60 Gy
Full-tolerance C_1-BED	94.3 Gy_3	N/A	94.3 Gy_3	111.4 Gy_2
Formula for C_2-BED	129 % Full-tolerance C_1-BED – C_1-BED	135 Gy_2 – C_1-BED	Full-tolerance C_1-BED – 50 % C_1-BED	$\frac{C_2\text{-BED}}{\text{Full tolerance } C_1\text{-BED}} = \left(1 - \frac{C_1\text{-BED}}{\text{Full tolerance } C_1\text{-BED}}\right)^{\frac{1}{r+1}}$
Ref tolerance BED	121.6 Gy_3	135 Gy_2	94.3 Gy_3	111.4 Gy_2
C_1 dose	50 Gy	50 Gy	50 Gy	50 Gy
C_1-BED	73.8 Gy_3	85.7 Gy_2	73.8 Gy_3	85.7 Gy_2
Tolerable C_2-BED	47.8 Gy_3	49.3 Gy_2	57.4 Gy_3	86.6 Gy_2
Tolerable C_2 dose	*34 Gy*	*32 Gy*	*39 Gy*	*48 Gy*

The α/β ratios for the various models were taken from their original publications

animals, as well as the type and the site of the normal tissue damaged.

The above provides a rough guidance for clinicians to estimate the dose permitted at re-irradiation. Table 1 shows the maximum tolerable re-irradiation dose according to the different models assuming that the 100 % tolerance dose for an OAR by a single course is 60 Gy, the dose received at the primary course was 50 Gy, and the numbers of fractions are 35 and 30 for the first and second courses respectively. The maximum tolerable dose varied from 32 to 48 Gy (assuming that the treatment gap between the two courses is 2 years). An even higher dose can be applied if the maximum dose points of the two courses do not overlap. However, one must be cautious that the models were based on rather limited clinical data; detailed dose distributions within the OARs are often not known in these studies. Accurate prediction is difficult given the complex interplay of multiple factors and the wide range of individual susceptibility to radiation injury. Furthermore, if protection of normal tissues will compromise the adequacy of tumor coverage, patients should be duly informed of the risk and the grave consequence of salvage failure, the target dose should be given top priority if patients accept the extra risk.

Besides the total dose, the dose per fraction is another important factor affecting the risk of late toxicities. Large fractional doses incur higher risk; hyperfractionation schedule (Karam et al. 2015) is worth considering; the schedule currently used in our center is 1.2Gy per fraction, twice daily, at least 6 h apart to a total dose of 64.8 Gy.

5.3 Technical Factors

Treatment techniques for recurrent disease reflect the technological development of radiotherapy delivery in the past few decades. Initial studies mostly employed 2D external RT (Wang 1987; Lee et al. 1997; Teo et al. 1998) and/or brachytherapy (Leung et al. 2000a). Brachytherapy as sole treatment was mainly confined to superficial mucosal recurrence; salvage rate of 60 % and above had been reported for rT1 or limited rT2 disease using interstitial implants with either radioactive gold grains (Kwong et al. 2001) or iridium mold (Law et al. 2002). However, severe late soft tissue and bony complications were not uncommon. More recently, image-guided brachytherapy approach has been studied, but preliminary results by Shen et al. (2015) only achieved a median survival time of 18 months for a cohort of 30 patients treated with CT-guided permanent implantation of iodine-125 seeds.

Conformal radiotherapy gradually replaced 2D RT in the 1990s as dosimetry allows not only better tumor coverage but also better sparing of OARs (Zheng et al. 2005; Li et al. 2006; Luo et al. 2010). Available reports showed encouraging local control, but no significant reduction in late toxicities. The study by Zheng et al. (2005) using 3D conformal technique to a median dose of 68 Gy reported a very encouraging 5-year local salvage rate of 71 %. However, the 5-year OS only improved to 40 % because of serious late toxicities (all patients developed one or more late ≥ grade 3 toxicities and treatment mortality was 13 %).

In the modern era, either IMRT or stereotactic technique is used. Stereotactic radiosurgery/radiotherapy is advantageous due to the rapid dose falloff and geometric precision. Encouraging results of stereotactic treatment have been reported with local salvage rates ranging from 53 to 86 % (Chua et al. 1999 and 2009; Chen et al. 2001; Leung et al. 2009; Ozyigit et al. 2011; Dizman et al. 2014). However, very high radiation dose given per fraction could induce severe damage of normal tissues leading to torrential hemorrhage with fatal outcome (Chua et al. 1999; Ozyigit et al. 2011). Stereotactic radiosurgery should be avoided in patients with tumor encasing the carotid artery.

Currently, IMRT is the most commonly used method. Most series aimed to deliver radiation dose ≥60 Gy to recurrent gross tumor volume (GTV). Encouraging local control rate ranging from 52 to 86 % have been reported (Chua et al. 2005a; Han et al. 2012; Hua et al. 2012; Qiu et al. 2012 and 2014; Chen et al. 2013; Tian et al. 2014). However, late complications and treatment-related death varied significantly among different series. Important issues such as optimal total dose, fractionation schedule, and dose constraint for OARs remain to be defined.

Development of intensity-modulated proton therapy (IMPT) lead to further improvement in physical dose distribution: its unique beam properties (the Bragg peak, rapid distal falloff, and potentially sharper penumbra) could facilitate better sparing of OARs (Widesott et al. 2008). A recent study by Lin et al. (1999) using IMPT to doses of 59.4–70.2 cobalt gray equivalent in a cohort of 16 recurrent NPC patients (12 of whom had rT4 disease) reported 50 % OS and locoregional PFS. More importantly, the doses to critical OARs were low (0–22 Gy), and no CNS side effects were observed with a mean follow-up of 24 months.

5.4 Integration with Systemic Treatment

Despite the lack of high-level evidence, induction and concurrent chemotherapy is often employed with re-irradiation. In particular, induction chemotherapy could reduce the recurrent tumor bulk, potentially leading to better sparing of adjacent OARs especially for rT3–4 disease, and eradicate micrometastasis. Extrapolating from the experience of primary treatment, concurrent chemotherapy may be more potent for improving tumor control; the main concern is whether this would further aggravate the risk of late toxicities.

Various chemotherapy combinations have been studied including cisplatin (Poon et al. 2004; Koutcher et al. 2010), 5-fluorouracil (Poon et al. 2004; Ngan et al. 2015), gemcitabine (Chua et al. 2005), and taxane (Ngan et al. 2015). Other novel agents such as anti-EGFR agents (Lartigau et al. 2013; Ngan et al. 2015; Vargo et al. 2015) and anti-angiogenic agents (Seiwert et al. 2008) have been tested in recurrent head and neck cancer. However, data on recurrent NPC are relatively sparse (Xu et al. 2016), and the risk of bleeding should be duly considered for drugs targeting on angiogenesis (Hui et al. 2011).

6 Prognostic Factors

The most important prognostic factor is the stage of disease and GTV at the time of recurrence (Han et al. 2012; Chen et al. 2013; Tian et al. 2015; Xiao et al. 2015). Advanced recurrent

T stage, especially extensive intracranial extension, is associated with worse prognosis (Leung et al. 2000b; Chua et al. 2005a; Han et al. 2012; Qiu et al. 2012). Larger recurrent tumors had poorer outcome not only because of proximity to critical structures limiting the RT dose but also of increasing risk of radioresistance due to hypoxia. The study by Xiao et al. (2015) on 291 patients with locally recurrent NPC showed that the 5-year OS rates were 63.1 % and 20.8 % for patients with tumor volume <22 cm^3 and ≥22 cm^3, respectively. Those with tumor volume ≥22 cm^3 also had higher incidence of distant metastasis and radiation-induced toxicities.

The latency is another prognostic factor (Lee et al. 1999; Qiu et al. 2012). The study by Lee et al. (1999) on 847 recurrent NPC showed that those with long latency had better prognosis due to lower risk of distant failure: the 5-year distant failure-free rates for recurrence ≤2 years, 2–5 years, and ≥5 years were 57 %, 67 %, and 83 %, respectively. Histological type has also been shown to be an independent prognostic factor: Hwang et al. (1998) reported that patients with undifferentiated carcinoma had significantly better 5-year locoregional progression-free rate and survival than those with keratinizing type.

7 Treatment Outcomes

Table 2 summarizes the results achieved by re-irradiation using IMRT. These studies can be divided into two groups based on the dose employed in the second course of irradiation.

Studies from North America (Koutcher et al. 2010; Karam et al. 2015) and Hong Kong (Chua et al. 2005b; Ngan et al. 2015), using re-irradiation dose of around 60 Gy combined with systemic chemotherapy, achieved OS of around 60 %. Major late complication rates were variable. A recent phase 2 study by the Hong Kong NPC Study Group explored the possibility of improving outcome for rT3-4 tumor by integrating re-irradiation with more intensive systemic therapy using triplet induction consisting of docetaxel, cisplatin, and 5-fluorouracil (TPF), followed by re-irradiation with concurrent weekly docetaxel and cetuximab (Ngan et al. 2015). Preliminary outcome in 32 recruited patients showed encouraging 2-year OS of 67 %, but the toxicity rate was high [eight temporal lobe necrosis (TLN) and two fatal epistaxis were observed]. In addition, the tolerance to induction TPF was poor in this cohort of recurrent patients (five patients withdrew after the first cycle of TPF due to fatigue; and ≥ grade 3 neutropenia and hyponatremia occurred in 38 % and 28 %, respectively).

Table 2 Efficacy and late toxicities of re-irradiation by intensity-modulated radiotherapy

Author	Pt. no.	rT1–2 (%)	Dose (Gy)	Chemo.	Yr.	L-FFR (%)	OS (%)	Brain necrosis (%)	Massive bleeding (%)	RT-related death (%)
Chua (2005a)	31	25	50–60	68 %	1	56	63	7	NR	NR
Karam (2015)	27	78	40–60 (1.1–1.4 Gy/fr BID)	85 %	3	53	57	0	0	0
Koutcher (2010)	29	45	45–59	93 %	5	52	60	22	NR	NR
Ngan (2015)	32	0	60	100 %	2	75	68	35	13	13
Qiu (2012)	70	53	Median 70	44 % (I) ± 18 % (C)	3	49	52	NR	9	9
Han (2012)	239	25	61.7–78.7	49 %	5	86	45	28	NR	35
Chen (2013)	54	20	49.8–76.6	52 %	2	64	44	19	11	24
Tian (2014)	117	21	65.4–73.1	0 %	5	64–71	37	21	25	32

Abbreviation: *L-FFR* local failure-free rate, *OS* overall survival, *I* induction, *C* concurrent, *NR* not reported

Four studies from China used re-irradiation dose of around 70 Gy. The largest study was reported by Han et al. (2012): a total of 239 patients (25 % rT1–2) were re-irradiated, and the mean total dose to GTV was 69.94 Gy and the mean dose per fraction was 2.31 Gy. The 5-year local relapse-free survival was 85 %, but the OS rate was only 45 % with 35 % who died of treatment-related death toxicities. Chen et al. (2013) showed similar findings in 54 recurrent NPC patients treated to an average GTV dose of 69.96 Gy. The 2-year local failure-free survival was 64 %, but the OS rate was only 44 % with 48 % of patients suffering from severe late toxicities, and 25 % died of treatment complications. Similarly, in the randomized phase 2 study reported by Tian et al. (2014) on two different fractionation schemes (60 Gy in 27 fractions vs. 68 Gy in 34 fractions), high incidence of treatment-related death was noted in both arms (24 % vs. 41 %). Furthermore, OS was in fact better for the group receiving 60 Gy in 27 fractions due to lower rate of treatment-related death.

8 Treatment Complications

Late toxicities are the main prohibitory factor for re-irradiation of NPC. Figure 1 illustrates some of the possible late treatment complications after re-irradiation. Other common toxicities include xerostomia, hearing impairment, trismus, cranial nerve palsy, and hypopituitarism. Detailed studies on structured QOL measurements are lacking.

8.1 Carotid Blowout

Carotid blowout is the most daunting complication among all and is the main cause of treatment-related death. Literature-based systematic review by McDonald et al. (2012) on 1554 patients reported a crude rate of carotid blowout after re-irradiation of the head and neck (H&N) region of 2.6, and 76 % of them died. But the reported hemorrhage rate following re-irradiation for NPC varied widely; the incidence following IMRT or SRT ranged from 0 to 25 % (Seo et al. 2009; Ozyigit et al. 2011; Chen et al. 2013; Benhaim et al. 2014). The total re-irradiation dose is the significant aggravating factor. In a phase 2 randomized study by Tian et al. (2014) comparing two IMRT dose regimens in recurrent NPC, the massive hemorrhage rate at a median follow-up of 25 months was 19 % in the group re-irradiated to 60 Gy in 27 fractions compared to 31 % in the group with 68 Gy in 34 fractions. Whether this is aggravated by combining RT with intensive systemic therapy is uncertain, interim analysis of the prospective phase 2 study by the Hong Kong NPC Study Group mentioned above reported a 14 % bleeding rate following 60 Gy plus intensive induction-concurrent therapy (Ngan et al. 2015).

8.2 Temporal Lobe Necrosis

TLN is another potentially life-threatening late toxicity. While some may be asymptomatic especially at early phase of development, others may suffer from debilitating symptoms (including headache, dizziness, memory loss, epilepsy, pressure symptoms, changes in conscious level, and occasional intracranial hemorrhage) (Lee et al. 2002). The incidence is much higher in cohorts after re-irradiation than single-course RT, ranging from 7 to 35 % (Chua et al. 2005a; Koutcher et al. 2010; Han et al. 2012; Chen et al. 2013; Tian et al. 2014; Ngan et al. 2015). Risk of TLN depends on fractional dose, cumulative dose, RT techniques, and time interval between two courses of RT (Lee et al. 1998; Bakst et al. 2011; Chen et al. 2011; Zhou et al. 2014). The study by Liu et al. (2014) on over 200 recurrent NPC patients re-irradiated to around 70 Gy revealed a 31 % risk of TLN with a median latency period of only 15 months; a maximum summated dose of less than 125Gy EQD2 and interval between courses of at least 2 years is recommended.

8.3 Mucosal Necrosis and Skull Base Osteoradionecrosis (ORN)

Soft tissue and bone necrosis is a common problem following re-irradiation. Clinical features

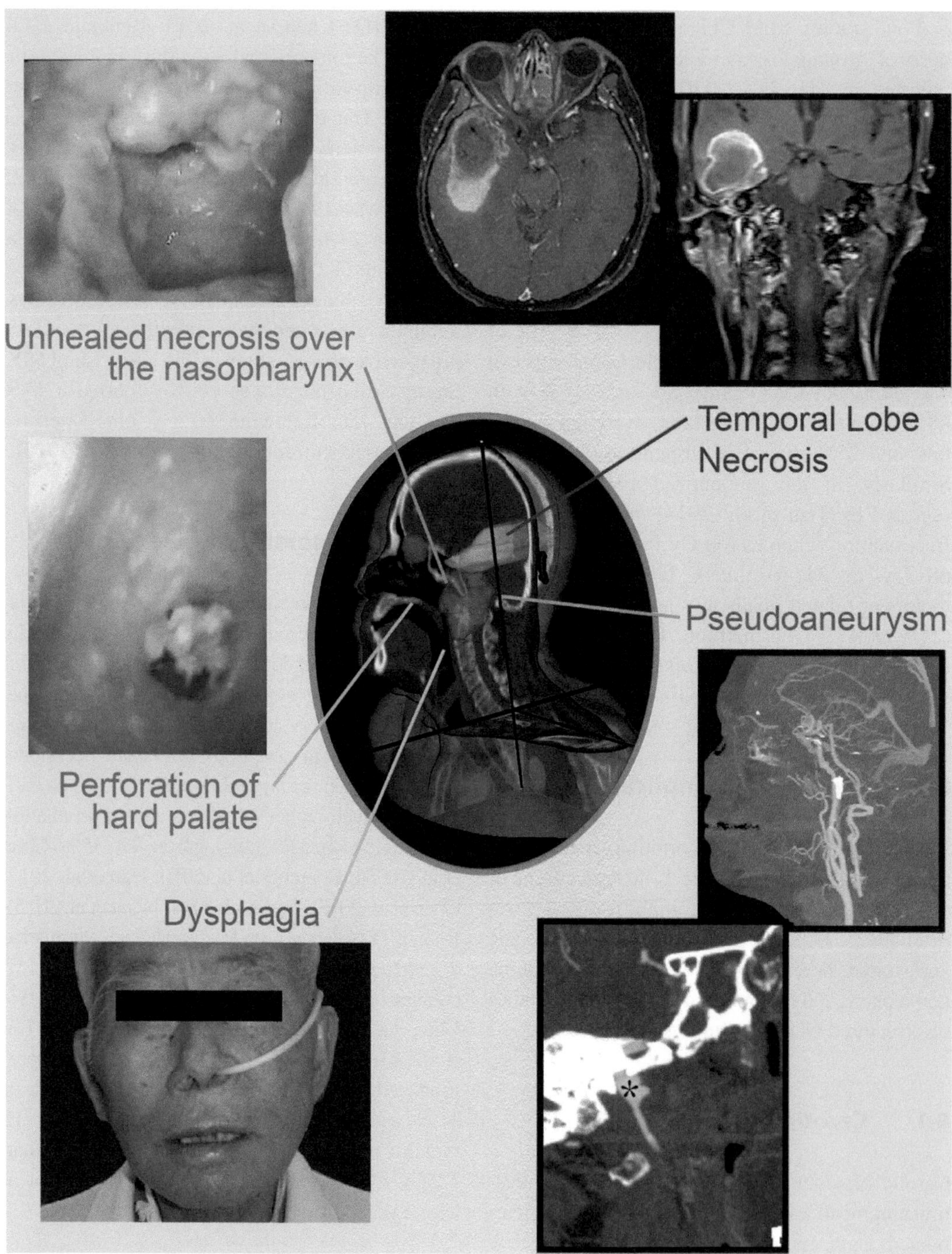

Fig. 1 Potential late complications due to re-irradiation: pseudoaneurysm (*black asterisk*)

include foul odor, intense headache, and even profuse bleeding. Crust, necrotic tissue, and exposed bones can be found in endoscopic examination. The reported incidence ranged from 6.3 to 40.6 % (Han et al. 2012; Qiu et al. 2012; Chen et al. 2013; Tian et al. 2014). Huang et al. (2006) observed a latent period of 7–24 months from re-irradiation to onset of ORN.

8.4 Swallowing Impairment

Trismus, impaired pharyngeal peristalsis, and lower cranial nerve neuropathy can all lead to swallowing problems leading to malnutrition and aspiration. Chen et al. (2013) reported that 20 % of patients had feeding difficulty after re-irradiation resulting in permanent nasogastric tube or gastrostomy feeding. Severe trismus rate reported was around 17 % (Koutcher et al. 2010; Qiu et al. 2012; Tian et al. 2014).

8.5 Hearing Impairment

Hearing loss can be sensorineural (due to damage of cochlear hair cells or eighth nerve), conductive (due to auditory canal osteoradionecrosis or middle ear pathology), or a mixture of both in nature. High-tone sensorineural hearing loss (≥30 dB loss) can reach up to 35 % even after a single course of chemoradiotherapy; the incidence is expected to be much higher after re-irradiation as the mean cochlear dose correlated with the incidence of sensorineural hearing impairment (Chan et al. 2009). Majority of reports were based on clinical grading rather than detailed pure-tone audiogram assessment, and reported incidence ranged from 12 to 22 % (Han et al. 2012; Qiu et al. 2012; Tian et al. 2014).

8.6 Treatment-Related Mortality

The reported treatment mortality rate ranged from 9 % up to an alarming rate of 35 % (Han et al. 2012; Qiu et al. 2012; Chen et al. 2013; Tian et al. 2014; Ngan et al. 2015). Treatment-induced deaths are commonly related to carotid blowout and brain and/or mucosal/bone necrosis. However, some treatment deaths are more subtle, like pneumonia caused by silent aspiration. A careful balance between the treatment toxicities and local control should be taken, and the possible morbid and fatal toxicities must be discussed in detail before treatment.

9 Concluding Remarks and Future Direction

Basing on currently available data, the following key observations can be summarized:

- Aggressive salvage is indicated for patients with locoregional recurrence. Re-irradiation with/without chemotherapy is an effective method, but incurred substantial risk of severe late toxicities, and surgical resection should be considered especially for rT1–2 disease if expertise is available.
- Treatment outcomes are closely related to the stage at detection of recurrence, the tumor bulk and the latency.
- Local control depends on the re-irradiation dose, while late toxicity is related to cumulative doses from both the primary and the re-treatment courses. High re-irradiation dose can improve local salvage, but may not necessarily translate into higher survival due to excessive treatment-related deaths; an optimal balance is needed.
- The most conformal technique should be used for better protection of normal tissues, but high incidence of serious late toxicities still occurs even with IMRT or SRT; more novel technique should be explored. IMPT has physical advantages over photon therapy allowing a better avoidance of OARs. Long-term survival and toxicity outcome is awaited.
- Different models have been proposed for estimating the maximum tolerable doses, but most were based on past treatment without accurate information on doses at various OARs. Uncertainties of various parameters remain, and further studies on tolerance doses, optimization of dose constraints, and dose fractionation are warranted.
- In addition to the total dose, the dose per fraction at re-irradiation is also important; high fractional dose incurs higher risk of life-threatening toxicities, including neurological damage, vascular damage, and soft tissue and bone necrosis. SRT at large fractional dose should be avoided particularly for tumors encasing the carotid vessel. Hyperfractionation schedule is worth considering.

- Ideally treatment regimen should be tailored to individual risk pattern, radiosensitivity, and tolerance. Radiogenomics emerges as a new research direction to identify potential genetic determinants of adverse reactions to RT. Genome-wide association studies (GWAS) are now underway to identify potential genetic variations that affect radiosensitivity. It is hoped that large-scale GWAS can identify genetic signatures to help selecting patients suitable for re-irradiation (Barnett et al. 2012; Rattay and Talbot 2014).
- No study has yet been conducted to assess the exact contribution of adding chemotherapy. Past studies on targeted therapy did not show promising efficacy. Further studies to explore for more potent and less toxic systemic therapy are needed. Immunotherapy has emerged as a new armament in cancer management. A recent phase I study using a PD1 inhibitor achieved a 22 % response rate in a cohort of heavily pretreated recurrent or metastatic NPC, with a remarkable PFS of 11 months (Hsu et al. 2015). Further exploration on the value of immunotherapy is warranted.

Acknowledgment The authors wish to thank Dr. Michael C. H. Lee (Department of Medical Physics, Pamela Youde Nethersole Eastern Hospital) for his contributions on the section of "radiobiological factors."

References

Ang KK, Price RE, Stephens LC, Jiang GL, Feng Y, Schultheiss TE et al (1993) The tolerance of primate spinal cord to re-irradiation. Int J Radiat Oncol Biol Phys 25:459–464

Bakst RL, Lee N, Pfister DG, Zelefsky MJ, Hunt MA, Kraus DH et al (2011) Hypofractionated dose-painting intensity modulated radiation therapy with chemotherapy for nasopharyngeal carcinoma: a prospective trial. Int J Radiat Oncol Biol Phys 80:148–153

Barnett GC, Coles CE, Elliott RM, Baynes C, Luccarini C, Conroy D et al (2012) Independent validation of genes and polymorphisms reported to be associated with radiation toxicity: a prospective analysis study. Lancet Oncol 13:65–77

Benhaim C, Lapeyre M, Thariat J (2014) Stereotactic irradiation in head and neck cancers. Cancer Radiother 18:280–296

Cao CN, Luo JW, Gao L, Yi JL, Huang XD, Wang K et al (2013) Clinical outcomes and patterns of failure after intensity-modulated radiotherapy for T4 nasopharyngeal carcinoma. Oral Oncol 49:175–181

Chai SJ, Pua KC, Saleh A, Yap YY, Lim PV, Subramaniam SK et al (2012) Clinical significance of plasma Epstein-Barr Virus DNA loads in a large cohort of Malaysian patients with nasopharyngeal carcinoma. J Clin Virol 55:34–39

Chan JY (2014) Surgical management of recurrent nasopharyngeal carcinoma. Oral Oncol 50:913–917

Chan SH, Ng WT, Kam KL, Lee MC, Choi CW, Yau TK et al (2009) Sensorineural hearing loss after treatment of nasopharyngeal carcinoma: a longitudinal analysis. Int J Radiat Oncol Biol Phys 73:1335–1342

Chan YW, Chow VL, Wei WI (2012) Quality of life of patients after salvage nasopharyngectomy for recurrent nasopharyngeal carcinoma. Cancer 118:3710–3718

Chen HJ, Leung SW, Su CY (2001) Linear accelerator based radiosurgery as a salvage treatment for skull base and intracranial invasion of recurrent nasopharyngeal carcinomas. Am J Clin Oncol 24:255–258

Chen J, Dassarath M, Yin Z, Liu H, Yang K, Wu G (2011) Radiation induced temporal lobe necrosis in patients with nasopharyngeal carcinoma: a review of new avenues in its management. Radiat Oncol (London, England) 6:128

Chen HY, Ma XM, Ye M, Hou YL, Xie HY, Bai YR (2013) Effectiveness and toxicities of intensity-modulated radiotherapy for patients with locally recurrent nasopharyngeal carcinoma. PLoS One 8, e73918

Chua DT, Sham JS, Hung KN, Kwong DL, Kwong PW, Leung LH (1999) Stereotactic radiosurgery as a salvage treatment for locally persistent and recurrent nasopharyngeal carcinoma. Head Neck 21:620–626

Chua DT, Sham JS, Kwong PW, Hung KN, Leung LH (2003) Linear accelerator-based stereotactic radiosurgery for limited, locally persistent, and recurrent nasopharyngeal carcinoma: efficacy and complications. Int J Radiat Oncol Biol Phys 56:177–183

Chua DT, Sham JS, Leung LH, Au GK (2005a) Re-irradiation of nasopharyngeal carcinoma with intensity-modulated radiotherapy. Radiother Oncol 77:290–294

Chua DT, Sham JS, Au GK (2005b) Induction chemotherapy with cisplatin and gemcitabine followed by reirradiation for locally recurrent nasopharyngeal carcinoma. Am J Clin Oncol 28:464–471

Chua DT, Wu SX, Lee V, Tsang J (2009) Comparison of single versus fractionated dose of stereotactic radiotherapy for salvaging local failures of nasopharyngeal carcinoma: a matched-cohort analysis. Head Neck Oncol 1:13

Dizman A, Coskun-Breuneval M, Altinisik-Inan G, Olcay GK, Cetindag MF, Guney Y (2014) Reirradiation with robotic stereotactic body radiotherapy for recurrent nasopharyngeal carcinoma. Asian Pacific J Cancer Prevent 15:3561–3566

Han F, Zhao C, Huang SM, Lu LX, Huang Y, Deng XW et al (2012) Long-term outcomes and prognostic factors of re-irradiation for locally recurrent nasopharyngeal carcinoma using intensity-modulated radiotherapy. Clin Oncol (R Coll Radiol) 24:569–576

Hao SP, Tsang NM, Chang KP (2004) Monitoring tumor recurrence with nasopharyngeal swab and latent membrane protein-1 and epstein-barr nuclear antigen-1 gene detection in treated patients with nasopharyngeal carcinoma. Laryngoscope 114:2027–2030

Hong RL, Lin CY, Ting LL, Ko JY, Hsu MM (2004) Comparison of clinical and molecular surveillance in patients with advanced nasopharyngeal carcinoma after primary therapy: the potential role of quantitative analysis of circulating Epstein-Barr virus DNA. Cancer 100:1429–1437

Hong J, Yao Y, Zhang Y, Tang T, Zhang H, Bao D et al (2013) Value of magnetic resonance diffusion-weighted imaging for the prediction of radiosensitivity in nasopharyngeal carcinoma. Otolaryngol Head Neck Surg 149:707–713

Hou X, Zhao C, Guo Y, Han F, Lu LX, Wu SX et al (2011) Different clinical significance of pre- and post-treatment plasma Epstein-Barr virus DNA load in nasopharyngeal carcinoma treated with radiotherapy. Clin Oncol (R Coll Radiol) 23:128–133

Hsu CL, Chan SC, Chang KP, Lin TL, Lin CY, Hsieh CH et al (2013) Clinical scenario of EBV DNA follow-up in patients of treated localized nasopharyngeal carcinoma. Oral Oncol 49:620–625

Hsu C, Lee SH, Ejadi S, Even C, Cohen R, Le Tourneau C, Mehnert J (2015) Antitumor activity and safety of pembrolizumab in patients with PD-L1-positive nasopharyngeal carcinoma: Interim results from a phase 1b study positive nasopharyngeal carcinoma. Ann Oncol 26(suppl 9):ix94

Hua YJ, Han F, Lu LX, Mai HQ, Guo X, Hong MH et al (2012) Long-term treatment outcome of recurrent nasopharyngeal carcinoma treated with salvage intensity modulated radiotherapy. Eur J Cancer 48: 3422–3428

Huang XM, Zheng YQ, Zhang XM, Mai HQ, Zeng L, Liu X et al (2006) Diagnosis and management of skull base osteoradionecrosis after radiotherapy for nasopharyngeal carcinoma. Laryngoscope 116:1626–1631

Hui EP, Ma BB, King AD, Mo F, Chan SL, Kam MK et al (2011) Hemorrhagic complications in a phase II study of sunitinib in patients of nasopharyngeal carcinoma who has previously received high-dose radiation. Ann Oncol 22:1280–1287

Hwang JM, Fu KK, Phillips TL (1998) Results and prognostic factors in the retreatment of locally recurrent nasopharyngeal carcinoma. Int J Radiat Oncol Biol Phys 41:1099–1111

Jiang F, Jin T, Feng XL, Jin QF, Chen XZ (2015) Long-term outcomes and failure patterns of patients with nasopharyngeal carcinoma staged by magnetic resonance imaging in intensity-modulated radiotherapy era: The Zhejiang Cancer Hospital's experience. J Cancer Res Ther 11(Suppl 2):C179–C184

Jones B, Grant W (2014) Retreatment of central nervous system tumours. Clin Oncol (R Coll Radiol) 26:407–418

Karam I, Huang SH, McNiven A, Su J, Xu W, Waldron J et al (2015) Outcomes after reirradiation for recurrent nasopharyngeal carcinoma: North American experience. Head Neck

Kong FF, Ying H, Du CR, Huang S, Zhou JJ, Hu CS (2014) Effectiveness and toxicities of intensity-modulated radiation therapy for patients with T4 nasopharyngeal carcinoma. PLoS One 9, e91362

Koutcher L, Lee N, Zelefsky M, Chan K, Cohen G, Pfister D et al (2010) Reirradiation of locally recurrent nasopharynx cancer with external beam radiotherapy with or without brachytherapy. Int J Radiat Oncol Biol Phys 76:130–137

Kwong DL, Nicholls J, Wei WI, Chua DT, Sham JS, Yuen PW et al (1999) The time course of histologic remission after treatment of patients with nasopharyngeal carcinoma. Cancer 85:1446–1453

Kwong DL, Wei WI, Cheng AC, Choy DT, Lo AT, Wu PM et al (2001) Long term results of radioactive gold grain implantation for the treatment of persistent and recurrent nasopharyngeal carcinoma. Cancer 91:1105–1113

Lai V, Li X, Lee VH, Lam KO, Chan Q, Khong PL (2013) Intravoxel incoherent motion MR imaging: comparison of diffusion and perfusion characteristics between nasopharyngeal carcinoma and post-chemoradiation fibrosis. Eur Radiol 23:2793–2801

Lam JW, Chan JY, Ho WK, Tsang RK (2015) Use of transoral nasopharyngeal brush biopsy for Epstein-Barr virus DNA detection of local recurrence of nasopharyngeal carcinoma after radiotherapy. Head Neck. doi: 10.1002/hed.24216. [Epub ahead of print]

Lartigau EF, Tresch E, Thariat J, Graff P, Coche-Dequeant B, Benezery K et al (2013) Multi institutional phase II study of concomitant stereotactic reirradiation and cetuximab for recurrent head and neck cancer. Radiother Oncol 109:281–285

Law SC, Lam WK, Ng MF, Au SK, Mak WT, Lau WH (2002) Reirradiation of nasopharyngeal carcinoma with intracavitary mold brachytherapy: an effective means of local salvage. Int J Radiat Oncol Biol Phys 54:1095–1113

Lee AW, Foo W, Law SC, Poon YF, Sze WM, O SK et al (1997) Reirradiation for recurrent nasopharyngeal carcinoma: factors affecting the therapeutic ratio and ways for improvement. Int J Radiat Oncol Biol Phys 38:43–52

Lee AW, Foo W, Chappell R, Fowler JF, Sze WM, Poon YF et al (1998) Effect of time, dose, and fractionation on temporal lobe necrosis following radiotherapy for nasopharyngeal carcinoma. Int J Radiat Oncol Biol Phys 40:35–42

Lee AW, Foo W, Law SC, Poon YF, Sze WM, O SK et al (1999) Recurrent nasopharyngeal carcinoma: the puzzles of long latency. Int J Radiat Oncol Biol Phys 44:149–156

Lee AW, Foo W, Law SC, Peters LJ, Poon YF, Chappell R et al (2000) Total biological effect on late reactive tissues following reirradiation for recurrent nasopharyngeal carcinoma. Int J Radiat Oncol Biol Phys 46:865–872

Lee AW, Kwong DL, Leung SF, Tung SY, Sze WM, Sham JS et al (2002) Factors affecting risk of symptomatic temporal lobe necrosis: significance of fractional dose and treatment time. Int J Radiat Oncol Biol Phys 53:75–85

Lee AW, Fee WE Jr, Ng WT, Chan LK (2012) Nasopharyngeal carcinoma: salvage of local recurrence. Oral Oncol 48:768–774

Lee AW, Ng WT, Chan LL, Hung WM, Chan CC, Sze HC et al (2014) Evolution of treatment for nasopharyngeal cancer--success and setback in the intensity-modulated radiotherapy era. Radiother Oncol 110:377–384

Leung TW, Tung SY, Sze WK, Sze WM, Wong VY, O SK (2000a) Salvage brachytherapy for patients with locally persistent nasopharyngeal carcinoma. Int J Radiat Oncol Biol Phys 47:405–412

Leung TW, Tung SY, Sze WK, Sze WM, Wong VY, Wong CS et al (2000b) Salvage radiation therapy for locally recurrent nasopharyngeal carcinoma. Int J Radiat Oncol Biol Phys 48:1331–1338

Leung SF, Lo YM, Chan AT, To KF, To E, Chan LY et al (2003) Disparity of sensitivities in detection of radiation-naive and postirradiation recurrent nasopharyngeal carcinoma of the undifferentiated type by quantitative analysis of circulating Epstein-Barr virus DNA1,2. Clin Cancer Res 9:3431–3434

Leung SF, Zee B, Ma BB, Hui EP, Mo F, Lai M et al (2006) Plasma Epstein-Barr viral deoxyribonucleic acid quantitation complements tumor-node-metastasis staging prognostication in nasopharyngeal carcinoma. J Clin Oncol 24:5414–5418

Leung TW, Wong VY, Tung SY (2009) Stereotactic radiotherapy for locally recurrent nasopharyngeal carcinoma. Int J Radiat Oncol Biol Phys 75:734–741

Li JC, Hu CS, Jiang GL, Mayr NA, Wang JZ, He XY et al (2006) Dose escalation of three-dimensional conformal radiotherapy for locally recurrent nasopharyngeal carcinoma: a prospective randomised study. Clin Oncol (R Coll Radiol) 18:293–299

Li JX, Lu TX, Huang Y, Han F (2012) Clinical characteristics of recurrent nasopharyngeal carcinoma in high-incidence area. Sci World J 719754

Liang SB, Sun Y, Liu LZ, Chen Y, Chen L, Mao YP et al (2009) Extension of local disease in nasopharyngeal carcinoma detected by magnetic resonance imaging: improvement of clinical target volume delineation. Int J Radiat Oncol Biol Phys 75:742–750

Lin R, Slater JD, Yonemoto LT, Grove RI, Teichman SL, Watt DK et al (1999) Nasopharyngeal carcinoma: repeat treatment with conformal proton therapy--dose-volume histogram analysis. Radiology 213:489–494

Lin JC, Wang WY, Chen KY, Wei YH, Liang WM, Jan JS et al (2004) Quantification of plasma Epstein-Barr virus DNA in patients with advanced nasopharyngeal carcinoma. New Engl J Med 350:2461–2470

Liu S, Lu T, Zhao C, Shen J, Tian Y, Guan Y et al (2014) Temporal lobe injury after re-irradiation of locally recurrent nasopharyngeal carcinoma using intensity modulated radiotherapy: clinical characteristics and prognostic factors. J Neuro Oncol 119:421–428

Luo W, Ye L, Yu Z, He Z, Li F, Liu M (2010) Effectiveness of three-dimensional conformal radiotherapy for treating early primary nasopharyngeal carcinoma. Am J Clin Oncol 33:604–608

Mason KA, Withers HR, Chiang CS (1993) Late effects of radiation on the lumbar spinal cord of guinea pigs: re-treatment tolerance. Int J Radiat Oncol Biol Phys 26:643–648

Mayer R, Sminia P (2008) Reirradiation tolerance of the human brain. Int J Radiat Oncol Biol Phys 70: 1350–1360

McDonald MW, Moore MG, Johnstone PA (2012) Risk of carotid blowout after reirradiation of the head and neck: a systematic review. Int J Radiat Oncol Biol Phys 82:1083–1089

Ngan RK, Ng WT, Kwong D, Tung S, Yau CC, Leung SF, Chan WY, Lung M, Lee A (2015) Preliminary results of HKNPC-1001 trial to evaluate the role of induction TPF followed by weekly docetaxel and cetuximab in combination with intensity modulated radiotherapy for locally advanced nasopharyngeal carcinoma. Ann Oncol 26(Suppl 9):ix93–ix102

Nieder C, Grosu AL, Andratschke NH, Molls M (2005) Proposal of human spinal cord reirradiation dose based on collection of data from 40 patients. Int J Radiat Oncol Biol Phys 61:851–855

Nieder C, Grosu AL, Andratschke NH, Molls M (2006) Update of human spinal cord reirradiation tolerance based on additional data from 38 patients. Int J Radiat Oncol Biol Phys 66:1446–1449

Ozyigit G, Cengiz M, Yazici G, Yildiz F, Gurkaynak M, Zorlu F et al (2011) A retrospective comparison of robotic stereotactic body radiotherapy and three-dimensional conformal radiotherapy for the reirradiation of locally recurrent nasopharyngeal carcinoma. Int J Radiat Oncol Biol Phys 81:e263–e268

Poon D, Yap SP, Wong ZW, Cheung YB, Leong SS, Wee J et al (2004) Concurrent chemoradiotherapy in locoregionally recurrent nasopharyngeal carcinoma. Int J Radiat Oncol Biol Phys 59:1312–1318

Pryzant RM, Wendt CD, Delclos L, Peters LJ (1992) Re-treatment of nasopharyngeal carcinoma in 53 patients. Int J Radiat Oncol Biol Phys 22:941–947

Qiu S, Lin S, Tham IW, Pan J, Lu J, Lu JJ (2012) Intensity-modulated radiation therapy in the salvage of locally recurrent nasopharyngeal carcinoma. Int J Radiat Oncol Biol Phys 83:676–683

Qiu S, Lu J, Zheng W, Xu L, Lin S, Huang C et al (2014) Advantages of intensity modulated radiotherapy in recurrent T1-2 nasopharyngeal carcinoma: a retrospective study. BMC Cancer 14:797

Rattay T, Talbot CJ (2014) Finding the genetic determinants of adverse reactions to radiotherapy. Clin Oncol (R Coll Radiol) 26:301–308

Ruifrok AC, Kleiboer BJ, van der Kogel AJ (1992) Reirradiation tolerance of the immature rat spinal cord. Radiother Oncol 23:249–256

Seiwert TY, Haraf DJ, Cohen EE, Stenson K, Witt ME, Dekker A et al (2008) Phase I study of bevacizumab added to fluorouracil- and hydroxyurea-based concomitant chemoradiotherapy for poor-prognosis head and neck cancer. J Clin Oncol 26:1732–1741

Seo Y, Yoo H, Yoo S, Cho C, Yang K, Kim MS et al (2009) Robotic system-based fractionated stereotactic radiotherapy in locally recurrent nasopharyngeal carcinoma. Radiother Oncol 93:570–574

Setton J, Han J, Kannarunimit D, Wuu YR, Rosenberg SA, DeSelm C et al (2015) Long-term patterns of relapse and survival following definitive intensity-modulated radiotherapy for non-endemic nasopharyngeal carcinoma. Oral Oncol 53:67–73

Shen X, Li Y, Zhang Y, Kong J, Li Y (2015) An analysis of brachytherapy with computed tomography-guided permanent implantation of Iodine-125 seeds for recurrent nonkeratin nasopharyngeal carcinoma. Onco Targets Ther 8:991–997

Sulman EP, Schwartz DL, Le TT, Ang KK, Morrison WH, Rosenthal DI et al (2009) IMRT reirradiation of head and neck cancer-disease control and morbidity outcomes. Int J Radiat Oncol Biol Phys 73:399–409

Sun X, Su S, Chen C, Han F, Zhao C, Xiao W et al (2014) Long-term outcomes of intensity-modulated radiotherapy for 868 patients with nasopharyngeal carcinoma: an analysis of survival and treatment toxicities. Radiother Oncol 110:398–403

Teo PM, Kwan WH, Chan AT, Lee WY, King WW, Mok CO (1998) How successful is high-dose (> or = 60 Gy) reirradiation using mainly external beams in salvaging local failures of nasopharyngeal carcinoma? Int J Radiat Oncol Biol Phys 40:897–913

Tian YM, Zhao C, Guo Y, Huang Y, Huang SM, Deng XW et al (2014) Effect of total dose and fraction size on survival of patients with locally recurrent nasopharyngeal carcinoma treated with intensity-modulated radiotherapy: a phase 2, single-center, randomized controlled trial. Cancer 120:3502–3509

Tian YM, Xiao WW, Bai L, Liu XW, Zhao C, Lu TX et al (2015) Impact of primary tumor volume and location on the prognosis of patients with locally recurrent nasopharyngeal carcinoma. Chin J Cancer 34:247–253

Tsang RK, Ho WK, Wei WI, Chan JY (2013) Transoral robotic assisted nasopharyngectomy via a lateral palatal flap approach. Laryngoscope 123:2180–2183

van der Kogel AJ (1993) Retreatment tolerance of the spinal cord. Int J Radiat Oncol Biol Phys 26:715–717

Vargo JA, Ferris RL, Ohr J, Clump DA, Davis KS, Duvvuri U et al (2015) A prospective phase 2 trial of reirradiation with stereotactic body radiation therapy plus cetuximab in patients with previously irradiated recurrent squamous cell carcinoma of the head and neck. Int J Radiat Oncol Biol Phys 91:480–488

Wang CC (1987) Re-irradiation of recurrent nasopharyngeal carcinoma--treatment techniques and results. Int J Radiat Oncol Biol Phys 13:953–956

Wang WH, Lin YC, Chen WC, Chen MF, Chen CC, Lee KF (2012) Detection of mucosal recurrent nasopharyngeal carcinomas after radiotherapy with narrow-band imaging endoscopy. Int J Radiat Oncol Biol Phys 83:1213–1219

Wang R, Wu F, Lu H, Wei B, Feng G, Li G et al (2013) Definitive intensity-modulated radiation therapy for nasopharyngeal carcinoma: long-term outcome of a multicenter prospective study. J Cancer Res Clin Oncol 139:139–145

Wei J, Pei S, Zhu X (2015) Comparison of (18)F-FDG PET/CT, MRI and SPECT in the diagnosis of local residual/recurrent nasopharyngeal carcinoma: A meta-analysis. Oral Oncol

Widesott L, Pierelli A, Fiorino C, Dell'oca I, Broggi S, Cattaneo GM et al (2008) Intensity-modulated proton therapy versus helical tomotherapy in nasopharynx cancer: planning comparison and NTCP evaluation. Int J Radiat Oncol Biol Phys 72:589–596

Wong CS, Poon JK, Hill RP (1993) Re-irradiation tolerance in the rat spinal cord: influence of level of initial damage. Radiother Oncol 26:132–138

Xiao W, Liu S, Tian Y, Guan Y, Huang S, Lin C et al (2015) Prognostic significance of tumor volume in locally recurrent nasopharyngeal carcinoma treated with salvage intensity-modulated radiotherapy. PLoS One 10, e0125351

Xu T, Ou X, Shen C, Hu C (2016) Cetuximab in combination with chemoradiotherapy in the treatment of recurrent and/or metastatic nasopharyngeal carcinoma. Anticancer Drugs 27:66–70

Yau TK, Sze WM, Lee WM, Yeung MW, Leung KC, Hung WM et al (2004) Effectiveness of brachytherapy and fractionated stereotactic radiotherapy boost for persistent nasopharyngeal carcinoma. Head Neck 26: 1024–1030

Yen RF, Hung RL, Pan MH, Wang YH, Huang KM, Lui LT et al (2003) 18-fluoro-2-deoxyglucose positron emission tomography in detecting residual/recurrent nasopharyngeal carcinomas and comparison with magnetic resonance imaging. Cancer 98:283–287

Yu KH, Leung SF, Tung SY, Zee B, Chua DT, Sze WM et al (2005) Survival outcome of patients with nasopharyngeal carcinoma with first local failure: a study by the Hong Kong Nasopharyngeal Carcinoma Study Group. Head Neck 27:397–405

Zheng XK, Chen LH, Chen YQ, Deng XG (2004) Three-dimensional conformal radiotherapy versus intracavitary brachytherapy for salvage treatment of locally persistent nasopharyngeal carcinoma. Int J Radiat Oncol Biol Phys 60:165–170

Zheng XK, Ma J, Chen LH, Xia YF, Shi YS (2005) Dosimetric and clinical results of three-dimensional conformal radiotherapy for locally recurrent nasopharyngeal carcinoma. Radiother Oncol 75:197–203

Zhou X, Ou X, Xu T, Wang X, Shen C, Ding J et al (2014) Effect of dosimetric factors on occurrence and volume of temporal lobe necrosis following intensity modulated radiation therapy for nasopharyngeal carcinoma: a case–control study. Int J Radiat Oncol Biol Phys 90:261–269

Lung Cancer

Branislav Jeremić, Francesc Casas, Sherif Abdel-Wahab, Nikola Cihoric, Pavol Dubinsky, Ana Mena Merino, and Luhua Wang

Contents

Abstract

In spite of recent advances in both biology and technology of diagnosis and treatment of lung cancer, the overall results remain dismal. After initial treatment, irrespective of stage and histology of the disease, local/regional recurrence is a frequent type of failure. While it is virtually unknown which proportion of patients initially treated with chest radiotherapy undergo reirradiation during the natural course of the disease, there are more reports documenting outcome of reirradiation in recent years. The majority of available studies are retrospective in nature and of limited size. External beam radiation therapy has been used to treat local/regional intrathoracic recurrences after previous radiation therapy for lung cancer, mostly non-small cell histology. In most cases, the aim of the treatment was palliation of symptoms. However, the increasing availability of new technology such as intensity-modulated and stereotactic radiotherapy has resulted in promising outcome

The original version of this chapter was revised. An erratum to this chapter can be found at 10.1007/978-3-319-41825-4_78.

B. Jeremić (✉)
Department of Radiation Oncology, Institute of Pulmonary Diseases, Sremska Kamenica, Serbia

BioIRC Centre for Biomedical Research, Kragujevac, Serbia
e-mail: nebareje@gmail.com

F. Casas
Department of Radiation Oncology, University Clinic, Barcelona, Spain

S. Abdel-Wahab
Department of Clinical Oncology, Ain Shams University, Cairo, Egypt

N. Cihoric
Department of Radiation Oncology, Inselspital, Bern, Switzerland

P. Dubinsky
Department of Radiation Oncology, Eastern Slovakia University, Kosice, Slovakia

A.M. Merino
Department of Radiation Oncology, University of Palma de Majorca, Palma, Spain

L. Wang
Department of Radiation Oncology, Chinese Medical Academy of Science, Beijing, China

Med Radiol Radiat Oncol (2016)
DOI 10.1007/174_2016_61, © Springer International Publishing Switzerland
Published Online: 07 May 2016

after these more aggressive regimens. While endobronchial brachytherapy remains useful in palliating symptomatic recurrences, it is used less frequently in recent years. Although no guideline exists, likely due to considerable variety in first-line radiation therapy parameters, different planning and retreatment characteristics, and lack of validated prognostic factors, current wisdom calls for setting up objectives upfront and making prudent use of available technology.

1 Introduction

Lung cancer is one of the major challenges for health care systems worldwide. It was estimated that in the USA in 2014 there were 224.210 new cases and estimated 159.260 deaths of lung cancer (Siegel et al. 2009), therefore being the major cancer killer in both sexes. The most recent data from the International Agency for the Research of Cancer (IARC) showed that in 2012 there was an estimated total of 1.825 millions of lung cancer cases (1.242 million in men and 0.583 million in women) with an estimated 1.59 millions of deaths (1.099 million in men and 0.41 million in women) worldwide (IARC 2012). This huge burden is especially visible in less-developed regions with limited resources where lung cancer occurs more frequently and causes more deaths than in well-developed countries.

To improve global success in the fight against lung cancer, many novel diagnostic and treatment approaches have been implemented in clinical practice in recent decades, such as novel molecular oncology approaches which led to refinements in histological criteria and definitions of lung cancer subtypes; and positron emission tomography (PET) – computed tomography (CT) which is extensively used nowadays to diagnose and stage lung cancer patients (Vanuytsel et al. 2000; Videtic et al. 2008), but also used to optimize radiotherapy (RT) treatment planning (Nestle et al. 1999 and 2006; Faria et al. 2008; Schaefer et al. 2008; MacManus et al. 2009; Grgic et al. 2009; Hanna et al. 2010; Riegel et al. 2010; Wu et al. 2010). PET may also enable monitoring of metabolic responses during RT and improve adaptive RT (ART) planning. Recent years also brought massive introduction of innovative RT techniques (intensity-modulated radiotherapy-IMRT, stereotactic ablative radiotherapy-SABR, ART, protons) and novel agents (targeted drugs) in daily clinical practice.

Disappointingly, the vast majority of non-small cell lung cancer (NSCLC) patients and almost all with small cell lung cancer (SCLC) are presenting with disease not amenable to surgical resection. In such cases, RT and chemotherapy (CHT), given either alone or combined, are practiced worldwide. In spite of promising novel biological and technological opportunities, major leaps in the treatment of this disease are lacking, with recurrence still being a dominating and bitter event after treatment, irrespective of histologies (NSCLC vs. SCLC), stages (early versus locally advanced versus metastatic), treatments (surgery, RT, CHT, or any combination of these), or timing of appearance of recurrence (soon after the initial treatment or years later). All recurrences can be separated into three groups: local (e.g., lung parenchyma, bronchial stump, or chest wall), regional (e.g., mediastinal lymph nodes), and distant (brain, liver, adrenal glands, bones, or contralateral lung), but any combination of these may occur in a patient. Once occurring, recurrences present as almost universally fatal event and only rarely efforts with treatment led to cure, irrespective of patient- and/or tumor-related characteristics as well as (re)treatments administered. Not to be forgotten, recurrence usually brings substantially distressing symptoms, which mandates additional supportive treatment. Finally, quality of life of patients experiencing a recurrence is substantially decreased.

Recurrences may appear in anatomically different compartments of the thorax including those located in lung parenchyma (ipsilateral or contralateral lung) alone. It is, therefore, of paramount importance to differentiate between the distinct features of a second metachronous primary lung cancer and those of recurrence in lung parenchyma, the latter occurring after the initial treatment. The diagnosis and the definition of the second primary metachronous primary lung cancer appearing after initial treatment of the primary lung cancer requests particular criteria being necessary for differentiating it from recurrence or from metastatic disease. As proposed by Martini and Melamed (1975), a tumor can be defined as a second metachronous primary lung cancer if it has the following features: (I) with different histology or (II) with the same histology as initial lung cancer but if (a) free interval between the occurrence of cancers was at least 2 years, (b) second cancer originated from a carcinoma in situ, or (c) second cancer was in different lobe or lung, but neither cancer in lymphatics common to both cancers, nor extrapulmonary metastases were found at the time of diagnosis. While second metachronous primary lung cancer will not be discussed here, accumulated data (Jeremic et al. 2001; Kawaguchi et al. 2006) clearly show that lung cancer survivors continue to be at increasing risk of developing second lung cancer. For these patients, RT represents an important treatment option (Jeremic et al. 2001).

A necessary introduction to the overall problem of reirradiation is the rather basic question: to treat a recurrence or not to treat it at all? In an era of modern medicine having an imperative of prolongation of patient's life, especially in the Western civilization, this question seems an outdated one. This is especially so since studies showed that active treatment offers better outcome than pure supportive care, as recently reconfirmed by Hung et al. (2009). They have reconfirmed earlier observation of Sugimura et al. (2007) who investigated 390 recurrent patients out of 1073 patients initially treated with surgery. Median time from surgical resection to recurrence was 11.5 months, and median postrecurrence survival was 8.1 months. Recurrence was intrathoracic in 171 patients, extrathoracic in 172, and a combination of both in 47. Treatments after recurrence included surgery in 43 patients, CHT in 59, RT in 73, and a combination in 96. All patients who received treatment survived longer than those who received no treatment. If one accepts an active oncological approach, i.e., to treat a recurrence, then the next logical step would include a question about the treatment intent, i.e., whether to treat it with curative or palliative intent. Due to important advances in both surgical and radiotherapeutic approaches, all based on novel technologies, more curative approaches seem to have been preferred. However, one must clearly emphasize the lack of established prognostic factors, which may have contributed to a specific decision-making process in this setting, largely due to small number of subjects in many studies. The situation seems changed with the recent introduction of SABR. While stage of the recurrent disease and performance status dictated treatment choice with more conventional RT approaches (mostly limiting the dose given in an reirradiation attempt), with SABR, emphasis moved away from pure palliation to merely control symptoms of an incurable disease towards more radical approaches, aiming towards prolonging patient's life.

Concerning RT for locoregional postsurgical recurrences of NSCLC, this approach was used to treat local/regional recurrences located at various intrathoracic sites. They were usually divided into chest wall/pleural, parenchymal, bronchial stump, and mediastinal lymph node recurrences, but could include any combination of these. Numerous reports showed its effectiveness (Green and Kern 1978; Kopelson and Choi 1980; Law et al. 1982; Shaw et al. 1992; Curran et al. 1992; Yano et al. 1994; Leung et al. 1995; Emami et al. 1997; Kagami et al. 1998; Kono et al. 1998; Jeremic et al. 1999a, b). These studies indicated that there is a dose–response favoring higher doses as well as they indicated that location may influence treatment outcome. In particular, bronchial stump recurrences seem to fare much better than recurrences located in chest wall/pleura or mediastinal lymph nodes. When Jeremic and Bamberg (2002) pooled the data from the literature on bronchial stump cases with no other intrathoracic component, the median survival time (MST) was estimated to be approximately 28.5 months and 5-year survival to be about 31.5 %. These results clearly establish external beam radiation therapy (EBRT) as a treatment of choice in this patient population. In a small ($n=7$) subset of "early" (i.e., stage I: T2N0) bronchial stump recurrences in the study of Jeremic et al. (1999b), an excellent survival (5-year: 57 %) with high-dose EBRT (≥60 Gy) was achieved, approaching that obtainable with surgery alone in newly diagnosed NSCLC of the same stage (Mountain 1986;

Naruke et al. 1988). An interesting and still unexplained fact is that their survival seems much better than that of patients with newly diagnosed NSCLC of a similar stage when treated with high-dose standard or hyperfractionated RT (Ono et al. 1991; Morita et al. 1997; Jeremic et al. 1997; Sibley et al. 1998; Hayakawa et al. 1999; Jeremic et al. 1999a). The findings of the study of Law et al. (1982) who also provided data on patients having "more extensive" bronchial or tracheal component of the disease further support the effectiveness of EBRT in bronchial stump recurrence. These patients achieved a MST of 19 months and 1- and 3-year survival of 75 %, and 12.5 %, respectively, showing that more extensive but still localized disease (no nodal metastases present) may also benefit from RT. When stump recurrence was accompanied by other sites, such as nodal, inferior survival was clearly documented (Curran et al. 1992; Jeremic et al. 1999b; Kagami et al. 1998; Kono et al. 1998).

The past decade brought reconfirmation of these observations. Kelsey et al. (2006) treated 29 patients with either definitive RT ($n=14$) or RT-CHT ($n=15$) for recurrent NSCLC after surgical resection. Most patients had mediastinal adenopathy ($n=19$), while seven patients had disease confined to the surgical stump and three had hilar adenopathy with ($n=2$) or without ($n=1$) a stump recurrence. The median RT dose was 66 Gy (range, 46–74). The MST after RT was 17 months. Actuarial local control and overall survival at 2 years were 62 % and 38 %, respectively. Similarly, Sugimura et al. (2007) found that while the overall MST for local recurrence was 9.8 months, nonsurgical treatment (RT and/or CHT) of recurrence in the lung increased survival time to 13.4 months. Finally, SABR was used to treat postsurgical locoregional recurrences. Coon et al. (2008) reported on a fractionated SABR approach using a CyberKnife. For all ($n=12$) patients with postsurgical recurrent tumors, a dose of 60 Gy was given in 3 fractions. While in the majority of patients pretreatment PET-CT scans were performed to aid in delineation of tumor volume, all patients were followed up regularly, including CT or PET-CT imaging. Overall response rate was 75 %. One of 12 patients (8 %) recurred locally after 7 months. Overall a total of 9 patients (75 %) experienced local, regional, or distant progression, with a median time to disease progression of 3 months (range, 2–7 months). At a median follow-up of 11 months, the local control rate at the site treated was 92 % and overall survival was 67 %. Figure 1 shows an example of CyberKnife dose distributions. Most recently, Agolli et al. (2015) treated 28 patients with 30 lesions and observed an overall response rate of 86 %. Local progression was observed in three patients. Regional relapse occurred in five patients. Distant progression occurred in 10 patients. The 2-year overall survival and disease-free survival were 57.5 % and 36.6 %, respectively. Authors indicated that SABR could have

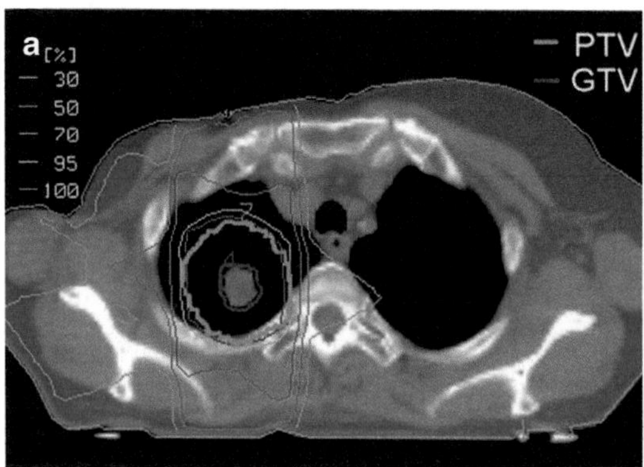

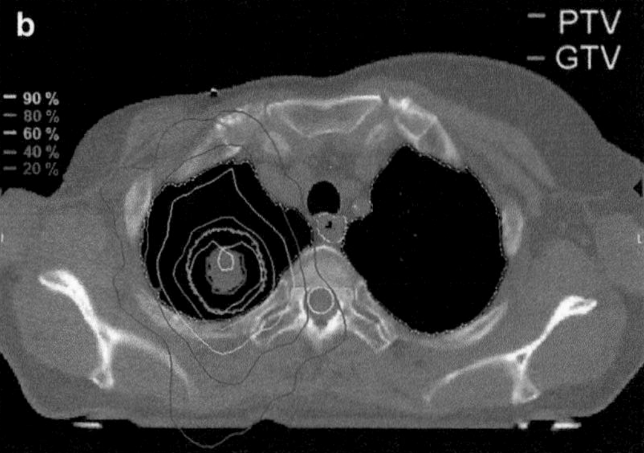

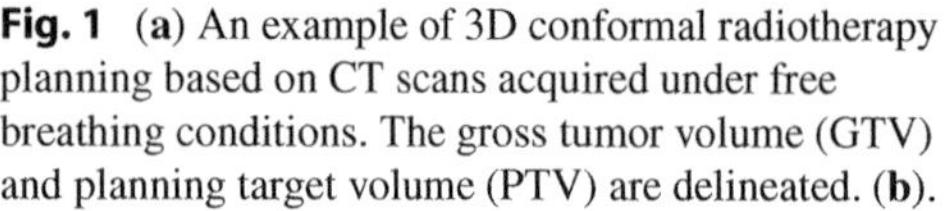

Fig. 1 (**a**) An example of 3D conformal radiotherapy planning based on CT scans acquired under free breathing conditions. The gross tumor volume (GTV) and planning target volume (PTV) are delineated. (**b**). The same patient is planned for CyberKnife treatment. Note the smaller margin from GTV to PTV. The PTV is surrounded by the 80 % isodose line

an alternative role in isolated locoregional relapse in patients unfit or resistant to other therapies.

2 EBRT for Local/Regional Intrathoracic Recurrences After Previous EBRT

EBRT was also used to treat local/regional intrathoracic recurrences after previous EBRT for lung cancer, mostly NSCLC. Currently, there seems to be a total of 13 reports (Tables 1, 2, and 3) in the English literature with only 435 patients reported, so far, using radiotherapy techniques other than SABR. They cover the time period of more than three decades (1982–2015). In spite of existing reports and gradually documented effectiveness of RT in this setting, it is still questionable which proportion of patients initially treated with chest RT eventually undergo reirradiation during the natural course of the disease. To investigate this issue, Estall et al. (2007) examined the proportion of patients who received more than one series of RT for lung cancer. Although the initial RT utilization rate has been estimated to be 76 % (Delaney et al. 2003) accounting for the first RT episode delivered, in the study of Estall et al. (2007) it was 52 %. While initial RT was delivered to local disease in the chest in most cases (79 %), the second (22 %) and third (21 %) RT treatments were offered much less frequently. As the number of treatment episodes increased, the mean duration between each episode decreased. The total dose and number of fractions also decreased, possibly as reflection of deteriorating performance status (PS) and worsening prognosis of patients in the end stage of their disease and their life. Unfortunately, the study covered the data from 2 years (1993 and 1996) and not prolonged periods of time, limiting our understanding and applicability of the results. Additionally, there is a general lack of data provided from other regions/institutions. It is certainly possible that in different settings institutions would have different initial RT utilization rates as well as reirradiation rates.

Reirradiation represents a challenge due to several reasons. There are limited data available to establish its efficacy (Tables 1, 2, and 3). The adequate dose/fractionation and duration of RT to achieve specific goals (cure, palliation) is still not well known. Neither are there clear data about the side effects reirradiation can cause, especially when previous high-dose radical RT was followed by high-dose reirradiation. In spite of these challenging aspects, feasibility and efficacy of reirradiation was clearly documented in several early reports on treatment of recurrent lung cancer (Green and Melbye 1982; Jackson and Ball 1987; Montebello et al. 1993). These studies were all retrospective and besides patients with parenchymal recurrences being reirradiated, sometimes included mixture of patients such as those with postsurgical relapses, postoperatively irradiated patients, those with metastasis, and those with second primary lung cancer. While doses of the initial course of RT ranged from 25 to 80 Gy, those administered at the time of recurrence ranged from 6 to 70 Gy, with cumulative doses ranging from 43 to 150 Gy. Occasionally, a few patients underwent a third course of RT (second reirradiation). RT treatment portals used during the initial course of RT usually included more or less of uninvolved (prophylactic) nodal regions, while those used at the time of reirradiation were obviously limited, in general only including visible recurrence with a safety margin of 1–2 cm (Green and Melbye 1982; Jackson and Ball 1987; Montebello et al. 1993; Gressen et al. 2000; Okamoto et al. 2002). It is likely that the fear of excessive toxicity, which primarily may have occurred in lung and spinal cord, clearly influenced the choice of both total dose and treatment fields used during the reirradiation. Symptom relief, rather than the prolongation of life, was the main goal of reirradiation. In a comprehensive review published 15 years ago (Gressen et al. 2000), clinical data of original articles were summarized. They indicated a beneficial effect of reirradiation on symptom control: control of hemoptysis was observed in 83 %, cough in 65 %, dyspnea in 60 %, and pain in 64 % of cases. Reirradiation carried a merely 5 % complication rate (Green and Melbye 1982; Jackson and Ball 1987; Montebello et al. 1993; Gressen et al. 2000; Okamoto et al. 2002), the most frequent event

Table 1 Patient and tumor characteristics (non-SABR studies)

Author (year)	*N* pts	Sex (M/F)	Age range (median)	Initial tumor staging, % of pts	Histology, % of pts	PS at re-RT, range (median)	Time interval in months from first to second RT (median)
Green and Melbye (1982)	29	23/6	35–85 (57)	n.s.	SCC-66 % ADC-14 % LC-14 % SCLC-6 %	n.s.	3–40 (10)
Jackson and Ball (1987)	22	21/1	45–76 (62)	n.s.	SCC-50 % ADC-36 % other-14 %	n.s.	5.7–48.5 (15)
Montebello et al. (1992)	30	18/12	45–83 (62)	I–II-23 %; IIIA-47 %	SCC-53 %; ADC-27 % LC-10 % Other-10 %	KPS 40–100 (60)	n.s.
Gressen et al. (2000)	23	13/10	47–87 (66)	n.s.	SCC-35 % ADC-30 % LC-9 % Other-27 %	n.s.	3–156 (15)
Okamoto et al. (2002)	34	29/5	38–85 (69)	I–II-9 % IIIA-29 % IIIB-53 % IV-9 %	SCC-50 % ADC-18 % LC-6 % Other-24 %	PS0-1 = 41 % PS ≥2 = 59 %	5–87 (23)
Wu et al. (2003)	23	21/2	43–79 (68)	II-30 % III-70 %	SCC-40 % ADC-30 % SCLC-30 %	KPS 70–100	6–42 (13)
Kramer et al. (2004)	28	27/1	52–83 (68)	n.s.	all NSCLC	n.s.	6–72 (17)
Tada et al. (2005)	19	17/2	49–84 (64)	IIIA = 21 % IIIB = 79 %	SCC-74 % ADC-21 % LC-5 %	PS0-1 = 42 % PS2-3 = 58 %	5–60 (16)
Ebara et al. (2007)	44	n.s.	49–86 (71)	n.s.	SCC-43 % ADC-27 % SCLC-20 % Other-10 %	PS0-1 = 86 % PS2-3 = 14 %	5.8–47.2 (12.6)
Cetingoz et al. (2009)	38	35/3	33–80 (58)	IIB = 5 % IIIA = 10 % IIIB = 84 %	SCC-61 % ADC-13 % Other-26 %	n.s.	1–47 (9)

Ohguri et al. (2012)	33	30/3	45–85 (68)	IB: 2 (6 %) IIB: 4 (12 %) IIIA : 7 (21 %) IIIB: 10 (30 %) IV: 4 (12 %) Postoperative recurrence: 6 (18 %)	SCC: 16 (48 %) ADC: 15 (45 %) Other: 2 (6 %)	PS0 : 3 (9 %) PS1: 21 (64 %) PS2: 9 (27 %) (median, PS1)	1.1–28.2 (7.9)
Yoshitake et al. (2013)	17	15/2	69–88 (81)	Medically inoperable or refusing surgery (all early NSCLC)	SCC: 9 (53 %) ADC: 3 (18 %) NSCLC, NOS: 1 (6 %) Unknown: 4 (24 %)	PS0: 3 (18 %) PS1: 8 (47 %) PS2: 5 (29 %) PS3: 1 (6 %) (median, PS1)	6.3–35.5 (12.4)
Kruser et al. (2014)	48	29/19	40–81 (61)	I: 2 (4 %) II: 5 (10 %) III:20 (42 %) IV:10 (21 %) SCLC: 11 (23 %)	SCC: 17 (35 %) Non-SCC: 15 (31 %) NSCLC NOS: 5 (10 %) SCLC: 11 (23 %)	n.s.	n.s. (19.1)
Tetar et al. (2015)	30	16/14	44–80 (63)	n.s.	n.s.	PS 0-2 (1)	5–189 (30)

M male, *F* female, *KPS* Karnofsky performance status, *PS* WHO/ECOG performance status, *RT* radiotherapy, *n.s.* not stated, *SCC* squamous cell carcinoma, *ADC* adenocarcinoma, *LC* large cell carcinoma, *SCLC* small cell lung cancer, *NSCLC NOS* non-small cell lung cancer not otherwise specified, *other* include at least two other histologies

Adapted with permission from Elsevier from the journal "International Journal of Radiation Oncology, Biology and Physics"

Table 2 Treatment characteristics (non-SABR studies)

Author	Initial RT dose Gy (median)	Re-RT dose Gy (median)	Cumulative RT dose Gy (median)	RT fields and/or volume	RT field size in cm^2 (median)	% pts receiving CHT
Green and Melbye (1982)	40–65 (53)	6–54 (35)	60–166[a] (82)	Tumor only = 76 % Uninvolved mediastinum = 24 %	average, 80	24
Jackson and Ball (1987)	50–61 (55)	20–30 (30)	70–90 (85)	Volume encompassing the disease causing symptoms	n.s.	n.s.
Montebello et al. (1992)	28–66 (60)	15–57 (30)	43–122[a] (88)	Large fields[b] = 4–25 pts Tumor only = 30 pts	(96) (85)	23 %
Gressen et al. (2000)	25–66 (59)	6–40 (30)	60–101 (86)	Tumor + 1–2 cm	30–315 (81)	61 %
Okamoto et al. (2002)	30–80 (66)	10–70 (50)	56.5–150 (110)	Radical = tumor only Palliative = affected region	20–238 (65)	47 %
Wu et al. (2003)	30–78 (66)	46–60 (51)	n.s.	Tumor + 1.5–2.0 cm	42–210 (104)	100 %
Kramer et al. (2004)	40–60 (n.s.)	16 (16)	56–76 (n.s.)	"Limited RT"	n.s.	n.s.
Tada et al. (2005)	50–70 (n.s.)	50–60 (50)	n.s.	"Limited RT"	30–204 (64)	6 %
Ebara et al. (2007)	50–70-(60)	30–60 (40)	80–130 (102)	Tumor + 5–10 mm	n.s.	57 %
Cetingoz et al. (2009)	29–67 (30)	5–30 (25)	n.s.	Tumor + 1–2 cm	25–245 (89)	24 %
Ohguri et al. (2012)	30–85 (70)	29–70 (50)	70–146 (115)	3D PTV = GTV + 7–20 mm	24–386 (112)	15 (45 %)
Yoshitake et al. (2013)	48–60 (48)	60–70 (60)	168–189.6 (Gy_{10}) (177.6)	3D and 4D Tumor only	n.s.	4 (23.5 %)
Kruser et al. (2014)	30–80.5 (57)	12–60 (30)	42–140.5 (87)	3D, IMRT PTV = GTV + 5–11 mm	n.s.	12 (32 %)
Tetar et al. (2015)	24–70 (60)	39–66 (60)	63–136 (120)	4D-IMRT n.s.	n.s.	20 (67 %)

RT radiotherapy, *CHT* chemotherapy, *n.s.* not stated, *3D* three-dimensional RT, *4D* four-dimensional RT, *GTV* gross tumor volume, *PTV* planning target volume, *IMRT* intensity-modulated RT

[a]Includes patients reirradiated twice

[b]Includes various field sizes including ipsilateral hilum, contralateral hilum, mediastinum, and ipsilateral supraclavicular fossa

Adapted with permission from Elsevier from the journal "International Journal of Radiation Oncology, Biology and Physics"

Table 3 Treatment outcome from reirradiation (non-SABR studies)

Author	MST months (range)	OS in years for % pts shown	% of pts showing symptom improvement					% of pts with high-grade (≥3) toxicities indicated
			Hemoptysis	Cough	Chest pain	Dyspnea	Overall	
Green and Melbye (1982)	5 (1–54)	1 year =14 % 5 years=3 %	33 %	55 %	n.s.	44 %	48 %	Rib fracture – 3 % Pneumonitis – 3 %
Jackson and Ball (1987)	5.4 (n.s)	1 year=38 % 2 years=15 %	83 %	50 %	40 %	67 %	50 %	Myelopathy – 5 %
Montebello et al. (1992)	5 (n.s.)	n.s.	89 %	64 %	77 %	53 %	70 %	Esophagitis – 20 % Skin-13 % 13 % Pneumonitis – 3 % Skin – 13 % Pneumonitis – 3
Gressen et al. (2000)	4.9 (n.s.)	1 year=13 %	100 %	60 %	80 %	73 %	72 %	Grade 5 (fatal) – 4 %
Okamoto et al. (2002)	8 (n.s.)	1 year=43 % 2 years=27 %	n.s	n.s	n.s	n.s	75 %	G2 pneumonitis – 35 % G3 pneumonitis – 21 % G2 esophagitis – 12 % G3 esophagitis – 6 %
Wu et al. (2003)	14 (2–37)	1 year=59 % 2 years=21 %	n.s	n.s	n.s	n.s	n.s	G1-2 esophagitis – 9 % G1-2 pneumonitis – 22 % 2 years=21 % G1-2 pneumonitis – 22 %
Kramer et al. (2004)	5.6 (n.s.)	1 year=18 %	100 %	67 %	n.s.	35 %	71 %	G2 esophagitis – 4 %
Tada et al. (2005)	7.1 (n.s.)	1 year=26 % 2 years=11 %	n.s.	n.s.	80 %	100 %	n.s.	G3 pneumonitis – 5 % G2 esophagitis – 16 %
Ebara et al. (2007)	6.5 (n.s.)	1 year=27.7 %	n.s.	n.s.	n.s.	n.s.	81 %	G2 pneumonitis-7 % G3 pneumonitis-7 %
Cetingoz et al. (2009)	3 (n.s.)	1 year=8.7 % 2 years=5.8 %	86 %	77 %	60 %	69 %	78 %	G1-2 esophagitis – 77 % G3 esophagitis – 4 %
Ohguri (2012)	n.s. (18.1)	1 year: 62 % (est.)	100 %	100 %	100 %	100 %	16/17 (94 %) of all tumor-related symptoms	Platelets G3: 1 (3 %) Pleuritis G3: 1 (3 %) Brachial plexopathy G3: 1 (3 %)
Yoshitake (2013)	n.s. (17)	1 year: 74.7 %	n.s.	n.s.	n.s.	n.s.	n.s.	No G3-5 toxicity
Kruser (2014)	n.s. (5.1)	1 year: 22 %	n.s.	n.s.	n.s.	n.s.	75 %	No G3-5 toxicity
Tetar (2015)	n.s. (13.5)	2 years: 23 %	n.s.	n.s.	n.s.	n.s.	n.s.	Bleeding G5: 5 (17 %) Subcutaneous and mediastinal emphysema : 1 (3 %) Bronchial stenosis and oxygen dependency: 1 (3 %)

MST median survival time, *OS* overall survival, *n.s.* not stated, *G* grade, *est.* estimated from available survival curve

Adapted with permission from Elsevier from the journal "International Journal of Radiation Oncology, Biology and Physics"

being radiation pneumonitis appearing in 3 % of cases, while radiation myelopathy and rib fracture were rare events. Although higher incidence of RT pneumonitis was noted in a recent study (Okamoto et al. 2002), described as grade 2 (moderate) and occurring after cumulative radiation doses of 12–150 Gy, in that study a somewhat different policy was instituted, resulting in not only symptomatic, but also asymptomatic patients being reirradiated. This has given the authors an opportunity to use higher RT doses. Patients received a median RT dose of 45 Gy. While symptomatic response in earlier studies ranged from 48 to 72 % with an average cumulative dose of 30 Gy (Green and Melbye 1982; Jackson and Ball 1987; Montebello et al. 1993; Gressen et al. 2000), in that study (Okamoto et al. 2002) palliation was achieved in 75 %. Again, this may indicate that higher doses may lead to higher palliation rate at no cost of increased high-grade (≥3) pneumonitis. Indeed, whereas earlier reports achieved MST of approximately 5 months (Green and Melbye 1982; Jackson and Ball 1987; Gressen et al. 2000), this study (Okamoto et al. 2002) reported a MST of 8 months and a 2-year survival of 27 %, being as high as 15 months and 51 %, respectively, for patients treated with curative intent and higher RT doses. Of additional importance is that it was also observed no difference in the treatment outcome between patients <70 years and those ≥70 years (Gressen et al. 2000), indicating greater applicability of EBRT in this disease, in particular when palliative intention is pursued and when severe late effects become less important. Kramer et al. (2004) confirmed this observation, using 2 fractions of 8 Gy given with 1 week split, a practical and comfortable palliative regimen for both patients and hospitals. The MST was 5.6 months and 71 % of patients had partial or complete relief of one or more of their symptoms. Relief of dyspnea, hemoptysis, and cough was observed in 35 %, 100 %, and 67 %, respectively. Karnofsky performance status (KPS) improved in 45 % patients. The overall median duration of symptom relief was 4 months. Figure 2 shows an example of palliative reirradiation.

Contrary to Kramer et al. (2004), Tada et al. (2005) used more radical approaches with curative intent in 19 patients with stage III NSCLC (50 Gy in 25 daily fractions, including one patient treated with 60 Gy in 30 daily fractions). The overall 1-year and 2-year survival rates were 26 % and 11 %, respectively, and the MST was 7.1 months. However, for 14 patients who received the prescribed dose, it was 10.5 months. Reirradiation alleviated the symptoms in all symptomatic patients except for the one with chest pain. In the recent study of Wu et al. (2003), seemingly the first prospective phase I–II study, the median dose of the first course was 66 Gy (range, 30–78 Gy). Reirradiation was carried using a 3D conformal technique to deliver a median dose of 51 Gy (range, 46–60 Gy), using standard fractionation. The MST was 14 months and the 2-year survival rate was 21 %, while 2-year locoregional progression-free survival was 42 %.

In addition to this pioneering study, more than 10 years ago, Beavis et al. (2005) provided the first report on the use of IMRT, in the retreatment of a patient with NSCLC. With the conventional technique, the target coverage was clearly inferior to that offered by the IMRT plan. With the widespread use of IMRT in cases when it can be of a significant advantage (e.g., shape and location of the tumor as well as in cases of reirradiation), it was expected that this technique might play an important role in reirradiation of lung cancer.

Several recent studies (Ohguri et al. 2012; Yoshitake et al. 2013; Kruser et al. 2014; Tetar et al. 2015) used either three-dimensional (3D) or four-dimensional (4D) or IMRT (Tables 1, 2, and 3) and showed that all techniques allowed consistent use of higher reirradiation (and, therefore, total cumulative) dose of RT. Relatively limited fields also allowed for higher percentage of patients receiving additional CHT. It is, therefore, not surprising that somewhat higher MST (13.5–18.1 months) and 1-year survival rates of 60–70 % were observed. Interestingly, except the study of Ohguri et al. (2012), other studies did not report on symptom control, which may perhaps indicate a shift in philosophy of the treatment towards more curative (and less palliative) outcome. These reports provided evidence of the safety of such approaches, although

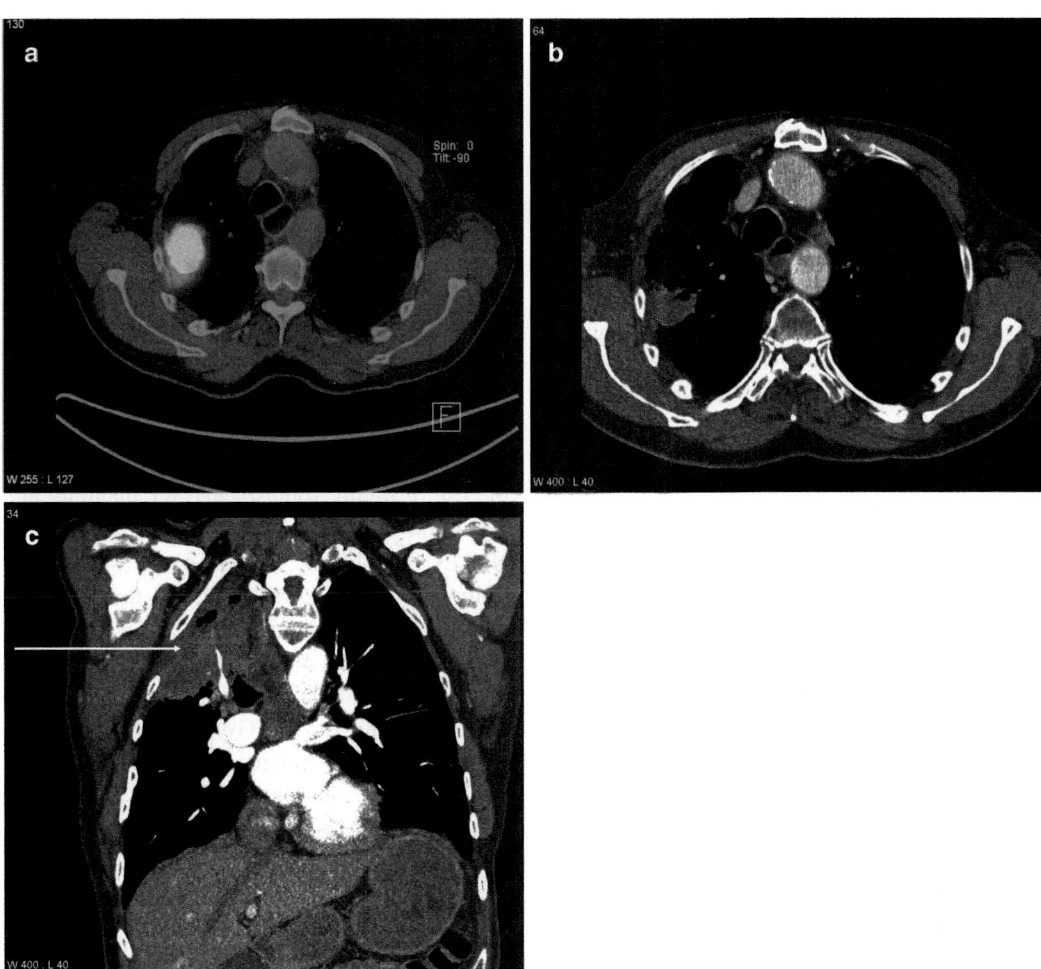

Fig. 2 A 70-year-old male patient was diagnosed with asymptomatic squamous cell cancer in the right lung during surveillance approximately 12 years after he had been cured from two simultaneous squamous cell cancers in the left and right lung, respectively (initial surgical resection, no adjuvant therapy). When he developed this new primary tumor, his lung function was severely compromised and further surgery was not possible. PET-CT showed no lymph node metastases (**a**). He was referred for high-dose radiotherapy and received 3D conformal treatment to the primary lesion only with 2.2 Gy per fraction in October 2008. During treatment, he developed increasing neck pain, and further CT scans showed bone metastasis in the first thoracic vertebra. This metastasis was not detected on the initial PET-CT. In the light of this new finding, radiation treatment to the primary tumor was stopped after 52.8 Gy. The patient refused systemic chemotherapy. He was treated with palliative radiotherapy to the thoracic vertebra. Follow-up CT scans showed a partial remission of the lung tumor (**b**). However, in August 2009, i.e., 10 months after radiotherapy, the patient experienced increasing chest pain and dyspnea. His performance status was ECOG 2. New CT scans revealed local tumor progression and atelectasis (**c**), as well as two small lung metastases. As the patient continued to refuse chemotherapy and was considered ineligible for brachytherapy based on the disease extent, palliative external beam reirradiation was offered (10 fractions of 3 Gy, 2D anterior-posterior opposing fields, the previous course had not resulted in close to tolerance doses to any organ at risk). Clinical improvement was obtained in the absence of acute grade 2 or higher toxicity. Late toxicity could not be assessed because survival was limited to 3.5 months. In the light of this survival outcome, the administration of a different even more hypofractionated regimen might have been a reasonable choice

the study of Tetar et al. (2015) stands as an exemption to this rule. They reported on mortality of 17 % due to bleeding or respiratory failure, likely as a consequence of overlapping high-dose regions of the first and the second RT course in patients with more centrally located tumors.

Observations coming from the literature, especially when more recent studies using highly sophisticated planning and delivery techniques (other than SABR) are taken into account, include but are not limited to the following facts: (1) a great variety of RT characteristics exists regarding the total dose, the dose per fraction and dose prescriptions used, due to different techniques used, including algorithms used to address inhomogeneities, (2) a tendency towards the use of smaller margins during treatment planning exists, although it is still unknown whether this was deliberately done due to special case of recurrent tumor or could perhaps be seen as a consequence of novel techniques being used, (3) a tendency for better reporting of toxicity occurring during and after reirradiation using different toxicity scoring systems was observed, (4) there seems to be a shift in treatment intention, moving away from pure palliation of symptoms towards more radical approaches, with an unfortunate lack of reporting of symptom control in the most recent high-technology studies (Yoshitake et al. 2013; Kruser et al. 2014; Tetar et al. 2015), and (5) time intervals between the initial RT and reirradiation were specified more frequently in the past decade (Okamoto et al. 2002; Wu et al. 2003; Tada et al. 2005; Cetingoz et al. 2009; Oghuri et al. 2012; Yoshitake et al. 2013, Tetar et al. 2015), but not always (Kruser et al. 2014). The latter may well be the crucial issue due to several implications: better understanding of the natural history of the disease, discussing potential prognostic factors as well as the occurrence and timing of anticipated toxicity. Reirradiation started as early as 1–6 months after the first RT course and was as late as 39–189 months after it, with similar median values of 13–16 months (Wu et al. 2003; Tada et al. 2005). Exceptions were the studies by Cetingoz et al. (2009) where it was 8.5 months and Okamoto et al. (2002) and Tetar et al. (2015) where it was 23 and 30 months, respectively. Influence of time interval between the first and the second irradiation was documented by Tada et al. (2005) who showed that in addition to PS, time interval was an important factor influencing treatment outcome. The MST associated with time intervals of less than 12 months, 12–18 months, and more than 18 months were 2.1, 7.1, and 11.5 months, respectively. However, Gressen et al. (2000) did not observe this influence. Cetingoz et al. (2009) showed that time interval between the first and second irradiation was the only independent prognosticator influencing overall survival in multivariate analysis. While these findings may imply less aggressive behavior of tumors reirradiated later, they may also indicate willingness of radiation oncologists to use higher reirradiation doses with prolonged time intervals between first and second irradiation.

Recent years brought a number of reports on the use of highly sophisticated RT planning and execution in cases of reirradiation of, mostly, NSCLC (Tables 4, 5, and 6). It seems that Poltinnikov et al. (2005) were the first to report on the use of hypofractionated SABR in patients previously treated with concurrent RT-CHT. The median dose of the hypofractionated schedule was 32 Gy (range, 4–42 Gy), with a median fraction size of 4 Gy (range, 2.5–4.2 Gy) delivered 3–5 times per week. Five patients also received concurrent CHT. Radiologic response was observed in five (29 %) and stable disease in another five (29 %) patients. The MST from the start of reirradiation was 5.5 months. Symptom resolution was observed in 85 % of symptomatic patients. No grade 3 or higher side effects were observed. Chang et al. (2008) reported on the use of 4D planning to deliver 40–50 Gy to 14 patients with either isolated recurrent tumors previously treated with definitive RT with or without CHT or surgical resection before SABR. With a median follow-up of 17 months, the crude local control at the treated site was 100 % for patients treated to 50 Gy. Four (29 %) patients developed grade 2 pneumonitis. In 38 patients reirradiated with different techniques, other side effects were observed too (Binkley et al. 2015). These included vocal cord paralysis ($n=2$), brachial plexopathy ($n=1$), and Horner's syndrome ($n=1$). No grade ≥4 toxicity was observed.

In the past few years, there were several reports on SABR used in reirradiation of lung recurrences after initial RT (Tables 4, 5, and 6). The number of patients ranged from as low as 8

Table 4 Patient and tumor characteristics (SABR studies)

Author (year)	*N* pts	Sex (M/F)	Age range (median)	Initial tumor staging, % of pts	Histology, % of pts	PS at re-RT, range (median)	Time interval in months from first to second RT (median)
Poltinnikov et al. (2005)	17	10/7	45–79 (66)	n.s.	SCC-35 % ADC-59 % Other-6 %	KPS 60–90 (80)	2–39 (13)
Kelly et al. (2010)	36	16/20	52–92 (67.5)	Stage I–II: 16 (44 %) Stage III: 17 (47 %) Stage IV: 3 (8 %)	ADC: 14 (39 %) SQC: 12 (33 %) NSCLC NOS: 8 (22 %) Other: 2 (6 %)	KPS: 60–100 (80)	0–92 (22)
Seung et al. (2011)	8	2/6	50–85 (71)	I: 3 II: 3 III: 1 LD SCLC: 1	NSCLC: 7 SCLC: 1	KPS 70–100 (90)	8–57 (36.5)
Liu et al. (2012)	72	47/25	44–89 (67)	T1-2: 37 T3-4: 25 N0-2: 48 N3: 14	ADC: 31 (43 %) SQC: 20 (28 %) NSCLC, NOS: 20 (28 %) Other: 1 (1 %)	PS0-1: 54 (75 %) PS2-3: 18 (25 %)	0–106 (21)
Trakul et al. (2012)	15	8/9	49–92 (66)	n.s.	n.s.	n.s.	5–80 (16)
Meijneke et al. (2013)	20	14/6	50–80 (71)	Stage I: 10 Stage II: 1 Stage IV: 9	ADC: 1 SQC: 2 Clear cell: 1 Small cell: 2 No pathology: 14 (Non-lung: 3)	n.s.	2–33 (17)
Valakh et al. (2013)	9	n.s.	59–83 (74)	Stage I: 5 Stage II: 1 Stage III: 2 Stage IV: 1	ADC: 1 SQC: 4 NSCLC, NOS: 3 ADC (metastatic): 1	n.s.	n.s.

(continued)

Table 4 (continued)

Author (year)	*N* pts	Sex (M/F)	Age range (median)	Initial tumor staging, % of pts	Histology, % of pts	PS at re-RT, range (median)	Time interval in months from first to second RT (median)
Kilburn et al. (2014)	33	19/14	45–80 (66)	Stage IA: 5 Stage IB: 4 Stage IIA: 2 Stage IIB: 2 Stage IIIA: 8 Stage IIIB: 5 Stage IV 3: Non-lung: 4	ADC : 12 SQC : 11 SCLC: 4 NSCLC: 1 ADC and SQC: 1 Non-lung: 4	PS0: 7 PS1: 19 PS2: 6	6–61 (18)
Trovo et al. (2014)	17	14/3	40–88 (66)	IIIA: 14 IIIB: 3	SQC: 9 ADC: 8	PS0-1: 9 PS2: 8	1–60 (18)
Patel et al. (2015)	26	7/19	42–87 (68)	I–II: 8 III: 15 IV: 3	NSCLC: 23 Non-NSCLC: 3	n.s.	3–26 (8)

SABR stereotactic ablative radiotherapy, *M* male, *F* female, *KPS* Karnofsky performance status, *PS* WHO/ECOG performance status, *RT* radiotherapy, *n.s.* not stated, *SCC* squamous cell carcinoma, *ADC* adenocarcinoma, *LC* large cell carcinoma, *SCLC* small cell lung cancer, *NSCLC NOS* non-small cell lung cancer not otherwise specified

Table 5 Treatment characteristics (SABR studies)

Author (year)	Initial RT dose Gy (median)	Re-RT dose Gy (median)	Cumulative RT dose (median)	RT fields and/or volume	RT field size in cm^2 (median)	% pts receiving CHT
Poltinnikov et al. (2007)	50–66 (52)	4–42 (32)	n.s.	SABR	95 (30–189) GTV + 5 mm	29 %
Kelly et al. (2010)	30–79.2 (61.5)	40–50 (50)	59.4–134.6 (81.5)	SABR	CTV = iGTV + 8 mm PTV = CTV + 3 mm	n.s.
Seung et al. (2011)	50–68 (61.5)	48–60 (n.a.)	100–126 (113)	SABR	PTV = ITV + 3–5 mm	0
Liu et al. (2012)	30–79.2 (63)	50 (50)	80–129.2 (113)	SABR	CTV = iGTV + 8 mm PTV = CTV + 3 mm	0
Trakul et al. (2012)	60–112.5 (BED) (87.5)	60–112.5 (BED) (80)	n.a. (157.6) (BED)	SABR	GTV = CTV PTV = ITV + 5 mm	n.s.
Meijnke et al. (2013)	30–60 (60) 44–150 (Gy_{10}) (133) (Gy_{10})	20–60 (48) 23–150 (Gy_{10}) (83) (Gy_{10})	78–120 (93) 67–300 (Gy_{10}) (216) (Gy_{10})	SABR: 18 3D: 2	n.s.	2 (10 %)
Valakh et al. (2013)	30–60 (60) 60–180 (BED_{10}) (132) (BED_{10})	30–60 (60) 60–180 (BED_{10}) (132) (BED_{10})	60–120 (116) 120–360 (BED_{10}) (264) (BED_{10})	SABR after 1st SABR	PTV = ITV + 3 mm	n.s.
Kilburn et al. (2014)	45–80.5 (66) (EBRT) 22.6–60 (50) (SBRT)	20–54 (50) (SBRT) 66–70.2 (70) (EBRT)	Summed composite max dose: 74–130 (103); Max dose (EQD2): 118–507 (209)	EBRT- SABR: 23 SABR – SABR: 7 SABR -EBRT: 3	3D-EBRT: GTV + 10 mm 3D-SBRT: GTV +5–10 mm 4D-EBRT: ITV + 5 mm 4D-SBRT: ITV + 5 mm	n.s.
Trovo et al. (2014)	50–60 (n.a.)	30 (37.5–40) (BED)	87.5–90 (n.a.)	SABR	PTV = GTV + 5 mm	n.s.
Patel et al. (2015)	30–70.4 (61.2)	15–50 (30)	45–120.4 (91.2)	SABR	PTV = CTV + 5 mm	13 (50 %)

SABR stereotactic ablative radiotherapy, *RT* radiotherapy, *CHT* chemotherapy, *n.s.* not stated, *3D* three-dimensional RT, *4D* four-dimensional RT, *GTV* gross tumor volume, *CTV* clinical target volume, *PTV* planning target volume, *EBRT* external beam RT, *IMRT* intensity-modulated RT, *ITV* internal target volume, *iGTV* internal GTV, *BED* biologically equivalent dose, *EQD2* dose equivalent to total dose when given in 2 Gy fractions

Table 6 Treatment outcome from reirradiation (SABR studies)

Author (year)	MST months (range)	OS in years for % pts shown	% of pts showing symptom improvement					% of pts with high-grade (≥3) toxicities indicated
			Hemoptysis	Cough	Chest pain	Dyspnea	Overall	
Poltinnikov et al.	5.5 (2.5–30)	n.s.	n.s.	n.s.	n.s.	n.s.	65 %	No G3-5 toxicity G2 esophagitis- 24 % G1 pneumonitis- 6 %
Kelly et al. (2010)	26 (est)	2 year: 59 %	n.s.	n.s.	n.s.	n.s.	n.s.	G3 Cough: 1 (3 %) G3 Pneumonitis: 7 (28 %) G3 Esophagitis: 3 (8 %) G3 Skin: 2 (6 %) G3 Chest wall pain: 6 (17 %)
Seung et al. (2011)	18	1 year: 87 %	n.s.	n.s.	n.s.	n.s.	n.s.	No G3-5 toxicity
Liu et al. (2012)	n.s.	2 years: 74.4 %	n.s.	n.s.	n.s.	n.s.	n.s.	Pneumonitis G3 = 14 (19 %) Pneumonitis G 5 = 1 (1 %)
Trakul et al. (2012)	21	1 year: 80 %	n.s.	n.s.	n.s.	n.s.	n.s.	No G3-5 toxicity
Meijneke et al. (2013)	15	2 years: 33 %	n.s.	n.s.	n.s.	n.s.	n.s.	No G3-5 toxicity
Valakh et al. (2013)	22	2 years: 68.6 %	n.s.	n.s.	n.s.	n.s.	n.s.	G3 late lung: 2 (22 %) G3 late chest pain: 1 (11 %)
Kilburn et al. (2014)	21	2 years: 45 %	n.s.	n.s.	n.s.	n.s.	n.s.	Dyspnea G3: 1 (3 %) Bleeding G5: 1 (3 %)
Trovo et al. (2014)	19	2 years: 29 %	n.s.	n.s.	n.s.	n.s.	n.s.	Pneumonitis G3: 4 (23 %) Pneumonitis G5: 1 (5 %)
Patel et al. (2015)	14	2 years: 27 %	n.s.	n.s.	n.s.	n.s.	n.s.	No G3-5 toxicity

SABR stereotactic ablative radiotherapy, *MST* median survival time, *OS* overall survival, *n.s.* not stated, *G* grade, *est.* estimated from available survival curve to as high as 72 in rather elderly populations (total age range, 40–92 years; median values, range 66–74), while the majority of patients had good PS (either KPS 80–90 or PS 0-1). Time interval from the first RT course to the reirradiation with SABR varied from short (0–2 months) to long (92–106 months), similarly to its historic predecessors. While earlier reports (Poltinnikov et al. 2007; Kelly et al. 2010; Seung et al. 2011; Liu et al. 2012) specified only total doses of initial RT and SABR course, respectively, using total doses delivered, more recent reports (Trakul et al. 2012; Meijeneke et al. 2013; Valakh et al. 2013; Kilburn et al. 2014; Trovo et al. 2014) used biologically equivalent doses (BED) to incorporate more contemporary radiobiological calculations for the sake of considerations of both tumor control and toxicity in normal tissues. Majority of studies used existing ICRU specifications for the dose prescription on specified volumes, but not all specified whether concurrent CHT was used. As expected, owing to higher BED doses given with this approach, results were promising. Except the study of Poltinnikov et al. (2007), which achieved MST of 5.5 months and with no 1- to 2-year survival reported, only Liu et al. (2012) did not report on MST, but they reported impressive 2-year survival of 74 %. Other studies also reported excellent results, with MST ranging from 14 to 26 months and 2-year survival rates as high as 59–69 % in selected populations (Tables 4, 5 , and 6). These results were accompanied with acceptable and rather low toxicity. However, some reports included an occasional patient experiencing grade 5 (fatal) toxicity, either lung or bleeding. A total of three such patients have been encountered among the total of 253 (1 %) treated in the 10 studies we tabulated here. It must, however, be clearly acknowledged that most series did not report on the use of elastic deformation, making an accurate assessment of the cumulative radiation doses to the organs at risk impossible. On the other hand, it was consistently observed that the majority if not all, grade 5 toxicities occurred in centrally located recurrences. Finally and disappointingly, except Poltinnikov et al. (2007) who provided total symptom relief (but not specified per symptom), not a single study using SABR reported symptom relief like older nonstereotactic studies did. One of the possible reasons may well be found in higher BED doses investigators used, shifting the treatment intention from pure palliation to a more curative setting with expected prolongation of life. Indeed, such a shift may have been rewarded by results which significantly surpass those obtained with traditionally used techniques such as 3D RT, aiming at simple and fast palliation in this setting.

Finally, availability of proton facilities in several countries also meant that sporadic reports on its use in reirradiation of recurrent lung cancer started to appear in the literature. Berman et al. (2013) preliminarily reported on a multi-institutional trial in NSCLC. Twenty-four patients were reirradiated, with 12 on a prospective trial of proton RT for reirradiation. Median age was 69 years (51–89). Median prior dose was 62.4 Gy (30.6–80). Concurrent CHT (platinum-based or erlotinib) was given in 63 %. Median proton RT dose was 66.6 Gy (36–74). Follow-up was >60 days in 17 pts. There was one in-field and four other thoracic recurrences, and nine deaths. These results showed promising early outcomes and acceptable toxicity in low volume patients, but due to the toxicity seen in high volume patients, additional exclusion criteria were needed and have been added for NSCLC patients in the ongoing trial. McAvoy et al. (2013) reported on 33 such patients who initially underwent RT with a variety of treatment techniques that ranged from conventional through 3D, IMRT, and SABR to protons between 1979 and 2010. Interval between initial RT course and reirradiation ranged from 1 to 376 months (median, 36 months). Initial median RT dose was 63 Gy (range 40–74 Gy) in a median 33 fractions (range 4–59 fractions), with a median dose per fraction of 2 Gy (range 1.18–12.5 Gy). Median BED for initial RT was 93 Gy_4 (range 62–206 Gy_4) while median dose equivalent to the dose given in 2 Gy fractions (EQD2) was 62.2 Gy (range 39–155 Gy). The median dose delivered was

66 Gy (relative biological effectiveness – RBE) (range 16.4–75 Gy (RBE)) delivered in a median of 32 fractions (range 9–58 fractions) resulting in a median dose per fraction of 2 Gy (RBE) (range 1.2–7 Gy (RBE)). For patients who completed proton RT as planned, the median BED was 99 Gy_4 (RBE) (range 57–192 Gy_4 (RBE)). Median EQD2 was 66 Gy (RBE) (range 38–140 Gy (RBE)). The MST was 11.1 months and 2-year overall survival was 33 %. One patient developed grade 4 esophagitis, and two patients developed grade 4 lung toxicity, making the total high-grade toxicity acceptable. With more centers embarking on the use of protons due to its superior dose distribution versus photons, it is not unrealistic to expect more such reports in the near future.

In small cell lung cancer (SCLC), RT was not frequently used to treat locoregional recurrence. In a recent review article by Drodge et al. (2014) including 13 studies with a total of 421 patients with lung cancer, only 42 had SCLC, merely 10 %. Due to this small number of patients, unfortunately, no separate data for SCLC histology were provided. Scarce data on reirradiated limited disease were likely due to previous treatment with a combined RT-CHT approach, because of the fear that reirradiation may add only toxicity without clear benefit for patients (Fig. 3). For extensive disease, RT became frequently practiced only in recent years. Hence, majority of data on reirradiation at the time of recurrence was after initial CHT. Retrospective studies (Ihde et al. 1979; Ochs et al. 1983; Salazar et al. 1991) used doses ranging from 21 to 60 Gy in patients harboring recurrences from both limited and extensive disease SCLC. Although response rates observed within the RT field were 52–77 %, the MST reached only 3–4 months, likely as a result of early systemic progression, too. Nevertheless, the wide range of doses used gave an opportunity to the authors to speculate about higher doses (≥40 Gy) producing better palliation, an important but unresolved matter in patients with limited remaining lifetime. With recent success of RT in extensive disease and prolonged survival of such patients, it is expected that reirradiation may be instituted more frequently in the near future.

3 Endobronchial (Endoluminal) Brachytherapy for Locoregionally Recurrent Lung Cancer

Endobronchial brachytherapy was also used to treat recurrent lung cancer, particularly when previous EBRT has been given. Here as well, the vast majority of reports include a mixture of histologies with only a minority of patients having SCLC. First reports more than 25 years ago provided data of endobronchial brachytherapy using different sources combined with low-dose EBRT to treat recurrent lung cancer (Mendiondo et al. 1983) and achieved satisfactory palliative results. Since then, a number of studies of endobronchial brachytherapy using different dose rate were published. The vast majority of reports included the use of high dose rate (HDR) brachytherapy (Seagren et al. 1985; Mehta et al. 1989; Bedwinek et al. 1991; Sutedja et al. 1992; Gauwitz et al. 1992; Gustafson et al. 1995; Micke et al. 1995; Delclos et al. 1996; Ornadel et al. 1997; Hatlevoll et al. 1999; Kelly et al. 2000; Zorlu et al. 2008; Hauswald et al. 2010). In the majority of reports, median doses of previous EBRT mostly ranged between 54 and 58 Gy (Bedwinek et al. 1991; Sutedja et al. 1992; Gauwitz et al. 1992; Gustafson et al. 1995; Micke et al. 1995; Hauswald et al. 2010), although in the study of Zorlu et al. (2008) the median total dose was 30 Gy (range, 30–70 Gy). In some studies, a single fraction of endobronchial RT of either 10 Gy (Seagren et al. 1985; Hatlevoll et al. 1999; Zorlu et al. 2008) or 15 Gy (Zorlu et al. 2008) or 20–30 Gy (Mehta et al. 1989) was used; however, the majority of other authors prescribed 2–3 fractions given in weekly intervals. The dose per fraction/session mostly ranged from 6 to 15 Gy, while in two German studies (Micke et al. 1995; Hauswald et al. 2010) it was 5 Gy per fraction, delivered 2–4 times. Subjective response to treatment was observed in 66–94 %, and it was of a similar magnitude (per symptom) than that of palliative

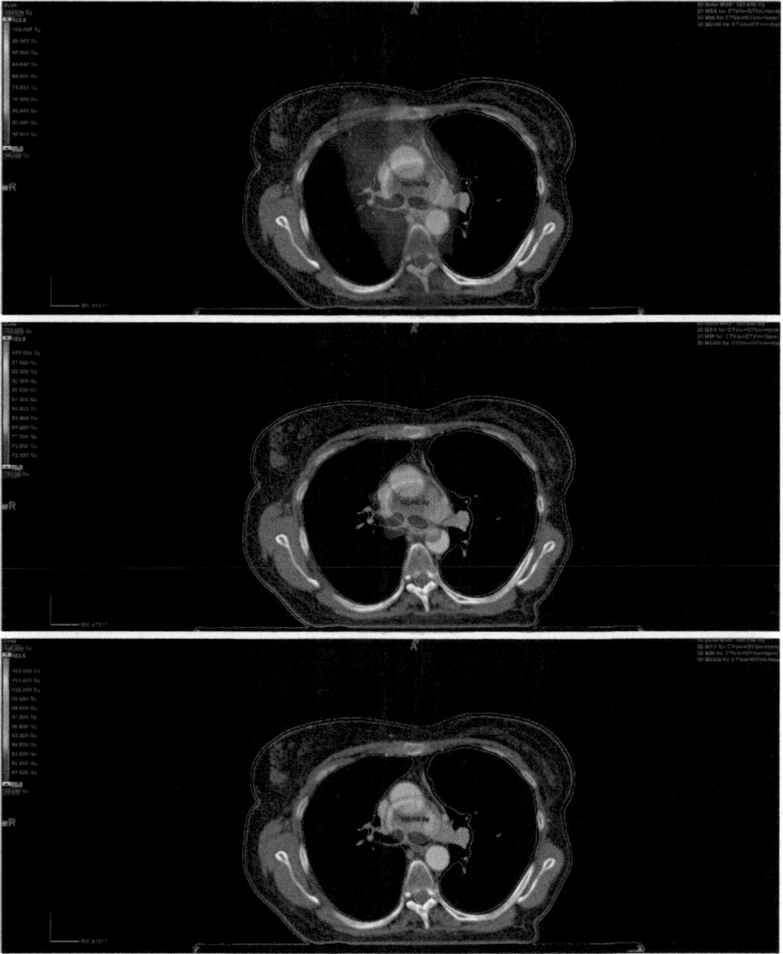

Fig. 3 A 60-year-old female patient was diagnosed with small cell lung cancer centrally in the right hilum with N2 nodal disease, stage IIIA. She had previously received adjuvant radiotherapy for left-sided breast cancer, 15 years ago. She was treated with concomitant chemoradiation, cisplatin/etoposide, and radiotherapy (45 Gy in 30 fractions, 1.5 Gy bid, 3-D conformal) between the second and third cycle, followed by prophylactic cranial irradiation. One year later, an isolated mediastinal in-field relapse was diagnosed (PET-CT, positive biopsy from endoscopic bronchial ultrasound, gross tumor volume 1.2 cc). She was reirradiated (57 Gy, 1.5 Gy bid, 3-D conformal, no uninvolved nodes or levels included, concomitant cisplatin/etoposide). Cumulative isodoses are shown below (50, 70, and 90 Gy; Varian Eclipse™). Despite low esophageal reirradiation dose (mean 9.7 Gy, V50<3 %), she developed temporary acute grade 3 esophagitis. The esophagus had received the full prescription dose earlier at this level. Hematological toxicity was severe, too. Mean lung dose was 4 Gy (reirradiation) and 14.5 Gy, respectively. Current follow-up of 6 months is too short to judge other side effects

EBRT. However, in some studies (Zorlu et al. 2008), the mean period of palliation was disappointingly low, 45 days (range, 0–9 months). On the other side, the period of palliation was significantly longer in patients with high KPS (≥80) at the initial evaluation. Hauswald et al. (2010) showed that relief of symptoms was excellent in 12 % of patients and good in 46 % of patients. Complete remission was observed in 15 % of patients, and partial response in 58 % of patients. In other studies, objective response measured by bronchoscopy was observed in 72–100 % of patients, while radiologic documentation of reaeration was observed in 64–88 % patients. Duration of response ranged from 4.5 to 6.5 months. Actuarial local control rates were rarely reported, being in the most recent study of Hauswald et al. (2010) 17 % at 1 year and 3 % at 2 years, respectively. In that study, the median local progression-free survival time was 4 months (range, 1–23 months). Survival was reported with increasing frequency in recent years, being approximately 25 % at 1 year (Bedwinek et al. 1991), while Kelly et al. (2000) and Hauswald et al. (2010) both achieved survival of 18 % and 7 % at 1 and 2 years, respectively. The MST ranged from 5 to 9 months (Bedwinek et al. 1991; Gauwitz et al. 1992; Delclos et al. 1996; Micke et al. 1995; Kelly et al. 2000; Zorlu et al. 2008; Hauswald et al. 2010) with two studies reporting identical findings of the MST of 7 months for responders (Sutedja et al. 1992; Kelly et al. 2000). Although a number of different treatment-related complications have been observed, the most feared was fatal bleeding. Contrary to initial reports (Seagren et al. 1985; Bedwinek et al. 1991; Sutedja et al. 1992) which documented an incidence of severe pulmonary bleeding of 25–32 %, those reported in the last decades (Gauwitz et al. 1992; Gustafson et al. 1995; Delclos et al. 1996; Kelly et al. 2000; Zorlu et al. 2008; Hauswald et al. 2010) reported significantly lower incidence of this complication (range, 0–7 %). Although a number of risk factors were investigated, different nature of reporting (crude versus actuarial) and frequently lacking pretreatment patient and tumor characteristics make firm conclusions difficult. Prior laser resection was identified as the major factor contributing to the risk of fatal hemoptysis in the study by Ornadel et al. (1997) (20 % at 2 years). Detailed analysis of other side effects has been provided by Hauswald et al. (2010). They included tissue necrosis, pneumothorax causing dyspnea, bronchomediastinal fistulas, or mild hemoptysis not requiring transfusion and called for detailed documentation of any side effect occurring during and after the treatment as to put it into a perspective of cost-benefit analysis, especially when single-fraction HDR is considered.

Conclusions

Recurrence is a frequent observation during the history of lung cancer, regardless of its initial treatment. Recent advances in both biology and technology of diagnosis and treatment of lung cancer offer hope for more successful treatment. This, paradoxically, may also increase the number of patients experiencing a recurrence after the end of treatment, maybe later during follow-up. With close follow-up, earlier detection may allow for effective treatment.

Also, novel technologies, such as SABR, may allow for successful dose escalation, thereby providing a basis for reirradiating locoregional recurrences. Technological advances such as CyberKnife, protons, or carbon ions may become an indispensable tool in treating these patients with more success. It is important to discriminate between curative and palliative intention. Factors to consider include stage of the disease and PS as well as time interval between the two RT courses and, definitely, radiobiological calculations of the total dose (expressed in biological equivalents) of the initial and second RT course. Recurrences not suitable for more aggressive treatment may require either palliative RT and/or best supportive care. While no established guidelines can be expected to appear soon, due to great variety in initial RT parameters, different planning and execution characteristics (including different reirradiation tools used), and the lack of prognostic factors, current wisdom calls for prudent use of available technology, with clear objectives set up front.

Finally, as is the case with other tumor entities, the best way to ask important questions and get answers, which may be used in the clinic, is to perform prospective clinical studies.

References

Agolli L, Valeriani M, Carnevale A, Falco T, Bracci S, De Sanctis V, Minniti G, Enrici RM, Osti MF (2015) Role of salvage stereotactic body radiation therapy in post-surgical loco-regional recurrence in a selected population of non-small cell lung cancer patients. Anticancer Res 35:1783–1789

Beavis AW, Abdel-Hamid A, Upadhyay S (2005) Re-treatment of a lung tumour using a simple intensity-modulated radiotherapy approach. Br J Radiol 78: 358–361

Bedwinek J, Petty A, Bruton C, Sofield J, Lee L (1991) The use of high dose rate endobronchial brachytherapy to palliate symptomatic endobronchial recurrence of previously irradiated bronchogenic carcinoma. Int J Radiat Oncol Biol Phys 22:23–30

Berman AT, Ciunci, CA, Lin H, Both S, Langer CJ, Varillo K, Rengan R, Hahn SM, Fagundes MD, Hartsell W (2013) Multi-institutional prospective study of reirradiation with proton beam radiotherapy for non-small cell lung cancer. J Clin Oncol 31(suppl; abstr 7578)

Binkley MS, Hiniker SM, Chaudhuri A, Maxim PG, Diehn M, Loo BW Jr, Shultz DB (2015) Dosimetric factors and toxicity in highly conformal thoracic reirradiation. Int J Radiat Oncol Biol Phys. pii: S0360-3016(15)26844-7. doi:10.1016/j.ijrobp.2015.12.007

Cetingoz R, Arikan-Alicikus Z, Nur-Demiral A, Durmak-Isman B, Bakis-Altas B, Kinay M (2009) Is re-irradiation effective in symptomatic local recurrence of non small cell lung cancer patients? A single institution experience and review of the literature. J BUON 14:33–40

Chang JY, Balter PA, Dong L, Yang Q, Liao Z, Jeter M, Bucci MK, McAleer MF, Mehran RJ, Roth JA, Komaki R (2008) Stereotactic body radiation therapy in centrally and superiorly located stage I or isolated recurrent non-small-cell lung cancer. Int J Radiat Oncol Biol Phys 72:967–971

Coon D, Gokhale AS, Burton SA, Heron DE, Ozhasoglu C, Christie N (2008) Fractionated stereotactic body radiation therapy in the treatment of primary, recurrent, and metastatic lung tumors: The role of Positron Emission Tomography/Computed Tomography-based treatment planning. Clin Lung Cancer 9:217–221

Curran WJ Jr, Herbert SH, Stafford PM, Sandler HM, Rosenthal SA, McKenna WG, Hughes E, Dougherty MJ, Keller S (1992) Should patients with post-resection locoregional recurrence of lung cancer receive aggressive therapy? Int J Radiat Oncol Biol Phys 24:25–30

Delaney G, Barton M, Jacob S, Jalaludin B (2003) A model for decision making for the use of radiotherapy in lung cancer. Lancet Oncol 4:120–128

Delclos ME, Komaki R, Morice RC, Allen PK, Davis M, Garden A (1996) Endobronchial brachytherapy with high-dose-rate remote afterloading for recurrent endobronchial lesions. Radiology 201:279–282

Drodge CS, Ghosh S, Fairchild A (2014) Thoracic reirradiation for lung cancer: a literature review and practical guide. Ann Palliat Med 3:75–91

Ebara T, Tanio N, Etoh T, Shichi I, Honda A, Nakajima N (2007) Palliative reirradiation for in-field recurrence after definitive radiotherapy in patients with primarylung cancer. Anticancer Res 27(1):531–534

Emami B, Graham MV, Deedy M, Shapiro S, Kucik N (1997) Radiation therapy for intrathoracic recurrence of non-small cell lung cancer. Am J Clin Oncol (CCT) 20:46–50

Estall V, Barton MB, Vinod SK (2007) Patterns of radiotherapy re-treatment in patients with lung cancer: a retrospective, longitudinal study. J Thorac Oncol 2:531–536

Faria SL, Menard S, Devic S, Sirois C, Souhami L, Lisbona R, Freeman CR (2008) Impact of FDG-PET/CT on radiotherapy volume delineation in non-small-cell lung cancer and correlation of imaging stage with pathologic findings. Int J Radiat Oncol Biol Phys 70:1035–1038

Gauwitz M, Ellerbroek N, Komaki R, Putnam JB Jr, Ryan MB, DeCaro L, Davis M, Cundiff J (1992) High dose endobronchial irradiation in recurrent bronchogenic carcinoma. Int J Radiat Oncol Biol Phys 23:397–400

Green N, Kern W (1978) The clinical course and treatment results of patients with postresection locally recurrent lung cancer. Cancer 42:2478–2482

Green N, Melbye RW (1982) Lung cancer: Retreatment of local recurrence after definitive irradiation. Cancer 49:865–868

Gressen EL, Werner-Wasik M, Cohn J, Topham A, Curran WJ Jr (2000) Thoracic reirradiation for symptomatic relief after prior radiotherapeutic management for lung cancer. Am J Clin Oncol (CCT) 23:160–163

Grgic A, Nestle U, Schaefer-Schuler A, Kremp S, Ballek E, Fleckenstein J, Rübe C, Kirsch CM, Hellwig D (2009) Nonrigid versus rigid registration of thoracic 18F-FDG PET and CT in patients with lung cancer: an intraindividual comparison of different breathing maneuvers. J Nucl Med 50:1921–1926

Gustafson G, Vicini F, Freedman L, Johnston E, Edmudson G, Sherman S, Pursel S, Komic M, Chen P, Borrego JC, Seidman J, Martinez A (1995) High dose rate endobronchial brachytherapy in the management of primary and recurrent bronchogenic malignancies. Cancer 75:2345–2350

Hanna GG, McAleese J, Carson KJ, Stewart DP, Cosgrove VP, Eakin RL, Zatari A, Lynch T, Jarritt PH, Young VA, O'Sullivan JM, Hounsell AR (2010) (18)F-FDG PET-CT simulation for non-small-cell lung cancer: effect in patients already staged by PET-CT. Int J Radiat Oncol Biol Phys 77:24–30

Hatlevoll R, Karlsen KO, Skovlund E (1999) Endobronchial radiotherapy for malignant bronchial obstruction or recurrence. Acta Oncol 38:999–1004

Hauswald H, Stoiber E, Rochet N, Lindel K, Grehn C, Becker HD, Debus J, Harms W (2010) Treatment of recurrent bronchial carcinoma: the role of high-dose-rate endoluminal brachytherapy. Int J Radiat Oncol Biol Phys 77:373–377

Hayakawa K, Mitsuhashi N, Saito Y, Nakayama Y, Furuta M, Sakurai H, Kawashima M, Ohno T, Nasu S, Niibe H (1999) Limited field irradiation for medically inoperable patients with peripheral stage I non-small cell lung cancer. Lung Cancer 26:137–142

Hung JJ, Hsu WH, Hsieh CC, Huang BS, Huang MH, Liu JS, Wu YC (2009) Post-recurrence survival in completely resected stage I non-small cell lung cancer with local recurrence. Thorax 64:192–196

Ihde DC, Bilek FS, Cohen MH (1979) Response to thoracic radiotherapy in patients with small cell carcinoma of the lung after failure of combination chemotherapy. Radiology 132:443–446

International Agency for Research on Cancer (IARC): http://globocan.iarc.fr (2012)

Jackson MA, Ball DL (1987) Palliative retreatment of locally recurrent lung cancer after radical radiotherapy. Med J Aust 147:391–394

Jeremic B, Bamberg M (2002) External beam radiation therapy for bronchial stump recurrence of non-small-cell lung cancer after complete resection. Radiother Oncol 64:251–257

Jeremic B, Shibamoto Y, Acimovic LJ, Milisavljevic S (1997) Hyperfractionated radiotherapy alone for clinical stage I nonsmall cell lung cancer. Int J Radiat Oncol Biol Phys 38:521–525

Jeremic B, Shibamoto Y, Acimovic LJ, Milisavljevic S (1999a) Hyperfractionated radiotherapy for clinical Stage II nonsmall cell lung cancer. Radiother Oncol 51:141–145

Jeremic B, Shibamoto Y, Milicic B, Milisavljevic S, Nikolic N, Dagovic A, Aleksandrovic J, Radosavljevic-Asic G (1999b) External beam radiation therapy alone for loco-regional recurrence of non-small-cell lung cancer after complete resection. Lung Cancer 23: 135–142

Jeremic B, Shibamoto Y, Acimovic L, Nikolic N, Dagovic A, Aleksandrovic J, Radosavljevic-Asic G (2001) Second cancers occurring in patients with early stage non-small cell lung cancer treated with chest radiation therapy alone. J Clin Oncol 19:1056–1063

Kagami Y, Nishio M, Narimatsu N, Mjoujin M, Sakurai T, Hareyama M, Saito A (1998) Radiotherapy for locoregional recurrent tumours after resection of non-small cell lung cancer. Lung Cancer 20:31–35

Kawaguchi T, Matsumura A, Iuchi K, Ishikawa S, Maeda H, Fukai S, Komatsu H, Kawahara M (2006) Second primary cancers in patients with stage III non-small cell lung cancer successfully treated with chemo-radiotherapy. Jpn J Clin Oncol 36:7–11

Kelly JF, Delclos ME, Morice RC, Huaringa A, Allen PK, Komaki R (2000) High-dose-rate endobrobchial brachytherapy effectively palliates symptoms due to airway tumors: the 10-year M.D. Anderson Cancer Center experience. Int J Radiat Oncol Biol Phys 48:697–702

Kelly P, Balter PA, Rebueno N, Sharp HJ, Liao Z, Komaki R, Chang JY (2010) Stereotactic body radiation therapy for patients with lung cancer previously treated with thoracic radiation. Int J Radiat Oncol Biol Phys 78:1387–1393

Kelsey CR, Clough RW, Marks LB (2006) Local recurrence following initial resection of NSCLC: salvage is possible with radiation therapy. Cancer J 12:283–288

Kilburn JM, Kuremsky JG, Blackstock AW, Munley MT, Kearns WT, Hinson WH, Lovato JF, Miller AA, Petty WJ, Urbanic JJ (2014) Thoracic re-irradiation using stereotactic body radiotherapy (SBRT) techniques as first or second course of treatment. Radiother Oncol 110:505–510

Kono K, Murakami M, Sasaki R (1998) Radiation therapy for non-small cell lung cancer with postoperative intrathoracic recurrence. Nippon Igaku Hoshasen Gakkai Zasshi 58:18–24

Kopelson G, Choi NCH (1980) Radiation therapy for postoperative local-regionally recurrent lung cancer. Int J Radiat Oncol Biol Phys 6:1503–1506

Kramer GWPM, Gans S, Ullmann E, van Meerbeck JP, Legrand C, Leer JWH (2004) Hypofractionated external beam radiotherapy as retreatment for symptomatic non-small-cell lung carcinoma: an effective treatment? Int J Radiat Oncol Biol Phys 58:1388–1393

Kruser TJ, McCabe BP, Mehta MP, Khuntia D, Campbell TC, Geye HM, Cannon GM (2014) Reirradiation for locoregionally recurrent lung cancer: outcomes in small cell and non-small cell lung carcinoma. Am J Clin Oncol 37:70–76

Law MR, Henk JM, Lennox SC, Hodson M (1982) Value of radiotherapy for tumour on the bronchial stump after resection of bronchial carcinoma. Thorax 37: 496–499

Leung J, Ball D, Worotniuk T, Laidlaw C (1995) Survival following radiotherapy for post-surgical locoregional recurrence of non-small cell lung cancer. Lung Cancer 13:121–127

Liu H, Zhang X, Vinogradskiy YY, Swisher SG, Komaki R, Chang JY (2012) Predicting radiation pneumonitis after stereotactic ablative radiation therapy in patients previously treated with conventional thoracic radiation therapy. Int J Radiat Oncol Biol Phys 84:1017–1023

MacManus M, Nestle U, Rosenzweig KE, Carrio I, Messa C, Belohlavek O, Danna M, Inoue T, Deniaud-Alexandre E, Schipani S, Watanabe N, Dondi M, Jeremic B (2009) Use of PET and PET/CT for radiation therapy planning: IAEA expert report 2006-2007. Radiother Oncol 91: 85–94

Martini N, Melamed MR (1975) Multiple primary lung cancers. J Thorac Cardiovasc Surg 70:606–612

McAvoy SA, Ciura KT, Rineer JM, Allen PK, Liao Z, Chang JY, Palmer MB, Cox JD, Komaki R, Gomez DR (2013) Feasibility of proton beam therapy for reirradiation of locoregionally recurrent non-small cell lung cancer. Radiother Oncol 109:38–44

Mehta MP, Shahabi S, Jarjour NN, Kinsella TJ (1989) Endobronchial irradiation for malignant airway obstruction. Int J Radiat Oncol Biol Phys 17:847–851

Mendiondo OA, Dillon M, Beach LJ (1983) Endobronchial brachytherapy in the treatment of recurrent bronchogenic carcinoma. Int J Radiat Oncol Biol Phys 9: 579–582

Meijneke TR, Petit SF, Wentzler D, Hoogeman M, Nuyttens JJ (2013) Reirradiation and stereotactic radiotherapy for tumors in the lung: dose summation and toxicity. Radiother Oncol 107:423–427

Micke O, Prott FJ, Schäfer U, Wagner W, Pötter R (1995) Endoluminal HDR brachytherapy in the palliative treatment of patients with the recurrence of a non-small-cell bronchial carcinoma after prior radiotherapy. Strahlenther Onkol 171:554–559

Montebello JF, Aron BS, Manatunga AK, Horvath JL, Peyton FW (1993) The reirradiation of recurrent bronchogenic carcinoma with external beam irradiation. Am J Clin Oncol 16:482–488

Morita K, Fuwa N, Suzuki Y, Nishio M, Sakai K, Tamaki Y, Niibe H, Chujo M, Wada S, Sugawara T, Kita M (1997) Radical radiotherapy for medically inoperable non-small cell lung cancer in clinical stage I: retrospective analysis of 149 patients. Radiother Oncol 42:31–36

Mountain CF (1986) A new international staging system for lung cancer. Chest 89:225S–233S
Naruke T, Goya T, Tsuchiya R, Suemasu K (1988) Prognosis and survival in resected lung carcinoma based on the new international staging system. J Thorac Cardiovasc Surg 96:440–447
Nestle U, Walter K, Schmidt S, Licht N, Nieder C, Motaref B, Hellwig D, Niewald M, Ukena D, Kirsch CM, Sybrecht GW, Schnabel K (1999) 18F-deoxyglucose positron emission tomography (FDG-PET) for the planning of radiotherapy in lung cancer: high impact in patients with atelectasis. Int J Radiat Oncol Biol Phys 44:593–597
Nestle U, Kremp S, Grosu AL (2006) Practical integration of [18F]-FDG-PET and PET-CT in the planning of radiotherapy for non-small cell lung cancer (NSCLC): the technical basis, ICRU-target volumes, problems, perspectives. Radiother Oncol 81:209–225
Ochs JJ, Tester WJ, Cohen MH, Lichter AS, Ihde DC (1983) Salvage radiation therapy for intrathoracic small cell carcinoma of the lung progressing on combination chemotherapy. Cancer Treat Rep 67: 1123–1126
Ohguri T, Imada H, Yahara K, Moon SD, Yamaguchi S, Yatera K, Mukae H, Hanagiri T, Tanaka F, Korogi Y (2012) Re-irradiation plus regional hyperthermia for recurrent non- small cell lung cancer: a potential modality for inducing long-term survival in selected patients. Lung Cancer 77:140–145
Okamoto Y, Murakami M, Yoden E, Sasaki R, Okuno Y, Nakajima T, Kuroda Y (2002) Reirradiation for locally recurrent lung cancer previously treated with radiation therapy. Int J Radiat Oncol Biol Phys 52:390–396
Ono R, Egawa S, Suemasu K, Sakura M, Kitagawa T (1991) Radiotherapy in inoperable stage I lung cancer. Jpn J Clin Oncol 21:125–128
Ornadel D, Duchesne G, Wall P, Ng A, Hetzel M (1997) Defining the roles of high dose rate endobronchial brachytherapy and laser resection for recurrent bronchial malignancy. Lung Cancer 16:203–213
Patel NR, Lanciano R, Sura K, Yang J, Lamond J, Feng J, Good M, Gracely EJ, Komarnicky L, Brady L (2015) Stereotactic body radiotherapy for re-irradiation of lung cancer recurrence with lower biological effective doses. J Radiat Oncol 4:65–70
Poltinnikov IM, Fallon K, Xiao Y, Reiff JE, Curran WJ Jr, Werner-Wasik M (2005) Combination of longitudinal and circumferential three-dimensional esophageal dose distribution predicts acute esophagitis in hypofractionated reirradiation of patients with non-small-cell lung cancer treated in stereotactic body frame. Int J Radiat Oncol Biol Phys 62:652–658
Riegel AC, Bucci MK, Mawlawi OR, Johnson V, Ahmad M, Sun X, Luo D, Chandler AG, Pan T (2010) Target definition of moving lung tumors in positron emission tomography: correlation of optimal activity concentration thresholds with object size, motion extent, and source-to-background ratio. Med Phys 37:1742–1752
Salazar OM, Yee GJ, Slawson RG (1991) Radiation therapy for chest recurrence following induction chemotherapy in small cell lung cancer. Int J Radiat Oncol Biol Phys 21:645–650
Schaefer A, Kremp S, Hellwig D, Rübe C, Kirsch CM, Nestle U (2008) A contrast-oriented algorithm for FDG-PET-based delineation of tumour volumes for the radiotherapy of lung cancer: derivation from phantom measurements and validation in patient data. Eur J Nucl Med Mol Imaging 35:1989–1999
Seagren SL, Harrell JH, Horn RA (1985) High dose rate intraluminal irradiation in recurrent endobronchial carcinoma. Chest 88:810–814
Seung SK, Matthew SM (2011) Salvage SBRT for previously irradiated lung cancer. J Cancer Ther 2:190–195
Shaw EG, Brindle JS, Creagan ET, Foote RL, Trastek VF, Buskirk SJ (1992) Locally recurrent non-small-cell lung cancer after complete surgical resection. Mayo Clin Proc 67:1129–1133
Sibley GS, Jamieson TA, Marks LB, Anscher MS, Prosnitz LR (1998) Radiotherapy alone for medically inoperable stage I non-small-cell lung cancer: The Duke experience. Int J Radiat Oncol Biol Phys 40:149–154
Siegel R, Ma J, Zou Z, Jemal A (2009) Cancer Statistics, 2014. CA Cancer J Clin 64:9–29
Sugimura H, Nichols FC, Yang P, Allen MS, Cassivi SD, Deschamps C, Williams BA, Pairolero PC (2007) Survival after recurrent nonsmall-cell lung cancer after complete pulmonary resection. Ann Thorac Surg 83:409–417
Sutedja G, Baris G, Schaake-Koning C, van Zandwijk N (1992) High dose rate brachytherapy in patients with local recurrences after radiotherapy of non-small cell lung cancer. Int J Radiat Oncol Biol Phys 24:551–553
Tada T, Fukuda H, Matsui K, Hirashima T, Hosono M, Takada Y, Inoue Y (2005) Non-small-cell lung cancer: reirradiation for loco-regional relapse previously treated with radiation therapy. Int J Clin Oncol 10: 247–250
Tetar S, Dahele M, Griffioen G, Slotman B, Senan S (2015) High-dose conventional thoracic re-irradiation for lung cancer: updated results. Lung Cancer 88:235–236
Trakul N, Harris JP, Le QT, Hara WY, Maxim PG, Loo BW Jr, Diehn M (2012) Stereotactic ablative radiotherapy for reirradiation of locally recurrent lung tumors. J Thorac Oncol 7:1462–1465
Trovo M, Minatel E, Durofil E, Polesel J, Avanzo M, Baresic T, Bearz A, Del Conte A, Franchin G, Gobitti C, Rumeileh IA, Trovo MG (2014) Stereotactic body radiation therapy for re-irradiation of persistent or recurrent non-small cell lung cancer. Int J Radiat Oncol Biol Phys 88:1114–1119
Vanuytsel LJ, Vansteenkiste JF, Stroobants SG, De Leyn PR, De Wever W, Verbeken EK, Gatti GG, Huyskens DP, Kutcher GJ (2000) The impact of (18)F-fluoro-2-deoxy-D-glucose positron emission tomography (FDG-PET) lymph node staging on the radiation treatment volumes in patients with non-small cell lung cancer. Radiother Oncol 55:317–324
Valakh V, Miyamoto C, Micaily B, Chan P, Neicu T, Li S (2013) Repeat stereotactic body radiation therapy for patients with pulmonary malignancies who had previously received SBRT to the same or an adjacent tumor site. J Cancer Res Ther 9:680–685

Videtic GM, Rice TW, Murthy S, Suh JH, Saxton JP, Adelstein DJ, Mekhail TM (2008) Utility of positron emission tomography compared with mediastinoscopy for delineating involved lymph nodes in stage III lung cancer: insights for radiotherapy planning from a surgical cohort. Int J Radiat Oncol Biol Phys 72:702–706

Wu KL, Jiang G-L, Qian H, Wang L-J, Yang H-J, Fu X-L, Zhao S (2003) Three-dimensional conformal radiotherapy for locoregionally recurrent lung carcinoma after external beam irradiation: a prospective phase I-II clinical trial. Int J Radiat Oncol Biol Phys 57: 1345–1350

Wu K, Ung YC, Hornby J, Freeman M, Hwang D, Tsao MS, Dahele M, Darling G, Maziak DE, Tirona R, Mah K, Wong CS (2010) PET CT thresholds for radiotherapy target definition in non-small-cell lung cancer: how close are we to the pathologic findings? Int J Radiat Oncol Biol Phys 77:699–706

Yano T, Hara N, Ichinose Y, Asoh H, Yokoyama H, Ohta M, Hata K (1994) Local recurrence after complete resection for nonsmall-cell carcinoma of the lung. Significance of local control by radiation treatment. J Thorac Cardiovasc Surg 10:8–12

Yoshitake T, Shioyama Y, Nakamura K, Sasaki T, Ohga S, Shinoto M, Terashima K, Asai K, Matsumoto K, Hirata H, Honda H (2013) Definitive fractionated re-irradiation for local recurrence following stereotactic body radiotherapy for primary lung cancer. Anticancer Res 33:5649–5653

Zorlu AF, Selek U, Emri S, Gurkayanak M, Akyol FH (2008) Second line palliative endobronchial radiotherapy with HDR Ir 192 in recurrent lung carcinoma. Yonsei Med J 49:620–624

Re-irradiation for Esophageal Cancer

Stefano Arcangeli and Vittorio Donato

Contents

Abstract

While recurrent esophageal cancer is a common clinical scenario, limited data exist regarding management approaches that include re-irradiation. Tremendous technological advances in the treatment planning and delivery of radiotherapy pave the way to evaluate the appropriateness of re-irradiation in the management of radio-recurrent esophageal cancer. Patients with radio-recurrent esophageal cancer may still be selected for a potentially curative treatment, especially those in good clinical condition, who may experience prolonged survival and good symptom control rates. None of the different therapeutic options is carried out without potentially life-threatening treatment-related toxicities in a relevant proportion of the patients. In this scenario, patient selection performed on individual basis could help to identify the most appropriate treatment modality, including re-irradiation with cutting-edge techniques. Enrollment of these patients in clinical trials is highly warranted.

1 Introduction

Locoregional recurrence is still the major type of treatment failure in patients with esophageal cancer after definitive radiotherapy (RT) or radiochemotherapy (RCT). The recurrence rate after

The original version of this chapter was revised. An erratum to this chapter can be found at 10.1007/978-3-319-41825-4_78.

S. Arcangeli (✉) • V. Donato
Department of Radiation Oncology,
S. Camillo and Forlanini Hospitals, Rome, Italy
e-mail: stefano.arcangeli@yahoo.it;
vdonato@scamilloforlanini.rm.it

Med Radiol Radiat Oncol (2016)
DOI 10.1007/174_2016_77, © Springer International Publishing Switzerland
Published Online: 14 Aug 2016

radical RT, RCT, and surgery is more than 70 % (Fujita et al. 1994; Stahl et al. 2005) with in-field relapse after RCT in more than 20 % of patients (Haefner et al. 2015; Ordu et al. 2015). Once recurrence occurs, the 5-year survival rate drops dramatically down (Yano et al. 2006; Shioyama et al. 2007). Current NCCN guidelines recommend palliative/best supportive care (BSC) in this setting (NCCN guidelines Version 2.2016). Due to its disappointing outcomes, chemotherapy has only a palliative role and it is associated to a median survival of 5 months (Sudo et al. 2014). Salvage surgical resection can result in favorable local control (95 %) and overall survival (up to 59 months), but is hampered by high rates of anastomotic leakage (17–39 %), pulmonary complications (17–30 %), intensive care unit readmission (17–22 %), and postoperative mortality (3–15 %) (Swisher et al. 2002; Marks et al. 2012, 2014; Sudo et al. 2013, 2014), which makes this choice highly demanding and limited to a carefully selected patient population (Marks et al. 2012).

2 Re-irradiation

Salvage re-irradiation largely depends on the location of local failure in relation to the prior radiation field, but it is often discouraged because it infringes the basic, long-standing principle that once definitive RT has been administered, further RT cannot be given because it would likely exceed normal tissue tolerances. Indeed, with external beam radiation therapy (EBRT), it is often difficult to avoid organs that already have received tolerance doses of radiation with the primary treatment. Although re-irradiation has been proven to be feasible and effective in other tumors (Zwicker et al. 2011; Zerini et al. 2015), the advantage of this approach in the management of local tumor bed recurrence after definitive RCT remains uncertain. Advances in the treatment planning and delivery of RT have aroused interest in assessing the appropriateness of re-irradiation for various anatomical sites (Mantel et al. 2013). However, experiences with advanced forms of radiotherapy – intensity-modulated radiation therapy (IMRT) and stereotactic body radiotherapy (SBRT) – are sparse and limited to case reports, while only few studies have been published on salvage re-irradiation for locoregional recurrence after primary radical RCT (Yamaguchi et al. 2011; Kim et al. 2012; Zhou et al. 2015). Yamaguchi et al. (2011) reported on 31 patients with recurrent or persistent squamous cell carcinoma of the esophagus treated with re-irradiation to a dose of 36–40 Gy in 2-Gy fractions using 3-dimensional conformal RT. Among them, 27 patients received concurrent chemotherapy, and 14 patients underwent regional hyperthermia during the re-irradiation course. Despite the lower radiation doses used, severe toxicities were not uncommon, with 6 patients (20 %) who suffered from grade 3 esophageal perforation. Zhou et al. (2015) reported on the largest studied cohort retrospectively analyzing a total of 114 patients with locally recurrent esophageal squamous cell carcinoma after initial radical RCT. Fifty-five patients underwent salvage RT with a median dose of 54 Gy (range 18–66 Gy), 1.8–2.0 Gy per fraction, 5 days/week, and 59 patients received BSC only. After a median follow-up period of 20 months (range 8–70 months), those who received the active treatment reported a 6-month and 1-year survival rate after recurrence of 41.8 % and 16.4 %, respectively. The same features in the non-salvage cohort were 11.9 % and 3.4 %, respectively ($p<0.001$). However, treatment-related toxicity was relevant, with 3 (5.5 %) and 11 (20.0 %) patients from the active group who experienced ≥ grade 3 radiation pneumonitis and esophageal fistula/perforation, respectively, compared to none and 8 patients (13.6 %) from the BSC group. At multivariate analysis, a salvage radiation dose >50 Gy and late recurrence (>12 months) were associated with a better prognosis. Due to its intrinsic dose distribution, brachytherapy (BT) may be considered in place of EBRT to restore the integrity of the lumen by the use of appropriate applicators which can decrease an excessive dose deposition on mucosal surfaces (Harms et al. 2005). Nevertheless, also salvage BT is carried out with significant risk of severe (grade ≥ 3) toxicities, mainly consisting in perforation, hemorrhage, and fistula formation, observed in up to 30 % of the patients (Homs et al. 2004). A further option in this patient population is represented by proton therapy (PT), which may offer an advantage over photon therapy, as the proton beam deposits most of its energy at a specific depth, so the radiation dose beyond that target is negligible. Fernandes et al. (2016) reported on a series of 14 patients with a history of thoracic radiation and newly diagnosed or locally recurrent esophageal cancer who were offered proton beam re-irradiation on a prospective trial. The median re-irradiation prescription dose was 54.0 Gy (relative biological effectiveness [RBE]) (50.4–61.2 Gy [RBE]), and the median interval between radiation courses was 32 months (10–307 months). Eleven patients received concurrent chemotherapy. After a median follow-up of 10 months (2–25 months), the median overall survival was 14 months and among the 10 patients who presented with symptomatic disease, 4 had complete resolution of symptoms, and 4 had diminished or stable symptoms. Late grade 3 toxicities and late grade 5 esophageal ulcer occurred in four and one patients, respectively. Although the differential diagnosis between tumor progression and late adverse reactions appears difficult, it is undeniable that treatment-related toxicities may occur in spite of the use of such advanced forms of RT.

Conclusions

In conclusion, several points can be gleaned from these limited data:

1. Tremendous technological advances in the treatment planning and delivery of EBRT pave the way to evaluate the appropriateness of re-irradiation in the management of radio-recurrent esophageal cancer.
2. Patients with radio-recurrent esophageal cancer may still be selected for a potentially curative treatment, especially those in good clinical condition, who may experience prolonged survival and good symptom control rates.
3. Active therapeutic options include salvage surgery, endoscopic procedures – including BT – and chemotherapy. None of them is carried out without life-threatening treatment-related toxicities in a relevant proportion of the patients.
4. PT may offer an advantage over photon therapy and should be considered in this setting, allowing for a better sparing of organs at risk such as the spinal cord, heart, and lung, provided that treatment-related toxicities are still possible.

In this scenario, patients selection performed on individual basis could help to identify the most appropriate treatment modality, including re-irradiation with cutting-edge techniques. Enrollment of these patients in clinical trials is highly warranted.

References

Fernandes A, Berman AT, Mick R et al (2016) A prospective study of proton beam reirradiation for esophageal cancer. Int J Radiat Oncol Biol Phys 95:483–487

Fujita H, Kakegawa T, Yamana H et al (1994) Lymph node metastasis and recurrence in patients with a carcinoma of the thoracic esophagus who underwent three-field dissection. World J Surg 18:266–272

Haefner MF, Lang K, Krug D et al (2015) Prognostic factors, patterns of recurrence and toxicity for patients with esophageal cancer undergoing definitive radiotherapy or chemo-radiotherapy. J Radiat Res 56:742–749

Harms W, Krempien R, Grehn C et al (2005) Daytime pulsed dose rate brachytherapy as a new treatment option for previously irradiated patients with recurrent oesophageal cancer. Br J Radiol 78:236–241

Homs MY, Steyerberg EW, Eijkenboom WM et al (2004) Single-dose brachytherapy versus metal stent placement for the palliation of dysphagia from oesophageal cancer: multicentre randomised trial. Lancet 364: 1497–1504

Kim YS, Lee CG, Kim KH et al (2012) Re-irradiation of recurrent esophageal cancer after primary definitive radiotherapy. Radiat Oncol J 30:182–188

Mantel F, Flentje M, Guckenberger M (2013) Stereotactic body radiation therapy in the re-irradiation situation – a review. Radiat Oncol 8:7

Markar SR, Karthikesalingam A, Penna M et al (2014) Assessment of short-term clinical outcomes following salvage esophagectomy for the treatment of esophageal malignancy: systematic review and pooled analysis. Ann Surg Oncol 21:922–931

Marks JL, Hofstetter W, Correa AM et al (2012) Salvage esophagectomy after failed definitive chemoradiation for esophageal adenocarcinoma. Ann Thorac Surg 94:1126–1133

NCCN Guidelines Version 2.2016 Updates Esophageal and Esophagogastric Junction Cancers Available online

Ordu AD, Nieder C, Geinitz H et al (2015) Radio(chemo) therapy for locally advanced squamous cell carcinoma of the esophagus: long-term outcome. Strahlenther Onkol 191:153–160

Shioyama Y, Nakamura K, Ohga S et al (2007) Radiation therapy for recurrent esophageal cancer after surgery: clinical results and prognostic factors. Jpn J Clin Oncol 37:918–923

Stahl M, Stuschke M, Lehmann N et al (2005) Chemoradiation with and without surgery in patients with locally advanced squamous cell carcinoma of the esophagus. J Clin Oncol 23:2310–2317

Sudo K, Taketa T, Correa AM et al (2013) Locoregional failure rate after preoperative chemoradiation of esophageal adenocarcinoma and the outcomes of salvage strategies. J Clin Oncol 31:4306–4310

Sudo K, Xiao L, Wadhwa R et al (2014) Importance of surveillance and success of salvage strategies after definitive chemoradiation in patients with esophageal cancer. J Clin Oncol 32:3400–3405

Swisher SG, Wynn P, Putnam JB et al (2002) Salvage esophagectomy for recurrent tumors after definitive chemotherapy and radiotherapy. J Thorac Cardiovasc Surg 123:175–183

Yamaguchi S, Ohguri T, Imada H et al (2011) Multimodal approaches including three-dimensional conformal re-irradiation for recurrent or persistent esophageal cancer: preliminary results. J Radiat Res 52:812–820

Yano M, Takachi K, Doki Y et al (2006) Prognosis of patients who develop cervical lymph node recurrence following curative resection for thoracic esophageal cancer. Dis Esophagus 19:73–77

Zerini D, Jereczek-Fossa BA, Fodor C et al (2015) Salvage image-guided intensity modulated or stereotactic body reirradiation of local recurrence of prostate cancer. Br J Radiol 88:20150197

Zhou Z, Zhen C, Bai W et al (2015) Salvage radiotherapy in patients with local recurrent esophageal cancer after radical radiochemotherapy. Radiat Oncol 10:54

Zwicker F, Roeder F, Thieke C et al (2011) IMRT reirradiation with concurrent cetuximab immunotherapy in recurrent head and neck cancer. Strahlenther Onkol 187:32–38

Re-irradiation for Locally Recurrent Breast Cancer

Andrew O. Wahl and William Small Jr.

Contents

The original version of this chapter was revised. An erratum to this chapter can be found at 10.1007/978-3-319-41825-4_78.

A.O. Wahl, MD (✉)
Department of Radiation Oncology,
University of Nebraska Medical Center,
Buffett Cancer Center, 987521 Nebraska Medical,
Omaha, NE 68198-7521, USA
e-mail: awahl@unmc.edu

W. Small Jr., MD, FACRO, FACR, FASTRO
Department of Radiation Oncology,
Loyola University, Cardinal Bernardin Cancer Center,
Maguire Center – Room 2944, 2160 S. 1st Ave.,
Maywood, IL 60153, USA
e-mail: wmsmall@lumc.edu

Abstract

Locally recurrent breast cancer occurs in 5–15% of patients after breast conservation therapy and after mastectomy with adjuvant radiotherapy. Ipsilateral breast tumor recurrences may be salvaged with mastectomy; however, outcomes from repeat breast-conserving surgery and breast re-irradiation are promising. Chest wall recurrence generally portends a worse prognosis than in-breast local recurrences. A subset of patients may be long-term survivors in the absence of metastasis. Persistent chest wall disease can be symptomatic, and in previously irradiated patients, treatment options are limited. Experiences with chest wall re-irradiation have shown excellent response rates with acceptable late toxicity, but follow-up is limited.

1 Re-irradiation of the Intact Breast

Following breast-conserving surgery and external beam radiotherapy, local recurrence rates are 2–10% at 5 years and 5–15% at 10 years (Fourquet et al. 1989; Bartelink et al. 2001; Fisher et al. 2002; Veronesi et al. 2002). Distant metastases are diagnosed in 5–10% of patients with an ipsilateral breast cancer recurrence (Fourquet et al. 1989; Touboul et al. 1999). Predictors of distant metastasis include skin involvement, recurrent tumor size >10 mm, lymph node status, and grade of primary

DOI 10.1007/174_2016_75, © Springer International Publishing Switzerland
Published Online: 14 Aug 2016

disease (Voogd et al. 1999). A prolonged time interval between initial diagnosis and recurrent tumor is a favorable prognostic indicator (Kurtz et al. 1990). Patients with late local failure have similar long-term survivals to 5-year survivors who have never failed locally. Approximately 40% of local recurrences may be considered new primary tumors versus recurrent disease, which have different natural histories and implications for treatment (Smith et al. 2000; Huang et al. 2002). Single nucleotide polymorphism arrays have been used to distinguish new primary tumors from recurrent disease and may outperform clinical determination (Bollet et al. 2008).

1.1 Salvage Mastectomy of an Ipsilateral Breast Cancer Recurrence

Salvage mastectomy is generally considered to be the standard of care of a locally recurrent breast cancer previously treated with breast-conserving surgery and adjuvant breast radiotherapy, as there traditionally have been concerns about re-irradiation of the breast and poor cosmetic outcome (Kurtz et al. 1988; Kennedy and Abeloff 1993; Osborne and Simmons 1994; Huston and Simmons 2005). The local control rate of salvage mastectomy ranges from 51 to 85% (Kurtz et al. 1988; Cajucom et al. 1993; Osborne and Simmons 1994), and 5-year disease-free survival is 52–72% (Kurtz et al. 1991; Abner et al. 1993; Cajucom et al. 1993; Osborne and Simmons 1994; Alpert et al. 2005).

Mastectomy is associated with increased psychological distress compared to lumpectomy. The degree of difficulty with body image and clothing are more pronounced with mastectomy versus partial mastectomy; however, quality of life and mood assessment are generally equivalent 1 year after surgical intervention (Ganz et al. 1992). Younger women may be more susceptible to increased psychological distress after mastectomy than older women. About 66% of mastectomy patients under age 40 had high-psychological distress compared to 13% of partial mastectomy patients, $p=0.027$ (Maunsell et al. 1989). Lumpectomy has less negative impact on sex life compared to mastectomy, 30% versus 45% (Rowland et al. 2000).

1.2 Salvage Breast-Conserving Surgery Alone

Salvage breast-conserving surgery may be preferable to patients who wish to preserve their breast; however, there is limited published data on this approach (Table 1). A review of 50 patients who underwent salvage lumpectomy revealed a second local failure rate of 32% and a median survival following salvage surgery of 33 months. Patients who developed a recurrence 5 years after their initial therapy had 92% local control after salvage breast conservation surgery compared to 49% for failures occurring within 5 years of diagnosis ($p=0.01$). There was no statistical difference between salvage lumpectomy and mastectomy in locoregional control in patients with late local failures (96% versus 78%, $p=0.18$). Positive or indeterminate resection margins resulted in higher local failure rates than negative margins (47% versus 24%, $p<0.01$) (Kurtz et al. 1990, 1991).

Alpert et al. utilized salvage breast-conserving surgery in 30 patients with tumor size <3 cm, ≤3 positive lymph nodes, no skin involvement, and no lymphovascular space invasion. These patients were compared to a cohort of patients with ipsilateral breast cancer recurrence treated with salvage mastectomy. With a median follow-up

Table 1 Results of salvage breast-conserving surgery without repeat radiotherapy

First author	Year	*N*	Follow-up (years)	Local control (%)
Alpert	2005	30	13.8	93
Abner	1993	16	3.25	69
Kurtz	1991	50	4.25	62
Komoike	2003	30	3.6	70
Salvadori	1999	57	6.1	86
Gentilini	2007	161	3.6	79
Dalberg	1998	14	13	50
Ishitobi	2014	130	4.8	81
Voogd	1999	16	4.3	62

Abbreviations: *N* number of patients

after salvage surgery of 13.8 years, local control was 93%. After a second local failure, mastectomy was performed for repeat salvage surgery. There was no difference in distant metastasis, cause-specific survival, or overall survival between the repeat lumpectomy and mastectomy groups. In the cohort who underwent salvage mastectomy for local recurrence, 24% had multicentric disease on pathologic review. Multicentric disease was identified preoperatively on physical exam or mammography in all patients (Alpert et al. 2005).

Abner et al. reviewed 16 patients who refused mastectomy and received excisional biopsy alone for recurrent breast cancer. The local failure rate was 31% (Abner et al. 1993). The Milan group performed a review of their repeat lumpectomy patients ($n=57$) and salvage mastectomy ($n=134$) with a median follow-up of 73 months. In the lumpectomy alone group, local control and 5-year overall survival were 86 and 85%, respectively, compared to 97 and 70% in the mastectomy group. No difference was seen with regard to the disease-free survival between patients who underwent mastectomy and those who had repeat excision (Salvadori et al. 1999). A review of 14 patients who received salvage breast-conserving surgery reported a local failure rate of 50% (Dalberg et al. 1998).

As noted above, local recurrence rates following repeat breast-conserving surgery range from 10 to 50%, with most reports in the 30–35% range. Interpretation of these results is limited by the fact that the use of breast imaging and margin status are not uniformly reported. The local control rate of salvage lumpectomy is similar to that seen in prospective trials of newly diagnosed breast cancer patients treated with lumpectomy without adjuvant radiation. The addition of repeat irradiation may lead to a decrease in local failure after salvage lumpectomy similar to that seen at initial treatment.

1.3 Salvage Breast-Conserving Surgery with Breast Re-irradiation

Despite the belief that previous breast or mantle irradiation is considered a contraindication to breast conservation surgery and repeat breast irradiation, several investigators have reported their clinical experience or performed prospective trials. The general treatment approach has utilized partial breast irradiation or accelerated partial breast irradiation. Technological advances in radiotherapy delivery have aided in the delivery of radiation to a portion of the breast over a shorter period of time compared to standard whole breast radiotherapy. In the case of repeat breast radiotherapy, delivering radiation to a portion of the breast has the advantage of limiting the possible toxicity of re-irradiation. Partial breast irradiation can be delivered using conformal external beam radiation therapy, interstitial brachytherapy, intracavitary brachytherapy, electron therapy, or intraoperative orthovoltage therapy (Harms et al. 2016).

Chadha et al. reported the results of a prospective phase I/II trial of partial breast low-dose-rate interstitial brachytherapy after salvage lumpectomy. The median prior external beam dose to the breast was 60 Gy (Chadha et al. 2008). The first six patients received 30 Gy and after a minimum follow-up of 12 months, there was no unacceptable toxicity. For the next nine patients, the repeat radiation dose was increased to 45 Gy to the lumpectomy cavity plus a 1–2 cm margin. The skin dose was limited to ≤20 Gy. At a median follow-up of 36 months, overall survival is 100%, and local disease-free survival is 89%. One patient developed a local recurrence at 27 months after re-irradiation, underwent salvage mastectomy, and is without evidence of disease. Three patients developed skin pigmentation at catheter entry/exit sites with no grade 3 or 4 fibrosis. No infection was noted. No adverse cosmetic outcomes were noted on serial follow-up examinations with the exception of breast asymmetry present prior to re-irradiation.

The Allegheny group published their results of 26 patients treated with salvage breast-conserving surgery followed by repeat breast irradiation with brachytherapy with a median follow-up of 38 months from re-irradiation (Trombetta et al. 2009). The previous radiotherapy was 45–60.4 Gy, with one patient treated with mantle irradiation and the remainder treated for breast cancer. A total of 22 patients were treated with interstitial low-dose-rate brachytherapy to the tumor bed plus 1 cm margin to 45–50 Gy. Four patients were treated with intracavitary balloon brachytherapy to 34 Gy in ten fractions given twice daily. Local control was 96 %. Cosmetic outcome was graded according to the National Surgical Adjuvant Breast and Bowel Project cosmesis scale. Two patients had grade III cosmesis, and no grade IV cosmesis was seen. In a separate study, this same group treated 18 patients with balloon-based brachytherapy to 34 Gy in 3.4 Gy fractions twice daily. At a median follow-up of 39.6 months, 11 % experienced a local failure treated with salvage mastectomy. One patient developed a chronic infection in the balloon tract which required a mastectomy (Trombetta et al. 2014).

In a prospective trial from Vienna University, 17 patients with small (0.5–2.5 cm) breast recurrences underwent a second breast-conserving surgery and breast re-irradiation (Resch et al. 2002). The prior dose to the breast was 50–60 Gy. In the pilot phase of the trial, eight patients were treated. They received 30 Gy external beam radiotherapy and a 12.5 Gy pulsed-dose-rate brachytherapy to the tumor bed plus 2 cm margin. The next seven patients were treated with decreasing the external beam dose while increasing the dose delivered via brachytherapy. The final nine patients received 40.2–50 Gy pulsed-dose-rate brachytherapy alone. After a median follow-up of 59 months, 24 % (four patients) developed a second local recurrence. A total of 12 patients were alive and free of local tumor, with bone metastasis in two patients. Toxicity was limited to grade 1–2 fibrosis. There were no issues with wound healing. No patients developed unacceptable cosmesis. As a follow-up to this pilot, the authors conducted a prospective protocol of repeat radiotherapy after breast-conserving therapy using multi-catheter accelerated PDR brachytherapy to 50.1 Gy to the tumor bed plus 2 cm (Kauer-Dorner et al. 2012). The EQD2 to the late-responding tissue was calculated to be 63.4 Gy for the PDR brachytherapy. The prior whole breast radiotherapy dose was 50 Gy with a boost given to 28 %. At 57 months mean follow-up, local control was 93 % with late grade $\geq$3 side effects in 16 % in the 24 women with detailed data on late side effects. Seventy-six percent had excellent to fair cosmesis.

Investigators from two institutions in France reported the largest series of breast re-irradiation with interstitial LDR brachytherapy in 69 patients who declined salvage mastectomy (Hannoun-Levi et al. 2004). The mean dose to the breast at diagnosis was 60.5 Gy. After second lumpectomy, repeat irradiation was delivered to the tumor bed plus 2 cm to a dose of 50 and 30 Gy in Marseilles and Nice, respectively. A cumulative dose (first-course dose plus second-course dose) greater than 100 Gy was administered to the breast in 62 patients. The median follow-up was 50.2 months. Freedom from a second local recurrence at 5 years was 77.4 %, and freedom from metastasis after local recurrence at 5 years was 86.7 %. Grade 2 (toxicity requiring medical treatment) and grade 3 (toxicity requiring surgical intervention) late complications were experienced by 11.6 and 10.2 % of the study patients, respectively. When the cumulative radiotherapy dose was greater than 100 Gy, the rate of grade 2 or 3 complications was higher (4 % versus 32.5 %, $p=0.005$). When the re-irradiation dose was greater than 46 Gy, the rate of grade 2 or 3 toxicity was 36 % compared to 13.6 % when the re-irradiation dose was less than 46 Gy ($p=0.007$).

A series of 42 patients who underwent a second lumpectomy followed by interstitial HDR brachytherapy was performed by the investigators in Nice (Hannoun-Levi et al. 2011). A dose of 34 Gy in 10 fractions over 5 consecutive days was prescribed to the tumor bed plus 1 cm. Median follow-up was 21 months. Local control was 97 % and late toxicities were grade 1, 28 %; grade 2, 19 %; and grade 3, 3 %. Most toxicities were cutaneous and subcutaneous fibrosis. However, pain, telangiectasias, and rib fractures were observed in 28, 21, and 2 %.

A multi-institutional retrospective review of 217 patients who received a second lumpectomy and repeat radiotherapy using interstitial partial breast brachytherapy was performed from eight European radiation oncology departments (Hannoun-Levi et al. 2013). Five- and 10-year local failure rates were 5.6 and 7.2 %, respectively. Five- and 10-year metastasis rates were

Table 2 Results of salvage breast-conserving surgery and partial breast re-irradiation

First author	Year	*N*	Technique	Prior RT dose (Gy)	Re-RT dose (Gy)	Local control (%)
Chadha	2008	15	LDR PBI	60	30–45	89
Hannoun-Levi	2004	69	LDR PBI	60.5	30–50	77
Maulard	1995	38	LDR PBI	65	30–70	79
Resch	2002	17	Mixed	50–60	40–50	76
Trombetta	2009	26	LDR/HDR PBI	45–60.4	45–50 LDR; 34 HDR	96
Trombetta	2014	18	HDR PBI	NR	34	89
Guix	2010	36	HDR	NR	30	89
Hannoun-Levi	2011	42	HDR	45–66	34	97
Kauer-Dorner	2012	39	PDR	50–61.8	50.1	93

Abbreviations: *RT* radiation therapy, *Re-RT* re-irradiation, *LDR* low-dose-rate brachytherapy, *HDR* high-dose-rate brachytherapy, *EBRT* external beam radiation therapy, *PDR* pulsed-dose-rate brachytherapy, *N* number of patients, *NR* not reported

9.6 and 19.1 %, respectively. Grades 3–4 late toxicity rate was 11 %.

Limited data is available on intraoperative radiotherapy for repeat breast radiotherapy. The first publication included 15 patients treated with a single dose of 14.7–20 Gy 50 kV X-rays to the applicator surface with Intrabeam (Kraus-Tiefenbacher et al. 2007). Local control was 100 % at a median follow-up of 26 months and no late grade 3 or 4 toxicities were seen.

Most reports of repeat partial breast irradiation have utilized interstitial brachytherapy as opposed to external beam radiation therapy (Table 2). Deutsch published a review of 39 patients with recurrent breast cancer ($n=38$) or ductal carcinoma in situ ($n=8$) who underwent repeat breast-conserving surgery and external beam re-irradiation (Deutsch 2002). All patients received prior whole breast radiation to 45–50 Gy followed by a boost to the tumor bed (unreported dose) in 21 patients. Margins were positive in 13 % after salvage lumpectomy. Repeat irradiation was performed using electrons to the tumor bed to 50 Gy in 25 fractions. Local control was 79 %, with the second local recurrence developing in the same quadrant in three of the eight local failures. Nine patients had a fair to poor cosmetic result.

The NRG Oncology/Radiation Therapy Oncology Group has completed a prospective phase II trial evaluating salvage lumpectomy and re-irradiation using three-dimensional conformal radiation therapy. Eligible patients must meet the following criteria: recurrent tumors ≤3 cm, no evidence of multicentric disease on MRI and breast imaging, no distant metastasis, no skin involvement, ≤3 positive axillary nodes. Previous lumpectomy and adjuvant breast radiotherapy must be completed at least 1 year prior to enrollment. The treatment technique generally uses three, four, or five non-coplanar beam arrangements to meet dose constraints (Table 3) (Baglan et al. 2003; Formenti et al. 2004; Kozak et al.

Table 3 Normal tissue constraints for repeat partial breast irradiation according to RTOG 1014

Normal tissue	Constraint
Uninvolved normal breast	<60 % of whole breast receives ≥50 % of prescription dose and <35 % of whole breast receives prescribed dose
Contralateral breast	<3 % receives prescription dose
Ipsilateral lung	<15 % receives 30 % of prescription dose
Contralateral lung	<15 % receives 5 % of prescription dose
Heart (right-sided recurrence)	<5 % receives 5 % of prescription dose
Heart (left-sided recurrence)	Volume of receiving 5 % of prescription dose <40 %
Thyroid	Maximum point dose of 3 % of prescription dose

Abbreviations: *RTOG* radiation therapy oncology group

2006a&b). The target volumes are defined as follows:

- Clinical target volume (CTV) is defined as the tumor bed with uniform expansion of 15 mm. The CTV is limited to 5 mm from skin surface and excludes the posterior chest wall structures.
- Planning target volume (PTV) is defined as the CTV with a uniform 10 mm expansion. The PTV is used to define the appropriate block margin.
- PTV_EVAL is defined as the PTV excluding portion of PTV that extend outside the breast and first 5 mm of tissue beneath the skin and posterior extent of the breast. PTV_EVAL is used for dose volume histogram analysis.

A hyperfractionated regimen of 45 Gy in 1.5 Gy twice-daily fractions is prescribed to the PTV. Study endpoints include toxicity outcomes, cosmesis, local control and freedom from mastectomy rate, disease-free survival, and overall survival. For the first 55 patients at 1-year follow-up, skin, fibrosis, and/or breast pain adverse events were grade 1 in 63 %, grade 2 in 7 %, and grade ≥3 in <2 % (Arthur et al. 2015). Recurrence endpoints have not been published and longer follow-up is needed.

1.4 Chest Wall Re-irradiation Alone

An early publication on chest wall re-irradiation from the University of Washington suggested that repeat radiotherapy was feasible (Laramore et al. 1978). A total of 13 patients were re-irradiated after postmastectomy radiotherapy was given at diagnosis, after a mean disease-free interval of 5.9 years. The initial radiation therapy dose to the chest wall was 40–50 Gy, with the details of prior radiation unknown in four patients. The dose of the chest wall re-irradiation was 36–60 Gy in 2 Gy fractions. Cumulative radiotherapy doses were 80–100 Gy. At a mean follow-up of 20 months, the local disease-free survival was 62 %. Acute toxicity appeared tolerable with one patient requiring a treatment break due to moist desquamation. Late toxicity was not reported.

A total of 13 patients from Memorial Sloan-Kettering Cancer Center received chest wall repeat radiation therapy (Wagman et al. 2002). At initial diagnosis, 12 patients underwent lumpectomy and adjuvant breast radiotherapy to 45–50.4 Gy followed by a tumor bed boost of 6–20 Gy. One patient received preoperative radiotherapy 22 Gy in four fractions followed by mastectomy. The median disease-free interval was 46 months to first recurrence, when three patients had repeat radiotherapy. Ten patients had re-irradiation at second local recurrence. Treatment was given with conformal electron fields to a dose of 7.5–64.4 Gy (median 50.4 Gy). The median follow-up from re-irradiation was 20 months. The 2-year local recurrence-free survival was 85 % and 2-year overall survival was 85 %. Grade 3 skin toxicity was noted in 46 %,

Table 4 Results of chest wall re-irradiation

First author	Year	*N*	F/U (mo)	RT 1 (Gy)	RT 2 (Gy)	Cumulative dose (Gy)	HT	CR (%)	LC (%)
Laramore	1978	13	20	40–50	36–60	80–100	No	62	62
Wagman	2002	13	20	60.8	50.4	111.2	No	–	85
Jones	2005	39	–	–	30–66	–	Yes	68	–
van der Zee	1999	13	21	45	32	77	Yes	71	74
Oldenborg	2010	78	64	65	32	97	Yes	–	78
Dragovic	1989	30	–	50	32	82	Yes	57	43
Phromratanapongse	1991	44	–	59.7	29.4[a]	89.1	Yes	41	67
Wahl	2008	81	12	60	48	108	54 %	57	66
Li	2004	41	–	58	43	101	Yes	56	–
Kouloulias	2002	15	–	60	30.6	90.6	Yes	20	–

Abbreviations: *N* number of patients, *RT 1* dose of first course of radiotherapy, *RT 2* dose of second course of radiotherapy, *HT* hyperthermia, *LC* local control, *mo* months, *F/U* follow-up

[a]A variety of fractionation regimens used

with 38 % requiring a treatment break. Late toxicities include a rib fracture and pericarditis.

1.5 Chest Wall Re-irradiation with Hyperthermia or Chemotherapy

Response rates and local disease-free survival rates vary widely after repeat radiotherapy, with complete response rate of 20–70 % (Table 4). Adding concurrent chemotherapy and/or hyperthermia may improve response rates (Datta et al. 2016). A randomized trial of radiation therapy with or without concurrent hyperthermia in superficial tumors demonstrated an improved complete response rate in the hyperthermia arm (Jones et al. 2005). Approximately, 60 % of patients enrolled in that trial had a breast cancer diagnosis. A superior complete response rate from radiotherapy and hyperthermia was seen in previously irradiated patients compared to previously unirradiated patients (68 % versus 24 %, respectively). A meta-analysis of five randomized trials of radiation therapy and hyperthermia revealed that previously irradiated patients who had concurrent hyperthermia and re-irradiation had a statistically significant improvement in complete response rate compared to re-irradiation alone, 57 % versus 31 %, respectively (OR 4.7, 95 % CI 2.4–5.9) (Vernon et al. 1996). A multi-institutional retrospective review of chest wall re-irradiation demonstrated a trend toward improved response rate with the addition of hyperthermia; however, it was not significant (67 % versus 39 %, $p=0.08$) (Wahl et al. 2008). Despite the poor prognosis of chest wall recurrences, a complete response to therapy enhances the quality of life and hyperthermia appears to improve response rates.

Investigators from the Netherlands re-irradiated patients with positive margins after resection or inoperable recurrent tumor (van der Zee et al. 1999). The repeat radiotherapy schedule consisted of 32 Gy in eight fractions, two fractions per week with hyperthermia. In patients with macroscopic tumors, a 71 % complete response rate was seen. In the subset with a complete response, in-field tumor regrowth was noted in 36 %. The median duration of local control was 31 months. A total of 14 patients developed chest wall ulcerations; however, nine patients had ulceration prior to repeat radiation therapy. Persistent ulceration without tumor was present in five patients. Bone necrosis, fracture, or brachial plexopathy were not observed. A similar re-irradiation fractionation regimen of 32 Gy in eight fractions with hyperthermia was used in a prospective phase II trial of 30 patients (Dragovic et al. 1989). The median dose of the first radiation course was 50 Gy. About 57 % of patients achieved a complete response. Complete response rate in tumors <5 cm was 81 % and ≥5 cm was 29 % ($p<0.001$). The local control was 43 %, and 2-year overall survival rate was 30 %. Other studies have shown improved response rates with smaller tumor sizes. A review from the University of Wisconsin of 44 patients undergoing chest wall re-irradiation with concurrent hyperthermia demonstrated a complete response rate of 65 % with a tumor size of ≤6 cm and 26 % with a tumor size >6 cm ($p=0.013$) (Phromratanapongse et al. 1991). The overall complete response rate was 41 %.

There is little data to support the routine use of concurrent radiosensitizing chemotherapy with re-irradiation, although it could potentially improve response rates. Liposomal doxorubicin was given with 30.6 Gy of chest wall repeat radiotherapy and hyperthermia (Kouloulias et al. 2002). All patients had prior chest wall irradiation to 60 Gy. Although the 20 % complete response rate is lower than other experiences, the trial had a small number of patients. The addition of radiosensitizing chemotherapy did not improve complete response rates in a retrospective review of chest wall re-irradiation (Wahl et al. 2008). However, of the patients who did receive chemotherapy, 86 % had gross disease at the time of re-irradiation compared to 53 % who did not receive chemotherapy ($p=0.01$). More studies are required to determine the effects of concurrent chemotherapy.

1.6 Chest Wall Re-irradiation Techniques

A variety of techniques may be used for repeat radiotherapy. Most published studies use electrons

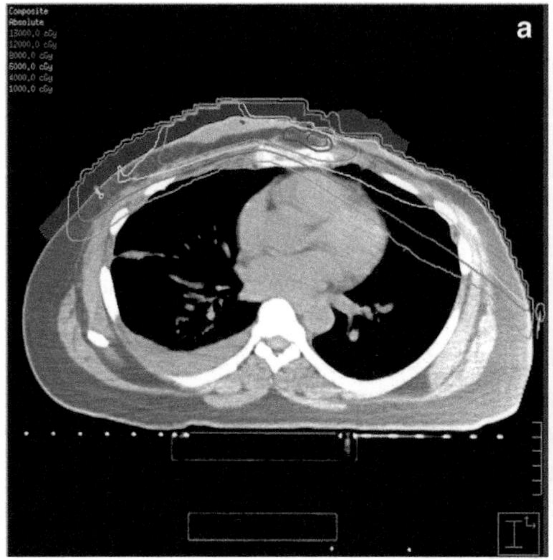

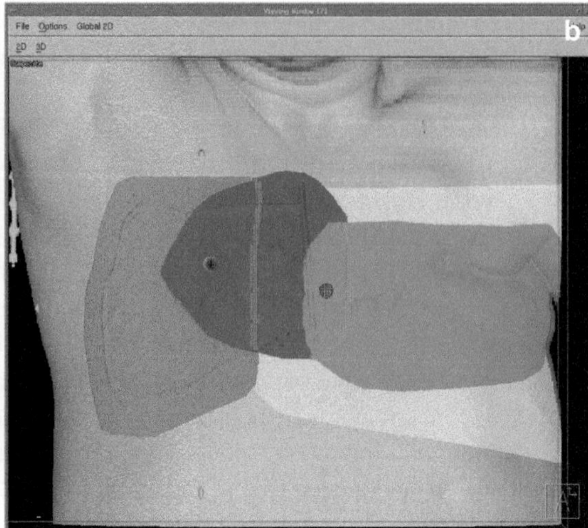

Fig. 1 A patient underwent bilateral mastectomies for locally advanced left breast cancer. She received previous left chest wall radiotherapy via tangents to 50.4 Gy plus a 9 Gy scar boost. The patient failed medially to the initial tangent fields and developed diffuse bilateral chest wall recurrences. (**a**) Axial CT slice with isodose lines reconstructing the previous radiotherapy dose with the re-irradiation dose. (**b**) Skin surface rendering of the left-sided tangent fields with two right chest wall re-irradiation fields

to treat chest wall recurrences (Laramore et al. 1978; van der Zee et al. 1999; Dragovic et al. 1989; Phromratanapongse et al. 1991, Fig. 1). In order to adequately treat the skin surface, bolus may be needed. Tangents with megavoltage photons may also be used to treat large recurrences or to treat the entire chest wall (Kouloulias et al. 2002). In the multi-institutional review of repeat irradiation, 80% of patients were treated with photons only, 14% with electrons only, and 6% with combined electrons and photons (Wahl et al. 2008). Limiting the radiotherapy field to the area of gross and potentially microscopic disease may limit potential morbidity in patients with an extremely poor prognosis; however, the recurrence rate may be higher than treatment fields that include the uninvolved chest wall. If the regional lymph nodes have not been irradiated, they should be included during the chest wall re-irradiation course (Halverson et al. 1990). There is little data regarding repeat radiotherapy of the regional lymphatics, and given the potential toxicity, this should rarely be considered. Published cumulative (first-course dose plus second-course dose) chest wall doses range from 90 to 110 Gy. In patients whose cumulative dose is greater than 120 Gy, there appeared to be acceptable late toxicities, although late toxicity data were available in only 12 patients (Wahl et al. 2008).

1.7 Chest Wall Re-irradiation Toxicity

Long-term follow-up of chest wall re-irradiation patients is limited, and toxicity data are not reported uniformly (Table 5). Li et al. (2004) re-irradiated 41 patients with concurrent hyperthermia using conventional radiotherapy to 40–50 Gy. Skin ulceration occurred in 14%, and two of these patients had cumulative doses >100 Gy. One patient died from persistent ulceration. In 81 patients re-irradiated to a median cumulative dose of 106 Gy (range 74.4–137.5 Gy), toxicities were retrospectively graded according to the National Cancer Institute's Common Terminology Criteria for Adverse Events, version 3.0 (Wahl et al. 2008). Late grade 3 toxicity was seen in 4%, and late grade 4 toxicity in 1% (dermatitis), and there were no treatment-related deaths. No late severe soft-tissue necrosis, osteonecrosis, fractures, brachial plexopathy, pneumonitis, or pericarditis were seen. Of the 25 patients followed for >20 months, no late grade 3 or 4

Table 5 Chest wall re-irradiation toxicity

First author	*N*	F/U (mo)	Median re-RT dose	Cumulative dose (Gy)	Interval between RT courses (mo)	Toxicity
Wahl et al. (2008)	81	12	48 Gy in 24 fractions	108	38	5 % late grade 3 or 4 toxicity
Oldenborg et al. (2010)	78	64	32 Gy in 8 fractions	97	58	43 % late grade 3 or 4 toxicity
van der Zee et al. (1999)	134	21	32 Gy in 8 fractions	77	41	Five patients with ulceration without tumor
Li et al. (2004)	41	–	40–50 Gy in 20–25 fractions	101	–	Six patients with skin ulceration, two with persistent ulceration, one death from ulceration
Dragovic et al. (1989)	30	–	32 Gy in 8 fractions	82		11 patients with skin ulceration, two patients with persistent ulceration

Abbreviations: *Re-RT* re-irradiation, *F/U* follow-up, *mo* months

toxicities were seen. About 35 % of patients experienced acute, non-skin-related toxicity, with 9 % requiring a treatment break. Concurrent hyperthermia was associated with a higher acute non-skin toxicity. Cumulative radiation dose, repeat radiotherapy dose, interval between radiotherapy courses, treatment modality, and concurrent chemotherapy were not associated with an increase in late toxicity.

In patients treated with cumulative doses of 82 Gy and a re-irradiation dose of 32 Gy in 4 Gy fractions with hyperthermia, 11 % of patients with a complete response developed nonhealing ulceration (Dragovic et al. 1989). In patients treated with the same regimen, 4 % developed chest wall ulceration without persistent tumor (van der Zee et al. 1999). The incidence of late grade 3 or greater toxicity was 40 % in a trial of chest wall re-irradiation using 32 Gy in 4 Gy fractions with concurrent hyperthermia (Oldenborg et al. 2010). Skin ulceration was the most common toxicity encountered, but osteonecrosis, rib fractures, cardiomyopathy, and brachial plexopathy were seen. No treatment deaths were observed. This trial is unique in that it has the longest published follow-up of 64 months from re-irradiation. The rate of toxicity is higher than other studies, which may be due to the longer follow-up with higher survival rates or the larger fraction size used. Patients with scar dehiscence or postoperative skin infection appeared to be more susceptible to skin toxicity.

Given the potential toxicity associated with repeat chest wall irradiation, identifying the appropriate patients for re-irradiation is important. Conclusions regarding toxicity are difficult to make given the limited follow-up, heterogeneous patient population, heterogeneous treatment regimens, and retrospective nature of most publications. Patients with widely metastatic disease and limited survival who have symptomatic local recurrences may receive palliative re-irradiation to improve malodorous tumors, bleeding, and pain. In patients with limited local recurrences in previously radiotherapy fields, re-irradiation should be used judiciously. Most reports of chest wall re-irradiation have a median time between radiotherapy courses of 38–58 months and median cumulative doses of 80–110 Gy (Wahl et al. 2008; Oldenborg et al. 2010). A short interval between radiation therapy courses may have a negative impact on late toxicity.

Conclusion

Repeat breast radiotherapy has generally been performed after salvage lumpectomy with treatment fields limited to the tumor bed plus a margin. Most publications utilized brachytherapy to deliver partial breast re-irradiation; however, there is an RTOG study using conformal external beam radiotherapy. Breast re-irradiation is not considered standard and should generally be used under the auspices of a clinical trial. Chest wall re-irradiation has been used to treat both residual microscopic disease and gross disease with or without metastatic disease. Hyperthermia should be used to improve the response rate for gross disease. There is little data on using concurrent chemotherapy and administering systemic therapy after re-irradiation. Biologic agents, such as antiangiogenic drugs, should be used carefully given the lack of toxicity data. Chest wall repeat radiotherapy should be used judiciously as the data on late toxicity is limited. In patients where chest wall re-irradiation may be indicated relatively soon after the initial radiotherapy course, caution is warranted as median time intervals between radiation courses is at least 38 months in the literature. In general, toxicity data suffer from short follow-up, heterogeneous treatment regimens, nonstandard reporting, and varied patient selection.

References

Abner AL, Recht A et al (1993) Prognosis following salvage mastectomy for recurrence in the breast after conservative surgery and radiation therapy for early-stage breast cancer. J Clin Oncol 11:44–48

Alpert TE, Kuerer HM et al (2005) Ipsilateral breast tumor cancer recurrence after breast conservation therapy: outcomes of salvage mastectomy vs. salvage breast-conserving surgery and prognostic factors for salvage breast preservation. Int J Radiat Oncol Biol Phys 63:845–851

Arthur DW, Winter K et al (2015) NRG Oncology/RTOG 1014: 1-year toxicity report from a phase II study of repeat breast preserving surgery and 3D conformal partial-breast reirradiation (PBrI) for in-breast recurrence. Int J Radiat Oncol Biol Phys 93:S58–S59

Baglan KL, Sharpe MB et al (2003) Accelerated partial breast irradiation using 3D conformal radiation therapy (3D-CRT). Int J Radiat Oncol Biol Phys 55:302–311

Bartelink H, Horiot JC et al (2001) Recurrence rates after treatment of breast cancer with standard radiotherapy with or without additional radiation. N Engl J Med 345:1378–1387

Beck TM, Hart NE et al (1983) Local or regionally recurrent carcinoma of the breast: results of therapy in 121 patients. J Clin Oncol 1:400–405

Bedwinek JM, Lee J et al (1981) Prognostic indicators in patients with isolated local-regional recurrence of breast cancer. Cancer 47:2232–2235

Bollet M, Servant N et al (2008) High-resolution mapping of DNA breakpoints to define true recurrences among ipsilateral breast cancers. J Natl Cancer Inst 100:48–58

Buzdar AU, Blumenschein GR et al (1979) Adjuvant chemoimmunotherapy following regional therapy for isolated recurrences of breast cancer (stage IV NED). J Surg Oncol 12:27–40

Cajucom CC, Tsangaris TN et al (1993) Results of salvage mastectomy for local recurrence after breast-conserving surgery without radiation therapy. Cancer 71:1774–1779

Chadha M, Feldman S et al (2008) The feasibility of a second lumpectomy and breast brachytherapy for localized cancer in a breast previously treated with lumpectomy and radiation therapy for breast cancer. Brachytherapy 7:22–28

Chu FC, Lin FJ et al (1976) Locally recurrent carcinoma of the breast. Results of radiation therapy. Cancer 37:2677–2681

Dahlstrom KK, Andersson AP et al (1993) Wide local excision of recurrent breast cancer in the thoracic wall. Cancer 72:774–777

Dalberg K, Mattsson A et al (1998) Outcome of treatment for ipsilateral breast tumor recurrence in early-stage breast cancer. Breast Cancer Res Treat 49:69–78

Datta NR, Puric E et al (2016) Hyperthermia and radiation therapy in locoregional recurrent breast cancers: a systematic review and meta-analysis. Int J Radiat Oncol Biol Phys 94:1073–1087

Deutsch M (2002) Repeat high-dose external beam irradiation for in-breast tumor recurrence after previous lumpectomy and whole breast irradiation. Int J Radiat Oncol Biol Phys 53:687–691

Deutsch M, Parsons JA et al (1986) Radiation therapy for local-regional recurrent breast carcinoma. Int J Radiat Oncol Biol Phys 12:2061–2065

Dragovic J, Seydel HG et al (1989) Local superficial hyperthermia in combination with low-dose radiation therapy for palliation of locally recurrent breast carcinoma. J Clin Oncol 7:30–35

Fisher B, Anderson S et al (2002) Twenty-year follow-up of a randomized trial comparing total mastectomy, lumpectomy, and lumpectomy plus irradiation for the treatment of invasive breast cancer. N Engl J Med 347:1233–1241

Formenti SC, Truong MT et al (2004) Prone accelerated partial breast irradiation after breast-conserving surgery: preliminary clinical results and dose-volume histogram analysis. Int J Radiat Oncol Biol Phys 60:493–504

Fourquet A, Campana F et al (1989) Prognostic factors of breast recurrence in the conservative management of early breast cancer: a 25-year follow-up. Int J Radiat Oncol Biol Phys 17:719–725

Ganz PA, Schag AC et al (1992) Breast conservation versus mastectomy. Is there a difference in psychological adjustment or quality of life in the year after surgery? Cancer 69:1729–1738

Gentilini O, Botteri E et al (2007) When can a second conservative approach be considered for ipsilateral breast tumour recurrence? Ann Oncol 18:468–472

Guix B, Lejárcegui JA et al (2010) Exeresis and brachytherapy as salvage treatment for local recurrence after conservative treatment for breast cancer: results of a ten-year pilot study. Int J Radiat Oncol Biol Phys 78:804–810

Halverson KJ, Perez CA et al (1990) Isolated local-regional recurrence of breast cancer following mastectomy: radiotherapeutic management. Int J Radiat Oncol Biol Phys 19:851–858

Halverson KJ, Perez CA et al (1992) Survival following locoregional recurrence of breast cancer: univariate and multivariate analysis. Int J Radiat Oncol Biol Phys 23:285–291

Hannoun-Levi JM, Houvenaeghel G et al (2004) Partial breast irradiation as second conservative treatment for local breast cancer recurrence. Int J Radiat Oncol Biol Phys 60:1385–1392

Hannoun-Levi JM, Castelli J et al (2011) Second conservative treatment for ipsilateral breast cancer recurrence using high-dose rate interstitial brachytherapy: preliminary clinical results and evaluation of patient satisfaction. Brachytherapy 10:171–177

Hannoun-Levi JM, Resch A et al (2013) Accelerated partial breast irradiation with interstitial brachytherapy as second conservative treatment for ipsilateral breast tumour recurrence: multicentric study of the GEC-ESTRO Breast Cancer Working Group. Radiother Oncol 108:226–231

Harms W, Budach W et al (2016) DEGRO practical guidelines for radiotherapy of breast cancer VI: therapy of locoregional breast cancer recurrences. Strahlenther Onkol 192:199–208

Huang E, Buchholz TA et al (2002) Classifying local disease recurrences after breast conservation therapy based on location and histology: new primary tumors have more favorable outcomes than true local disease recurrences. Cancer 95:2059–2067

Huston TL, Simmons RM (2005) Locally recurrent breast cancer after conservation therapy. Am J Surg 189: 229–235

Ishitobi M, Komoike S (2011) Repeat lumpectomy for ipsilateral breast tumor recurrence after breast-conserving treatment. Oncology 81:381–386

Ishitobi M, Okumura Y et al (2014) Repeat lumpectomy for ipsilateral breast tumor recurrence (IBTR) after breast-conserving surgery: the impact of radiotherapy on second IBTR. Breast Cancer Tokyo Jpn 21: 754–760

Jones EL, Oleson JR et al (2005) Randomized trial of hyperthermia and radiation for superficial tumors. J Clin Oncol 23:3079–3085

Kauer-Dorner D, Pötter R et al (2012) Partial breast irradiation for locally recurrent breast cancer within a second breast conserving treatment: Alternative to mastectomy? Results from a prospective trial. Radiother Oncol 102:96–101

Kennedy MJ, Abeloff MD (1993) Management of locally recurrent breast cancer. Cancer 71:2395–2409

Komoike Y, Motomura K et al (2003) Repeat lumpectomy for patients with ipsilateral breast tumor recurrence after breast-conserving surgery. Preliminary results. Oncology 64:1–6

Kouloulias VE, Dardoufas CE et al (2002) Liposomal doxorubicin in conjunction with reirradiation and local hyperthermia treatment in recurrent breast cancer: a phase I/II trial. Clin Cancer Res 8:374–382

Kozak KR, Doppke KP et al (2006a) Dosimetric comparison of two different three-dimensional conformal external beam accelerated partial breast irradiation techniques. Int J Radiat Oncol Biol Phys 65:340–346

Kozak KR, Katz A et al (2006b) Dosimetric comparison of proton and photon three-dimensional, conformal, external beam accelerated partial breast irradiation techniques. Int J Radiat Oncol Biol Phys 65:1572–1578

Kraus-Tiefenbacher U, Bauer L et al (2007) Intraoperative radiotherapy (IORT) is an option for patients with localized breast recurrences after previous external-beam radiotherapy. BMC Cancer 7:178

Kurtz JM, Amalric R et al (1988) Results of salvage surgery for mammary recurrence following breast-conserving therapy. Ann Surg 207:347–351

Kurtz JM, Spitalier JM et al (1990) The prognostic significance of late local recurrence after breast-conserving therapy. Int J Radiat Oncol Biol Phys 18:87–93

Kurtz JM, Jacquemier J et al (1991) Is breast conservation after local recurrence feasible? Eur J Cancer 27:240–244

Laramore GE, Griffin TW et al (1978) The use of electron beams in treating local recurrence of breast cancer in previously irradiated fields. Cancer 41:991–995

Li G, Mitsumori M et al (2004) Local hyperthermia combined with external irradiation for regional recurrent breast carcinoma. Int J Clin Oncol 9:179–183

Maulard C, Housset M et al (1995) Use of perioperative or split-course interstitial brachytherapy techniques for salvage irradiation of isolated local recurrences after conservative management of breast cancer. Am J Clin Oncol 18:348–352

Maunsell E, Brisson J et al (1989) Psychological distress after initial treatment for breast cancer: a comparison of partial and total mastectomy. J Clin Epidemiol 42:765–771

Nielsen HM, Overgaard M et al (2006) Study of failure pattern among high-risk breast cancer patients with or without postmastectomy radiotherapy in addition to adjuvant systemic therapy: long-term results from the Danish Breast Cancer Cooperative Group DBCG 82 b and c randomized studies. J Clin Oncol 24:2268–2275

Oldenborg S, Van Os RM et al (2010) Elective re-irradiation and hyperthermia following resection of persistent locoregional recurrent breast cancer: a retrospective study. Int J Hyperthermia 26:136–144

Osborne MP, Simmons RM (1994) Salvage surgery for recurrence after breast conservation. World J Surg 18:93–97

Overgaard M, Hansen PS et al (1997) Postoperative radiotherapy in high-risk premenopausal women with breast cancer who receive adjuvant chemotherapy. Danish Breast Cancer Cooperative Group 82b trial. N Engl J Med 337:949–955

Overgaard M, Jensen MB et al (1999) Postoperative radiotherapy in high-risk postmenopausal breast-cancer patients given adjuvant tamoxifen: Danish Breast Cancer Cooperative Group DBCG 82c randomised trial. Lancet 353:1641–1648

Phromratanapongse P, Steeves RA et al (1991) Hyperthermia and irradiation for locally recurrent previously irradiated breast cancer. Strahlenther Onkol 167:93–97

Ragaz J, Olivotto IA et al (2005) Locoregional radiation therapy in patients with high-risk breast cancer receiving adjuvant chemotherapy: 20-year results of the British Columbia randomized trial. J Natl Cancer Inst 97:116–126

Resch A, Fellner C et al (2002) Locally recurrent breast cancer: pulse dose rate brachytherapy for repeat irradiation following lumpectomy—a second chance to preserve the breast. Radiology 225:713–718

Rowland JH, Desmond KA et al (2000) Role of breast reconstructive surgery in physical and emotional outcomes among breast cancer survivors. J Natl Cancer Inst 92:1422–1429

Salvadori B, Marubini E et al (1999) Reoperation for locally recurrent breast cancer in patients previously treated with conservative surgery. Br J Surg 86:84–87

Schwaibold F, Fowble BL et al (1991) The results of radiation therapy for isolated local regional recurrence after mastectomy. Int J Radiat Oncol Biol Phys 21:299–310

Smith TE, Lee D et al (2000) True recurrence vs. new primary ipsilateral breast tumor relapse: an analysis of clinical and pathologic differences and their implications in natural history, prognoses, and therapeutic management. Int J Radiat Oncol Biol Phys 48:1281–1289

Touboul E, Buffat L et al (1999) Local recurrences and distant metastases after breast-conserving surgery and radiation therapy for early breast cancer. Int J Radiat Oncol Biol Phys 43:25–38

Trombetta M, Julian TB et al (2009) Long-term cosmesis after lumpectomy and brachytherapy in the management of carcinoma of the previously irradiated breast. Am J Clin Oncol 32:314–318

Trombetta M, Hall M et al (2014) Long-term follow-up of breast preservation by re-excision and balloon brachytherapy after ipsilateral breast tumor recurrence. Brachytherapy 13:488–492

van der Zee J, van der Holt B et al (1999) Reirradiation combined with hyperthermia in recurrent breast cancer results in a worthwhile local palliation. Br J Cancer 79:483–490

Vernon CC, Hand JW et al (1996) Radiotherapy with or without hyperthermia in the treatment of superficial localized breast cancer: results from five randomized controlled trials. International Collaborative Hyperthermia Group. Int J Radiat Oncol Biol Phys 35: 731–744

Veronesi U, Cascinelli N et al (2002) Twenty-year follow-up of a randomized study comparing breast-conserving surgery with radical mastectomy for early breast cancer. N Engl J Med 347:1227–1232

Vicini FA, Recht A et al (1992) Recurrence in the breast following conservative surgery and radiation therapy for early-stage breast cancer. J Natl Cancer Inst Monogr 11:33–39

Voogd AC, van Tienhoven G et al (1999) Local recurrence after breast conservation therapy for early stage breast carcinoma: detection, treatment, and outcome in 266 patients. Dutch study group on local recurrence after breast conservation (BORST). Cancer 85:437–446

Wagman R, Katz M et al (2002) Re-irradiation of the chest wall for recurrent breast cancer. Int J Radiat Oncol Biol Phys 54:237–238

Wahl AO, Rademaker A et al (2008) Multi-institutional review of repeat irradiation of chest wall and breast for recurrent breast cancer. Int J Radiat Oncol Biol Phys 70:477–484

Prostate Cancer

Max Peters, Metha Maenhout, Steven Frank, and Marco van Vulpen

Contents

The original version of this chapter was revised. An erratum to this chapter can be found at 10.1007/978-3-319-41825-4_78.

M. Peters (✉) • M. Maenhout • S. Frank
M. van Vulpen
Department of Radiotherapy, University Medical Center Utrecht, Heidelberglaan 100, Utrecht 3584CX, The Netherlands
e-mail: M.Peters-10@umcutrecht.nl; M.Maenhout@umcutrecht.nl; sjfrank@mdanderson.org; M.vanvulpen@umcutrecht.nl

Abstract

Salvage radiotherapy for locally recurrent prostate cancer after primary radiation is generally performed using brachytherapy. Only a limited amount of small studies has been performed so far. In these studies the rate of severe toxicity, requiring operative reintervention, was high and cancer control outcome was disappointing. Furthermore, it is unclear whether salvage treatment will improve disease-specific or overall survival. For these reasons, salvage brachytherapy is not popular and usually only performed in large tertiary centers. Salvage can currently be considered in patients with a pathology-proven local recurrence with an interval of at least 2–3 years after primary treatment, together with a limited and nonaggressive tumor presentation at time of salvage. Currently, experienced groups recommend at least equal doses used in primary treatment, together with targeting the entire prostate. Diagnostic developments in magnetic resonance imaging (MRI) and positron emission tomography (PET) and biopsy techniques such as transperineal and MRI-targeted biopsies provide the possibility to localize the macroscopic recurrent tumor in the prostate. This enables a shift to focal salvage techniques which can be expected to reduce severe toxicity rates while maintaining cancer control.

DOI 10.1007/174_2016_56, © Springer International Publishing Switzerland
Published Online: 01 May 2016

1 Introduction

Re-irradiation in prostate cancer after primary curative radiotherapy or prostatectomy is generally called a salvage treatment and will further be referred to as salvage in this entire chapter. In addition, salvage here refers to the post-radiotherapy setting only. Salvage radiotherapy post prostatectomy falls outside the scope of this chapter.

The treatment of patients suffering from radio-recurrent prostate cancer is a significant clinical problem worldwide (Ward et al. 2008). It has been calculated that in the United States approximately 31,680 men per year will be at risk for failure after primary radiotherapy (Ward et al. 2008). Owing to the rising incidence of prostate cancer and the increasing use of radiotherapy, this number is likely to increase in the future (Dutch cancer society 2010). Other sources suggest that up to 60 % of patients undergoing radiotherapy as a primary treatment option may experience a recurrence within 10 years after treatment (Brachman et al. 2000; Agarwal et al. 2008; Zelefsky et al. 2007; Heidenreich et al. 2008). Even in the era of dose escalation (≥78 Gy) for primary prostate cancer, biochemical recurrences occur in approximately 10 % of low-risk, 23 % of intermediate-risk, and 44 % of high-risk patients after 8 years (Zumsteg et al. 2015). Even though, following primary treatment, it is difficult to differentiate between locally recurrent disease and distant metastases when the prostate-specific antigen (PSA) level increases, many of these patients will harbor organ-confined disease (Pound et al. 2001). Some expect even over two-thirds of patients to have locally recurrent disease (Menard et al. 2015; Cellini et al. 2002; Pucar et al. 2008; Arrayeh et al. 2012). Others state most men with a rising PSA after treatment will harbor micrometastatic disease and only a minority would have a true local recurrence only and could potentially benefit from a salvage treatment (Ward et al. 2005; Nguyen et al. 2007a, b; Huang et al. 2007; Leibovici et al. 2012).

For patients diagnosed with recurrent prostate cancer after primary radiotherapy, different salvage treatment methods with a curative intend exist: salvage radical prostatectomy, salvage brachytherapy, salvage external beam radiotherapy, salvage high-intensity focused ultrasound (HIFU), and salvage cryosurgery (Nguyen et al. 2007a, b; Moman et al. 2009; Alongi et al. 2013; Peters et al. 2013). These procedures are associated with high failure and high severe toxicity rates and are therefore unpopular (Moman et al. 2009; Peters et al. 2013). This probably explains the absence of large prospective trials in the literature. Most data are derived from retrospective evaluation of a limited number of patients, which are often heterogeneous before salvage treatment regarding prognostic characteristics. The only palliative treatment alternative is hormonal therapy or androgen deprivation therapy (ADT), which is associated with often significant cardiovascular, metabolic, and even mental side effects (Heidenreich et al. 2014; Nguyen et al. 2015). In the case of a biochemical recurrence after radiotherapy for prostate cancer, hormonal therapy is the worldwide most applied treatment, with approximately 98 % of patients being treated in this manner (Moman et al. 2009; Tran et al. 2014).

The high failure rates after prostate cancer salvage are probably related to inaccurate patient selection, as many of these patients will have early distant metastases (Haider et al. 2008; Nguyen et al. 2007a, b). The high severe toxicity rate might be related to the fact that current salvage treatments are directed at the entire prostatic volume. This is required because of a lack of accurate localization possibilities and blind systematic biopsies to detect a local recurrence. Currently, new MRI and PET-imaging modalities are adopted, which provide more accurate localization information (Barentsz et al. 2012; Umbehr et al. 2013; Fütterer et al 2015; Hamoen et al. 2015; Evangelista et al. 2013; de Rooij et al. 2015). In addition, template prostate mapping biopsies and MRI-targeted biopsies provide additional information regarding location and the presence of clinically significant disease (Siddiqui et al. 2015; Valerio et al. 2015; Moore et al. 2013). These modalities will be used in the near future for focal salvage treatment planning of prostate cancer recurrences (Moman et al.

2010; Peters et al. 2014), which can be expected to have limited severe toxicity rates.

This chapter will first discuss the possibilities and difficulties with regard to detecting a local recurrence and will provide current internationally used selection criteria to identify patients for salvage. Next, the results of prostate cancer salvage will be discussed when comparing different salvage methods. Further, technical details of current radiotherapy salvage techniques will be described, followed by new developments, most importantly focal salvage.

2 Detecting a Patient with a Local Recurrence Only

As prostate cancer salvage has a high risk of treatment failure, it is essential to perform proper patient selection before treatment. Only patients with a true local recurrence will be able to benefit from any salvage treatment. Each detection tool has several specific pitfalls in prostate cancer recurrence assessment, and these will be discussed below. This will result in a list of internationally accepted patient selection criteria for prostate cancer salvage.

PSA is currently used for follow-up of prostate cancer treatment. The independent prognostic value of PSA pre-primary treatment has been well established. Pre-salvage, the PSA value also seems to be a prognostic factor in many studies using varying modalities (Chade et al. 2012; Wenske et al. 2013; Murat et al. 2009). However, the definition of a normal PSA value after primary treatment remains problematic and differs between different primary treatment modalities. The lowest PSA value after treatment is called the nadir value. Different from the situation after radical prostatectomy, patients following radiotherapy will still have a prostate gland and therefore are not expected to achieve an undetectable nadir. Still, post-radiation PSA values are lower compared to the pretreatment values as irradiated prostates show atrophy and a reduction of size and gland tissue (Grignon and Hammond 1995). There are potentially three sources of PSA which contribute to the nadir: (1) remaining normal prostate gland tissue, (2) remaining local prostate cancer cells, and (3) subclinical metastases. Of course, serum PSA measurements cannot differentiate between any of these three PSA sources. Therefore, changes in PSA over time are evaluated. The longer the time to nadir, the more likely it is that remaining benign prostate tissue is the source of the residual PSA (Huang et al. 2011). Furthermore, PSA from benign residual prostate tissue will not show a clear rise. Early distant metastases will also produce PSA and will eventually "overgrow" the PSA decline after the local treatment, mostly in the first few years after treatment. Also, these patients usually will have a higher nadir PSA (Zietman et al. 1996). A slow PSA rise many years after treatment will probably be due to a local recurrence as these prostate cancer cells first would have to recover the damage from the prostate cancer treatment (Zumsteg et al. 2015). A PSA rise after treatment can further be attributed to PSA from cancer cells or a PSA bounce. This last phenomenon is a temporary rise of PSA followed by a PSA decline back to nadir levels and is not associated with cancer progression. Bounces may occur in up to 40 % of patients (Akyol et al. 2005; Roach et al. 2006). To date, no conclusive evidence-based explanation for the bouncing behavior of PSA exists. Precipitating factors such as ejaculation or instrumentation are known to cause some PSA fluctuation (Das et al. 2002). Also the physiological variability of PSA assays in healthy test subjects was found to be considerable (Prestigiacomo and Stamey 1996). Lastly, PSA bounces after therapy have been associated with an increase in biochemical recurrence-free, prostate cancer-specific, and overall survival after brachytherapy using multivariable analyses (Hinnen et al. 2012). It is hypothesized that a delayed wave of cell destruction due to radiation effects is responsible for the bounce phenomenon and therefore possibly leads to an increase in survival. A small fraction of bounces may be caused by these factors; however, they fail to provide a complete explanation. In clinical practice a PSA rise, therefore, needs differentiation between PSA bounce and cancer progression. For this reason different guidelines have been developed of which the

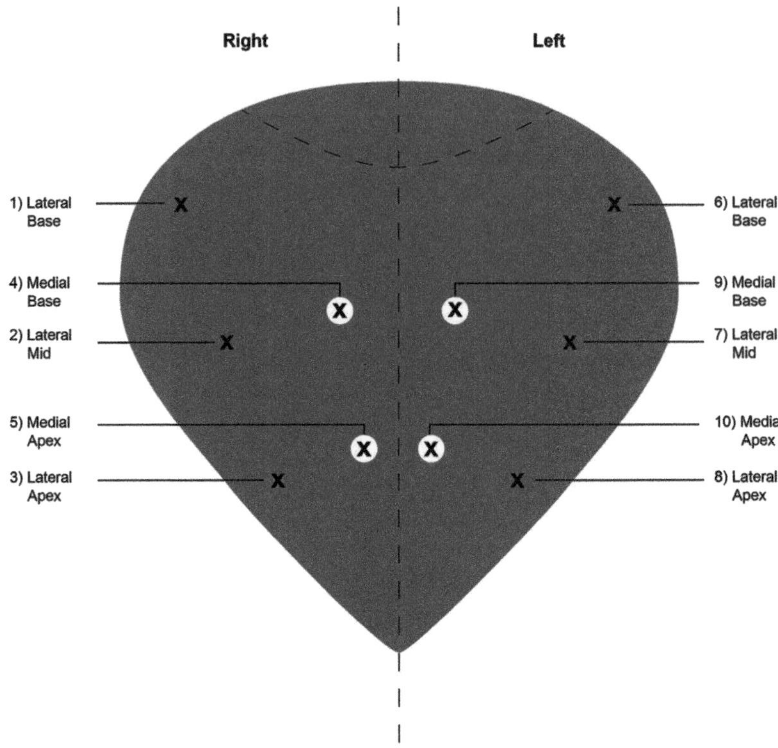

Fig. 1 Example of an internationally used systematic biopsy scheme which can be used to prove a local recurrence. The number of cores depicted here is 10

most commonly used are the ASTRO definition (Cox et al. 1997) and the Phoenix definition (Roach et al. 2006). The ASTRO definition required three rises of more than 50 % with at least an interval of 3 months and the moment of failure is subsequently backdated to midway between the nadir and the first rise. However, this definition seemed to have a high false-positive rate of approximately 20 % after the use of adjuvant hormonal treatment (Roach et al. 2006). Therefore, currently, the Phoenix definition is the internationally accepted approach. A biochemical relapse is considered any PSA rise of 2 ng/ml above nadir. This definition does not suffer in terms of accuracy with ADT use (Buyyounouski et al. 2005). In clinical practice, outcome is worse if the PSA level at the time of salvage is higher than 10 ng/ml (Izawa et al. 2002; de la Taille et al. 2000; Wenske et al. 2013; Chade et al. 2012), the PSA doubling time should be ideally more than 12 months (Zelefsky et al. 2005; Nguyen et al. 2007a, b), and the interval to PSA failure should be at least 3 years (Nguyen et al. 2007a, b). Of course, these tumor characteristics will somehow reflect the amount of tumor and the tumor aggressiveness and thus the risk of already having metastases (Freedland et al. 2005).

Of course, each local recurrence should be pathology proven. Usually this is performed by systematic transrectal ultrasound (TRUS)-guided biopsies (Fig. 1). Crook et al. (1995) routinely performed prostate biopsies post treatment and found that 19 % of patients with an initially negative biopsy later had a positive biopsy for cancer. Systematic biopsy schedules have a high chance of spatially missing tumor (sampling error), especially as local radio-recurrent tumor is hardly visible on TRUS (Crook et al. 1993). As the chance of a successful local salvage treatment will depend on the amount of tumor in the prostate at the time of salvage, it is obvious that currently used systematic biopsy schedules will detect most recurring tumor in a rather advanced state. Newer biopsy techniques have a higher accuracy in detecting localized recurrences and furthermore in assessing clinically significant disease. Transperineal template prostate mapping (TTPM) biopsies are taken with a brachytherapy grid, usually with 5 mm spacing. With TTPM, a large part of the prostate is sampled, usually subdivided in 24 Barzell zones (Barzell and Whitmore 2003). This technique leads to the detection of approximately 30 % more clinically significant tumors over systematic transrectal biopsies alone (Onik et al. 2009; Sivaraman et al. 2015). This is mainly due to the higher amount of cores taken but also because the anterior part of the prostate is sampled, which is undersampled with transrectal biopsies. A limitation of TTPM is the detection of more clinically insignificant tumors. However, these lesions are often eligible for active surveillance, which shows excellent results regarding (cancer-specific) survival (Klotz et al. 2010, 2015). In addition, MRI-guided biopsies to a suspicious lesion can lead to an increase in detecting clinically significant disease while not increasing or even decreasing the detection rate of insignificant lesions (Siddiqui et al. 2015; Moore et al. 2013).

Next, the evaluation of the biopsies is difficult. In early reports, little was known about the rate of histological clearance of irradiated tumor, and failures were determined on biopsies even 6 months after radiotherapy (Scardino 1983). More recent analyses have shown that early biopsies have a high chance of being false positive. Radiation causes postmitotic cell death. Therefore, fatally damaged cells may even survive a limited number of cell divisions before dying off (Mostofi et al. 1992). As there is no visible difference between these dying cells and viable tumor cells, it is impossible for a pathologist to predict whether visible tumor cells are really clonogenic and need treatment (Crook et al. 1997). Approximately 30 % of biopsies positive in the first year after radiation treatment will be negative for tumor in 24–30 months (Crook et al. 1995, 2000). Crook et al. (1995) therefore determined that the optimal time to biopsy would be 30–36 months post radiotherapy. Of course, even 36 months after treatment biopsies may be false positive, although chances are reduced at that moment. As postradiation pathology is difficult to interpret, experienced uropathologists are required to evaluate these biopsies. An extra difficulty is the interpretation of biopsies. The currently used Gleason system is based on the glandular pattern of the tumor seen at relatively low magnification. As an irradiated prostate will show a significantly changed anatomy, especially on glandular level, Gleason score seems less useful after radiation treatment. Still, to evaluate the possibilities for salvage, it will be required to have some information on the potential aggressiveness of the visible tumor cells. Pathologists will need to be cautious here as one of the problems with evaluating carcinomas that have been treated with radiotherapy is that the grade often appears higher (Bostwick et al. 1982). Although post-RT prostate biopsies are burdened with problems of timing, interpretation, and sampling error, they are required as evidence before radical local salvage for radiation failure is considered.

Imaging to visualize the local recurrence is regularly performed using TRUS. Unfortunately, sensitivity is very poor for the primary setting (Crook et al. 1993; Onur et al. 2004). In radio-recurrent disease, accuracy may even be further decreased due to fibrosis of the prostatic tissue. Therefore, current clinical practice lacks a proper imaging tool to detect a local recurrence. Promising local imaging techniques still under development are dynamic contrast-enhanced magnetic resonance imaging (DCE-MRI) and ^{18}F or ^{11}C-choline positron emission tomography (PET) (Rouviere et al. 2004; Haider et al. 2008; Moman et al. 2010; Wang et al. 2009; Breeuwsma et al. 2010; Barentsz et al. 2012; de Rooij et al. 2015; Umbehr et al. 2013). More recent developments have provided prostate-specific membrane antigen (PSMA) PET-CT using various tracers (Jadvar 2015; Rybalov et al. 2014). However larger series evaluating these techniques and assessment with the pathology reference standard is needed. Recent diagnostic meta-analyses have shown that the use of MRI (using the prostate imaging reporting and data system (PI-RADS)) can help in assessing localized disease, capsular extension, and the exclusion of clinically significant disease with a negative predictive value up to 95 %

(Hamoen et al. 2015; Fütterer et al. 2015; de Rooij et al. 2015).

Imaging to exclude possible distant metastases should be performed when evaluating the possibilities for salvage. But as a bone scan, pelvic computed tomography (CT), and MRI need a significant tumor load to show metastases (Hovels et al. 2008; Abuzallouf et al. 2004), it is unlikely they will detect small metastases present in patients being selected for salvage treatment, e.g., with a PSA less than 10 ng/ml (Zagars and Pollack 1997; Nguyen et al. 2007a, b). Next, a pelvic lymph node dissection may be performed to exclude metastases. As a limited pelvic node dissection of the obturator fossa will only detect approximately 30 % of lymph node metastases, the value of a lymph node dissection is questioned (Heesakkers et al. 2008). For early metastases detection in the future, the role of choline PET with various tracers (Breeuwsma et al. 2010) and magnetic nanoparticles in MRI (Barentsz et al. 2007) needs to be further evaluated. PET-CT imaging seems to be able to provide more accurate assessment of metastatic disease and assessment of prostate-confined recurrences. Recent overviews have shown promising results regarding lymph node involvement, prostate-confined recurrences, and distant metastatic disease (pooled sensitivity and specificity of 85.6 and 92.6 % for all three sites) (Evangelista et al. 2013). However, the spread across series is still large and standardization is necessary to achieve this high diagnostic accuracy in every center.

Of course, clinical patient characteristics before primary treatment and salvage are of importance when evaluating the possibility of successful salvage. Patients with a high initial chance of developing distant metastases are unlikely to have a local recurrence only (Nguyen et al. 2007a, b). An initial high Gleason score, high T-stage, high PSA value, and high PSA kinetics (before primary treatment) are possibly also risk factors post treatment to evaluate the likelihood of effective salvage. Therefore, salvage especially is advocated in primary low-risk clinical features (Nguyen et al. 2007a, b). However, evidence in this area from multivariable models is generally lacking and pre-salvage characteristics seem to have the highest predictive ability for cancer control outcomes (Chade et al. 2011, 2012; Wenske et al. 2013; Murat et al. 2009). From these larger salvage series, it seems pre-salvage PSA, PSADT, and pre-salvage Gleason score are most often associated with cancer control outcomes.

Next, the chance of having toxicity from a local salvage treatment will be increased if a patient had severe toxicity during or after primary radiation treatment. Also, other additional treatments may attribute to the possible toxicity from salvage, like a transurethral resection (TURP), high-intensity focussed ultrasound (HIFU) treatment, or ADT use. These treatments will produce extra scar tissue and, therefore, will reduce the repair capacity of normal tissue in case of re-irradiation of the prostate. So far, however, no current salvage re-irradiation literature exists, which models these characteristics in a multivariable manner to the probability of developing toxicity.

Based on the above, a list of preliminary selection criteria for local salvage can be completed. Still, it is of major importance to use such a list reasonably, as many clinical aspects, like age, medical history, and performance score contribute in the decision for a local salvage treatment. The list below partially uses the criteria as described in the currently active radiation therapy oncology group (RTOG) trial 0526 (principle investigator: J. Crook, MD). These selection criteria were also mostly verified in a recent international collaboration on selection for salvage treatment (van den Bos et al. 2015).

- Biopsy-proven local recurrence at least 3 years after primary radiation treatment
- Posttreatment PSA <10 ng/ml, PSA doubling time (PSADT) >12 months
- Bone scan and CT abdomen or lymph node dissection without evidence of metastases
- Primary tumor characteristics preferably low to intermediate risk
- Acceptable toxicity of primary radiation treatment
- No other prostate treatments performed (like TURP, HIFU, etc.)

- Additional to RTOG: verification of tumor localization with multiparametric MRI (consisting at least of a 1.5 Tesla T_2-weighted, dynamic contrast-enhanced, and diffusion-weighted imaging sequence). Exclusion of metastatic disease using PET-CT (^{18}F or 11C choline PET or Ga-68-PSMA)

3 General Results of Prostate Cancer Salvage

Different salvage treatment modalities are currently clinically practiced. Radical prostatectomy, external beam radiotherapy, cryosurgery, additional I125/Pd103 or Ir192 brachytherapy, and HIFU are used (Pisters et al. 2000; Lee et al. 2008; Grado et al. 1999; Murat et al. 2009; van der Poel et al. 2007; Nguyen et al. 2007a, b; Chade et al. 2011, 2012, Paparel et al. 2009 Wenske et al. 2013, Williams et al. 2011, Spiess et al. 2010, Chen et al. 2013, Peters et al. 2013, Burri et al. 2010; Henríquez et al. 2014; Yamada et al. 2014). Literature is scarce and shows discordant results in terms of treatment effect and toxicity. Furthermore, few large series have been published; most studies are retrospective and contain less than 100 patients. No head-to-head comparisons have been performed. As a consequence, current treatment decisions often depend on patients' and doctors'/institutional preferences. An overview of the literature is presented below.

Salvage radical prostatectomy has been described in several articles and has been performed in these series since the 1960s. Five-year biochemical no evidence of disease (bNED) ranges from 50 to 60 % (Nguyen et al. 2007a, b, Chade et al. 2012). In most series pre-salvage PSA was <10 ng/ml. Only a few rather large series have been described. Chade et al. (2011) described the largest salvage radical prostatectomy series with 404 radio-recurrent prostate cancer patients, treated since 1985. Ward et al. (2005) described the results of 199 patients, treated since 1967. In addition, Paparel et al. (2009) described 146 patients from a single institution. Finally, Stephenson et al. (2004) described results of 100 patients (Stephenson et al. 2004). The other published studies contain between 6 and 51 patients (Sanderson et al. 2006; van der Poel et al. 2007; Vaidya and Soloway 2000). The definition of bNED after prostatectomy was most commonly defined as a rise in PSA of >0.2 ng/ml. It was concluded that patients with a pre-salvage PSA of <10 ng/ml did significantly better compared to patients with a PSA >10 ng/ml (Ward et al. 2005; Bianco et al. 2005). In addition, a lower pre-salvage Gleason score was shown to improve biochemical disease-free survival and reduced the development of metastases in multivariable analysis (Chade et al. 2011). Multivariable analysis was not performed for mortality in this largest series. However, these factors were associated with prostate cancer-specific survival after multivariable analysis in the series of Paparel et al. (2009). Neoadjuvant hormonal therapy did not seem to improve outcome (Ward et al. 2005; van der Poel et al. 2007). Also a cystoprostatectomy did not seem to improve oncologic outcome compared to a radical prostatectomy alone (Ward et al. 2005). Although preoperative morbidity, lasting from the previous radiotherapy treatment, was low, urinary incontinence had a weighted average of 41 %, bladder neck strictures of 24 %, and rectal injury of approximately 5 % (Nguyen et al. 2007a, b).

Salvage cryotherapy studies have been described with patients treated since the 1990s (Nguyen et al. 2007a, b). Five larger series have been published. The largest series describes 797 patients from 6 tertiary centers, of the basis of which a pretreatment nomogram to predict biochemical recurrence was created (Spiess et al. 2010). Wenske et al. (2013) described 328 patients after either primary EBRT ($n = 259$), primary I-125 brachytherapy ($n = 49$), or primary cryotherapy ($n = 20$). Furthermore, Williams et al. described 187 patients, Izawa et al. (2002) showed outcomes of 131 patients, and Chin et al. (2001) described results of 125 patients. Other studies contained 59 patients or less (Bahn et al. 2003). Most series used a double freeze-thaw therapy (Izawa et al. 2002; Chin et al. 2001; Bahn et al. 2003, Williams et al. 2011). Unfortunately, the series published on salvage cryotherapy used different definitions for a relapse after salvage, which hampers a decent comparison. In addition, there were also large differences in prognostic characteristics between cohorts. From their overview Nguyen et al. (2007a, b) concluded that outcome of salvage cryotherapy is comparable with the outcome reported from the prostatectomy data above. This is confirmed in the larger series, although the spread across series remains significant. Toxicity again is severe, with a weighted average of urinary incontinence of 36 %, urinary sloughing 11 %, bladder neck stricture or retention 36 %, perineal pain 44 %, and fistulas approximately 3 % (Nguyen et al. 2007a, b).

Salvage brachytherapy series also describe patients treated since the 1990s (Nguyen et al. 2007a, b). Compared to the salvage prostatectomy and salvage cryotherapy series, far less and smaller brachytherapy series have been published. The largest I-125 salvage brachytherapy study contained 49 patients (Grado et al. 1999). Recently, Chen et al. (2013) reported on their HDR-salvage brachytherapy patients ($n=52$), and the results of a somewhat larger combined I-125 salvage brachytherapy ($n=37$) and HDR-salvage brachytherapy ($n=19$) cohort have been published (Henríquez et al. 2014). In addition, a phase II study of salvage HDR brachytherapy ($n=42$) has recently been reported (Yamada et al. 2014). Other series reported 31 patients or less (Nguyen et al. 2007b; Wallner et al. 1990; Beyer 1999; Lee et al. 2008; Battermann 2000; Moman et al. 2010). Again, varying definitions of PSA relapse after treatment hamper comparison between the different series. Still, midterm outcomes can be considered comparable to salvage prostatectomy and salvage cryotherapy series (Nguyen et al. 2007a, b). However, multivariable analyses do not provide uniform parameters associated with biochemical failure or survival due to insufficient sample size and sometimes methodological limitations. Weighted incontinence rate was 6 % and other grade 3–4 toxicities were weighted 6 % for the gastrointestinal (GI) tract and 17 % for the genitourinary (GU) tract. Fistulas averaged 3 % (Nguyen et al. 2007a, b). Table 1 shows an overview of published salvage brachytherapy series.

Data on other modalities for local salvage are very limited. One study on HIFU has a mean follow-up of 15 months and showed an incontinence rate of 7 %, bladder neck stenosis 17 %, and fistulas 6 % (Gelet et al. 2004). A more recent and larger series in 290 patients has shown a 5-year biochemical recurrence-free rate in 43, 22, and 17 % in D'Amico low-, intermediate-, and high-risk patients, respectively. Grade 3 urinary incontinence occurred in approximately 10 % of patients; 46 % of patients had a bladder outlet obstruction for which intervention was needed, of which four patients (1.3 %) required urinary diversion. Rectourethral fistulas occurred in 2 % and pubic osteitis in 2.7 % (Crouzet et al. 2012).

Ferromagnetic thermal ablation has been described in 14 patients (Master et al. 2004) and external beam radiotherapy (30.6–50 Gy) combined with external hyperthermia (5–8 treatments) in three patients (Kalapurakal et al. 2001). Of course, further more extensive studies are required to be able to judge these new developments regarding tumor control and toxicity.

In the studies above outcome is mainly described as bNED. Still, survival data are required to judge whether salvage is worthwhile performing. Salvage is often performed in an older patient population. Because of the competing risks in these patients, the potential survival benefit is therefore not automatically derived from the benefit in bNED. However, ADT use can be postponed or prevented with postponing the moment of biochemical failure, thereby reducing side effects from this palliative strategy and possibly increasing cost-effectiveness. Therefore, a generally accepted primary goal of a salvage approach can be to postpone hormonal therapy. This leads to a discussion whether also patients with oligo-metastases in slowly progressing disease might benefit from a local salvage treatment.

The high severe toxicity rates of the varying salvage modalities make salvage unpopular and this probably causes the absence of large randomized studies. Still, these are required to evaluate whether salvage has a future. A randomized study would preferably consist of comparing hormonal treatment alone to one type of salvage and

Table 1 Overview of clinical outcome and severe toxicity of published series on salvage brachytherapy

Reference	iPSA (ng/ml)	*N*	HDR/seeds	HT (%)	FU (months)	bNED, Kaplan-Meier estimates	% GI ≥ grade 3	% GU ≥ grade 3
Yamada et al. (2014)	Median 3.5	42	HDR	+ (43)	Median 36	69 % (5-year)	0	8
Henríquez (2014)	Median 3.7	56	HDR (n=19), seeds (n=37)	+ (27)	Median 48	77 % (5-year)[a,b]	4	23
Chen et al. (2013)	Median 9.3	52	HDR	+ (46)	Median 60	51 % (5-year)[a]	0	2
Burri et al. (2010)	Median 5.6	37	Seeds	+ (84)	Median 86	54 % (10-year)	3	8
Moman et al. (2010)	Mean 11.4	31	Seeds	+ (16)	Mean 110	20 % (5-year)[a]	0	6
Lee et al. (2008)	Median 3.8	21	Seeds	NA	Median 36	38 % (5-year)[b]	0	0
Nguyen et al. (2007a, b)	Median 7.5	25	Seeds	–	Median 47	70 % (4-year)[a]	24	16
Lee et al. (2007)	Median 5.9	21	HDR	+ (52)	Median 19	89 % (2-year)[b]	0	14
Wong et al. (2006)	Median 4.7	17	Seeds	+ (88)	Median 44	75 % (4-year)[b]	6	47
Lo et al. (2005)	NA	30	Seeds	–	Median 59	57 % (5-year)[b]	3	10
Koutrouvelis et al. (2003)	NA	31	Seeds	+	Median 30	87 % (3-year)[b]	5	13
Grado et al. (1999)	Median 5.6	49	Seeds	+ (16)	Median 64	34 % (5-year)[c]	4	20
Beyer (1999)	Median 2.2	17	Seeds	+ (47)	Median 62	53 % (5-year)[b]	0	24
Loening and Turner (1993)	NA	31	Seeds	–	Median 23	67 % (2-year)[c]	0	0

Different PSA failure definitions have been used

N number of patients, *HT* hormonal therapy neoadjuvantly before salvage; no, –; yes, +, %. *bNED* percentage biochemical no evidence of disease including year of measurement, *NA* not available, *iPSA* initial PSA, *HDR* high dose rate (brachytherapy), *FU* follow-up, *GI* gastrointestinal, *GU* genitourinary

[a]Phoenix (nadir + 2 ng/ml)

[b]ASTRO (three successive PSA rises >50 %)

[c]Other definitions

would have to prove a gain in survival. Next to toxicity scoring, quality of life will be essential to monitor (Nguyen et al. 2009) to judge the actual influence of severe toxicities and compare the difference between ADT use and salvage therapy.

4 Re-irradiation of Prostate Cancer

Post-radiotherapy local salvage is historically performed by brachytherapy (LDR, PDR, or HDR) or EBRT (Kimura et al. 2010). There is a preference for brachytherapy, as it can be expected that the surrounding area which receives a relatively high dose will be larger after EBRT, and therefore EBRT can be expected to cause more severe toxicity. This explains why there is hardly any literature on EBRT for recurrent local disease after primary radiotherapy. In a national disease registry, the Cancer of the Prostate Strategic Urologic Research Endeavor (CaPSURE), 935 men were described who received a salvage treatment after primary EBRT. Of these men only eight received salvage by EBRT (Agarwal et al. 2008). In their article, Agarwal et al. (2008) did not notice any survival benefit for any particular combination of primary and salvage therapy. The inability to protect the bladder and the anterior rectal wall without blocking a part of the prostate/tumor was largely caused by the limitations of the EBRT technique. Current EBRT techniques have improved enormously, e.g., by daily position verification techniques (van der Heide et al. 2007) and by the introduction of intensity-modulated radiotherapy (IMRT). Passive-scattering proton therapy has recently been associated with a potential increase in GI toxicity in a large propensity score-matched analysis (Sheets et al. 2012). Advanced forms of proton therapy delivery with intensity-modulated proton therapy (IMPT) may provide better salvage outcome and toxicity data, but IMPT will need IGRT and daily position verification. Although most articles and textbooks discourage the use of EBRT for salvage after primary radiotherapy, these new techniques indeed might lead to comparable results as described above. But as the current standard salvage techniques already show hardly acceptable severe toxicity rates, the further evaluation of EBRT for this purpose seems not the way forward.

In salvage brachytherapy permanent seeds are commonly used. Both I125 and Pd103 have been described (Wallner et al. 1990; Beyer 1999; Grado et al. 1999; Koutrouvelis et al. 2003; Lee et al. 2008; Battermann 2000; Nguyen et al. 2007b; Moman et al. 2010). More recently, HDR brachytherapy is being adopted in the salvage setting (Chen et al. 2013; Henríquez et al. 2014; Yamada et al. 2014). Again, comparison in outcome is hampered by differences in study populations, treatment methods, and the definition of failure (Nguyen et al. 2007a, b). In patients who meet the criteria described in part 2, it can be expected to achieve a 5-year bNED rate of approximately 50–70% (Table 1). Five-year overall survival rates ranging from 80 to 90% have been described (Beyer 1999; Lee et al. 2008). Still, the severe toxicity rate is high, up to approximately 10–30% for GU and GI combined (Moman et al. 2010; Nguyen et al. 2007b, Peters et al. 2013). Currently, an RTOG trial (no. 0526) is ongoing for the prospective evaluation of brachytherapy after EBRT. The results of this trial can be expected to give more insight in the toxicity risk profiles of patients receiving salvage brachytherapy. This can improve patient selection and may augment the benefit/risk ratio (Nguyen et al. 2007a, b; Moman et al. 2010).

As all studies showed a rather large proportion of patients with severe toxicity, specific dose constraints for salvage are essential. Many different doses have been applied, but most groups used regular doses, which are also applied for a primary treatment, e.g., 120–145 Gy in I125 implants and 100–120 Gy in Pd103. Recent research has suggested dose constraints for whole-gland salvage I-125 brachytherapy for the urethra, bladder, and rectal wall (Peters et al. 2015, 2016). These constraints are, however, based on 28 salvage patients without the use of multivariable modeling, taking into account other important prognostic characteristics related to toxicity. In essence, these dose constraints therefore represent a univariable association between dosimetry and late severe GU and GI toxicity for salvage patients. However, it was shown that these restrictions were all set lower than in the primary brachytherapy setting, indicating increased sensitivity of these structures after a primary course of radiation.

From the salvage prostatectomy data, a learning curve has been described (Ward et al. 2005), with less severe toxicity over time. This also seems likely for permanent seed salvage. The technical performance of LDR salvage treatment after primary radiotherapy should, therefore, probably be performed in agreement with current brachytherapy guidelines (Kovacs et al. 2005). Still, technical difficulties remain, e.g., how to perform post-salvage dosimetry after a primary seed implant.

Most experience in salvage re-irradiation has been developed in permanent seed (LDR) brachytherapy (Battermann 2000), but HDR might also be of use for salvage. Currently only scarce literature exists on this topic (Table 1). The problem with HDR is that primary treatment often is performed in several fractions and that catheters retract during treatment, and therefore, it seems prone to more severe toxicity and a poorer outcome. Still, current clinical practice is actively working toward a single-fraction primary HDR treatment. Furthermore, current brachytherapy groups have developed on-line MRI guidance techniques. With these techniques a single-fraction HDR treatment for salvage can be developed. Current results of HDR brachytherapy in terms of cancer control and late toxicity are promising and seem to be favorable compared to previous LDR brachytherapy (Table 1) (Morton et al. 2013).

5 Focal Salvage, the Near Future

Several studies have shown that for salvage after primary radiotherapy, the rate of treatment-related toxicity is high (Nguyen et al. 2007a, b; Moman et al. 2010, Peters et al. 2013). Multiple factors will contribute to the fact that toxicity rates after salvage are greater compared to primary treatment, e.g., the cumulated radiotherapy dose and the patient's age and comorbidities. Most likely, the area of normal tissue which receives a significant radiation dose is too large. This probably is caused by the fact that local salvage always is performed on the entire prostate, as the spatial accuracy of current biopsy and imaging is poor (Moman et al. 2010). If the location of the local recurrence could be determined with better accuracy, treatment of the macroscopic tumor alone would result in reduced normal tissue exposure. This could be expected to reduce the rate of severe toxicity (Moman et al. 2010).

Evidence is emerging that local recurrences are located predominantly at the primary lesion site (GTV) (Cellini et al. 2002; Pucar et al. 2008; Arrayeh et al. 2012; Menard et al. 2015). Apparently, the surviving macroscopic tumor received an insufficient radiation dose from the primary treatment. Minor secondary tumor lesions (CTV) probably will have received sufficient doses. This corresponds with the remarks above that the radiation dose should not be lowered, and this adds to the argument of reducing the target volume to the macroscopic lesion alone (Moman et al. 2010). This can be called focal salvage (Moman et al. 2010; Peters et al. 2014).

There are several new imaging techniques, which may contribute to a spatially accurate detection of a local recurrence in the prostate. 18F-fluorocholine PET-guided target volume delineation for partial prostate re-irradiation in locally recurrent prostate cancer has already been described (Wang et al. 2009). However, PET seems to have a larger role in excluding lymph node and distant metastases (Umbehr et al. 2013; Evangelista et al. 2013). As resolution of MRI is better, more groups use advanced functional MRI techniques to localize the recurrence in the prostate (Ahmed et al. 2012; Peters et al. 2014; Menard et al. 2015). Dynamic contrast-enhanced (DCE)-MRI shows blood perfusion. After radiation treatment a large part of the prostate will be fibrotic and a normal T_2-weighted image cannot differentiate between fibrosis and tumor. DCE-MRI will be able to visualize a high blood perfusion, caused by neovascularization of the recurring tumor, in a fibrotic prostate bed. A sensitivity of 70–74%

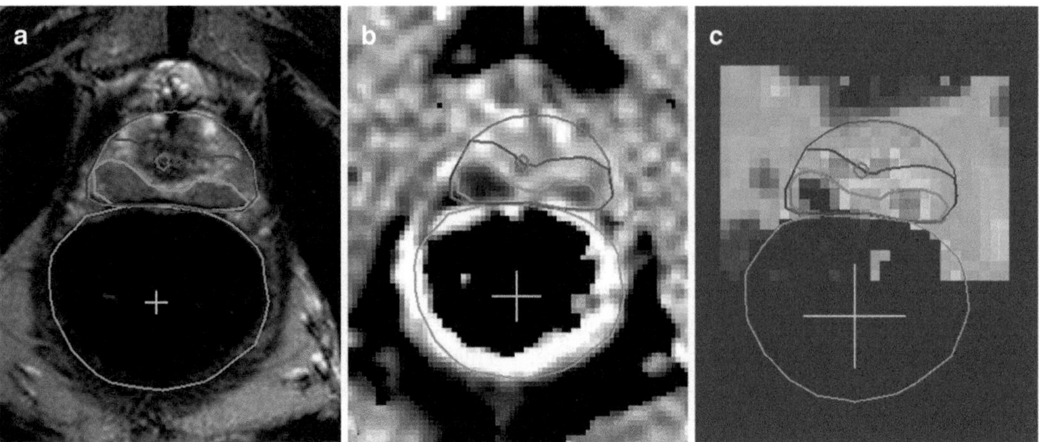

Fig. 2 Multiparametric MRI used for tumor delineation. (**a**) Transversal T2-weighted image, (**b**) transversal ADC, (**c**) transversal K-trans

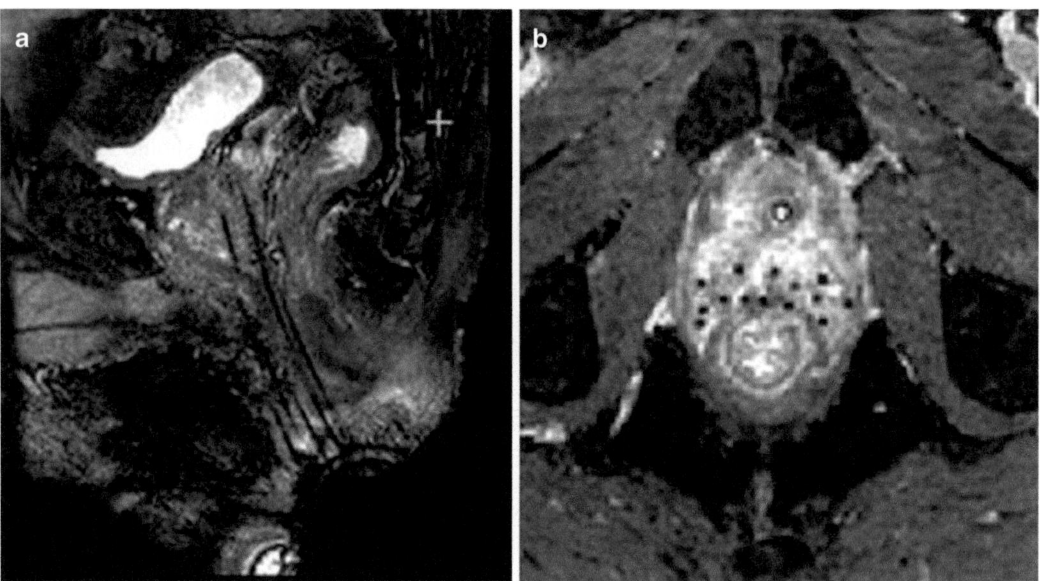

Fig. 3 Catheter visualization on MRI. (**a**) Sagittal SPIR image, (**b**) transversal SPAIR image

and a specificity of 73–85 % have been described (Rouviere et al. 2004; Haider et al. 2008). Recent diagnostic meta-analyses have shown mp-MRI (DCE-MRI in combination with diffusion-weighted imaging and/or MR spectroscopy) to be of importance in several aspects of prostate cancer staging, and a negative predictive value of 95 % for clinically significant disease can be achieved with standardized assessment (using PIRADS). However, these studies pertain to the primary setting (Hamoen et al. 2015; Fütterer et al. 2015; de Rooij et al. 2015; Barentsz et al. 2012). An example of the combination of T_2-weighted, DCE-MRI, and DWI-MRI for salvage planning is depicted in Fig. 2. The intraoperative MRI-based catheter reconstruction is depicted in Fig. 3. Finally, Fig. 4 shows the same MRI sequences and planning for a patient who underwent focal salvage HDR after radiotherapy failure. Lastly, each suspicious lesion on MRI should

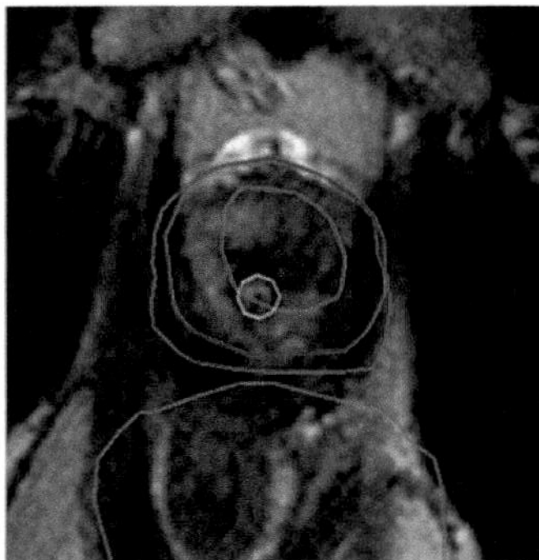
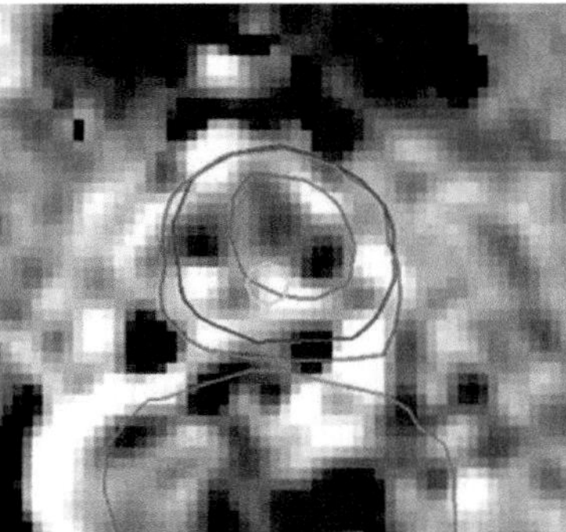
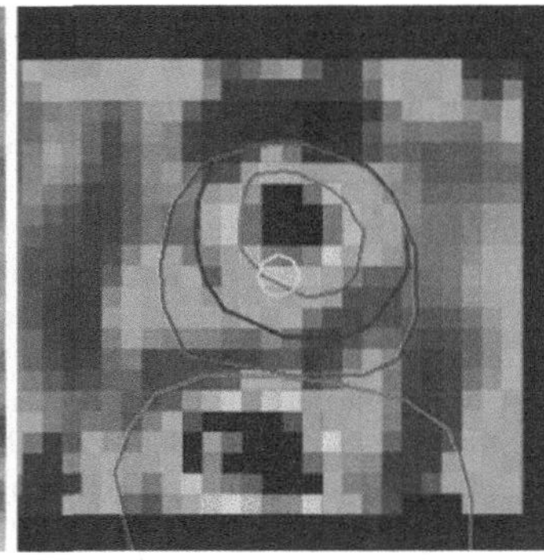

Fig. 4 *From left to right*: transversal T2-weighted, DWI and DCE-MRI for a locally recurrent prostate tumor after primary radiotherapy. This MR is an example of a 67-year-old male, with a prostate cancer recurrence 3 years after primary I-125 brachytherapy treatment. PSA before salvage treatment was 5.4 ng/ml. After salvage treatment, PSA decreased to 1.0 ng/ml

always be confirmed by biopsies, preferably MRI guided (Siddiqui et al. 2015; Moore et al. 2013).

Eggener et al. (2007) already proposed a set of criteria for primary focal therapy using multiple clinical, biopsy, and imaging characteristics that results in the exclusion of high-risk patients. Moman et al. (2010) did the same for focal salvage in a planning study. Ideally, multivariable prediction models are needed to provide the optimal set of selection criteria for both whole-gland and focal salvage. Larger series in the future are needed to attain this goal.

Focal salvage has been performed using several modalities, most importantly cryotherapy (Eisenberg and Shinohara 2008; de Castro Abreu et al. 2013; Bomers et al. 2013; Li et al. 2015), HIFU (Ahmed et al. 2012; Baco et al. 2014), and I125 brachytherapy (Peters et al. 2014; Hsu et al. 2013). In these cohorts toxicity indeed seemed reduced, while cancer control seemed to be maintained. One-, 2-, 3-, and 5-year BDFS ranges were 83–100 %, 49–100 %, 50–91 %, and 46.5–54.4 %, respectively, for these focal salvage modalities, which seems comparable to whole-gland salvage cancer control outcomes. Toxicity was mostly self-limiting or handled by medication in these series. Salvage brachytherapy showed a biochemical recurrence-free rate of approximately 60 % after 3 years with only one grade three urethral stricture in a combined set of 42 patients (Peters et al. 2014; Hsu et al. 2013; Sasaki et al. 2013). Currently, the FORECAST trial is under way for focal salvage cryotherapy and HIFU, and results can be expected in the next few years (Kanthabalan et al. 2015).

These focal salvage strategies also started a discussion on cure versus chronic disease. As doubling time of prostate cancer generally is very slow and patients evaluated for salvage only have low- to intermediate-risk features and probably an advanced age, it remains questionable whether salvage will be able to improve survival. Most of these patients would probably not die from their prostate cancer. If acceptable toxicity rates could be achieved with focal salvage, re-treatment would be possible if, during follow-up, another area of locally recurrent disease would be diagnosed. In this way, ADT could be postponed or even prevented in a subset of patients. This could turn recurrent prostate cancer into a more chronic disease and have a positive effect on the quality of life of recurrent prostate cancer patients.

References

Abuzallouf S, Dayes I, Lukka H (2004) Baseline staging of newly diagnosed prostate cancer: a summary of the literature. J Urol 171:2122–2127

Agarwal PK, Sadetsky N, Konety BR, Resnick MI, Carroll PR (2008) Treatment failure after primary and salvage therapy for prostate cancer: likelihood, patterns of care, and outcomes. Cancer 112:307–314

Ahmed HU, Cathcart P, McCartan N et al (2012) Focal salvage therapy for localized prostate cancer recurrence after external beam radiotherapy: a pilot study. Cancer 118:4148–4155

Akyol F, Ozyigit G, Selek U et al (2005) PSA bouncing after short term androgen deprivation and 3D-conformal radiotherapy for localized prostate adenocarcinoma and the relationship with the kinetics of testosterone. Eur Urol 48:40–45

Alongi F, De Bari B, Campostrini F et al (2013) Salvage therapy of intraprostatic failure after radical external-beam radiotherapy for prostate cancer: a review. Crit Rev Oncol Hematol 88:550–563

American Society for Therapeutic Radiology and Oncology Consensus Panel (1997) Consensus statement: Guidelines for PSA following radiation therapy. Int J Radiat Oncol Biol Phys. 37:1035–1041

Arrayeh E, Westphalen AC, Kurhanewicz J et al (2012) Does local recurrence of prostate cancer after radiation therapy occur at the site of primary tumor? Results of a longitudinal MRI and MRSI study. Int J Radiat Oncol Biol Phys 82:787–793

Baco E, Gelet A, Crouzet S et al (2014) Hemi salvage high-intensity focused ultrasound (HIFU) in unilateral radiorecurrent prostate cancer: a prospective two-centre study. BJU Int 114:532–540

Bahn DK, Lee F, Silverman P et al (2003) Salvage cryosurgery for recurrent prostate cancer after radiation therapy: a seven-year follow-up. Clin Prostate Cancer 2:111–114

Barentsz JO, Fütterer JJ, Takahashi S (2007) Use of ultrasmall superparamagnetic iron oxide in lymph node MR imaging in prostate cancer patients. Eur J Radiol 63:369–372

Barentsz JO, Richenberg J, Clements R et al (2012) ESUR prostate MR guidelines 2012. Eur Radiol 22:746–757

Barzell WE, Whitmore WF (2003) Transperineal template guided saturation biopsy of the prostate: rationale, indications, and technique. Urol Times 31: 41–42

Battermann JJ (2000) Feasibility of permanent implants for prostate cancer after previous radiotherapy in the true pelvis. Radiother Oncol 73:297–300

Beyer DC (1999) Permanent brachytherapy as salvage treatment for recurrent prostate cancer. Urology 54:880–883

Bianco FJ Jr, Scardino PT, Stephenson AJ et al (2005) Long-term oncologic results of salvage radical prostatectomy for locally recurrent prostate cancer after radiotherapy. Int J Radiat Oncol Biol Phys 62: 448–453

Bomers JG, Yakar D, Overduin CG et al (2013) MR imaging-guided focal cryoablation in patients with recurrent prostate cancer. Radiology 268:451–460

Bostwick DG, Egbert BM, Fajardo LF (1982) Radiation injury of the normal and neoplastic prostate. Am J Surg Pathol 6:541–551

Brachman DG, Thomas T, Hilbe J, Beyer DC (2000) Failure-free survival following brachytherapy alone or external beam irradiation alone for T1–2 prostate tumors in 2222 patients: results from a single practice. Int J Radiat Oncol Biol Phys 48:111–117

Breeuwsma AJ, Pruim J, van den Bergh AC, Leliveld AM, Nijman RJ, Dierckx RA, de Jong IJ (2010) Detection of local, regional, and distant recurrence in patients with psa relapse after external-beam radiotherapy using (11)C-choline positron emission tomography. Int J Radiat Oncol Biol Phys 77:160–164

Burri RJ, Stone NN, Unger P, Stock RG (2010) Long-term outcome and toxicity of salvage brachytherapy for local failure after initial radiotherapy for prostate cancer. Int J Radiat Oncol Biol Phys 77:1338–1344

Buyyounouski MK, Hanlon AL, Eisenberg DF, Horwitz EM, Feigenberg SJ, Uzzo RG et al (2005) Defining biochemical failure after radiotherapy with and without androgen deprivation for prostate cancer. Int J Radiat Oncol Biol Phys 63:1455–1462

Cellini N, Morganti AG, Mattiucci GC et al (2002) Analysis of intraprostatic failures in patients treated with hormonal therapy and radiotherapy: implications for conformal therapy planning. Int J Radiat Oncol Biol Phys 53:595–599

Chade DC, Shariat SF, Cronin AM et al (2011) Salvage radical prostatectomy for radiation-recurrent prostate cancer: a multi-institutional collaboration. Eur Urol 60:205–210

Chade DC, Eastham J, Graefen M et al (2012) Cancer control and functional outcomes of salvage radical prostatectomy for radiation-recurrent prostate cancer: a systematic review of the literature. Eur Urol 61:961–971

Chen CP, Weinberg V, Shinohara K et al (2013) Salvage HDR brachytherapy for recurrent prostate cancer after previous definitive radiation therapy: 5-year outcomes. Int J Radiat Oncol Biol Phys 86:324–329

Chin JL, Pautler SE, Mouraviev V et al (2001) Results of salvage cryoablation of the prostate after radiation: identifying predictors of treatment failure and complications. J Urol 165:1937–1941

Cox JD, Grignon DJ, Kaplan RS, Parsons JT, Schellhammer PF (1997) Consensus statement: guidelines for PSA following radiation therapy. American society for therapeutic radiology and oncology consensus panel. Int J Radiat Oncol Biol Phys 37:1035–1041

Crook J, Robertson S, Collin G et al (1993) Clinical relevance of trans-rectal ultrasound, biopsy, and serum prostate-specific antigen following external beam radiotherapy for carcinoma of the prostate. Int J Radiat Oncol Biol Phys 27:31–37

Crook JM, Perry GA, Robertson S et al (1995) Routine prostate biopsies following radiotherapy for prostate cancer: results for 226 patients. Urology 45:624–631

Crook J, Bahadur Y, Robertson S et al (1997) Evaluation of radiation effect, tumor differentiation, and prostate specific antigen staining in sequential prostate biopsies after external beam radiotherapy for patients with prostate carcinoma. Cancer 27:81–89

Crook J, Malone S, Perry G et al (2000) Postradiotherapy prostate biopsies: what do they really mean? Results for 498 patients. Int J Radiat Oncol Biol Phys 48: 355–367

Crouzet S, Murat FJ, Pommier P et al (2012) Locally recurrent prostate cancer after initial radiation therapy: early salvage high-intensity focused ultrasound improves oncologic outcomes. Radiother Oncol 105:198–202

Das P, Chen MH, Valentine K et al (2002) Using the magnitude of PSA bounce after MRI-guided prostate brachytherapy to distinguish recurrence, benign precipitating factors, and idiopathic bounce. Int J Radiat Oncol Biol Phys 54:698–702

de Castro Abreu AL, Bahn D, Leslie S et al (2013) Salvage focal and salvage total cryoablation for locally recurrent prostate cancer after primary radiation therapy. BJU Int 112:298–307

De la Taille A, Hayek O, Benson MC et al (2000) Salvage cryotherapy for recurrent prostate cancer after radiation therapy: the Columbia experience. Urology 55:79–84

de Rooij M, Hamoen EH, Witjes JA, Barentsz JO, Rovers MM (2015) Accuracy of magnetic resonance imaging for local staging of prostate cancer: a diagnostic meta-analysis. Eur Urol [epub ahead of print]

Dutch Cancer Society (2010) SCK rapport kanker in Nederland, pp 141–145. www.kwfkankerbestrijding.nl/index.jsp?objectid=kwfredactie:6419

Eggener SE, Scardino PT et al (2007) Focal therapy for localized prostate cancer: a critical appraisal of rationale and modalities. J Urol 178:2260–2267

Eisenberg ML, Shinohara K (2008) Partial salvage cryoablation of the prostate for recurrent prostate cancer after radiotherapy failure. Urology 72:1315–1318

Evangelista L, Zattoni F, Guttilla A et al (2013) Choline PET or PET/CT and biochemical relapse of prostate cancer: a systematic review and meta-analysis. Clin Nucl Med 38:305–314

Freedland SJ, Humphreys EB, Mangold LA et al (2005) Risk of prostate cancer-specific mortality following biochemical recurrence after radical prostatectomy. JAMA 294:433–439

Fütterer JJ, Briganti A, De Visschere P et al (2015) Can clinically significant prostate cancer be detected with multiparametric magnetic resonance imaging? A systematic review of the literature. Eur Urol 68: 1045–1053

Gelet A, Chapelon JY, Poissonnier L et al (2004) Local recurrence of prostate cancer after external beam radiotherapy: early experience of salvage therapy using high-intensity focused ultrasonography. Urology 63:625–629

Grado GL, Collins JM, Kriegshauser JS et al (1999) Salvage brachytherapy for localized prostate cancer after radiotherapy failure. Urology 53:2–10

Grignon DJ, Hammond EH (1995) College of American Pathologists Conference XXVI on clinical relevance of prognostic markers in solid tumors. Report of the prostate cancer working group. Arch Pathol Lab Med 119:1122–1126

Haider MA, Chung P, Sweet J et al (2008) Dynamic contrast-enhanced magnetic resonance imaging for localization of recurrent prostate cancer after external beam radiotherapy. Int J Radiat Oncol Biol Phys 70:425–430

Hamoen EH, de Rooij M, Witjes JA, Barentsz JO, Rovers MM (2015) Use of the prostate imaging reporting and data system (PI-RADS) for prostate cancer detection with multiparametric magnetic resonance imaging: a diagnostic meta-analysis. Eur Urol 67:1112–1121

Heesakkers RA, Hövels AM, Jager GJ, van den Bosch HC, Witjes JA, Raat HP, Severens JL, Adang EM, van der Kaa CH, Fütterer JJ, Barentsz J (2008) MRI with a lymph-node-specific contrast agent as an alternative to CT scan and lymph-node dissection in patients with prostate cancer: a prospective multicohort study. Lancet Oncol 9:850–856

Heidenreich A, Aus G, Bolla M et al (2008) EAU guidelines on prostate cancer. Eur Urol 53:68–80

Heidenreich A, Bastian PJ, Bellmunt J et al (2014) EAU guidelines on prostate cancer. Part II: treatment of advanced, relapsing, and castration-resistant prostate cancer. Eur Urol 65:467–479

Hinnen KA, Monninkhof EM, Battermann JJ et al (2012) Prostate specific antigen bounce is related to overall survival in prostate brachytherapy. Int J Radiat Oncol Biol Phys 82:883–888

Henríquez I, Sancho G, Hervás A et al (2014) Salvage brachytherapy in prostate local recurrence after radiation therapy: predicting factors for control and toxicity. Radiat Oncol 9:102–109

Hovels AM, Heesakkers RA, Adang EM et al (2008) The diagnostic accuracy of CT and MRI in the staging of pelvic lymph nodes in patients with prostate cancer: a meta-analysis. Clin Radiol 63:387–395

Hsu CC, Hsu H, Pickett B et al (2013) Feasibility of MR imaging/MR spectroscopy-planned focal partial salvage permanent prostate implant (PPI) for localized recurrence after initial PPI for prostate cancer. Int J Radiat Oncol Biol Phys 85:370–377

Huang WC, Kuroiwa K, Serio AM et al (2007) The anatomical and pathological characteristics of irradiated prostate cancers may influence the oncological efficacy of salvage ablative therapies. J Urol 177:1324–1329

Huang SP, Bao BY, Wu MT et al (2011) Impact of prostate-specific antigen (PSA) nadir and time to PSA nadir on disease progression in prostate cancer treated with androgen-deprivation therapy. Prostate 71:1189–1197

Izawa JI, Madsen LT, Scott SM et al (2002) Salvage cryotherapy for recurrent prostate cancer after radiotherapy: variables affecting patient outcome. J Clin Oncol 20:2664–2671

Jadvar H (2015) PSMA PET in prostate cancer. J Nucl Med 56:1131–1132

Kalapurakal JA, Mittal BB, Sathiaseelan V (2001) Re-irradiation and external hyperthermia in locally advanced, radiation recurrent, hormone refractory prostate cancer: a preliminary report. Br J Radiol 74:745–751

Kanthabalan A, Shah T, Arya M et al (2015) The FORECAST study – focal recurrent assessment and salvage treatment for radiorecurrent prostate cancer. Contemp Clin Trials [epub ahead of print]

Kimura M, Mouraviev V, Tsivian M, Mayes JM, Satoh T, Polascik TJ (2010) Current salvage methods for recurrent prostate cancer after failure of primary radiotherapy. BJU Int 150:191–201

Klotz L, Zhang L, Lam A, Nam R, Mamedov A, Loblaw A (2010) Clinical results of long-term follow-up of a large, active surveillance cohort with localized prostate cancer. J Clin Oncol 28:126–131

Klotz L, Vesprini D, Sethukavalan P et al (2015) Long-term follow-up of a large active surveillance cohort of patients with prostate cancer. J Clin Oncol 33:272–277

Koutrouvelis P, Hendricks F, Lailas N et al (2003) Salvage reimplantation in patient with local recurrent prostate carcinoma after brachytherapy with three dimensional computed tomography-guided permanent pararectal implant. Technol Cancer Res Treat 2:339–344

Kovacs G, Potter R, Loch T et al (2005) GEC/ESTRO-EAU recommendations on temporary brachytherapy using stepping sources for localised prostate cancer. Radiother Oncol 74:137–148

Lee B, Shinohara K, Weinberg V et al (2007) Feasibility of high-dose-rate brachytherapy salvage for local prostate cancer recurrence after radiotherapy: the University of California-San Francisco experience. Int J Radiat Oncol Biol Phys 67:1106–1112

Lee KL, Adams MT, Motta J (2008) Salvage prostate brachytherapy for localized prostate cancer failure after external beam radiation therapy. Brachytherapy 7:17–21

Leibovici D, Chiong E, Pisters LL et al (2012) Pathological characteristics of prostate cancer recurrence after radiation therapy: implications for focal salvage therapy. J Urol 188:98–102

Li YH, Elshafei A, Agarwal G, Ruckle H, Powsang J, Jones JS (2015) Salvage focal prostate cryoablation for locally recurrent prostate cancer after radiotherapy: initial results from the cryo on-line data registry. Prostate 75:1–7

Lo K, Stock RG, Stone NN (2005) Salvage prostate brachytherapy following radiotherapy failure. Int J Radiat Oncol Biol Phys 63:S290–S291

Loening SA, Turner JW (1993) Use of percutaneous transperineal 198Au seeds to treat recurrent prostate adenocarcinoma after failure of definitive radiotherapy. Prostate 23:283–290

Master VA, Shinohara K, Carroll PR (2004) Ferromagnetic thermal ablation of locally recurrent prostate cancer: prostate specific antigen results and immediate/intermediate morbidities. J Urol 172:2197–2202

Menard C, Iupati D, Publicover J et al (2015) MR-guided prostate biopsy for planning of focal salvage after radiation therapy. Radiology 274:181–191

Moman MR, Van der Poel HG, Battermann JJ, Moerland MA, van Vulpen M (2009) Treatment outcome and toxicity after salvage 125-I implantation for prostate cancer recurrences after primary 125-I implantation and external beam radiotherapy. Brachytherapy 9:119–125

Moman MR, van den Berg CA et al (2010) Focal salvage guided by T2 weighted and dynamic contrast enhanced magnetic resonance imaging for prostate cancer recurrences. Int J Radiat Oncol Biol Phys 76:741–746

Moore CM, Robertson NL, Arsanious N et al (2013) Image-guided prostate biopsy using magnetic resonance imaging-derived targets: a systematic review. Eur Urol 63:125–140

Morton GC, Hoskin PJ (2013) Brachytherapy: current status and future strategies – can high dose rate replace low dose rate and external beam radiotherapy? Clin Oncol (R Coll Radiol) 25:474–482

Mostofi F, Davis C, Sesterhenn I (1992) Pathology of carcinoma of the prostate. Cancer 70:235–253

Murat FJ, Poissonnier L, Rabilloud M et al (2009) Mid-term results demonstrate salvage high-intensity focused ultrasound (HIFU) as an effective and acceptably morbid salvage treatment option for locally radio-recurrent prostate cancer. Eur Urol 55(3):640–647

Nguyen PL, Chen MH, D'Amico AV et al (2007a) Magnetic resonance image-guided salvage brachytherapy after radiation in select men who initially presented with favorable-risk prostate cancer: a prospective phase 2 study. Cancer 110:4185–4192

Nguyen PL, D'Amico AV, Lee AK, Suh WW (2007b) Patient selection, cancer control, and complications after salvage local therapy for postradiation prostate-specific antigen failure: a systematic review of the literature. Cancer 110:1417–1428

Nguyen PL, Chen MH, Clark JA, Cormack RA, Loffredo M, McMahon E, Nguyen AU, Suh W, Tempany CM, D'Amico AV (2009) Patient-reported quality of life after salvage brachytherapy for radio-recurrent prostate cancer: a prospective phase II study. Brachytherapy 8:345–352

Nguyen PL, Alibhai SM, Basaria S et al (2015) Adverse effects of androgen deprivation therapy and strategies to mitigate them. Eur Urol 67:825–836

Onik G, Miessau M, Bostwick DG (2009) Three-dimensional prostate mapping biopsy has a potentially significant impact on prostate cancer management. J Clin Oncol 27:4321–4326

Onur R, Littrup PJ, Pontes JE, Bianco FJ Jr (2004) Contemporary impact of transrectal ultrasound lesions for prostate cancer detection. J Urol 172:512–514

Paparel P, Cronin AM, Savage C, Scardino PT, Eastham JA (2009) Oncologic outcome and patterns of recurrence after salvage radical prostatectomy. Eur Urol 55:404–410

Peters M, Moman MR, van der Poel HG et al (2013) Patterns of outcome and toxicity after salvage prostatectomy, salvage cryosurgery and salvage brachytherapy for prostate cancer recurrences after radiation therapy: a multi-center experience and literature review. World J Urol 31:403–409

Peters M, Maenhout M, van der Voort van Zyp JR et al. (2014) Focal salvage iodine-125 brachytherapy for prostate cancer recurrences after primary radiotherapy: a retrospective study regarding toxicity, biochemical outcome and quality of life. Radiother Oncol 112:77–82

Peters M, Van der Voort van Zyp J, Hoekstra C et al (2015) Urethral and bladder dosimetry of total and focal salvage Iodine-125 prostate brachytherapy: Late toxicity and dose constraints. Radiother Oncol 117(2):262–269

Peters M, Hoekstra C, van der Voort van Zyp J et al (2016) Rectal dose constraints for salvage iodine-125 prostate brachytherapy. Brachytherapy 15:85–93

Pisters LL, English SF, Scott SM et al (2000) Salvage prostatectomy with continent catheterizable urinary reconstruction: a novel approach to recurrent prostate cancer after radiation therapy. J Urol 163:1771–1774

Pound CR, Brawer MK, Partin AW (2001) Evaluation and treatment of men with biochemical prostate-specific antigen recurrence following definitive therapy for clinically localized prostate cancer. Rev Urol 3:72–84

Prestigiacomo AF, Stamey TA (1996) Physiological variation of serum prostate specific antigen in the 4.0 to 10.0 Ng/ml range in male volunteers. J Urol 155:1977–1980

Pucar D, Sella T, Schoder H (2008) The role of imaging in the detection of prostate cancer local recurrence after radiation therapy and surgery. Curr Opin Urol 18:87–97

Roach M III, Hanks G, Thames H Jr, Schellhammer P, Shipley WU, Sokol GH et al (2006) Defining biochemical failure following radiotherapy with or without hormonal therapy in men with clinically localized prostate cancer: recommendations of the RTOG-ASTRO Phoenix consensus conference. Int J Radiat Oncol Biol Phys 65:965–974

Rouviere O, Valette O, Grivolat S et al (2004) Recurrent prostate cancer after external beam radiotherapy: value of contrast-enhanced dynamic MRI in localizing intraprostatic tumor–correlation with biopsy findings. Urology 63:922–927

Rybalov M, Ananias HJK, Hoving HD (2014) PSMA, EpCAM, VEGF and GRPR as imaging targets in locally recurrent prostate cancer after radiotherapy. Int J Mol Sci 15:6046–6061

Sanderson KM, Penson DF, Cai J et al (2006) Salvage radical prostatectomy: quality of life outcomes and long-term oncological control of radiorecurrent prostate cancer. J Urol 176:2025–2031

Sasaki H, Kido M, Miki K et al (2013) Salvage partial brachytherapy for prostate cancer recurrence after primary brachytherapy. Int J Urol 21:572–577

Scardino PT (1983) The prognostic significance of biopsies after radiotherapy for prostatic cancer. Semin Urol 1:243–252

Sheets NC, Goldin GH, Meyer AM et al (2012) Intensity-modulated radiation therapy, proton therapy, or conformal radiation therapy and morbidity and disease control in localized prostate cancer. JAMA 307:1611–1620

Siddiqui MM, Rais-Bahrami S, Turkbey B et al (2015) Comparison of MR/ultrasound fusion-guided biopsy with ultrasound-guided biopsy for the diagnosis of prostate cancer. JAMA 313:390–397

Sivaraman A, Sanchez-Salas R, Barret E (2015) Transperineal template-guided mapping biopsy of the prostate. Int J Urol 22:146–151

Spiess PE, Katz AE, Chin JL et al (2010) A pretreatment nomogram predicting biochemical failure after salvage cryotherapy for locally recurrent prostate cancer. BJU Int 106:194–198

Stephenson AJ, Scardino PT, Bianco FJ et al (2004) Morbidity and functional outcomes of salvage radical prostatectomy for locally recurrent prostate cancer after radiation therapy. J Urol 172:2239–2243

Tran H, Kwok J, Pickles T, Tyldesley S, Black PC (2014) Underutilization of local salvage therapy after radiation therapy for prostate cancer. Urol Oncol 32:701–706

Umbehr MH, Muntener M, Hany T, Sulser T, Bachmann LM (2013) The role of 11C-choline and 18Ffluorocholine positron emission tomography (PET) and PET/CT in prostate cancer: a systematic review and meta-analysis. Eur Urol 64:106–117

Vaidya A, Soloway MS (2000) Salvage radical prostatectomy for radiorecurrent prostate cancer: morbidity revisited. J Urol 164:1998–2001

Valerio M, Anele C, Charman SC et al (2015) Transperineal template prostate mapping biopsies: an evaluation of different protocols in detection of clinically significant prostate cancer. BJU Int [epub ahead of print]

Van den Bos W, Muller BG, de Bruin DM (2015) Salvage ablative therapy in prostate cancer: international multidisciplinary consensus on trial design. Urol Oncol 33:495.e1–495.e7

Van der Heide UA, Dehnad H, Hofman P, Kotte ANTJ, Lagendijk JJW, Van Vulpen M (2007) Analysis of fiducial marker based position verification in the intensity-modulated radiotherapy of patients with prostate cancer. Radiother Oncol 82:38–45

Van der Poel HG, Beetsma DB, van Boven H et al (2007) Perineal salvage prostatectomy for radiation resistant prostate cancer. Eur Urol 51:1565–1571

Wallner KE, Nori D, Morse MJ et al (1990) 125iodine reimplantation for locally progressive prostatic carcinoma. J Urol 144:704–706

Wang H, Vees H, Miralbell R, Wissmeyer M, Steiner C, Ratib O, Senthamizhchelvan S, Zaidi H (2009) 18F-fluorocholine PET-guided target volume delineation techniques for partial prostate re-irradiation in local recurrent prostate cancer. Radiother Oncol 93:220–225

Ward JF, Sebo TJ, Blute ML et al (2005) Salvage surgery for radiorecurrent prostate cancer: contemporary outcomes. J Urol 173:1156–1160

Ward JF, Pagliaro LC, Pisters LL et al (2008) Salvage therapy for radiorecurrent prostate cancer. Curr Probl Cancer 32(6):242–271

Wenske S, Quarrier S, Katz AE (2013) Salvage cryosurgery of the prostate for failure after primary radiotherapy or cryosurgery: long-term clinical, functional, and oncologic outcomes in a large cohort at a tertiary referral centre. Eur Urol 64:1–7

Williams AK, Martinez CH, Lu C, Ng CK, Pautler SE, Chin JL (2011) Disease-free survival following salvage cryotherapy for biopsy-proven radio-recurrent prostate cancer. Eur Urol 60:405–410

Wong WW, Buskirk SJ, Schild SE et al (2006) Combined prostate brachytherapy and short-term androgen deprivation therapy as salvage therapy for locally recurrent prostate cancer after external beam irradiation. J Urol 176:2020–2024

Yamada Y, Kollmeier MA, Pei X et al (2014) A phase II study of salvage high-dose-rate brachytherapy for the treatment of locally recurrent prostate cancer after definitive external beam radiotherapy. Brachytherapy 13:111–116

Zagars GK, Pollack A (1997) Kinetics of serum prostate-specific antigen after external beam radiation for clinically localized prostate cancer. Radiother Oncol 44:213–221

Zelefsky MJ, Ben-Porat L, Scher HI et al (2005) Outcome predictors for the increasing PSA state after definitive external-beam radiotherapy for prostate cancer. J Clin Oncol 23:826–831

Zelefsky MJ, Kuban DA, Levy LB, Potters L, Beyer DC, Blasko JC et al (2007) Multi-institutional analysis of long-term outcome for stages T1–T2 prostate cancer treated with permanent seed implantation. Int J Radiat Oncol Biol Phys 67:327–333

Zietman AL, Tibbs MK, Dallow KC et al (1996) Use of PSA nadir to predict subsequent biochemical outcome following external beam radiation therapy for T1-2 adenocarcinoma of the prostate. Radiother Oncol 40:159–162

Zumsteg ZS, Spratt DE, Romesser PB et al (2015) The natural history and predictors of outcome following biochemical relapse in the dose escalation era for prostate cancer patients undergoing definitive external beam radiotherapy. Eur Urol 67:1009–1016

Rectal Cancer

Mariangela Massaccesi and Vincenzo Valentini

Contents

Abstract

Reirradiation combined with chemotherapy for patients developing recurrent rectal cancer after radiation or chemoradiation is feasible and provides high chances for cure and palliation. Nearly one-half of patients with resected disease achieve long-term control of pelvic disease, and up to 65% of them can have long-term (5-year) survival. Even in unresected patients, long-term control can be achieved in about 20% of cases with one out of five patients surviving after 5 years.

Acute and late toxicity are not prohibitive if proper attention is paid to both radiation technique and surgical technique. The use of small radiation fields, exclusion of the bowel and bladder, and the use of hyperfractionated radiation doses up to 40 Gy are recommended.

Since most of treatment failures occur within the radiation treatment field, future studies should investigate methods to further improve local control. In view of the fact that about one-half of surviving patients will develop distant metastases, innovative strategies for reduction of distant metastases should also be explored.

1 Introduction

Reirradiation for rectal cancer can be considered for two patient groups: patients who develop locoregional recurrence after previous pre- or

The original version of this chapter was revised. An erratum to this chapter can be found at 10.1007/978-3-319-41825-4_78.

M. Massaccesi • V. Valentini (✉)
Radiation Oncology Department – Gemelli ART, Università Cattolica del Sacro Cuore, Rome, Italy
e-mail: vincenzo.valentini@unicatt.it

Med Radiol Radiat Oncol (2016)
DOI 10.1007/174_2016_67, © Springer International Publishing Switzerland
Published Online: 26 Jul 2016

postoperative radiation, and patients with newly diagnosed rectal cancer who have received previous pelvic irradiation for other malignancies (e.g. prostate and gynaecological cancers). In this chapter we will focus on the reirradiation of local recurrence.

Locally recurrent rectal cancer (LRRC) is a devastating condition causing severe symptoms, including pelvic pain, bleeding and bowel obstruction in over two-third of patients. These distressful symptoms can cause a loss of quality of life (QoL). LRRC includes recurrence, progression or development of new sites of rectal tumour(s) within the pelvis after previous resection of rectal cancer (Beyond TME Collaborative 2013). Pelvic recurrence includes anastomotic recurrence, as well as recurrence within lymphatics such as residual mesorectal nodes and pelvic sidewall lymph nodes. Also included is inguinal node recurrence and disease manifesting along drain tracts and surgical scars (abdominal or perineal).

Local recurrence may be isolated or combined (local and metastasis). Patient prognosis is generally poor with a median overall survival without treatment of only 3.5–13.0 months (Saito et al. 2003).

The introduction of total mesorectal excision (TME) (Enker et al. 1995; Heald 1995; MacFarlane et al. 1993) together with neoadjuvant radio- and chemotherapy dramatically reduced LRRC rates from 20 to 30 % (Swedish Rectal Cancer Trial 1996; Goldberg et al. 1994) to 6–10 % (Rödel et al. 2015; Gérard et al. 2012). However, due to the high incidence of rectal cancer, still a high absolute number of patients present with recurrent rectal carcinomas. The management strategy in this cohort of patients is complex, with a number of options including surgery, with or without radiotherapy with either curative or palliative intent, with or without chemotherapy. Delay in diagnosis is common, and inequalities exist in referral patterns based on geography, with no clear clinical guidelines (Beyond TME Collaborative 2013).

Surgical excision of LRRC is the most significant measure used to improve survival. Particularly complete surgical resection (R0 resection) remains the only potentially curative treatment with reported 5-year survival rates in selected patients of up to 50 %. However, only 40–50 % of all patients with LRRC can undergo surgery with curative intent, and of those, 30–45 % will have R0 resection. Thus, only 20–30 % of all patients with LRRC have a potentially curative operation (Nielsen et al. 2011). Furthermore, to achieve cure most patients require extended, multivisceral, exenterative surgery, beyond conventional total mesorectal excision planes with high morbidity rates of 40–82 % (Haddock et al. 2011; Nielsen et al. 2012; Harji et al. 2013). Preoperative radiotherapy can provide higher chances of complete resection and local control (Vermaas et al. 2005; Rödel et al. 2000) potentially allowing less extensive surgical resections. In conjunction with fluoropyrimidine-based chemotherapy, preoperative radiotherapy is widely recognized as the most appropriate treatment option in patients with LRRC who have not received prior radiotherapy (Konski et al. 2012).

Although local recurrence rates have decreased, an increasing proportion of patients with LRRC have previously received high-dose pelvic radiotherapy as part of the primary multimodality treatment, either as preoperative short-course radiotherapy (5 × 5 Gy) or as chemoradiotherapy to 45–50 Gy (1.8–2.0 Gy/fraction). The prognosis for patients with LRRC seems to be worse in previously irradiated patients than in those without prior irradiation (Rombouts et al. 2015; van den Brink et al. 2004). Recurrences after neoadjuvant irradiation may represent a selection of patients with very unfavourable tumour characteristics. As an example, more than two-third of patients with LRRC after preoperative radiotherapy have also distant metastases at the time of recurrence as compared to less than half of patients with LRRC after surgery only (van den Brink et al. 2004). It has been observed that patients with LRRC who have received prior neoadjuvant radiotherapy and TME have a higher rate of incomplete resection of the recurrence (Alberda et al. 2014; van den Brink et al. 2004). In addition LRRC in patients treated with radiotherapy for the primary tumour may evolve from radiation-insensitive tumour deposits, rendering reirradiation less effective.

However, several recent observations and trials have demonstrated the safety and efficacy of reirradiation in patients with LRRC who previously underwent irradiation to the pelvis (Mohiuddin et al. 1993, 1997, 2002; Lingareddy et al. 1997; Valentini et al. 1999, 2006; Das et al. 2010; Sun et al. 2012; Koom et al. 2012; Ng et al. 2013; Bosman et al. 2014). Reirradiation might increase the rate of preservation of surrounding organs and radical (R0) resection and provide symptom palliation or long-term local control for inoperable tumours (Guren et al. 2014). However, reirradiation of infield recurrences can also aggravate the late radiation toxicities of adjacent tissue (including small bowel, bladder, etc.) and the complications of surgery. Therefore, the expected benefits in terms of achieving R0 surgery and long-term survival and/or symptom palliation should be weighed against the potential morbidity caused by retreatment.

Because LRRC presents a challenging problem, the international consensus statement by the Beyond TME Collaborative Group (2013) on the management of patients with LRRC clearly identified the need for referral of patients with LRRC to a specialist multidisciplinary team (MDT) for diagnosis, assessment and further management. The subspecialized MDT requires oncological, radiological, surgical and pathological expertise in pelvic exenteration.

2 Diagnosis and Staging of LRRC

Early diagnosis of the recurrence in potential surgical candidates is critical as it increases the likelihood of curative (R0) resection and prevention of dissemination; therefore, different follow-up strategies have been developed (Figueredo et al. 2003; Zitt et al. 2006). The timeframe for recurrence is typically within the first 2 years after resection of the primary tumour (Palmer et al. 2007). However in almost 30 % of patients with locally advanced rectal cancers treated by preoperative chemoradiation, the time to detection of local recurrence (LR) can be longer than 5 years (Coco et al. 2006). Existing nomograms to predict local recurrence can aid the selection of follow-up type and intensity (Valentini et al. 2011; van Gijn et al. 2015).

Regarding the pattern of LRRC in terms of location within the pelvis, in recent years, a subtle change has been observed. In general terms, in the pre-TME years, most recurrences were central, perianastomotic and anterior, whereas since the adoption of combined therapies, lateral and posterior (presacral) forms dominate (Enríquez-Navascués et al. 2011). With conventional surgical techniques, segments of the mesorectum could be left behind, and local recurrences in the remaining part were not uncommon, often being located in the anastomotic region (Palmer et al. 2007). After TME surgery, presacral LRs are the most common type of LR, and due to prior surgery, tumour growth is not confined to a specific compartment lined by fascias, because these fascias have been damaged during the primary surgery (Dresen et al. 2008). Furthermore it has been observed that while preoperative RT helps to prevent LRs at all sites, it is especially effective in preventing anastomotic recurrences (Mohiuddin and Marks 1993).

Many factors affect the risk of local recurrence. The involvement of circumferential resection margin (CRM) is the most important factor (Quirke et al. 1986). The pelvic recurrence rate is also tumour-stage dependent (Sagar and Pemberton 1996). The combination of risk factors is also important: in patients with T1-T2 stage, the incidence of LR is 1 % with a negative CRM but this rises to 12 % for a positive CRM, while for those with T3-T4 tumour, it is 15 % for a negative CRM but 25 % for a positive CRM (Kusters et al. 2010). A poor pathologic response and downstaging to preoperative chemoradiation is also a negative prognostic marker for LR (Rödel et al. 2005). Anatomical site of the tumour is also another critical factor; indeed LR is more likely with tumours in the lower third of the rectum (10–15 %) than in patients with tumours in either the middle third (5–10 %) or upper third (2–5 %) (MacFarlane et al. 1993; Kusters et al. 2010). The risk of LR is also related to the position of the tumour within the circumference of the rectum, being higher for tumours affecting the anterior side of the rectum than for other locations (Chan et al. 2006). Other factors that can influence the risk of local recurrence are the shape (exophytic versus non-exophytic) of the tumour, the presence or absence of budding, lymphatic, venous or perineural invasion, the presence of obstruction or perforation, the degree of tumour differentiation and the fixity of the tumour (Sagar and Pemberton 1996).

Clinical examination, tumour markers and radiologic modalities such as ultrasonography (US), computed tomography (CT), magnetic resonance (MR) and positron emission tomography (PET) are routinely used in follow-up. CT is the most commonly used modality for identification of pelvic recurrence, but it has poor accuracy in distinguishing between scar tissue and tumour (Grabbe and Winkler 1985), and this becomes even more difficult if radiotherapy has previously been applied (Heriot et al. 2006). Compared with CT, MR can more accurately differentiate recurrent cancer within a presacral scar, based on differences in signal intensity between tumour and fibrosis using T2-weighted sequences or contrast-enhanced imaging techniques (Dicle et al. 1999). Thus high-resolution MR with a sensitivity of 80–90 % and a specificity as high as 100 % (Lambregts et al. 2011) is generally regarded as the optimum modality for imaging the pelvis in patients with suspected LRRC. Differently from fibrosis, which appears hypointense on T2-weighted MR images, recurrent tumours typically display higher signal intensity than that of muscle. Moreover, tumours tend to have contrast enhancement greater than 40 % of the volume of a mass or a typical rim-enhancement pattern after gadolinium contrast material administration (Messiou et al. 2008).

However, benign fibrotic scarring, malignant local tumour recurrence and inflammation can all enhance after the administration of a gadolinium-based contrast agent (Tan et al. 2005). Furthermore, a tumour with significant fibrosis can cause low signal intensity on T2-weighted images. PET is an accurate diagnostic tool and may have advantages over CT and MR in discriminating fibrosis from cancer (Huebner et al. 2000), although false-negative results can occur in small deposits or in mucinous tumours. An increase in serum carcinoembryonic antigen (CEA) level may assist in reaching a diagnosis, although a spuriously high or low result can be confusing (Tan et al. 2009).

Given these limitations, the ideal for diagnosis of LRRC still remains tissue biopsy. Where tissue biopsy is not possible or is negative, serial enlargement of a lesion accompanied by either positive PET-CT or rising CEA level and specialist MDT opinion suggestive of malignancy can be accepted for diagnosis (Beyond TME Collaborative 2013).

The management of patients with LRRC mainly depends on the type and extent of recurrence. Therefore, radiologic assessments are used to determine whether recurrent disease is limited to the pelvis or has metastasized, and to outline the local extent of recurrent disease and its distribution within the pelvis to help surgeons determine the feasibility of resection and plan the optimal surgical approach.

A meta-analysis investigating the value of US, CT, MR and PET in detecting liver metastases demonstrated sensitivity of 63 %, 75 %, 81 % and 97 %, respectively, and high specificity (Floriani et al. 2010). Particularly PET with ^{18}F-fluoro-deoxy-glucose has been demonstrated to be highly accurate in the detection of disseminated disease (Ogunbiyi et al. 1997). PET has also been shown to have a high impact on the management of patients with suspected recurrent colorectal cancer (Kalff et al. 2002).

The identification of patients who can potentially achieve a R0 resection is crucial and extremely difficult. Resection margin status is an independent prognostic factor for re-recurrence rate and overall survival in surgically treated, locally recurrent rectal cancer. In the complete resection group, patients with tumour-free resection margins of 0–2 mm have a higher re-recurrence rate and a poorer overall survival than patients with tumour-free resection margins of >2 mm (Alberda et al. 2015). Preoperative imaging and clinical assessment are utilized in an effort to optimize the selection of patients in whom curative resection is considered possible. Although MR imaging has proved to be the preferred first-choice staging modality for primary rectal cancer, its performance for predicting tumour extent in patients with local recurrence could be impaired by the fibrosis after surgery and adjuvant therapies. In a retrospective analysis of 40 consecutive patients with locally recurrent rectal cancer, Dresen et al. (2010) found that although the positive predictive value of MR imaging was low (53–85 %) especially at the lateral pelvic side walls, MR was highly accurate for the prediction of the absence of tumour invasion into pelvic structures with negative predictive values of 93–100 %. Therefore, preoperative MR imaging in patients with LRRC could be a useful diagnostic tool for the identification of the absence of tumour invasion into pelvic structures.

2.1 Classification of LRRC

Although several classifications have been proposed to assess LRRC resectability (Table 1), at the moment no classification system is universally shared. Such a lack of a standard classification of LRRC strongly impairs the possibility of interpreting results and comparing between different series. Indeed, in addition to assisting decision-making regarding the potential for and the extent of resection, classification has also an important prognostic value.

In a recent prospective study by the Royal Marsden Hospital, a new classification is described based on the extent of tumour invasion in each of seven intrapelvic compartments, as seen on preoperative pelvic MR imaging (Georgiou et al. 2013). These correspond to the fascial boundaries and planes of dissection between the pelvic organs, and are described as central (C), posterior (P), inferior (I), anterior above (AA) and anterior below (AB) the peritoneal reflection and lateral (L) and peritoneal reflection (PR). Such a MR-based classification system is particularly promising, since it allows for better understanding of tumour invasion within the pelvis, hence contributing to optimal surgical planning.

3 The Role of Surgery in LRRC

Resectability in recurrent rectal cancer can be defined as the ability to complete a surgical resection with a microscopically clear margin (R0) and acceptable postoperative morbidity and mortality. According to the recent consensus statement by the Beyond TME Collaborative Group (2013), absolute contraindications to resectability include bilateral sciatic nerve involvement and circumferential bone involvement. Benefits of surgery are unclear when the tumour extends through the sciatic notch, or encases the external iliac vessels or involves the sacrum above the S2/3 junction or irresectable distant metastases are present.

There are three broad pelvic site patterns that determine resectability: (i) central recurrence, (ii) sacral recurrence and (iii) lateral recurrence. For central recurrences, if the recurrence does not involve any of the anterior genitourinary structures, an abdominoperineal resection (APR) of the anus and neorectum is occasionally possible. Where there is involvement of the anterior urogenital structures, an extended multivisceral resection is required to achieve a R0 resection. When posterior structures are involved, more extended radical resections are often necessary. Where bony invasion is present, an R0 resection is only possible with a sacral resection. Recurrence involving the lateral pelvic sidewall is associated with the poorest chance of achieving an R0 resection (Moore et al. 2004). Wound healing is frequently impaired after previous chemoradiotherapy, and in selected patients, optimal healing is best achieved using a variety of pedicled flaps.

A summary of outcomes of exenterative surgery for LRRC from contemporary studies has been recently provided by Renehan (2016). R0 resection rates are about 50 % (range 38–62 %) (Ferenschild et al. 2009; Bhangu et al. 2014; Nielsen et al. 2012) with almost half of patients requiring sacrectomy. Less than half of patients remain free from disease at long term, with reported 3-year disease-free survival of 22 % (Nielsen et al. 2012) and 50 % (Bhangu et al. 2014) in two different series.

Table 1 Classifications systems in use for locally recurrent rectal cancer

Study group	Classification	Definitions	
Mayo Clinic (Suzuki et al. 1996)	Symptoms	S0	Asymptomatic
		S1	Symptomatic without pain
		S2	Symptomatic with pain
	Degree and site of fixation	F0	No fixation
		F1	Fixation to 1 point
		F2	Fixation to 2 points
		F3	Fixation to > 2 points
Yamada et al. (2001)	Pattern of pelvic fixation	Localized	Invasion to the adjacent pelvic organs or tissue
		Sacral invasive	Invasion to lower sacrum (S3, S4, S5), coccyx, periosteum
		Lateral invasive	Invasion to sciatic nerve, greater sciatic foramen, lateral pelvic wall, upper sacrum (S1, S2)
Wanebo et al. (1999)	Five stages	TR1	Limited invasion of the muscularis
		TR2	Full-thickness penetration of the muscularispropria
		TR3	Anastomotic recurrences with full-thickness penetration beyond the bowel wall and into the perirectal soft tissue
		TR4	Invasion into adjacent organs without fixation
		TR5	Invasion of the bony ligamentous pelvic including sacrum, pelvic/sidewalls or sacrotuberous/ischial ligaments
Memorial Sloan-Kettering (Moore et al. 2004)	Anatomical region involved	Axial	Anastomotic, mesorectal, perirectal soft tissue, perineum (APER)
		Anterior	Genitourinary tract
		Posterior	Sacrum and presacral fascia
		Lateral	Soft tissues of the pelvic sidewall and the lateral bony pelvis

Leeds	Anatomical region involved	Central	Tumour confined to pelvic organs or connective tissue without contact with or invasion into the bone
		Sacral	Tumour present in the presacral space and abuts on to or invades into sacrum
		Sidewall	Tumour involving the structures on lateral pelvic sidewall, including greater sciatic foramen and sciatic nerve through to piriformis and gluteal region
		Composite	Sacral and sidewall recurrence combined
Royal Marsden Hospital (Georgiou et al. 2013)	MRI; planes of dissection	C	Rectum or neorectum, intraluminal recurrence, perirectal fat or mesorectum, extraluminal recurrence
		PR	Rectovesical pouch or rectouterine pouch of Douglas
		AA PR	Ureters and iliac vessels above the peritoneal reflection, sigmoid colon, small bowel and lateral sidewall fascia
		AB PR	Genitourinary system
		L	Ureters, external and internal iliac vessels, lateral pelvic lymph nodes, sciatic nerve, sciatic notch, S1 and S2 nerve roots, piriformis or obturator internus muscle
		P	Coccyx, presacral fascia, retrosacral space, sacrum up to the upper level of S1
		I	Levator ani muscles, external sphincter complex, perineal scar (APER), ischioanal fossa

Modified from the Beyond TME Collaborative (2013) Consensus

APER abdominoperineal resection, *MRI* magnetic resonance imaging, *C* central, *PR* peritoneal reflection, *AA* anterior above, *AB* anterior below, *L* lateral, *P* posterior, *I* inferior

The morbidity and mortality rate can be as high as 60 % (range 25–60 %) and 8 % (range 0–8 %), respectively.

The complication rate might be higher in patients who undergo multivisceral resection versus those having single organ resection (Gezen et al. 2012).

Morbidity and mortality rate might be higher for more extended surgical procedures. For example, sacrectomy (compared with other operations) was associated with significantly higher mean blood loss, longer duration of surgery and longer length of stay. Cystectomy (compared with no cystectomy) was associated with longer duration of surgery. Perineal flap reconstruction (compared with primary closure or nonflap reconstruction) was associated with a longer mean operating time and a longer mean length of stay (Bhangu et al. 2014).

Unfortunately, only one-third to one-half of LRRCs will be resectable with conventional surgical procedures; the rest will require extended radical resection with removal of surrounding organs, to achieve clean margins. Optimizing patients before multivisceral resection is vital to minimize perioperative morbidity, requires a multispecialist approach and may best be achieved by formal cardiopulmonary testing (Beyond TME Collaborative 2013).

4 The Role of Reirradiation in LRRC

Neoadjuvant external beam radiation up to a dose of 50.4 Gy with concurrent chemotherapy is the standard of care for patients with LRRC who have not received any radiotherapy, since it has been demonstrated to improve the local control (Vermaas et al. 2005; Dresen et al. 2008). Indeed neoadjuvant long-course chemoradiotherapy has the potential to increase the resectability rate of delayed surgery in LRRC from 29.2 to 64.9 % (Dresen et al. 2008) and, by downstaging the tumour, may theoretically allow for less-extended surgical operations. In general, recurrent rectal cancers are treatment-resistant tumours. In a recent study at the Royal Marsden Hospital, only 9 % of patients with LRRC had a pathologic complete response compared to 17 % of patients with locally advanced primary tumour after long-course chemoradiation (Yu et al. 2014). Recurrent rectal cancer after previous irradiation might be even more radio resistant due to the possible origin from radio-resistant clones. Reirradiation is also challenging, because the surrounding normal tissues may have already received doses near the organ- or endpoint-specific tolerance dose during the primary treatment. Therefore reirradiation has been generally discouraged for the fear of prohibitive normal tissue complications, particularly of the small intestine and bladder. However, there is increasing evidence in clinical studies that reirradiation is tolerable and yields good results. Particularly in a recently published study including a large number of patients with LRRC, reirradiated patients had almost the same R0 resection rate and long-term local disease control as those who received full-course irradiation for the first time. Furthermore, despite more extensive surgical procedures in the reirradiation group, reflecting more advanced disease, no significant difference was noted in the rate of complications between the two treatment groups (Bosman et al. 2014).

Intraoperative radiation therapy might also represent a useful technique for these patients, with the possibility of precisely delivering a large single dose (10–20 Gy) to the surgically defined recurrence site and avoiding the surrounding normal tissues (Gunderson et al. 1996; Mannaerts et al. 2001).

A recent systematic review suggests that only 40 % of unselected consecutive patients with locally recurrent rectal cancer are candidates for intentionally curative treatment (Tanis et al. 2013). Surgical resection should be evaluated in all instances of isolated LRRC. However, in some cases, a resection is not possible, or medical reasons such as concomitant illnesses restrain the surgeon from surgical interventions. In other cases, surgery is performed, but a gross resection is not possible, and macroscopic tumour remains, which requires adjuvant treatment. The remaining patients with isolated LRRC might benefit from image-guided stereotactic radiotherapy,

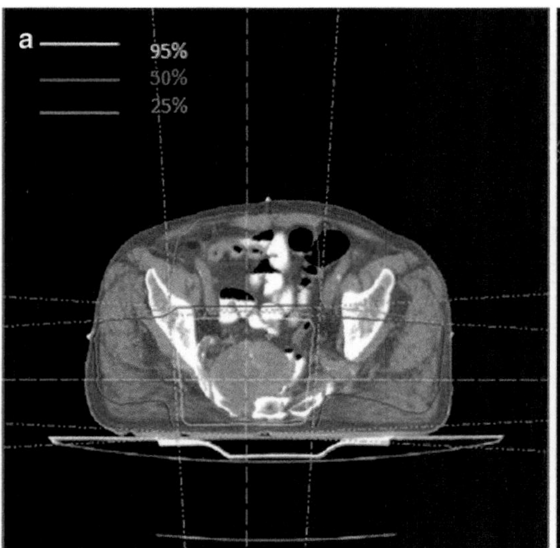

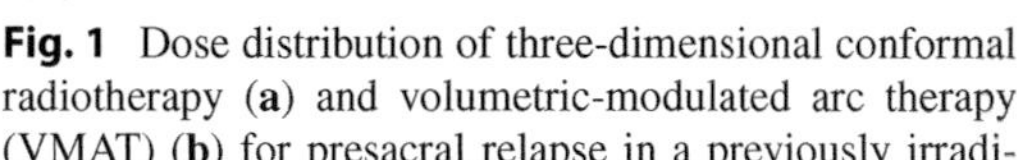
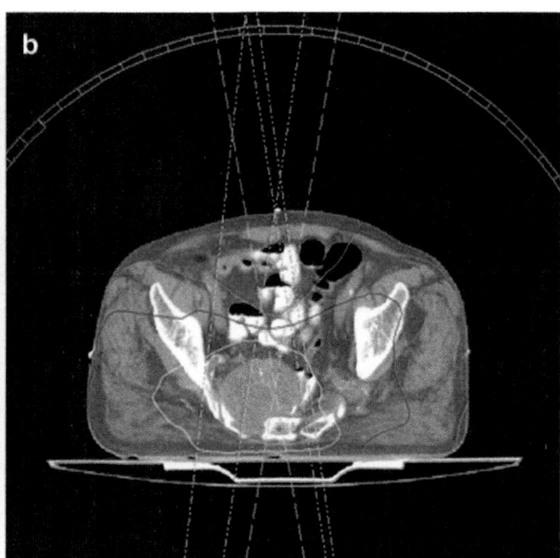

Fig. 1 Dose distribution of three-dimensional conformal radiotherapy (**a**) and volumetric-modulated arc therapy (VMAT) (**b**) for presacral relapse in a previously irradiated rectal cancer patient, showing small bowel sparing with VMAT

brachytherapy or particle beam radiotherapy with the aim of achieving both palliation and long-term local control (Combs et al. 2012).

4.1 Long-Course Reirradiation

The effects of conventional external beam reirradiation in terms of feasibility, toxicity and long-term outcomes in previously irradiated LRRCs were the subject of a recent systematic review (Guren et al. 2014) which included ten publications describing seven patient cohorts/ studies for a total of 375 patients (range 13–103) (Mohiuddin et al. 1993, 1997, 2002; Lingareddy et al. 1997; Valentini et al. 1999, 2006; Das et al. 2010; Koom et al. 2012; Sun et al. 2012; Ng et al. 2013). Most studies were retrospectively designed, with highly variable therapies, patient populations and duration of follow-up. Median time since previous RT in different series ranged between 8 and 30 months and was longer than 24 months in most series. Reirradiation for rectal cancer was mostly given with hyperfractionated chemoradiotherapy to total doses of 30–40 Gy, although higher doses have been explored (range 23.4–50.2 Gy). EQD2Gy ($\alpha/\beta = 3$ Gy) of previous irradiation ranged between 43.2 and 51.8 Gy3 with an estimated cumulative EQD2Gy with retreatment ranging between 71.9 and 101.7 Gy3 (Guren et al. 2014).

In older series, reirradiation was generally given by opposed lateral or three fields with a shrinking field technique, encompassing the presacral region or posterior pelvis (as prophylaxis for subclinical disease) and the gross tumour volume plus a margin of 1–4 cm (usually 2 cm) followed by a boost to the gross tumour volume (plus margin) only (Mohiuddin et al. 1993, 1997, 2002; Lingareddy et al. 1997; Valentini et al. 1999). In newer studies, reirradiation was delivered by multiple fields with a three-dimensional conformal or intensity-modulated technique, and the treatment volumes encompassed the gross tumour only with a 2-cm GTV to PTV margin (Valentini et al. 2006; Das et al. 2010; Koom et al. 2012; Sun et al. 2012; Ng et al. 2013).

Figure 1 shows the possibility of small bowel sparing with intensity-modulated techniques.

Disease control and survival outcomes in contemporary clinical trials of reirradiation (Valentini et al. 2006; Das et al. 2010; Koom et al. 2012; Sun et al. 2012; Ng et al. 2013; Milani et al. 2008; Bosman et al. 2014) are reported in Table 2. The proportion of patients who underwent resection after reirradiation varies widely (range 20–100%).

Table 2 Disease control and survival outcome in contemporary clinical trials of long-course reirradiation

Author, publication year and study design (inclusion period)	Patient n°	Previous radiation dose Gy, median value (range)	Reirradiation median total dose (range)/ fractionation	Technique	Concurrent chemotherapy	Tumour resection n (%)	Local control	Distant metastases-free survival	Median survival months	Overall survival
Bosman et al. (2014), retrospective (1994–2013)	135	15–55 Gy	30.6/1.8 or 30/2 Gy + IOERT boost 10 (R0), 12.5 (R1) or 15 (R2) Gy at the 90 % isodose	3-field or 3DCRT	Yes (86.7 %)	135/135 (100 %) 75/135 (55.7 %)	45.9 % (5-year)	56.6 % (5-year)	–	34.1 % (5-year)
Ng et al. (2013), retrospective (1997–2008)	56	50.4 Gy (21–64)	39.6 (20–39.6)/1.8 Gy	3DCRT or IMRT	5-FU	11/56 (20 %) R0:8/11 (72 %)	–	–	All, 19 Resected, 39 Unresected, 15	–
Sun et al. (2012), prospective (2004–2008)	72	<50 Gy (not reported)	30–36/1.2 Gy bid; nonresectable: redraw GTV, total 51.6–56.4 Gy	3DCRT	Capecitabine	18/72 (25 %) R0:16/18 (88 %)	–	–	All, 32	All, 45.1 % (3-year)
Koom et al. (2012), retrospective (2000–2007)	22	54 Gy (45–59.4 Gy)	50.2 Gy (30–66)/1.8–3 Gy	3DCRT or IMRT	Yes	5/22 (23 %)	All, 32 % (2-year)	–	All, 21	All, 50 % (2-year)
Das et al. (2010), retrospective (2001–2005)	50	47 Gy (25–70)	39Gy (if retreatment interval ≥ 1 year) or 30 (if retreatment interval < 1 year)/1.5 Gy bid +/– IORT, 5–10	3-field	Capecitabine	18/50 (36 %) R0:7/18 (38.8 %)	All, 33 % (3-year) Resected, 47 % Unresected, 21 %	–	All, 26 Resected, 60 Unresected, 16	All, 39 % (3-year) Resected, 66 % Unresected, 27 %

Milani et al. (2008), retrospective (2000–2005)	24	50.4 Gy (38.0–59.4 Gy)	39.6 Gy (30.0–45.0 Gy)/1.8 Gy	3–5 field	5-FU+ hyperthermia	0 %	–	–	–	–
Valentini et al. (2006), prospective (1997–2001)	59	50.4 (30–55)	30 Gy (+boost 10.8 Gy)/1.2 Gy bid	3DCRT	5-FU	30/59 (51 %) R0:21/30 (70 %)	All, 38.8 % (actuarial 5- year) Resected (R0), 69.0 %	42 % (actuarial 5 years)	All, 42	All, 39.3 % (5-year)
									Resected, 44	Resected (R0), 65.0 %
									Unresected, 14	Unresected (or partial tumour removal), 22.3 %

Differences in resection rates can be mainly explained by the fact that patients with unresectable disease or intraoperatively detected distant disease were not excluded from the initial study population in some studies. Furthermore, as previously said, the lack of a standard classification of LRRC negatively affects the possibility of comparing results between different series. Although pathological complete responses were rarely described, R0 resection was obtained in more than 70 % of operated patients in almost all series (range 39–89 %).

Median survival for all patients with LRRC ranged between 19 and 42 months. Unresected patients had median survival time of 14–16 months, whereas patients who underwent surgical removal of tumour had median survival of 39–60 months. Nearly one-half of patients, with resected LRRC treated with multimodality approach including reirradiation, achieved long-term control of pelvic disease, and up to 65 % of them had long-term (5-year) survival. Even in unresected patients, after preoperative long-course chemo-reirradiation, long-term control can be achieved in about 20 % of cases with a significant proportion of long-term (5-year) survivors (up to 22 %). About 50 % of patients developed distant metastases during follow-up (Valentini et al. 2006; Bosman et al. 2014).

Reirradiation is highly effective for palliation. Eighty-three to 94 % of reirradiated patients experienced partial pain relief, rectal bleeding completely resolved in 100 % of patients and rectal mass was palliated in more than 80 % of patients with a median duration of symptom relief of 9, 10 and 8 months, respectively, for each symptom (Guren et al. 2014).

Probably due to more conformal treatment and reduced volumes, there was a trend towards less acute and late toxicity in recent studies as compared to older trials (Guren et al. 2014). In modern series (Table 3), treatment break or termination due to toxicity infrequently occurred (less than 5 %). The most commonly observed grade 3–4 acute toxicities were diarrhoea (5–10 %) and skin reactions (5 %). The most frequently reported late toxicities were gastrointestinal and urinary complications such as small bowel obstruction or stricture in up to 14 % of patients, fistula, chronic diarrhoea, cystitis and impaired wound healing. In the series by Koom et al., a high rate (27 %) of ureter stricture was also reported.

A great proportion of late toxic events after multimodality treatment of LRRC is likely a consequence of surgery or local disease growth within the pelvis. It has already been said that the morbidity of surgery for LRRC can be as high as 60 %. Das and co-workers (2010) observed a trend towards a higher rate of grade 3–4 late toxicity in patients who had surgery than in patients who did not have surgery after reirradiation. More than half LRRCs re-recur or progress locally after treatment. In the series of Mohiuddin et al. (2002), small bowel obstruction without disease recurrence was seen in only 4 out of 15 (26.6 %) patients. Similarly in the series of Das et al. (2010), half of patients with small bowel obstruction also showed peritoneal carcinomatosis.

4.1.1 Prognostic Factors for Disease Control and Survival Outcomes After Long-Course Reirradiation

Several factors have been evaluated as potential prognostic determinants after reirradiation for LRRC. Response to chemo-reirradiation gives a better chance of achieving a R0 resection (Valentini et al. 2006).

A better local control was observed when R0 surgery was performed (Bosman et al. 2014; Valentini et al. 2006), when reirradiation doses higher than 30 Gy (Haddock et al. 2001) or 50 Gy_{10} (Koom et al. 2012) were delivered, or the interval between the primary treatment and recurrence was longer than 24 months (Valentini et al. 2006).

A better overall survival was observed in patients with good performance status (Karnofsky index ≥70), less-advanced stage of primary tumour (Mohiuddin et al. 2002), when the LRRC was completely resected (Bosman et al. 2014; Ng et al. 2013; Das et al. 2010; Valentini et al. 2006; Mohiuddin et al. 2002), when the interval between the primary treatment and recurrence was longer than 24 (Das et al. 2010) or 36 months (Bosman et al. 2014) or a reirradiation dose higher than 30 Gy was delivered (Mohiuddin et al. 2002).

Table 3 Toxicity in contemporary clinical trials of long-course reirradiation

Author, publication year, and study design (inclusion period)	Grade 3–4 acute toxicity (%)	Treatment break or termination (toxicity)	Follow-up time, months median (range)	Incidence of grade ≥ 3 late complication (%)						Surgical mortality (%)
				Small bowel obstructions	Fistula	Abscess	Wound dehiscence	Ureter	Bladder/urethra	
Bosman et al. (2014), retrospective (1994–2013)	Diarrhoea 5 Neutropenic sepsis 1	–		–	9.9[a]	15.9[a]	9.9[a]	–	10[a]	4.6
Ng et al. (2013), retrospective (1997–2008)	Skin 5 Gastrointestinal 9 Mucositis 2	Termination 4 %	15 (1–108)	1.7[b]	1.7[b]	3.5[b]	1.7[b]	–	3.5[b]	0
Sun et al. (2012), prospective (2004–2008)	Diarrhoea 10 Granulocytopenia 8	Termination 4 %	24 (10–57)	1.4	–	–	–	–	5.6	0
Koom et al. (2012), retrospective (2000–2007)	Diarrhoea 9	–		14	5	–	–	27	14	0
Das et al. (2010), retrospective (2001–2005)	Nausea/vomiting 4	–	25 (0–71)	4	4	4	4	4	–	0
Milani et al. (2008), retrospective (2000–2005)	Gastrointestinal 12.5	0	–	–	–	–	–	–	–	–
Valentini et al. (2006), prospective (1997–2001)	Gastrointestinal 5	Break 10 % Termination 3 %	36 (9–69)	3	–	–	–	–	4	2.6

[a]Thirty-day surgical complications
[b]Resected patients

4.1.2 Reirradiation Tolerance of the Pelvic Organs to Long-Course Reirradiation

Escalating the dose of reirradiation might improve the chance of local control and survival (Haddock et al. 2001; Mohiuddin et al. 2002; Koom et al. 2012). However, it is still unclear what the optimal dose of reirradiation is, since the tolerance of pelvic organs to reirradiation is poorly understood.

In the series of Bosman et al., there were no significant differences of incidence of acute toxicity between patients who were previously irradiated versus those who were not. This finding is in accordance with many clinical studies that have shown an almost complete recovery of acute responding tissue within a few months from irradiation (Langendijk et al. 2006; Würschmidt et al. 2008).

Much lesser is known about the reirradiation tolerance for late effects. The risk of late complications may depend on prior radiation dose. Das et al. (2010) observed a significantly higher incidence of late toxicity in patients who had received a radiation dose of ≥54 Gy than in those who had received a lower dose. The interval from the previous radiotherapy course might also have an impact. Long-term complications were reduced significantly in patients whose interval to reirradiation was longer than 24 months in the series of Mohiuddin et al. (2002).

Tumour location can be a predicting factor for toxicity risk too. In the series by Koom et al. (2012), patients with an axial or anterior tumour location had a significantly higher rate of grade 3 or 4 late toxicities than patients with a lateral or posterior tumour location (64 vs. 9 %).

Many of the published studies have employed hyperfractionated regimens in an attempt to minimize potential late toxicity. Mohiuddin et al. (2002) evaluated long-term results of reirradiation in 103 patients with recurrent rectal carcinoma. Patients were treated with either 1.8 Gy fractions daily or 1.2 Gy fractions twice daily, with a median dose of 34.8 Gy. Long-term complications were significantly reduced in patients receiving hyperfractionated radiation.

Reported late complications of long-course reirradiation occurred to the small bowel, urethra (incontinence, stenosis), bladder (cystitis), ureter (stricture, leakage) and skin (ulceration, fibrosis, delayed wound healing). Thus all these organs should be considered at risk of injury.

The most frequently reported late toxicity in clinical trials of pelvic reirradiation is small bowel obstruction or stricture. Despite hyperfractionation, early studies of reirradiation reported small bowel obstruction in nearly 15 % of patients (Mohiuddin et al. 1997, 2002; Lingareddy et al. 1997). Among older series only in the study by Das et al. (2010), the incidence of small bowel obstruction was particularly low (4 %), maybe because special efforts were made to limit the volume of small bowel in the field, and most patients were treated in a prone position with a belly board device for bowel displacement. The incidence of small bowel obstruction was also low (less than 4 %) in modern series where smaller radiation volumes defined on simulation CT and more conformal techniques were used (Bosman et al. 2014; Ng et al. 2013; Sun et al. 2012; Das et al. 2010; Valentini et al. 2006). Among contemporary studies, the highest incidence of late bowel obstruction (14 %) was reported by Koom et al., particularly in patients with an axial or anterior recurrent tumour, even if reirradiation was delivered to limited volumes with 3DCRT or IMRT. Differently from other modern series, in the study by Koom et al., hyperfractionation was not used; on the contrary, many patients received moderate hypofractionation (up to 3 Gy per fraction).

Fistula formation has been reported to have an incidence of 4 % after reirradiation. Similarly to bowel obstruction, fistula formation is often associated with disease persistence or recurrence (all patients in the series of Mohiuddin et al. 2002).

In the series published by Sun et al., the dose allowed for the small bowel located in the radiation field was 10 Gy for less than 50 % volume (Sun et al. 2012). No specific dose constraints for the small bowel were used in the other series. Therefore, in order to minimize the risk of late injury to the small bowel, it seems reasonable to recommend any efforts to limit the volume of the small bowel in the field and to use hyperfractionated schedule whenever the small bowel cannot be completely excluded.

Intraoperative technical problems or poor healing of surgical wound is among the major concerns discouraging preoperative reirradiation. In the series of Mohiuddin et al. (2002), although wound healing was slower, surgical morbidity was not dissimilar to patients treated without preoperative reirradiation, and there was no mortality. In contrast to previously published data that indicated significantly higher postoperative morbidity rates after preoperative radiotherapy, wound-healing complications or other complications after multimodality treatment were comparable to previously described results of surgery for nonirradiated recurrent rectal cancer (Bosman et al. 2014, Haddock et al. 2001).

4.2 Reirradiation with Intraoperative Radiotherapy (IORT)

IORT is a treatment modality that allows the delivery of high dose to the tumour bed while moving out from the radiation field the radiosensitive bowel and bladder. IORT can be given by three different techniques: electrons (IOERT), high-dose rate (HDR) brachytherapy and low-dose rate (LDR) brachytherapy using iodine 125 seeds.

Studies on IORT have now been published for nearly 30 years; however, still the effect of IORT in rectal cancer treatment is not clear, with some authors who have reported higher overall survival and lower LR rate with IORT in locally advanced/recurrent rectal cancer (Eble et al. 1998; Gunderson et al. 1997; Mannaerts et al. 2001), while others did not confirm such results (Dresen et al. 2008; Ferenschild et al. 2006; Masaki et al. 2008; Dubois et al. 2011).

IOERT 15–20 Gy to the 90 % isodose was used as the sole reirradiation modality in 43 patients with LRRC by Roeder et al., but results were disappointing in patients with incomplete resection with 5-year local control and overall survival rate of 19 % and 11 %, respectively (Roeder et al. 2012).

Similarly, in other series where IOERT was used as a boost after external beam reirradiation (Bosman et al. 2014; Pacelli et al. 2010), resection margin remained the strongest prognostic factor for LC and OS with R1 having worse outcomes than R0 resection. This finding means that IOERT does not thoroughly compensate for an incomplete resection. Although many series with IORT reported encouraging results of local control for patients with R0 resection, for this subset of patients, the added value of IORT remains still unclear (Roeder et al. 2012).

In the series of Pacelli et al. (2010), no differences were observed with and without IOERT in the incidence of complications despite patients in the IOERT group had more advanced disease, suggesting that IOERT itself had not increased the risks associated with surgery.

Data on late toxicity are scarce. Peripheral neuropathy seems to be the main dose-limiting toxicity of IORT.

Eight percent of patients in the series of Roeder et al. (2012) complained of peripheral neuropathy including severe chronic pain. Neuropathy was found in 11 % of the patients receiving IOERT doses of ≥15 Gy compared to 6 % in patients with <15 Gy, but this difference was not statistically significant. The incidence and severity of neuropathy were related to IOERT dose also in the series by Haddock et al. (2011), and the authors suggest that limiting the IOERT dose to 12.5 Gy may result in decreased peripheral nerve toxicity.

The risk of peripheral nerves damage seems to be lower with intraoperative LDR brachytherapy probably due to the continuous low-dose rate irradiation delivered by the ^{125}I seeds (Martinez-Monge et al. 1998).

Goes et al. (1997) reported on 30 patients who, after undergoing laparotomy and either radical or debulking surgical resection, were treated with brachytherapy involving the temporary or permanent implant of seeds of iridium-192 or iodine-125. Local control was 37 % in patients with gross residual disease, and 66 % with microscopic residual disease. These results suggest that intraoperative ^{125}I or ^{103}Pd seed implantation might improve local control, even in patients with noncuratively resected recurrent rectal carcinoma after surgery and EBRT.

Further studies are needed to assess the value of IORT for reirradiation. While IOERT may be not as effective to eradicate the residual disease after an incomplete resection, it could be more effective against a smaller amount of residual cancer cells, for example, it could be considered in patients with R0 resection but close resection margins that carry a higher risk of local recurrence (Alberda et al. 2015). Intraoperative implantation of iodine 125 seeds for LDR has been poorly investigated but might be a promising alternative in patients with incomplete resection.

4.3 Reirradiation with Stereotactic Radiotherapy

To date surgical resection remains the standard therapy for LRRC, with continuous advances in the surgical techniques. However, in some cases, resection is not possible or cannot be performed safely for medical reasons such as comorbidities. In patients who cannot undergo surgery due to medical or technical reasons, long-course chemo-reirradiation is very effective for symptom palliation but offers only a poor chance of long-term tumour control. Highly conformal treatment planning by the use of IMRT or volumetric-modulated arc therapy (VMAT) combined with daily image guidance that allows for tight safety margins can reduce incidental exposure of normal tissue to high irradiation doses, and thus potentially allowing for delivering of hypofractionated irradiation with high-dose per fraction. This is the concept of stereotactic radiation therapy (SRT). A short duration of treatment can be very convenient for the patient as retreatment often takes place in a palliative setting. Furthermore, since different mechanisms such as vascular damage in addition to DNA strand breaks and/or chromosome aberrations may be involved in response of tumours to high dose per fraction (Song et al. 2015), SRT might overcome the radioresistance of radio-recurrent tumours.

Preliminary results suggest that this approach may be a desirable option in patients with LRRC eligible for reirradiation (Defoe et al. 2011; Dewas et al. 2011; Abusaris et al. 2012; Dagoglu et al. 2015). Particularly in small series, OS and local control rates were comparable with those achieved in series of multimodality approach including surgery, whereas incidence of severe toxicity was remarkable lower (Table 4).

Due to limited experience with SRT for reirradiation in LRRC tumours, neither selection criteria for this approach nor total and fractional dose prescription and dosimetric constraints for the organs at risk can yet been clearly established.

Tumour volume varied widely among series ranging from 6.7 to 1114 cc. Defoe et al. (2011) only included presacral tumour recurrences, Dewas et al. (2011) treated lateral pelvic recurrences only, whereas Abusaris et al. (2012) and Dagoglu et al. (2015) also considered for SRT anterior and lateral recurrences.

A wide range of total and fractional dose was used. The local control in patients treated with a dose of more than 60 Gy_3 was significant better than in patients treated with lower stereotactic reirradiation dose in the series by Abusaris et al. (2012), although the differences in overall survival were not significant.

Also the reirradiation dose to the organs at risk varied widely. In the study by Abusaris et al. (2012), the cumulative maximum dose allowed for the rectum and bowel was 110 Gy_3 where a maximum volume of 10 cc bowel or rectum was allowed to receive a higher dose. The cumulative maximum dose allowed for the bladder was 120 Gy_3, where 10 cc of the bladder was allowed to get a higher dose. Even if the constraints were exceeded in some patients, no acute or late severe toxicity was observed in this study. Applying the principle of ALARA (as low as reasonably achievable) radiation dose to volumes of normal tissues as done by Dagoglu et al. (2015) seems therefore a reasonable approach in clinical trials of SRT for reirradiation of LRRC. All structures that could develop a late damage should be considered as organs at risk when calculating the treatment plan. In series of SRT reirradiation, late toxicity

Table 4 Disease control and survival outcome in clinical trials of stereotactic reirradiation

Author, publication year and study design (inclusion period)	Patient n°	Tumour volume cc median (range)	Previous radiation dose Gy, median value (range)	Reirradiation median total dose (range)/ fractionation	Technique	Median follow-up months (range)	Local control	Overall survival	Pain relief	Grade 3–4 toxicity
Dagoglu et al. (2015), retrospective (2006–2012)	18	90 (36.8–1029.4)	50.4 (25–100.4)	25 (24–40)/5 (3–6) to median isodose 78 % (69–86 %)	CyberKnife	38 (6–86)	68.7 % (2-year)	65.9 % (2-year)	[c]	16.6 % 1 small bowel perforation, 1 neuropathy, 1 hydronephrosis
Abusaris et al. (2012), retrospective (2005–2009)	22[a]	PTV 154 (6.7–1114.5).	EQD2 31–83 Gy10)	34 (8–60)/in 1–10 fractions to 70–85 % isodose	CyberKnife	15 (2–52)	53 % (2-year)	37 % (2-year)	95 % (at least partial relief)	0
Defoe et al. (2011), retrospective (2003–2008)	14[b]	52.5 (19–110)	50.4 (20–81)	36 Gy in 3 fractions, 2–3 times per week or single SBRT dose (12, 16 or 18 Gy) to the 80 % isodose	CyberKnife	16.5 (6–69)	68.2 % (2-year)	78.8 % (2-year)	57.1 % (complete relief)	0
Dewas et al. (2011), retrospective (2007–2010)	16[c]	Not reported	45 Gy (20–75 Gy)	36 Gy in 6 fractions over 3 weeks to the 80 % isodose	CyberKnife	10.6 (1.9–20.5).	51.4 % (1-year)	46 % (1-year)	50 % (partial relief)	0

[a]13 LRRC
[b]Presacral tumours only
[c]Lateral tumour only, 4 LRRC

occurred at the level of the small bowel (perforation), nerves (neuropathy with weakness and dumbness of the lower limb and pelvic pain) and ureter (ureteric fibrosis causing hydronephrosis) (Dagoglu et al. 2015).

All published series of SRT reirradiation for LRRC used the CyberKnife technology. Patient positioning and image guidance was performed with registration to the patient's spine and pelvic bones (Dewas et al. 2011) or real-time fiducial tracking (Dagoglu et al. 2015; Abusaris et al. 2012; Defoe et al. 2011). However, it is well known that the position of the organs at risk, particularly the small bowel and the bladder, can change during treatment delivery, thus potentially moving into the high-dose region. While two-dimensional localization systems cannot detect such inter- and intra-fractional movements, volumetric onboard image guidance systems such as onboard CT or MR potentially can, thus allowing a further minimization of the risk of severe injury.

4.4 Reirradiation with Brachytherapy

Interstitial brachytherapy might be an alternative in the treatment of LRRC in patients who cannot or choose not to undergo radical surgical resection. Particularly, percutaneous image-guided seed implantation, which can be performed without surgery or general anaesthesia, has attracted increasing attention. Indeed in contrast to EBRT and IORT, it has the advantage of delivering low-dose-rate radiation, which allows continuous DNA repair of sublethal damage to occur in the normal tissues while ensuring protracted cancer cell killing, and thus resulting in a wider therapeutic index. Another advantage of interstitial brachytherapy is the relatively rapid dose fall-off. These benefits allow higher cumulative doses to be delivered, which may provide better tumour control. However, there are few reports on CT-guided implantation of radioactive seeds in the treatment of localized pelvic recurrences (Table 5) (Wang et al. 2010, 2011; Bishop et al. 2015).

In all these reports, patients were selected based on the technical feasibility of performing brachytherapy, the size of the recurrent lesions and the proximity of the lesions to critical organs. Particularly in the series of Bishop et al., patients with less infiltrative and smaller lesions were selected over time, after initial results for patients with larger tumours were unsatisfactory.

Interestingly in the series of Wang et al. (2010), three patients had ever received radiotherapy twice.

In such selected populations of patients, CT-guided interstitial brachytherapy led to durable local control and long-term survival. Treatment was also well tolerated and symptomatic palliation was common.

4.5 Reirradiation with Particle Therapy

Particle therapy using protons (^{1}H) or carbon ions (^{12}C) offers physical and biological advantages compared to photon radiotherapy. With particle therapy the dose can be precisely applied while avoiding normal tissue irradiation due to the high local-dose deposition within the Bragg peak. Moreover, ions offer an increased relative biological effectiveness (RBE), which for ^{12}C in particular, can be calculated between 2 and 5 depending on the cell line as well as the endpoint analysed, due to an increased induction of clustered DNA double-strand breaks within the irradiated cells, which are difficult to repair by the cells' intrinsic repair mechanisms. This higher relative biological effectiveness (RBE) can translate into improved clinical results (Combs et al. 2012).

Preliminary results of the phase I/II German trial PANDORA using carbon ions for reirradiation of LRRC were recently published. Ninety-nine patients treated with ^{12}C reirradiation at the Heidelberg Ion-Beam Therapy Center (HIT) between 2010 and 2013 were included in this preliminary analysis. All patients had a history of surgery and pelvic radiotherapy of at least 50.4 Gy. Median dose was 36 Gy [relative biologic efficacy (RBE)] [range 36–51 Gy (RBE)],

Table 5 Disease control and survival outcome in clinical trials of interstitial LDR brachytherapy

Author, publication year and study design (inclusion period)	Patient n°	Tumour volume cc median (range)	Previous radiation dose Gy, median value (range)	Reirradiation median total dose (range)/ fractionation	Technique	Median follow-up months (range)	Local control (2-year)	Overall survival (2-year)	Pain relief	Grade 3–4 toxicity
Bishop et al. (2015), retrospective (2000–2012)	20	n.r.	90 (72–149)	80 Gy at a 1-cm margin or 120 Gy to 100 % of the GTV	CT-guided percutaneous seeds implantation (^{198}Au or ^{125}I)	23 (13–132)	60 %	62 %	69 %	1 patient ureteral stricture
Wang et al. (2011), retrospective (2006–2009)	20	Volume implanted 68.9 (26.9–97.3)	70 % of patients, 60 Gy (50–70)	Median minimal peripheral dose 120 Gy (range 100–160)	CT-guided percutaneous seeds implantation (^{125}I)	22 (3–34)	15 %	25 %	85 %	1 patient ureteral stricture
Wang et al. (2011), retrospective (2006–2009)	15	n.r.	n.r.	Median minimal peripheral dose 150 Gy (range 110–165)	CT-guided percutaneous seeds implantation (^{125}I or ^{103}Pd)	8 (4–50)	8.1 %	10.7 %	53.8 %	1 cutaneous fistula (tumour invasion of the perineal skin)

n.r. not reported

and median planning target volume was 456 ml (range 75–1,597 ml). After a median follow-up of 7.8 months, three patients (16 %) died, four patients (21 %) experienced local progression after RT and three patients (16 %) were diagnosed with distant metastases. No grade 3 or higher toxicities were observed.

Conclusions

For patients with isolated LRRC or primary locally advanced rectal cancer after previous pelvic irradiation, the complete surgical removal (R0 resection) of the tumour is the most important measure to achieve long-term local control of the disease and survival. Preoperative long-course chemo-reirradiation can improve the chance of R0 resection without adding unacceptable morbidity if proper caution is paid to both radiation and surgical techniques. The use of small radiation fields, exclusion of the bowel and bladder and the use of hyperfractionated radiation doses up to 40 Gy are recommended.

Although intraoperative delivery of reirradiation doses lower than 15 Gy is feasible, the added value of IORT is still unclear.

In patients who cannot undergo surgery due to medical or technical reasons, long-course chemo-reirradiation is very effective for symptom palliation but offers only a poor chance of long-term tumour control. Patients with small isolated LRRC who cannot undergo surgery due to medical or technical reason might benefit from image-guided stereotactic reirradiation with the aim of achieving both palliation and long-term local control. Percutaneous image-guided seed implantation for LDR interstitial brachytherapy can be also considered in this subset of patients, especially for LRRC that is very close to critical normal structures.

Particle therapy, due to its physical and biological characteristics, might offer a chance of cure in nonsurgical candidates with large isolated LRRC. However, the optimal dose applicable in this clinical situation as well as efficacy as reirradiation still has to be determined.

Since distant metastases are a major problem in surviving patients, the role of anticancer drugs in reducing distant recurrences should also be explored.

References

Abusaris H, Hoogeman M, Nuyttens JJ (2012) Re-irradiation: outcome, cumulative dose and toxicity in patients retreated with stereotactic radiotherapy in the abdominal or pelvic region. Technol Cancer Res Treat 11(6):591–597

Alberda WJ, Verhoef C, Nuyttens JJ, Rothbarth J, van Meerten E, de Wilt JH, Burger JW (2014) Outcome in patients with resectable locally recurrent rectal cancer after total mesorectal excision with and without previous neoadjuvant radiotherapy for the primary rectal tumor. Ann Surg Oncol 21(2):520–526. doi:10.1245/s10434-013-3306-x

Alberda WJ, Verhoef C, Schipper ME, Nuyttens JJ, Rothbarth J, de Wilt JH, Burger JW (2015) The importance of a minimal tumor-free resection margin in locally recurrent rectal cancer. Dis Colon Rectum 58(7):677–685

Beyond TME Collaborative (2013) Consensus statement on the multidisciplinary management of patients with recurrent and primary rectal cancer beyond total mesorectal excision planes. Br J Surg 100(8):E1–E33. doi:10.1002/bjs.9192

Bhangu A, Ali SM, Brown G, Nicholls RJ, Tekkis P (2014) Indications and outcome of pelvic exenteration for locally advanced primary and recurrent rectal cancer. Ann Surg 259(2):315e–322e

Bishop AJ, Gupta S, Cunningham MG, Tao R, Berner PA, Korpela SG et al (2015) Interstitial brachytherapy for the treatment of locally recurrent anorectal cancer. Ann Surg Oncol 22(Suppl 3):596–602

Bosman SJ, Holman FA, Nieuwenhuijzen GA, Martijn H, Creemers GJ, Rutten HJ (2014) Feasibility of reirradiation in the treatment of locally recurrent rectal cancer. Br J Surg 101(10):1280–1289

Chan CL, Bokey EL, Chapuis PH, Renwick AA, Dent OF (2006) Local recurrence after curative resection for rectal cancer is associated with anterior position of the tumour. Br J Surg 93(1):105–112

Coco C, Valentini V, Manno A, Mattana C, Verbo A, Cellini N et al (2006) Long-term results after neoadjuvant radiochemotherapy for locally advanced resectable extraperitoneal rectal cancer. Dis Colon Rectum 49:311–318

Combs SE, Kieser M, Habermehl D, Weitz J, Jäger D, Fossati P et al (2012) Phase I/II trial evaluating carbon ion radiotherapy for the treatment of recurrent rectal cancer: the PANDORA-01 trial. BMC Cancer 12:137

Dagoglu N, Mahadevan A, Nedea E, Poylin V, Nagle D (2015) Stereotactic body radiotherapy (SBRT) reirradiation for pelvic recurrence from colorectal cancer. J Surg Oncol 111(4):478–482

Das P, Delclos ME, Skibber JM, Rodriguez-Bigas MA, Feig BW, Chang GJ et al (2010) Hyperfractionated accelerated radiotherapy for rectal cancer in patients with prior pelvic irradiation. Int J Radiat Oncol Biol Phys 77:60–65

Defoe SG, Bernard ME, Rwigema JC, Heron DE, Ozhasoglu C, Burton S et al (2011) Stereotactic body radiotherapy for the treatment of presacral recurrences from rectal cancers. J Cancer Res Ther 7(4):408–411

Dewas S, Bibault JE, Mirabel X, Nickers P, Castelain B, Lacornerie T, Jarraya H, Lartigau E (2011) Robotic image-guided reirradiation of lateral pelvic recurrences: preliminary results. Radiat Oncol 6:77. doi:10.1186/1748-717X-6-77

Dicle O, Obuz F, Cakmakci H (1999) Differentiation of recurrent rectal cancer and scarring with dynamic MR imaging. Br J Radiol 72:11559

Dresen RC, Gosens MJ, Martijn H et al (2008) Radical resection after IORT-containing multimodality treatment is the most important determinant for outcome in patients treated for locally recurrent rectal cancer. Ann Surg Oncol 15:1937–1947

Dresen RC, Kusters M, Daniels-Gooszen AW, Cappendijk VC, Nieuwenhuijzen GA, Kessels AG et al (2010) Absence of tumor invasion into pelvic structures in locally recurrent rectal cancer: prediction with preoperative MR imaging. Radiology 256(1):143–150

Dubois JB, Bussieres E, Richaud P, Rouanet P, Becouarn Y, Mathoulin-Pélissier S et al (2011) Intraoperative radiotherapy of rectal cancer: results of the French multi-institutional randomized study. Radiother Oncol 98(3):298–303

Eble MJ, Lehnert T, Treiber M, Latz D, Herfarth C, Wannenmacher M (1998) Moderate dose intraoperative and external beam radiotherapy for locally recurrent rectal carcinoma. Radiother Oncol 49:169–174

Enker WE, Thaler HT, Cranor ML et al (1995) Total mesorectal excision in the operative treatment of carcinoma of the rectum. J Am Coll Surg 181:335–346

Enríquez-Navascués JM, Borda N, Lizerazu A, Placer C, Elosegui JL, Ciria JP et al (2011) Patterns of local recurrence in rectal cancer after a multidisciplinary approach. World J Gastroenterol 17(13):1674–1684. doi:10.3748/wjg.v17.i13.1674

Ferenschild FT, Vermaas M, Nuyttens JJ, Graveland WJ, Marinelli AW, van der Sijp JR (2006) Value of intraoperative radiotherapy in locally advanced rectal cancer. Dis Colon Rectum 49:1257–1265

Ferenschild FT, Vermaas M, Verhoef C et al (2009) Total pelvic exenteration for primary and recurrent malignancies. World J Surg 33(7):1502e–1508e

Figueredo A, Rumble RB, Maroun J, Earle CC, Cummings B, McLeod R et al (2003) Follow-up of patients with curatively resected colorectal cancer: a practice guideline. BMC Cancer 3:26

Floriani I, Torri V, Rulli E et al (2010) Performance of imaging modalities in diagnosis of liver metastases from colorectal cancer: a systematic review and meta-analysis. J Magn Reson Imaging 31:1931

Georgiou PA, Tekkis PP, Constantinides VA, Patel U, Goldin RD, Darzi AW et al (2013) Diagnostic accuracy and value of magnetic resonance imaging (MRI) in planning exenterative pelvic surgery for advanced colorectal cancer. Eur J Cancer 49:72–81

Gérard JP, Azria D, Gourgou-Bourgade S, Martel-Lafay I, Hennequin C, Etienne PL et al (2012) Clinical outcome of the ACCORD 12/0405 PRODIGE 2 randomized trial in rectal cancer. J Clin Oncol 30(36):4558–4565. doi:10.1200/JCO.2012.42.8771

Gezen C, Kement M, Altuntas YE, Okkabaz N, Seker M, Vural S et al (2012) Results after multivisceral resections of locally advanced colorectal cancers: an analysis on clinical and pathological t4 tumors. World J Surg Oncol 15(10):39. doi:10.1186/1477-7819-10-39

Goes RN, Beart RW Jr, Simons AJ, Gunderson LL, Grado G, Streeter O (1997) Use of brachytherapy in management of locally recurrent rectal cancer. Dis Colon Rectum 40:1177–1179

Goldberg PA, Nicholls RJ, Porter NH et al (1994) Long-term results of a randomised trial of short-course low-dose adjuvant preoperative radiotherapy for rectal cancer: reduction in local treatment failure. Eur J Cancer 30A:1602–1606

Grabbe E, Winkler R (1985) Local recurrence after sphincter-saving resection for rectal and rectosigmoid carcinoma. Value of various diagnostic methods. Radiology 155:305–310

Gunderson LL, Nelson H, Martenson JA et al (1996) Intraoperative electron and external beam irradiation with or without 5-fluorouracil and maximum surgical resection for previously unirradiated locally recurrent colorectal cancer. Dis Colon Rectum 39:1379–1395

Gunderson LL, Nelson H, Martenson JA, Cha S, Haddock M, Devine R (1997) Locally advanced primary colorectal cancer: Intraoperative electron and external beam irradiation ± 5-FU. Int J Radiat Oncol Biol Phys 37:601–614

Guren MG, Undseth C, Rekstad BL, Brændengen M, Dueland S, Spindler KL et al (2014) Reirradiation of locally recurrent rectal cancer: a systematic review. Radiother Oncol 113(2):151–157. doi:10.1016/j.radonc.2014.11.021

Haddock MG, Gunderson LL, Nelson H, Cha SS, Devine RM, Dozois RR, Wolff BG (2001) Intraoperative irradiation for locally recurrent colorectal cancer in previously irradiated patients. Int J Radiat Oncol Biol Phys 49:1267–1274

Haddock MG, Miller RC, Nelson H et al (2011) Combined modality therapy including intraoperative electron irradiation for locally recurrent colorectal cancer. Int J Radiat Oncol Biol Phys 79:143–150

Harji DP, Griffiths B, McArthur DR, Sagar PM (2013) Surgery for recurrent rectal cancer: higher and wider? Colorectal Dis 15:139–145

Heald RJ (1995) Total mesorectal excision is optimal surgery for rectal cancer: a Scandinavian consensus. Br J Surg 82:1297–1299

Heriot AG, Tekkis PP, Darzi A, Mackay J (2006) Surgery for local recurrence of rectal cancer. Colorectal Dis 8:73347. doi:10.1111/j.1463-1318.2006.01018.x

Huebner RH, Park KC, Shepherd JE et al (2000) A meta-analysis of the literature for whole-body FDG PET detection of recurrent colorectal cancer. J Nucl Med 41:117789

Kalff V, Hicks R, Ware R et al (2002) The clinical impact of 18F-FDG PET in patients with suspected or confirmed recurrence of colorectal cancer: a prospective study. J Nucl Med 43:492–499

Konski AA, Suh WW, Herman JM, Blackstock AW Jr, Hong TS, Poggi MM et al (2012) ACR appropriateness criteria® - recurrent rectal cancer. Gastrointest Cancer Res 5(1):3–12

Koom WS, Choi Y, Shim SJ, Cha J, Seong J, Kim NK et al (2012) Reirradiation to the pelvis for recurrent rectal cancer. J Surg Oncol 105:637–642

Kusters M, Marijnen CA, van de Velde CJ, Rutten HJ, Lahaye MJ, Kim JH et al (2010) Patterns of local recurrence in rectal cancer; a study of the Dutch TME trial. Eur J Surg Oncol 36(5):470–476

Lambregts DM, Cappendijk VC, Maas M, Beets GL, Beets-Tan RG (2011) Value of MRI and diffusion-weighted MRI for the diagnosis of locally recurrent rectal cancer. Eur Radiol 21(6):1250–1258

Langendijk JA, Kasperts N, Leemans CR, Doornaert P, Slotman BJ (2006) A phase II study of primary reirradiation in squamous cell carcinoma of head and neck. Radiother Oncol 78(3):306–312

Lingareddy V, Ahmad NR, Mohiuddin M (1997) Palliative reirradiation for recurrent rectal cancer. Int J Radiat Oncol Biol Phys 38:785–790

MacFarlane JK, Ryall RD, Heald RJ (1993) Mesorectal excision for rectal cancer. Lancet 341:457–460

Mannaerts GH, Rutten HJ, Martijn H et al (2001) Comparison of intraoperative radiation therapy-containing multimodality treatment with historical treatment modalities for locally recurrent rectal cancer. Dis Colon Rectum 44:1749–1758

Martinez-Monge R, Nag S, Martin EW (1998) 125Iodine brachytherapy for colorectal adenocarcinoma recurrent in the pelvis and paraortics. Int J Radiat Oncol Biol Phys 42:545–550

Masaki T, Takayama M, Matsuoka H, Abe N, Ueki H, Sugiyama M et al (2008) Intraoperative radiotherapy for oncological and function-preserving surgery in patients with advanced lower rectal cancer. Langenbecks Arch Surg 393(2):173–180

Messiou C, Chalmers AG, Boyle K, Wilson D, Sagar P (2008) Preoperative MR assessment of recurrent rectal cancer. Br J Radiol 81(966):468–473

Milani V, Pazos M, Issels RD, Buecklein V, Rahman S, Tschoep K et al (2008) Radiochemotherapy in combination with regional hyperthermia in preirradiated patients with recurrent rectal cancer. Strahlenther Onkol 184(3):163–168

Mohiuddin M, Marks G (1993) Patterns of recurrence following high-dose preoperative radiation and sphincter-preserving surgery for cancer of the rectum. Dis Colon Rectum 36(2):117–126

Mohiuddin M, Lingareddy V, Rakinic J, Marks G (1993) Reirradiation for rectal cancer and surgical resection after ultra high doses. Int J Radiat Oncol Biol Phys 27:1159–1163

Mohiuddin M, Marks GM, Lingareddy V, Marks J (1997) Curative surgical resection following reirradiation for recurrent rectal cancer. Int J Radiat Oncol Biol Phys 39:643–649

Mohiuddin M, Marks G, Marks J (2002) Long-term results of reirradiation for patients with recurrent rectal carcinoma. Cancer 95:1144–1150

Moore HG, Shoup M, Riedel E et al (2004) Colorectal cancer pelvic recurrences: determinants of resectability. Dis Colon Rectum 47(10):1599e–1606e

Ng MK, Leong T, Heriot AG, Ngan SY (2013) Once-daily reirradiation for rectal cancer in patients who have received previous pelvic radiotherapy. J Med Imaging Radiat Oncol 57:512–518

Nielsen MB, Laurberg S, Holm T (2011) Current management of locally recurrent rectal cancer. Colorectal Dis 13:732–742

Nielsen M, Rasmussen P, Lindegaard J, Laurberg S (2012) A 10-year experience of total pelvic exenteration for primary advanced and locally recurrent rectal cancer based on a prospective database. Colorectal Dis 14(9):1076e–1083e

Ogunbiyi O, Flanagan F, Dehdashti F et al (1997) Detection of recurrent and metastatic colorectal cancer: comparison of positron emission tomography and computed tomography. Ann Surg Oncol 4:613–620

Pacelli F, Tortorelli AP, Rosa F, Bossola M, Sanchez AM, Papa V, Valentini V, Doglietto GB (2010) Locally recurrent rectal cancer: prognostic factors and long-term outcomes of multimodal therapy. Ann Surg Oncol 17(1):152–162. doi:10.1245/s10434-009-0737-5

Palmer G, Martling A, Cedermark B, Holm T (2007) A population-based study on the management and outcome in patients with locally recurrent rectal cancer. Ann Surg Oncol 14(2):447–454

Quirke P, Durdey P, Dixon MF, Williams NS (1986) Local recurrence of rectal adenocarcinoma due to inadequate surgical resection. Histopathological study of lateral tumour spread and surgical excision. Lancet 2(8514):996–999

Renehan AG (2016) Techniques and outcome of surgery for locally advanced and local recurrent rectal cancer. Clin Oncol (R Coll Radiol) 28(2):103–115

Rödel C, Grabenbauer GG, Matzel KE, Schick C, Fietkau R, Papadopoulos T et al (2000) Extensive surgery after high-dose preoperative chemoradiotherapy for locally advanced recurrent rectal cancer. Dis Colon Rectum 43(3):312–319

Rödel C, Martus P, Papadoupolos T, Füzesi L, Klimpfinger M, Fietkau R et al (2005) Prognostic significance of tumor regression after preoperative chemoradiotherapy for rectal cancer. J Clin Oncol 23(34):8688–8696

Rödel C, Graeven U, Fietkau R, Hohenberger W, Hothorn T, Arnold D, et al., German Rectal Cancer Study Group (2015) Oxaliplatin added to fluorouracil-based preoperative chemoradiotherapy and postoperative chemotherapy of locally advanced rectal cancer (the German CAO/ARO/AIO-04 study): final results of the multicentre, open-label, randomised, phase 3 trial. Lancet Oncol 16(8):979–89. doi:10.1016/S1470-2045(15)00159-X

Roeder F, Goetz JM, Habl G, Bischof M, Krempien R, Buechler MW, Hensley FW et al (2012) Intraoperative Electron Radiation Therapy (IOERT) in the management of locally recurrent rectal cancer. BMC Cancer 12:592

Rombouts AJ, Koh CE, Young JM, Masya L, Roberts R, De-Loyde K et al (2015) Does radiotherapy of the primary rectal cancer affect prognosis after pelvic exenteration for recurrent rectal cancer? Dis Colon Rectum 58(1):65–73

Sagar PM, Pemberton JH (1996) Surgical management of locally recurrent rectal cancer. Br J Surg 83(3):293–304

Saito N, Koda K, Takiguchi N, Oda K, Ono M, Sugito M et al (2003) Curative surgery for local pelvic recurrence of rectal cancer. Dig Surg 20:192–199

Song CW, Lee YJ, Griffin RJ, Park I, Koonce NA, Hui S et al (2015) Indirect tumor cell death after high-dose hypofractionated irradiation: implications for stereotactic body radiation therapy and stereotactic radiation surgery. Int J Radiat Oncol Biol Phys 93(1):166–172

Sun DS, Zhang JD, Li L, Dai Y, Yu JM, Shao ZY (2012) Accelerated hyperfractionation field-involved re-irradiation combined with concurrent capecitabine chemotherapy for locally recurrent and irresectable rectal cancer. Br J Radiol 1011:259–264

Suzuki K, Dozois RR, Devine RM, Nelson H, Weaver AL, Gunderson LL et al (1996) Curative reoperations for locally recurrent rectal cancer. Dis Colon Rectum 39:730–746

Swedish Rectal Cancer Trial (1996) Local recurrence rate in a randomised multicentre trial of preoperative radiotherapy compared with operation alone in resectable rectal carcinoma. Eur J Surg 162:397–402

Tan PL, Chan CL, Moore NR (2005) Radiological appearances in the pelvis following rectal cancer surgery. Clin Radiol 60(8):846–855

Tan E, Gouvas N, Nicholls RJ, Ziprin P, Xynos E, Tekkis PP (2009) Diagnostic precision of carcinoembryonic antigen in the detection of recurrence of colorectal cancer. Surg Oncol 18:15–24

Tanis PJ, Doeksen A, van Lanschot JJ (2013) Intentionally curative treatment of locally recurrent rectal cancer: a systematic review. Can J Surg 56(2):135–144

Valentini V, Morganti AG, De Franco A et al (1999) Chemoradiation with or without intraoperative radiation therapy in patients with locally recurrent rectal carcinoma: prognostic factors and long-term outcome. Cancer 86:2612–2624

Valentini V, Morganti AG, Gambacorta MA et al (2006) Preoperative hyperfractionated chemoradiation for locally recurrent rectal cancer in patients previously irradiated to the pelvis: a multicentric phase II study. Int J Radiat Oncol Biol Phys 64:1129–1139

Valentini V, van Stiphout RG, Lammering G, Gambacorta MA, Barba MC, Bebenek M et al (2011) Nomograms for predicting local recurrence, distant metastases, and overall survival for patients with locally advanced rectal cancer on the basis of European randomized clinical trials. J Clin Oncol 29:3163–3172

van den Brink M, Stiggelbout AM, van den Hout WB et al (2004) Clinical nature and prognosis of locally recurrent rectal cancer after total mesorectal excision with or without preoperative radiotherapy. J Clin Oncol 22:3958–3964

van Gijn W, van Stiphout RG, van de Velde CJ, Valentini V, Lammering G, Gambacorta MA et al (2015) Nomograms to predict survival and the risk for developing local or distant recurrence in patients with rectal cancer treated with optional short-term radiotherapy. Ann Oncol 26:928–935

Vermaas M, Ferenschild FT, Nuyttens JJ, Marinelli AW, Wiggers T, van der Sijp JR et al (2005) Preoperative radiotherapy improves outcome in recurrent rectal cancer. Dis Colon Rectum 48(5):918–928

Wanebo HJ, Antoniuk P, Koness RJ et al (1999) Pelvic resection of recurrent rectal cancer: technical considerations and outcomes. Dis Colon Rectum 42:1438–1448

Wang JJ, Yuan HS, Li JN, Jiang YL, Tian SQ, Yang RJ (2010) CT-guided radioactive seed implantation for recurrent rectal carcinoma after multiple therapy. Med Oncol 27:421–429

Wang Z, Lu J, Liu L et al (2011) Clinical application of CT-guided (125) I seed interstitial implantation for local recurrent rectal carcinoma. Radiat Oncol 6:138

Würschmidt F, Dahle J, Petersen C, Wenzel C, Kretschmer M, Bastian C (2008) Reirradiation of recurrent breast cancer with and without concurrent chemotherapy. Radiat Oncol 3:28. doi:10.1186/1748-717X-3-28

Yamada K, Ishizawa T, Niwa K, Chuman Y, Akiba S, Aikou T (2001) Patterns of pelvic invasion are prognostic in the treatment of locally recurrent rectal cancer. Br J Surg 88:988–993

Yu SK, Bhangu A, Tait DM, Tekkis P, Wotherspoon A, Brown G (2014) Chemoradiotherapy response in recurrent rectal cancer. Cancer Med 3(1):111–117

Zitt M, Mühlmann G, Weiss H, Kafka-Ritsch R, Oberwalder M, Kirchmayr W et al (2006) Assessment of risk-independent follow-up to detect asymptomatic recurrence after curative resection of colorectal cancer. Langenbecks Arch Surg 391:369–375

Gynecological Malignancies

Jennifer Croke, Eric Leung, and Anthony Fyles

Contents

The original version of this chapter was revised. An erratum to this chapter can be found at 10.1007/978-3-319-41825-4_78.

J. Croke • A. Fyles (✉)
Radiation Medicine Program, Princess Margaret Cancer Centre, Toronto, ON, Canada

Department of Radiation Oncology, University of Toronto, Toronto, ON, Canada
e-mail: Anthony.Fyles@rmp.uhn.on.ca

E. Leung
Department of Radiation Oncology, Odette Cancer Center, Toronto, ON, Canada

Department of Radiation Oncology, University of Toronto, Toronto, ON, Canada

Abstract

Surgical, technical, and biological advancements in treatment have improved clinical outcomes for patients with gynecological malignancies. Despite this a significant proportion will relapse locally, requiring multidisciplinary management. Patients who received definitive radiotherapy as primary treatment are ideally treated with surgery; however, this is not always possible. Re-irradiation poses a therapeutic dilemma, as the desire for local control must be weighed against the potential risks associated with re-treatment. A patient's suitability for radical re-treatment is determined by multiple factors: clinical performance status, symptomatology, site of recurrence, previous radiotherapy delivery technique, dose/fractionation, radiation-related toxicities, and disease extent. With improvement in technologies, an aggressive approach is now feasible and worth pursuing in carefully selected patients, where not only palliation of local symptoms is possible but also long-term local control. In this review, the clinical, tumor, and radiobiological factors as well as technological considerations are highlighted. A treatment algorithm for patients presenting for consideration of re-irradiation for recurrent gynecological malignancy is also presented.

Med Radiol Radiat Oncol (2016)
DOI 10.1007/174_2016_47, © Springer International Publishing Switzerland
Published Online: 30 Mar 2016

1 Introduction

Gynecological malignancies are a diverse group of cancers originating from the female reproductive tract that include the ovaries, uterus, cervix, vagina, and vulva and are a significant global health concern. In 2012, cervical, endometrial, and ovarian cancers were the fourth, sixth, and seventh most common new cancer diagnoses, respectively, in women worldwide (Torre et al. 2015). Radiotherapy (RT) has a well-established, important, and evidence-based role in the radical and adjuvant treatment of gynecological malignancies.

Despite surgical, radiotherapeutic, and biological advances in the management of gynecological malignancies, locoregional recurrence remains an important and challenging issue. Studies show that locoregional recurrences occur in approximately 35 % of patients with cervical cancer (Chemoradiotherapy for Cervical Cancer Meta-analysis C 2010). It is estimated that ~10 % of all gynecological cancer patients who have received definitive treatment relapse solely in the pelvis without evidence of distant disease (Aalders et al. 1984; Fuller et al. 1989; Look and Rocereto 1990) and that ~80 % of relapses occur in previously irradiated areas (Potter et al. 1990; Thomas et al. 1993).

The management of locoregional recurrences is challenging as limited data exist to guide treatment and therapeutic options are often limited after definitive surgery and/or radiotherapy. Patients who present with locoregional recurrence after primary radiotherapy are ideally treated surgically, usually with exenteration. Some series report significant long-term survival rates (Sharma et al. 2005; Maggioni et al. 2009; Fotopoulou et al. 2010); however, the substantial and severe morbidity associated with such an approach cannot be ignored (Morley and Lindenauer 1976; Roberts et al. 1987; Anthopoulos et al. 1989). When this is not possible, re-irradiation must be considered. Improvements in clinical outcomes and an increase in the number of long-term survivors have also translated into increases in the rates of re-irradiation, although the current frequency is unknown. The idea of re-irradiation poses a therapeutic dilemma, as the desire for local control must be carefully weighed against the potential risks associated with re-treatment. Therefore, many radiation oncologists are reluctant to re-irradiate patients because of the fear of causing significant normal tissue toxicity. Rates of normal tissue repair have not been accurately elucidated, and dose constraints for organs at risk in the setting of re-irradiation are lacking. Incorporating systemic therapy is an attractive means to further improve outcomes, particularly concurrent cisplatin chemotherapy, similar to treatment in primary cervix cancer; however, this may also be associated with increased toxicity.

Modern technologies such as intensity-modulated radiotherapy (IMRT), image-guided radiotherapy (IGRT), and stereotactic radiotherapy make the concept of re-irradiation more appealing and plausible as a highly conformal dose is able to be delivered to the pelvic recurrence while limiting dose to surrounding normal tissue.

2 Basic Principles and Considerations

Patients who present with locoregional recurrence after definitive radiotherapy require a comprehensive multidisciplinary evaluation. Several important factors must be recognized and accounted for. Treatment intent is based on clinical, tumor, and radiobiological factors and determines whether the goal is palliation of symptoms, symptom prevention due to disease progression or cure in the setting of limited local recurrence and absence of metastases.

2.1 Clinical Considerations

A thorough review of the patient's history and clinical examination is prudent when considering re-irradiation. Important considerations include assessment of performance status, assessment of medical comorbidities, and a thorough evaluation of any tumor-related symptoms. The details of previous treatment and any chronic toxicity should be clearly documented. Imaging studies to restage for distant metastases that would impact clinical decision-making are important. Combining functional imaging using FDG-PET with routine radiologic studies, such as CT and MRI, increases sensitivity for detecting occult metastases. The presence of distant metastases impacts treatment intent.

It is important to exclude benign lesions which may mimic recurrence. Differential diagnoses include seroma, lymphocele, pelvic abscess, hematoma, and postradiation fibrosis. Imaging should be reviewed by a specialist in pelvic oncologic radiology. If possible, a biopsy should be done to confirm recurrent disease. Treatment intent (curative or palliative) should be defined early and supported by full staging investigations. The prognosis for patients who have both local and distant disease is usually limited, and therefore the goal of re-irradiation should be aimed at alleviating symptoms and maximizing patient quality of life. In contrast, patients who have localized disease and good performance status and who tolerated previous radiotherapy well are often good candidates for radical re-irradiation.

Particular attention to late normal tissue toxicity and tolerance of previous irradiation should be given. This can be supported by self- or physician-administered questionnaires, for example, the Late Effects in Normal Tissues-Subjective, Objective, Management, and Analytic (LENT-SOMA) or Radiation Therapy Oncology Group (RTOG) scoring systems. Re-irradiation of patients who have developed significant gastrointestinal (GI) or genitourinary (GU) toxicity should be approached with extreme caution and other treatment options explored as an alternative. Approximately 15–25 % of patients receiving whole pelvic radiotherapy develop grade 2 or higher late GI toxicity (Mundt et al. 2003; Chen et al. 2007). Although the majority of patients have mild symptoms, ~5–10 % experience severe toxicity which significantly impacts their quality of life, e.g., fistula or stricture formation and bowel obstruction (Ooi et al. 1999; Denton et al. 2000; Andreyev 2005). Genitourinary toxicity typically develops over a longer time course such that there is a risk of approximately 5 % of grade 3 or 4 urinary toxicity at 20 years (Eifel et al. 1995). This can manifest as ureteral stenosis, chronic hematuria, or vesicovaginal fistula formation. The presence of chronic radiotherapy-related toxicity must be considered as it will likely predict the tolerance for re-irradiation and their risk for developing severe toxicity.

2.2 Tumor-Related Considerations

The tumor histology, anatomic site of recurrence, and extent of recurrence are important tumor-related factors one must assess when considering re-irradiation. Accurate clinical gynecological examination is important to establish the site of recurrence, the extent of disease, and the state of normal tissues. The volume of recurrent disease should be assessed both clinically and radiologically using MRI, with particular attention to the proximity of surrounding normal structures. The site of the recurrence should be evaluated carefully with respect to the previous region of high-dose radiation. Large, bulky recurrences or multifocal recurrences are difficult to treat with radiotherapy alone because a large dose or volume is required. This will also increase doses to adjacent organs at risk, which increases the risk of severe late normal tissue damage. Furthermore, some histologies, such as sarcomas, are more radioresistant than others, and therefore the tumor type should also be considered when offering re-irradiation.

2.3 Radiobiological Considerations

Disease-free interval is one of the most significant prognostic factors associated with tumor re-irradiation response and patient survival (Prempree et al. 1984). Patients who experience an infield recurrence with a short disease-free interval have likely developed a radioresistant tumor population. Tumors which recur within 12 months of primary definitive treatment often indicate an aggressive growth pattern, and there must be a high index of suspicion for the presence of distant metastases. A long disease-free interval (>12 months) typically represents less aggressive tumors, and furthermore, recovery of normal tissues has been able to take place. These patients are better suited for re-irradiation.

Estimating previous doses to organs at risk (OARs) is important when considering re-irradiation. However, many patients with gynecological malignancies likely received brachytherapy initially, and there are inherent difficulties in calculating the sum biological effective dose when combining brachytherapy and external beam fractionation. As the biological effect produced from external beam radiation differs from that produced by brachytherapy, it is necessary to convert each of these physical doses into their equivalent biological doses (EQD2) before summing them. The GEC-ESTRO group has published recommendations on adding external beam and brachytherapy doses using the EQD2 formula and has developed a spreadsheet which is currently used for dose reporting in the EMBRACE international study (Kirisits et al. 2005; Potter et al. 2006; Potter et al. 2007). If patients received external beam radiotherapy initially, then their radiotherapy treatment plans should be evaluated and dose-volume histograms for organs at risk analyzed. Unfortunately, patients treated before the era of image-guided 3D conformal radiotherapy may not have previous dosimetric data available, and therefore only an estimate can be made.

After radiotherapy, there is recovery of normal tissues. Acutely responding tissues can recover much of their initial tolerance in months to years post-radiotherapy (De Crevoisier et al. 1998; Stewart and van der Kogel 1994). However, late-responding tissues take longer to recover, if they do at all. For example, preclinical data has shown that there is limited recovery of bladder post-radiotherapy (Stewart et al. 1990). Additionally, there is limited data on bowel recovery post-radiation. Therefore, it is difficult to accurately estimate repair for pelvic organs and dose constraints in the re-irradiation setting. As such, efforts to minimize dose to organs at risk are emphasized.

2.4 Technological Factors

Modern radiotherapy techniques, using CT-based planning and creation of dose-volume histograms, have made the idea of re-irradiation more feasible as previous doses to the target and OARs have been documented. Composite plans can be developed showing the predicted total dose delivered to both the tumor and OARs. This helps predict tumor response and OAR toxicity. Techniques such as stereotactic radiotherapy and interstitial brachytherapy allow for dose escalation and normal tissue sparing, which can potentially lead to improvements in local control and toxicity profiles. Image guidance permits the delivery of precise radiotherapy. Although newer techniques allow for more conformal treatment, accurate target delineation is crucial as marginal misses and out-of-field progression can occur. These techniques should be delivered at centers with high volume and expertise to ensure proper treatment delivery.

3 Techniques in Re-irradiation

3.1 Intensity-Modulated Radiotherapy

Highly conformal radiotherapy can be delivered using intensity-modulated radiotherapy (IMRT), volumetric modulated radiotherapy (VMAT), or stereotactic radiotherapy. OARs can be spared from high doses; however, there is an increase volume "splash" of low-dose irradiation that one must consider in the re-irradiation setting. Because the target volume is limited to gross tumor alone, image guidance and effective immobilization devices are helpful.

Dosimetric and clinical studies in gynecological malignancies demonstrate that IMRT is feasible with comparable clinical outcomes to 3D conformal techniques and decreased toxicities (Mundt et al. 2002; Portelance et al. 2001; Hasselle et al. 2011). Therefore, it seems appropriate to consider and exploit IMRT techniques when considering re-irradiation. However, the conformality of IMRT is still superseded by stereotactic techniques and brachytherapy, and one must consider these options when considering higher doses of re-irradiation.

3.2 Stereotactic Radiotherapy

Stereotactic radiotherapy (SBRT) allows a high degree of conformality, delivery of a high dose of radiation, and decreased overall treatment time using hypo-fractionated treatment regimens. The last factor is particularly important in the re-irradiation setting if the treatment is palliative. Lateral pelvic sidewall recurrences are typically not surgically resectable given the proximity to blood vessels and are difficult to treat with brachytherapy. Stereotactic radiotherapy can be used alone or in conjunction with external beam radiotherapy. A summary of published series evaluating the role of stereotactic radiotherapy for recurrent gynecological malignancies is summarized in Table 1.

Guckenberger et al. (2010) described the use of stereotactic radiotherapy in 19 patients with recurrent cervix and endometrial cancer; seven had received radiotherapy as part of their initial treatment. These recurrences were either central or pelvic sidewall and ranged in size from 1.5 to 6.5 cm. These patients were treated with stereotactic radiotherapy alone and were prescribed either 30 Gy in 3 fractions or 28 Gy in 4 fractions prescribed to the 65 % isodose line. Systemic

Table 1 Series demonstrating use of stereotactic radiation (SBRT) for re-irradiation

Series	Total patients	No. with prior RT	Dose and fractionation	Local control (LC)	Toxicity
Guckenberger et al. (2010)	19	7	Median dose: 15 Gy in 3 fractions prescribed to 65 % isodose	3-year LC: 81 % 3-year LC: 100 % (re-irradiation patients)	25 %: > grade 2 late
Deodato et al. (2009)	11	5	20–30 Gy in 4–5 fractions prescribed to the 95 % isodose line	2-year LC: 82 %	0 %: > grade 2 acute and late
Kunos et al. (2009)	5	5	15–24 Gy in 3 fractions	3 complete responses, 2 partial responses	1/5: grade 3 acute (fatigue)
Dewas et al. (2011)	16	16 (5 gyne)	36 Gy in 6 fractions over 3 weeks prescribed to 80 % isodose line	1-year LC: 51 % (for entire cohort)	0 %: ≥ grade 3
Kunos et al. (2008)	3	3	24 Gy in 3 fractions	PFS: 1–3 months (all out-of-field recurrence)	0 %: ≥ grade 3
Seo et al. (2014)	23	17	27–45 Gy in 3 fractions prescribed to 80 % isodose line	2-year LC: 65 % (entire cohort)	3/17: grade 4 (fistula)
Abusaris et al. (2012)	27 (8 gyne)	27 (8 gyne)	Median maximum SBRT dose EQD2 = 90 Gy (42–420 Gy)	1-year LC: 64 % 2-year LC: 53 % Median OS: 14 months	0 %: ≥ grade 3 acute 0 %: ≥ grade 3 late
Park et al. (2015)	85	71	Median dose: 39 Gy in 3 fractions prescribed to median 80 % isodose line (BED = 90 Gy)	2-year LC: 83 % 5-year LC: 79 %	5/85: ≥ grade 3 late (2 rectovaginal fistula)
Pontoriero et al. (2015)	5	5	15–20 Gy in 3–4 consecutive fractions, prescribed to median isodose line 72 % (BED = 83 Gy)	3 complete responses, 2 partial responses	0 %: ≥ grade 3 within 90 days of SBRT

failure was the main cause of death, occurring in 7/10 patients. There were also significant rates of late ≥ grade 2 toxicity at 25 %. Unfortunately, this study did not separate their results for patients who had received previous radiotherapy. The role of SBRT has also been investigated in patients specifically with recurrent cervical cancer. One study involved 11 patients, 5 of whom had previous radiotherapy (Deodato et al. 2009). The commonly used treatment regimen consisted of 5 fractions of 6 Gy prescribed to the 95 % isodose line (EQD2 = 40 Gy). After a median follow-up of 18 months, there were two local failures. Treatment was well tolerated as there was no ≥ grade 2 late toxicity reported. Another study retrospectively reviewed 23 patients with locally recurrent cervical cancer limited to the pelvic sidewall (Seo et al. 2014). Seventeen of these patients had prior radiotherapy. Stereotactic doses ranged from 27 to 45 Gy (median, 39 Gy) in 3 fractions prescribed to the 80 % isodose line. For the entire cohort, the 2-year overall survival and local control rates were 43 % and 65 %, respectively. Patients with tumor volumes <30 cm^3 did significantly better than those with larger tumors. There were three cases of rectovaginal fistula (grade 4 toxicity), which all occurred in patients with larger tumors. Seventy-one percent of patients were able to achieve an analgesic reduction of ≥50 % from baseline.

Kunos et al. (2009) described the first use of CyberKnife radiosurgery in three patients with recurrent squamous cell carcinoma of the vulva after primary radiotherapy. Treatment consisted of 3 fractions of 8 Gy prescribed to the 75 % isodose line (EQD2 57.6 Gy). All patients developed acute skin irritation and desquamating necrosis within the treatment field, although all healed and there were no late toxicities reported. Although all three patients responded locally, they all developed progressive disease within 3 months of radiosurgery. A similar study evaluating the role of CyberKnife SBRT for patients with recurrent or oligometastatic cervical cancer was conducted in 85 patients by the Korean Radiation Oncology Group. The sites treated with SBRT were within the prior radiotherapy field in 59 cases and partially overlapped in nine cases. With a median dose of 39 Gy in 3 fractions (BED = 90 Gy), the 2-year and 5-year local control rates were 83 % and 79 %, respectively. A disease-free survival interval >36 months was found to be significant for both local control and overall survival. Late grade 3–4 toxicity occurred in five patients with rectovaginal fistula occurring in two patients (Park et al. 2015).

In conclusion, stereotactic radiotherapy is safe and feasible for patients with gynecological malignancies receiving re-irradiation to the pelvis. Results are promising with respect to treatment tolerance and local control. The short treatment times are also beneficial for palliative patients. Future directions may include the use of adaptive replanning in clinical scenarios of rapid tumor regression and/or anatomical changes to help with dose escalation and OAR avoidance.

3.3 Intraoperative Radiotherapy

Intraoperative radiotherapy can be delivered by two techniques: electron beam radiotherapy delivered using a linear accelerator or HDR brachytherapy using interstitial catheters. Intraoperative radiotherapy is typically reserved for cases of microscopic disease after surgery. Its benefit is that a single high-dose fraction can be delivered during surgery when adjacent OARs can be mobilized away from the target. Organs at risk include the pelvic nerves and ureters. Potential complications of intraoperative radiotherapy include damage of these structures leading to neuropathic pain, motor deficits, and ureteral obstruction. A summary of published series evaluating the role of IORT for recurrent gynecological malignancies is summarized in Table 2.

Mahe et al. (1996) published on 70 patients who received IORT for pelvic recurrence after initial treatment with radiotherapy. These patients largely had pelvic side wall disease ± central disease. Surgery varied according to initial treatment and tumor size. At 15-month follow-up, the median survival was only 11 months, and local control was 21 %. Grade 2–3 toxicity was observed in 27 % of patients and included GI or urinary fistulas, infection, rectal stricture,

Table 2 Series demonstrating use of intraoperative radiotherapy (IORT) for re-irradiation

Series	Patients	Prior RT	IORT details	Local control	Toxicity
Martinez Monge et al. (1993)	26	14	Median cone size: 8 cm (5–12 cm) Median dose: 15 Gy (10–25 Gy); median electron beam energy: 9 MeV (6–15 MeV)	4-year LC: 33 %	≥ grade 3 GU: 1/14 ≥ grade 3 GI: 0 Chronic pain: 6/14
Mahe et al. (1996)	70	54	Mean cone size: 7.5 cm (4–9 cm) Mean dose: 18 Gy (10–25 Gy) Mean energy: 12 MeV (6–20 MeV)	Median LC: 21 %	14 % IORT-related complications (5 neuropathies, 4 ureteral obstructions, 1 rectal stricture)
Tran et al. (2007)	36	23	Mean cone size: 6 cm (2.85–10 cm) Mean dose: 11.5 Gy (6–17.5 Gy) Energy: 6–12 MeV	5-year LC: 44% for entire cohort	≥ grade 3: 28% for entire cohort
Gemignani et al. (2001)	17	14	Mean dose: 14 Gy (12–15 Gy)	3-year LC: 67 %	Grade 2–3 toxicity: 58 % No life-threatening toxicity
Stelzer et al. (1995)	22	11	Median cone size: 6 cm (6–15 cm) Median dose: 22 Gy (14–28 Gy) Median energy: 12 MeV (9–22 MeV)	5-year LC: 48 %	Most common toxicity neuropathy: 7/22 treatment related

neuropathy, and ureteral obstruction. Another study retrospectively evaluated the role of IORT for patients with recurrent gynecological malignancies. Of the 36 patients reviewed, 23 had previous radiotherapy. The 5-year local control rate was 44 % and rates of grade 3+ toxicity were 28 %. Multivariate analysis found that disease-free interval, tumor size, cervical cancer primary and previous surgery were significant prognostic factors (Tran et al. 2007). Gross tumor resection has also been found to be significant prognostic factor (Gemignani et al. 2001). A single institution retrospective review compared the addition of IORT to surgically treated patients, all of whom has previously received pelvic radiotherapy. It found that the addition of IORT did not improve clinical outcomes (Backes et al. 2014). It should be noted that the patients who received IORT tended to have poorer prognostic features, such as shorter disease-free interval and increased lateral tumor extension.

In summary, IORT has been shown to provide reasonable local control for patients with recurrent gynecological malignancies; however, rates of toxicity are not trivial. Careful patient selection is paramount.

3.4 Brachytherapy

Brachytherapy is a useful modality in the treatment of local recurrences, allowing dose escalation with a favorable therapeutic ratio. Late toxicity is reported as being less significant in patients re-irradiated with brachytherapy as opposed to EBRT (Russell et al. 1987), in part because of the rapid dose falloff that can be achieved around the target volume, limiting dose to normal tissues. Both HDR and LDR have been used in the radical setting with no difference in outcome or toxicity. Local control rates in the re-irradiation setting have ranged from 67 to 100 %

in some series, particularly in small recurrences (Xiang et al. 1998; Petignat et al. 2006). Toxicities have included severe vaginal stenosis and GI toxicity rates of up to 25 %.

Multichannel applicators typically use line sources not limited to the center of the applicator but also on the edges or surfaces of the cylinder. This allows for asymmetric and conformal dose distributions to be delivered sparing the rectum and bladder but increasing vaginal mucosa dose as compared to single-channel applicators (Tanderup and Lindegaard 2004). Selected brachytherapy series are shown in Table 3.

3.5 Interstitial Brachytherapy

Interstitial brachytherapy allows for highly conformal dose delivery to recurrent disease with the use of catheter needles directly inserted into the tumor. This allows for high-dose radiation treatment to vaginal or pelvic recurrences from gynecological cancers. Interstitial brachytherapy may be a reasonable alternative to surgical salvage in patients with medical comorbidities or when organ sparing is preferred. In cases where surgical salvage is not appropriate due to the location of the recurrent disease, such as the lateral pelvis, interstitial brachytherapy may also be an option. Both permanent interstitial implants and remote afterloading technologies have been employed. Interstitial treatment is not a new technique as it has been studied and available for decades. However, with the introduction of three-dimensional guided imaging, there have been major advancements in the precision of the treatment planning and radiation delivery, and thus the technique has become more readily implemented in many centers.

Single institutions have reported good results in terms of local control, particularly in patients with lower volume disease (Badakh and Grover 2009). With the ability to deliver high-dose re-irradiation directly into tumors, as expected, toxicities can be severe in cases with disease in close proximity to organs at risk. Grade 4 complications including vesicovaginal fistula, rectovaginal fistula, soft tissue necrosis, and chronic rectal bleeding have been seen with this technique.

Brabham and Cardenes (2009) described their experience with permanent interstitial re-irradiation with ^{198}Au. Median tumor volume was only 3.3 cm^3 (0.8–21.3 cm^3). With a median follow-up of 21 months, an impressive rate of complete responses of nearly 95 % was achieved and local control of over 75 %, while maintaining a low rate of grade 3 toxicity of 5.3 %.

A study from Poland evaluated HDR brachytherapy for the re-irradiation of cervical and vaginal cancer specifically assessing doses to organs at risk (Zolciak-Siwinska et al. 2014). Most patients were treated with an interstitial technique. The median EQD2 for re-irradiation was 48.8 Gy (range, 16.0–91.0 Gy), and cumulative EQD2 was 133.5 Gy (range, 96.8–164.2 Gy). After a median follow-up of 31 months, a complete response after re-irradiation was noted in 95 % of patients. The 3-year local control was 45 %. Grade 3+ toxicities were observed in 15 % of patients (3/20, two grade 3 late GU and one grade 3 late GI). A cumulative EQD2 to 2 cm^3 of the bladder and rectum of approximately 100 Gy was found to be safe. Adverse prognostic factors were <12-month interval from primary radiotherapy to re-irradiation and tumor diameter >3 cm.

Another study by Mabuchi et al. (2014) evaluated HDR interstitial brachytherapy in 52 patients with recurrent cervical cancer. A combination of 2D and 3D planning was used depending on the treatment year. A total dose of 42 Gy in 7 fractions over 4 days was administered. The median follow-up was 55 months. A complete response was noted in 56 % of patients, and the local control rate was 77 %. Grade 3+ toxicities were observed in 25 % of patients and consisted primarily of fistulas. Again, tumor size and treatment-free interval were found to be significantly associated with outcome. These factors can be used to guide patients suitable for curative treatment versus palliative.

4 Discussion

Although outcomes for patients with gynecological malignancies are improving, a significant proportion will develop locoregional recurrence.

Table 3 Series demonstrating the use of brachytherapy for re-irradiation

Series	Total patients	No. with prior RT	Dose and fractionation	Local control (LC)	Toxicity
Brachytherapy (BT)					
Xiang et al. (1998)	73	73	Radium therapy: 30–40 Gy in 3–5 fractions or HDR 20–35 Gy in 3–5 fractions over 3–4 weeks Followed by vaginal mold: 20–30 Gy in 4–6 fractions at 5 mm depth 30–40 Gy EBRT to involved vulva or groin	5-year LC: 67 %	Grade 4 toxicity: 24.6 %
Petignat et al. (2006)	22	2	Median HDR BT: 26 Gy (range, 8–48 Gy) in a median of 4 fractions (1–11)	5-year LC 100 %	> grade 2 acute: 0 % > grade 2 late GI: 18 % > grade 2 late vaginal: 50 %
Interstitial implants					
Brabham and Cardenes (2009)	19	19	Median dose: 50 Gy (range, 25–55 Gy)	21-month LC: 63 %	> grade 2: 5.3 %
Badakh and Grover (2009)	22	22	Median dose: 25.8 Gy (range, 12–45 Gy) delivered BID, 4–6 Gy per fraction	LC: 22.7 %	Grade 4 toxicity: 18 %
Jhingran et al. (2003)	91	34	Median dose: 75 Gy (range, 34–122 Gy)	5-year LC: 69 %	> grade 2 toxicity: 12.1 %
Gupta et al. (1999)	69	15	Median dose: 35 Gy (range, 25–55 Gy)	3-year LC: 49 %	Grade 4 toxicity: 14 %
Randall et al. (1993)	13	13	30–90 Gy (0.17–0.59 Gy/h)	2-year LC: 46 %	Grade 4 late: 1/13 (rectovaginal fistula)
Mabuchi et al. (2014)	52	52	42 Gy in 7 fractions, OD on day of implant then BID × 3 days	32-month LC: 77 %	> grade 3 late: 25 %
Zolciak-Siwinska et al. (2014)	20	20	Median EQD2 for re-irradiation: 48.8 Gy (range, 16.0–91.0 Gy)	3-year LC: 45 %	Grade 3+ toxicity: 15 %

Management of recurrent gynecological malignancies in the setting of previous pelvic radiotherapy is highly complex and should involve a multidisciplinary evaluation. Surgery, in the form of exenteration, is the preferred option for patients with good performance status, long disease-free interval, and small-volume recurrence; however, in nonsurgical candidates, re-irradiation may be considered. The potential risks of re-treatment must be weighed against the benefits and careful patient selection, and early delineation of treatment intent is critical.

The Brachytherapy Working Party of the British Institute of Radiology developed clinical and radiobiological guidelines for re-irradiation (Jones and Blake 1999). The group advocated selecting patients who had previously tolerated radiotherapy well, who had biopsy-proven disease recurrence, and in whom a detailed discussion had taken place between the patient/family and radiation oncologist regarding the expected benefits and the risks. The group also recommended determining the goals of treatment upfront as this would impact factors such as field size, beam direction, and dose-fractionation schedule. In a Canadian Patterns of Care study, nearly all of respondents (99 %) would offer re-irradiation with the intent of improving patient quality of life (Joseph et al. 2008). One third would offer re-irradiation with curative intent. The main factors taken into account when considering re-irradiation were disease-free interval, performance status, absence of distant metastases, and absence of late toxicity from previous radiotherapy. Those who would not offer re-treatment cited concerns of uncertainty around normal tissue tolerance and radiobiological issues and uncertainty about the benefits of re-irradiation. The volume of previous radiation was also a major factor in considering re-irradiation.

Advances in imaging and treatment planning techniques have enhanced the feasibility of offering re-treatment to patients with recurrent disease in a previously irradiated field. While treatment outcomes may be improved by dose escalation, so too is treatment-related morbidity. In addition, while highly conformal treatments may be able to control recurrent disease, this will not address out-of-field and distant disease progression. Therefore, treatment intent and target volume delineation are of great importance.

4.1 Decision-Making Process

No clear guidelines exist to aid in the selection of a safe but effective re-irradiation dose. Treatment intent should be defined early. Radiobiological factors to consider include the time interval since original radiotherapy and the estimated re-treatment tolerance of normal pelvic tissue. The original radiation EQD2 dose (EBRT + brachytherapy) must be calculated or estimated, keeping in mind the inherent inaccuracies in such a calculation due to the different biological effect and dose/fraction of both modalities. Table 4 describes possible re-irradiation schedules. The previously outlined patient, tumor, technological, and radiobiological factors should all be considered. The time schedule over which re-irradiation will be delivered, including twice-daily regimens, also warrants consideration. Extrapolating the data from squamous cell head and neck cancer trials, the use of hyperfractionated regimes to escalate the total tumoricidal dose while not increasing late toxicity (Bourhis et al. 2006), is theoretically a viable option for cervical squamous cell tumors. However, evidence is lacking. Finally, the volume to be treated may be reduced in some cases, in order to maximize local control while reducing risks of toxicity. Figure 1 describes an algorithm to assist in the decision-making process for patients requiring re-irradiation.

4.2 Future Directions

Protons have been shown to be dosimetrically superior to photons with respect to normal tissue sparing (St Clair et al. 2004). Their main advantage is OAR sparing through the elimination of exit dose and decreased entrance dose which maximizes the therapeutic ratio. As such, proton therapy may offer a significant clinical benefit in the re-irradiation setting. Currently, experience with protons is still maturing; limited to the

Table 4 Suggested re-irradiation fractionation schedules

Location of recurrence	Radical dose/fractionation schedules	Palliative dose/fractionation schedules
Pelvic sidewall	EBRT 50 Gy in 25 fractions 45 Gy in 25 fractions 40 Gy in 20 fractions	EBRT 40 Gy in 20 fractions 20 Gy in 5 fractions 25–30 Gy in 10–15 fractions
Vaginal vault	EBRT + brachytherapy 45–50 Gy in 25 fractions EBRT, followed by vaginal vault brachytherapy to total dose 65–75 Gy	N/A
	EBRT alone 45–50 Gy in 25 fractions 40 Gy in 20 fractions	EBRT 40 Gy in 20 fractions 30 Gy in 20 fractions BID 20 Gy in 5 fractions 25–30 Gy in 10–15 fractions
	Brachytherapy alone 20–30 Gy in 4–6 fractions HDR	Brachytherapy alone 21 Gy in 3 fractions HDR 20 Gy in 4 fractions HDR

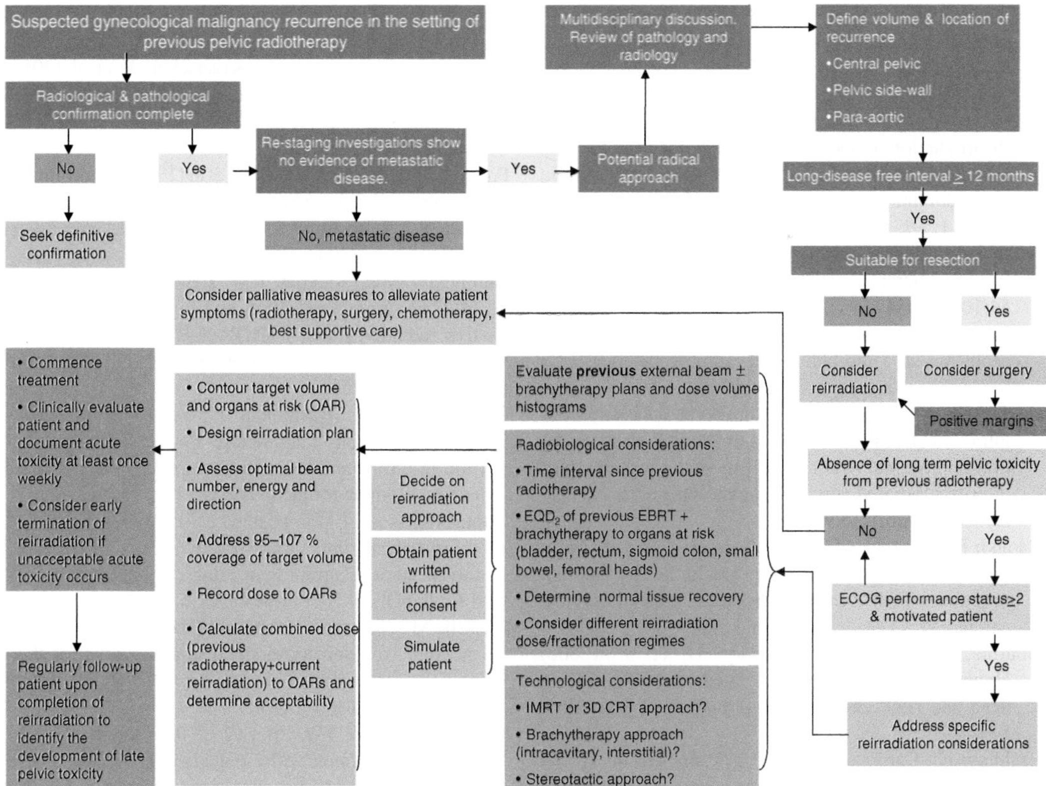

Fig. 1 Decision-making algorithm for re-irradiation for GYN malignancies

treatment of specific sites, such as prostate cancer and pediatric malignancies; and has limited accessibility. A recently published review article described the use of protons in the re-irradiation setting (Plastaras et al. 2014). No patients with gynecological malignancies were discussed, but as availability and experience increases, its use in gynecological malignancies and in the re-irradiation setting will increase.

Furthermore, the soundest way to evaluate the role of re-irradiation with respect to local control and toxicity is as part of a clinical trial. Studies assessing the role of re-irradiation in gynecological malignancies are necessary.

References

Aalders JG, Abeler V, Kolstad P (1984) Recurrent adenocarcinoma of the endometrium: a clinical and histopathological study of 379 patients. Gynecol Oncol 17:85–103

Abusaris H, Hoogeman M, Nuyttens JJ (2012) Re-irradiation: outcome, cumulative dose and toxicity in patients retreated with stereotactic radiotherapy in the abdominal or pelvic region. Technol Cancer Res Treat 11:591–597

Andreyev J (2005) Gastrointestinal complications of pelvic radiotherapy: are they of any importance? Gut 54:1051–1054

Anthopoulos AP, Manetta A, Larson JE et al (1989) Pelvic exenteration: a morbidity and mortality analysis of a seven-year experience. Gynecol Oncol 35:219–223

Backes FJ, Billingsley CC, Martin DD et al (2014) Does intra-operative radiation at the time of pelvic exenteration improve survival for patients with recurrent, previously irradiated cervical, vaginal, or vulvar cancer? Gynecol Oncol 135:95–99

Badakh DK, Grover AH (2009) Reirradiation with high-dose-rate remote afterloading brachytherapy implant in patients with locally recurrent or residual cervical carcinoma. J Cancer Res Ther 5:24–30

Bourhis J, Overgaard J, Audry H et al (2006) Hyperfractionated or accelerated radiotherapy in head and neck cancer: a meta-analysis. Lancet 368: 843–854

Brabham JG, Cardenes HR (2009) Permanent interstitial reirradiation with 198Au as salvage therapy for low volume recurrent gynecologic malignancies: a single institution experience. Am J Clin Oncol 32:417–422

Chemoradiotherapy for Cervical Cancer Meta-analysis C: reducing uncertainties about the effects of chemoradiotherapy for cervical cancer: individual patient data meta-analysis (2010) Cochrane Database Syst Rev CD008285

Chen MF, Tseng CJ, Tseng CC et al (2007) Clinical outcome in posthysterectomy cervical cancer patients treated with concurrent Cisplatin and intensity-modulated pelvic radiotherapy: comparison with conventional radiotherapy. Int J Radiat Oncol Biol Phys 67:1438–1444

De Crevoisier R, Bourhis J, Domenge C et al (1998) Full-dose reirradiation for unresectable head and neck carcinoma: experience at the Gustave-Roussy Institute in a series of 169 patients. J Clin Oncol 16:3556–3562

Denton AS, Bond SJ, Matthews S et al (2000) National audit of the management and outcome of carcinoma of the cervix treated with radiotherapy in 1993. Clin Oncol (R Coll Radiol) 12:347–353

Deodato F, Macchia G, Grimaldi L et al (2009) Stereotactic radiotherapy in recurrent gynecological cancer: a case series. Oncol Rep 22:415–419

Dewas S, Bibault JE, Mirabel X et al (2011) Robotic image-guided reirradiation of lateral pelvic recurrences: preliminary results. Radiat Oncol 6:77

Eifel PJ, Levenback C, Wharton JT et al (1995) Time course and incidence of late complications in patients treated with radiation therapy for FIGO stage IB carcinoma of the uterine cervix. Int J Radiat Oncol Biol Phys 32:1289–1300

Fotopoulou C, Neumann U, Kraetschell R et al (2010) Long-term clinical outcome of pelvic exenteration in patients with advanced gynecological malignancies. J Surg Oncol 101:507–512

Fuller AF Jr, Elliott N, Kosloff C et al (1989) Determinants of increased risk for recurrence in patients undergoing radical hysterectomy for stage IB and IIA carcinoma of the cervix. Gynecol Oncol 33:34–39

Gemignani ML, Alektiar KM, Leitao M et al (2001) Radical surgical resection and high-dose intraoperative radiation therapy (HDR-IORT) in patients with recurrent gynecologic cancers. Int J Radiat Oncol Biol Phys 50:687–694

Guckenberger M, Bachmann J, Wulf J et al (2010) Stereotactic body radiotherapy for local boost irradiation in unfavourable locally recurrent gynaecological cancer. Radiother Oncol 94:53–59

Gupta AK, Vicini FA, Frazier AJ et al (1999) Iridium-192 transperineal interstitial brachytherapy for locally advanced or recurrent gynecological malignancies. Int J Radiat Oncol Biol Phys 43:1055–1060

Hasselle MD, Rose BS, Kochanski JD et al (2011) Clinical outcomes of intensity-modulated pelvic radiation therapy for carcinoma of the cervix. Int J Radiat Oncol Biol Phys 80:1436–1445

Jhingran A, Burke TW, Eifel PJ (2003) Definitive radiotherapy for patients with isolated vaginal recurrence of endometrial carcinoma after hysterectomy. Int J Radiat Oncol Biol Phys 56:1366–1372

Jones B, Blake PR (1999) Retreatment of cancer after radical radiotherapy. Br J Radiol 72:1037–1039

Joseph KJ, Al-Mandhari Z, Pervez N et al (2008) Reirradiation after radical radiation therapy: a survey of patterns of practice among Canadian radiation oncologists. Int J Radiat Oncol Biol Phys 72:1523–1529

Kirisits C, Potter R, Lang S et al (2005) Dose and volume parameters for MRI-based treatment planning in intracavitary brachytherapy for cervical cancer. Int J Radiat Oncol Biol Phys 62:901–911

Kunos C, von Gruenigen V, Waggoner S et al (2008) Cyberknife radiosurgery for squamous cell carcinoma of vulva after prior pelvic radiation therapy. Technol Cancer Res Treat 7:375–380

Kunos C, Chen W, DeBernardo R et al (2009) Stereotactic body radiosurgery for pelvic relapse of gynecologic malignancies. Technol Cancer Res Treat 8:393–400

Look KY, Rocereto TF (1990) Relapse patterns in FIGO stage IB carcinoma of the cervix. Gynecol Oncol 38:114–120

Mabuchi S, Takahashi R, Isohashi F et al (2014) Reirradiation using high-dose-rate interstitial brachytherapy for locally recurrent cervical cancer: a single institutional experience. Int J Gynecol Cancer 24:141–148

Maggioni A, Roviglione G, Landoni F et al (2009) Pelvic exenteration: ten-year experience at the European Institute of Oncology in Milan. Gynecol Oncol 114:64–68

Mahe MA, Gerard JP, Dubois JB et al (1996) Intraoperative radiation therapy in recurrent carcinoma of the uterine cervix: report of the French intraoperative group on 70 patients. Int J Radiat Oncol Biol Phys 34:21–26

Martinez Monge R, Jurado M, Azinovic I et al (1993) Intraoperative radiotherapy in recurrent gynecological cancer. Radiother Oncol 28:127–133

Morley GW, Lindenauer SM (1976) Pelvic exenterative therapy for gynecologic malignancy: an analysis of 70 cases. Cancer 38:581–586

Mundt AJ, Lujan AE, Rotmensch J et al (2002) Intensity-modulated whole pelvic radiotherapy in women with gynecologic malignancies. Int J Radiat Oncol Biol Phys 52:1330–1337

Mundt AJ, Mell LK, Roeske JC (2003) Preliminary analysis of chronic gastrointestinal toxicity in gynecology patients treated with intensity-modulated whole pelvic radiation therapy. Int J Radiat Oncol Biol Phys 56:1354–1360

Ooi BS, Tjandra JJ, Green MD (1999) Morbidities of adjuvant chemotherapy and radiotherapy for resectable rectal cancer: an overview. Dis Colon Rectum 42:403–418

Park HJ, Chang AR, Seo Y et al (2015) Stereotactic body radiotherapy for recurrent or oligometastatic uterine cervix cancer: a cooperative study of the Korean radiation oncology group (KROG 14–11). Anticancer Res 35:5103–5110

Petignat P, Jolicoeur M, Alobaid A et al (2006) Salvage treatment with high-dose-rate brachytherapy for isolated vaginal endometrial cancer recurrence. Gynecol Oncol 101:445–449

Plastaras JP, Berman AT, Freedman GM (2014) Special cases for proton beam radiotherapy: re-irradiation, lymphoma, and breast cancer. Semin Oncol 41: 807–819

Pontoriero A, Iati G, Aiello D et al (2015) Stereotactic Radiotherapy in the Retreatment of Recurrent Cervical Cancers, Assessment of Toxicity, and Treatment Response: Initial Results and Literature Review. Technol Cancer Res Treat Sep 30. pii: 1533034615608740

Portelance L, Chao KS, Grigsby PW et al (2001) Intensity-modulated radiation therapy (IMRT) reduces small bowel, rectum, and bladder doses in patients with cervical cancer receiving pelvic and para-aortic irradiation. Int J Radiat Oncol Biol Phys 51:261–266

Potter ME, Alvarez RD, Gay FL et al (1990) Optimal therapy for pelvic recurrence after radical hysterectomy for early-stage cervical cancer. Gynecol Oncol 37:74–77

Potter R, Haie-Meder C, Van Limbergen E et al (2006) Recommendations from gynaecological (GYN) GEC ESTRO working group (II): concepts and terms in 3D image-based treatment planning in cervix cancer brachytherapy-3D dose volume parameters and aspects of 3D image-based anatomy, radiation physics, radiobiology. Radiother Oncol 78:67–77

Potter R, Dimopoulos J, Georg P et al (2007) Clinical impact of MRI assisted dose volume adaptation and dose escalation in brachytherapy of locally advanced cervix cancer. Radiother Oncol 83:148–155

Prempree T, Amornmarn R, Villasanta U et al (1984) Retreatment of very late recurrent invasive squamous cell carcinoma of the cervix with irradiation. II Criteria for patients' selection to achieve the success. Cancer 54:1950–1955

Randall ME, Evans L, Greven KM et al (1993) Interstitial reirradiation for recurrent gynecologic malignancies: results and analysis of prognostic factors. Gynecol Oncol 48:23–31

Roberts WS, Cavanagh D, Bryson SC et al (1987) Major morbidity after pelvic exenteration: a seven-year experience. Obstet Gynecol 69:617–621

Russell AH, Koh WJ, Markette K et al (1987) Radical reirradiation for recurrent or second primary carcinoma of the female reproductive tract. Gynecol Oncol 27:226–232

Seo Y, Kim MS, Yoo HJ et al (2014) Salvage stereotactic body radiotherapy for locally recurrent uterine cervix cancer at the pelvic sidewall: Feasibility and complication. Asia Pac J Clin Oncol May 30. doi:10.1111/ajco.12185

Sharma S, Odunsi K, Driscoll D et al (2005) Pelvic exenterations for gynecological malignancies: twenty-year experience at Roswell Park Cancer Institute. Int J Gynecol Cancer 15:475–482

St Clair WH, Adams JA, Bues M et al (2004) Advantage of protons compared to conventional X-ray or IMRT in the treatment of a pediatric patient with medulloblastoma. Int J Radiat Oncol Biol Phys 58:727–734

Stelzer KJ, Koh WJ, Greer BE et al (1995) The use of intraoperative radiation therapy in radical salvage for recurrent cervical cancer: outcome and toxicity. Am J Obstet Gynecol 172:1881–1886; discussion 1886–1888

Stewart FA, van der Kogel AJ (1994) Retreatment tolerance of normal tissues. Semin Radiat Oncol 4:103–111

Stewart FA, Oussoren Y, Luts A (1990) Long-term recovery and reirradiation tolerance of mouse bladder. Int J Radiat Oncol Biol Phys 18:1399–1406

Tanderup K, Lindegaard JC (2004) Multi-channel intracavitary vaginal brachytherapy using three-dimensional optimization of source geometry. Radiother Oncol 70:81–85

Thomas GM, Dembo AJ, Myhr T et al (1993) Long-term results of concurrent radiation and chemotherapy for carcinoma of the cervix recurrent after surgery. Int J Gynecol Cancer 3:193–198

Torre LA, Bray F, Siegel RL et al (2015) Global cancer statistics, 2012. CA Cancer J Clin 65:87–108

Tran PT, SU Z, Hara W et al (2007) Long-term survivors using intraoperative radiotherapy for recurrent gynecologic malignancies. Int J Radiat Oncol Biol Phys 69:504–511

Xiang EW, Shu-mo C, Ya-qin D et al (1998) Treatment of late recurrent vaginal malignancy after initial radiotherapy for carcinoma of the cervix: an analysis of 73 cases. Gynecol Oncol 69:125–129

Zolciak-Siwinska A, Bijok M, Jonska-Gmyrek J et al (2014) HDR brachytherapy for the reirradiation of cervical and vaginal cancer: analysis of efficacy and dosage delivered to organs at risk. Gynecol Oncol 132:93–97

Reirradiation for Soft Tissue Sarcomas

Michael S. Rutenberg and Daniel J. Indelicato

Contents

Abstract

The incidence of local recurrence after wide local excision and radiation of soft tissue sarcoma ranges from 5 to 20%. Up to 80% of these relapses will occur in the absence of metastatic disease. The optimal management of locally recurrent soft tissue sarcoma must be individualized and depends on prior therapy, the location of the recurrence, and the feasibility of conservative surgery. Following retreatment, the likelihood of ultimate local control ranges from 37 to 100% and is a reflection of well-known risk factors for de novo sarcomas such as the number of prior recurrences, high grade, positive margins, deep location, and non-extremity tumor site. Reirradiation as part of a multimodality retreatment strategy may improve the chance of local control and organ preservation, but its use must be balanced with the risk of severe treatment-related side effects. Various reirradiation techniques have been utilized for salvage treatment, each with unique risks and benefits.

1 Introduction

The incidence of soft tissue sarcoma (STS) has remained fairly constant over the past 30 years at approximately 7 cases per 100,000 adults (Siegel et al. 2016). It is estimated that in 2016,

The original version of this chapter was revised. An erratum to this chapter can be found at 10.1007/978-3-319-41825-4_78.

M.S. Rutenberg, MD, PhD • D.J. Indelicato, MD (✉)
Department of Radiation Oncology,
University of Florida College of Medicine,
2000 SW Archer Rd, Gainesville,
FL 32610-0385, USA

University of Florida Proton Therapy Institute,
2015 North Jefferson Street,
Jacksonville, FL 32206, USA
e-mail: dindelicato@floridaproton.org

Med Radiol Radiat Oncol (2016)
DOI 10.1007/174_2016_57, © Springer International Publishing Switzerland
Published Online: 07 May 2016

approximately 12,310 Americans will be diagnosed with STS (Siegel et al. 2016). Most of these patients are in the prime of their lives with a median age of 56 years old at diagnosis, and approximately one-fifth of patients are less than 35 years old (Horner et al. 1975–2006). Multimodality therapy is the accepted standard of care in the management of high-risk STS (National Comprehensive Cancer Network 2016). Multiple studies have demonstrated that limited surgery with adjuvant radiotherapy does not compromise survival, preserves functionality, and limits morbidity when compared to radical resection alone (Rosenberg et al. 1982; Kinsella et al. 1983; Wood et al. 1984; Suit et al. 1985; Karakousis et al. 1986; Zelefsky et al. 1990; Pisters et al. 1996; Yang et al. 1998). The incidence of local recurrence after organ-preserving treatment, however, remains as high as 20% in some series (Lindberg et al. 1981; Rosenberg et al. 1982; Mundt et al. 1995; Pisters et al. 1996; Yang et al. 1998), with the majority of local recurrences occurring within the first 2 years of treatment and thus still encompassing a relatively young population (Lindberg et al. 1981; Crago and Brennan 2015). Therefore, it is especially critical that salvage therapy considerations include not only survival but potentially decades of function, social productivity, and quality of life. As many as 80% of sarcoma relapses are isolated local recurrences (Ramanathan et al. 2001) and therefore justify aggressive curative management. While local recurrence of STS carries a negative prognosis, long-term control and survival are achievable with aggressive therapy (Essner et al. 1991; Stojadinovic et al. 2001; Ramanathan et al. 2001). Even with simultaneous isolated pulmonary metastases, there is a potential for long-term survival or cure (Casson et al. 1992; Verazin et al. 1992; van Geel et al. 1996; Rehders et al. 2007; Garcia Franco et al. 2009).

There remain no completed or ongoing prospective trials investigating reirradiation as part of salvage therapy for STS. Therefore, treatment recommendations are based on retrospective data often from small, single-institution series. These reports contain limitations common to all such series, such as selection bias, limited follow-up, and sparse details regarding complications and quality of life.

2 Repeat Conservative Surgery with Reirradiation

In the absence of metastatic disease, current national guidelines suggest that treatment decisions for patients with locally recurrent STS lesion should be made using the same algorithm as for patients at initial presentation (National Comprehensive Cancer Network 2016). Similar to STS management in the initial setting, there is no overall survival or disease-free survival benefit to radical surgery compared to limited resection and adjuvant radiotherapy (Giuliano et al. 1982; Stojadinovic et al. 2001). Therefore, the decision to pursue limited resection/organ preservation can be made based on the ability for adequate oncologic resection and preservation of organ function. If the recurrence is amenable to conservative salvage surgery, this often means planning for reoperation and reirradiation in a complex background of tissue fibrosis, ischemia, and gross anatomic distortion from prior treatment. However, data from multiple other tumor sites, including a large multi-institutional phase II head-and-neck study (Spencer et al. 2008), document that reirradiation following local tumor recurrence is feasible, albeit, potentially morbid (Valentini et al. 2006).

Historically, approximately 30% of STS patients with a local recurrence undergo conservative surgery with some form of reirradiation (Ramanathan et al. 2001), but peer-reviewed outcomes series are limited. Table 1 reviews the literature. Early attempts at conservative salvage treatment involved either preoperative or postoperative external-beam radiation. Essner et al. described 21 patients treated from 1972 to 1988 at the University of California, Los Angeles (UCLA), with isolated local recurrences of STS involving the extremities (Essner et al. 1991). The most common primary tumor site was the thigh, and the initial treatment course of resection and radiotherapy at diagnosis was heterogeneous among the group. The median follow-up was 3

Table 1 Literature review limited to patients treated with conservative surgery and reirradiation for recurrent soft tissue sarcoma (actuarial estimates provided when available)

Study	*N*	Study dates	Retreatment radiotherapy	Median follow-up (mo.)	5-year local control rate (%)	5-year overall survival rate (%)	Serious complications rate (%)	Amputation rate (%)
Nori et al. (1991)	40	1979–1988	BT	36	68	55–85	13	0
Essner et al. (1991)	21	1972–1988	EBRT	36	48	52	42	28
Graham et al. (1992)	5	1981–1987	EBRT	NR	50	40	>10	20
Catton et al. (1996)	10	1990–1995	BT and/or EBRT	31	100	NR	60	10
Pearlstone et al. (1999)	26	1990–1997	BT	16	52	52	15	0
Moureau-Zabotto et al. (2004)	16	1980–1994	BT or EBRT	59	37	NR	NR	NR
Torres et al. (2007)	37	1991–2004	BT or EBRT	72	58	66[a]	51	35
Indelicato et al. (2009)	5	1997–2004	BT and EBRT	3	40	0	80	80
Tinkle et al. (2015)	15	2000–2011	IORT	NR	55	NR	33	NR
Cambeiro et al. (2015)	10	1986–1999	IORT	NR	74	37	10	10
Cambeiro et al. (2015)	16	2001–2010	BT	NR	38	68	56	NR

Table borrowed and modified with permission from Indelicato et al. (2009)

Abbreviations: *BT* brachytherapy, *EBRT* external-beam radiation therapy, *f/u* follow-up, *mo month*, *IORT* intraoperative electron radiotherapy, *N* number of patients, *NR* not reported

[a]Disease-specific survival

years. Local control was achieved in 6 of 7 patients receiving preoperative salvage reirradiation (2800 cGy at 350 cGy/fx with intra-arterial doxorubicin) prior to surgical excision. However, in patients who received salvage surgery before postoperative reirradiation (5000 cGy at 200 cGy/fraction), local control was achieved in only 4 of 14 patients. Other than dose and fractionation, the external-beam radiation technique was similar between the two groups and involved opposing fields covering the entire region of the tumor, sparing only a strip of skin opposite the tumor bed. The surgical procedure for all patients was a wide local excision performed en bloc through "normal-appearing" tissues. Perineurium, periosteum, and vascular adventitia were removed en bloc if tumors were adjacent to these structures. No myocutaneous flaps or free flaps were utilized. Other series have included smaller groups of patients treated with external-beam radiation alone, either in the preoperative or postoperative setting. In these series, doses and fractionation are similar to the treatment in the primary setting (i.e., approximately 45–50 Gy preoperatively and 60–64 Gy postoperatively) (Catton et al. 1996; Torres et al. 2007; Indelicato et al. 2009).

A common concern regarding the administration of repeat external-beam irradiation for recurrent sarcomas is the fear of severe soft tissue necrosis and fibrosis. In the UCLA series described above, there were 3 serious complications in the 7 patients treated with preoperative reirradiation. Two of the 3 complications required reoperation, including 1 amputation as a result of the complication. In the 14 patients receiving postoperative reirradiation, there were 7 serious complications. Six of these required reoperation, including 1 amputation. Functional analysis was performed on all patients. The most common complication was edema requiring a support stocking, occurring in 29 % of the preoperative patients and 64 % of the postoperative group. No fractures of adjacent long bones or pain occurred in the preoperative reirradiation group, while 7 %

and 14 % in the postoperative reirradiation group experienced fracture or pain, respectively. Twenty-nine percent and 36 % required the use of external support (canes or braces) in the preoperative group and postoperative group, respectively. No instance of neuritis or compartment syndrome was observed despite the high cumulative radiation doses. Normal range of motion, defined as being 95 % of the uninvolved extremity, was present in 86 % of the preoperative patients and 36 % of the postoperative patients. The investigators from UCLA concluded that limb salvage was possible in the setting of an isolated local recurrence provided that external-beam radiation was delivered preoperatively in the manner described. For reasons of inferior local control and toxicity, they recommended against postoperative radiation.

In an attempt to further improve salvage therapy for local recurrences, some investigators have used brachytherapy for reirradiation. The largest series is from Memorial Sloan-Kettering Cancer Center (MSKCC; New York, NY) and includes 40 patients with recurrent extremity sarcoma treated from 1979 to 1988 (Nori et al. 1991). Seventy percent of patients had recurrent thigh lesions, and most had received external-beam irradiation as their initial treatment. For salvage, patients underwent conservative function-preserving surgery with brachytherapy alone via a temporary afterloaded iridium-192 (Ir-192) tumor bed implant. A median dose of 4500 cGy was delivered (range, 3000–4800 cGy) at a median dose rate of 40 cGy/h. The median follow-up was 3 years, which was sufficient to capture most local recurrences (Lindberg et al. 1981; Singer et al. 1992) and complications. The 5-year overall survival rate was 85 % and the 5-year local control rate was 68 %. The most important factor impacting the likelihood of local control following salvage was the number of prior local recurrences.

Another large experience involving salvage brachytherapy alone for sarcoma in a previously irradiated field was published in 1999 by Pearlstone et al. from MD Anderson Cancer Center (Houston, TX) (Pearlstone et al. 1999). This study included 26 patients with recurrent sarcoma treated from 1990 to 1997 with a diverse range of tumor sites including the extremities (55 %) as well as the trunk (27 %) and head-and-neck region (8 %). Sixty-five percent of patients had received external-beam irradiation as part of their initial treatment and the rest had received primary brachytherapy. For salvage, patients underwent conservative function-preserving surgery followed by brachytherapy alone via a single-plane afterloaded Ir-192 tumor bed implant. A mean dose of 4720 cGy was delivered (range, 1100–5000 cGy) at a median dose rate of 40 cGy/h. The median follow-up was 16 months. Five-year overall survival was 52 %, and 5-year local control was 52 %. As with the MSKCC experience, the most important factor impacting the likelihood of local control following salvage was the number of prior local recurrences. When patients with tumors located near joint spaces (notoriously difficult areas for brachytherapy) are excluded from the analysis, the local control rate was 82 %.

Brachytherapy alone for salvage offers several theoretical and practical advantages over external-beam reirradiation. By approaching the process of radiation as part of a team of physicians, the areas of highest risk can be directly identified and targeted in the operating room. Interstitial Ir-192 brachytherapy can be delivered in only a few days and commences approximately 1 week following surgery. This treatment option is in contrast to external-beam radiotherapy that typically lasts 6–7 weeks and cannot begin until at least 3–4 weeks following surgery or perhaps longer in tissue that has impaired wound healing from previous radiation. This prolonged postoperative period not only increases the social and economic burden of treatment but may delay the start of adjuvant chemotherapy if indicated. From a radiation delivery perspective, the rapid dose falloff of brachytherapy is such that very little previously irradiated normal tissue outside the target volume receives radiation. The MSKCC brachytherapy reirradiation series (Nori et al. 1991) reported five patients (12.5 %) who experienced serious complications (four patients had soft tissue necrosis and one had a long bone fracture). All patients recovered completely without amputation, functional loss, or disability. The group at MDACC reported a similar low rate of complications (15%) and no amputations (Pearlstone et al. 1999). All of the patients who experienced a perioperative complication underwent primary wound closure, and none of the patients who were reconstructed using a nonirradiated tissue flap experienced a perioperative complication. With a median follow-up of 16 months, however, events in this study may be underreported. In contrast to these series, a study from the Claudius Regaud Institute (Toulouse, France) with a median follow-up of 59 months reported significantly higher rates of late complications after reirradiation with brachytherapy (Moureau-Zabotto et al. 2004). Moureau-Zabotto et al. reported that 49% of patients developed one or more chronic grade 3 or 4 complications after salvage surgery and reirradiation.

A series from The University of Navarre (Pamplona, Spain) included 16 patients with locally recurrent STS treated for salvage with limited resection followed by brachytherapy beginning within 9 days of surgery (Cambeiro et al. 2015). Brachytherapy consisted of a single-plane catheter array covering the tumor bed plus a margin in 8–10 twice-daily treatments to a dose of 32 or 40 Gy for R0 and R1 resections, respectively. With a median follow-up in excess of 3 years, 5-year local-regional control, distant control, and overall survival rates were 38%, 44%, and 68%, respectively. Similar to the French series, these investigators reported high rates of treatment-related complications, with 56% of patients experiencing grade 3–4 complications, 50% of whom required reoperation. All acute and late complications were related to soft tissue injury (including wound dehiscence, infection/abscess, graft failure, necrosis).

Not surprisingly, there are striking differences between the disease control and toxicity outcomes among these retrospective single-institution reports using brachytherapy for reirradiation, which are likely related to differences in patient selection and treatment technique. Notably, the series from MSKCC and MDACC favored smaller and more accessible tumors for which one might expect better tumor control (Pearlstone et al. 1999; Zagars et al. 2003) and fewer complications. For example, the MSKCC series was limited to extremity tumors. Additionally, although recurrent sarcoma may be inherently aggressive from a biological standpoint, some reports indicate that brachytherapy is less effective for low-grade sarcomas, at least in the primary setting (Pisters et al. 1996).

Due to previous surgery and radiation, recurrent STS develop among disturbed tissue where fascial planes are obscured by fibrosis and lymphovascular drainage patterns are distorted. Disease may unpredictably extend well beyond the normal margins. In addition to physiologic remodeling, the anatomy itself is altered and challenges the geometry of brachytherapy implants (Torres et al. 2007). Supplementary external-beam radiotherapy has been utilized by some practitioners to essentially extend and compensate for the irregular dose distribution of brachytherapy.

The largest series describing outcomes following this approach of brachytherapy plus external-beam irradiation comes from the University of Florida. From 1976 to 2005, five patients who underwent primary conservative resection and irradiation developed an isolated local recurrence and were managed with preoperative external-beam radiation and then wide local excision followed by a brachytherapy boost. The external-beam radiation was 24 Gy delivered in a hyperfractionated manner at 1.2 Gy twice daily to minimize the late tissue effects. For the brachytherapy, eight to ten catheters were used, and the dose rate was 50–60 cGy/h prescribed to 5–10 mm from the single implant plane. The median interval between surgery and Ir-192 afterloading was 5 days. The median brachytherapy dose was 39 Gy (range, 26–42 Gy). The median total dose for retreatment was 63.5 Gy (range, 51.5–66.0 Gy). With a median follow-up of 3 years, the results were dismal. All five patients eventually died from their disease. This aggressive retreatment approach led to severe complications in four of five patients (all of which were chronic non-healing ulcers or other wound complications requiring amputation). Despite aggressive management, three patients ultimately developed another local recurrence before death.

Following a rationale similar to brachytherapy, several investigators have reported success using intraoperative electron-beam radiation therapy (IOERT) for reirradiation of STS (Azinovic et al. 2003; Cambeiro et al. 2015; Tinkle et al. 2015). IOERT applicators are desirable because they can directly visualize and access the surgical bed in the operating room and the dosimetry of the electrons may be easily customized. This strategy may decrease toxicity since dose-limiting normal tissues can be displaced or protected during IOERT (Willett et al. 2007). Like brachytherapy, IOERT might indirectly improve the quality of therapy by decreasing the overall treatment time. In the experience from the University of Navarre, ten patients with locally recurrent extremity STS or aggressive fibromatosis were treated with IOERT from 1986 to 1999 following limb-sparing surgery. The radiation therapy details of initial patient treatments were not available. For the IOERT course of reirradiation, electron energies between 6 and 15 MeV were utilized depending on the clinical scenario and the extent of residual disease. The IOERT reirradiation dose was between 10 and 20 Gy depending on the margin status. The 5-year actuarial local control, distant control, and overall survival rates were 58 %, 76 %, and 37 %, respectively. One severe toxicity (≥grade 3) occurred involving graft failure requiring amputation (Cambeiro et al. 2015).

A recent series from University of California, San Francisco, also utilized intraoperative radiotherapy for salvage of locally recurrent STS. Tinkle et al. (2015) described 26 patients with locally recurrent STS of the extremities treated with limited resection and IOERT. Of the 26 patients, 15 had previously received external-beam radiotherapy (EBRT; median dose, 63 Gy; range, 25–72 Gy) as part of their initial treatment course. The remaining 11 patients, who had received no prior radiotherapy, were treated with adjuvant EBRT (median dose, 52 Gy; range, 22–60 Gy) following limited resection and IOERT. Surgery consisted of limb-sparing surgery achieving a gross total resection and IOERT to 10–18 Gy (median dose, 15 Gy). With a median follow-up of 35 months, there was no major difference in 5-year actuarial local control in the reirradiation cohort compared to those with no prior radiotherapy, 55 % and 61 % ($p > 0.05$), respectively. In the reirradiation group, 20 % experienced ≥grade 3 acute toxicity, and 33 % experienced ≥grade 3 late toxicity, consisting of wound complications and limb/joint dysfunction.

3 Reirradiation Technique

As described above, there are limited published outcomes following reirradiation for STS, and most include few patients using varied patient selection methods. The information below represents guidelines based on the best available evidence and expert opinion. For all reirradiation cases, patients may benefit from referral to a high-volume center.

3.1 External-Beam Radiation (EBRT)

If possible, external-beam radiation should be delivered in the preoperative setting. Compared to postoperative RT, the lower dose of preoperative radiation is preferable for previously irradiated tissue. Preoperative reirradiation may allow for resection of the twice-irradiated soft tissue adjacent to the tumor bed and reconstructing with autologous nonirradiated tissue. The dose reported for preoperative reirradiation is typically 45–50 Gy with standard fractionation, although hyperfractionation has been utilized at some centers (Indelicato et al. 2009) in an effort to decrease late effects. The target for EBRT should include the tumor as imaged on contrast-enhanced computed tomography and magnetic resonance imaging plus radial and longitudinal margins of 1.5 cm and 3 cm, respectively, where possible. It is important to note that the principles of fascial containment might not apply in a setting of previously manipulated and irradiated tissue.

If preoperative radiation is to be followed by a brachytherapy boost, the external-beam dose should be approximately 24 Gy. Although neuropathy, fracture, edema, and soft tissue fibrosis and necrosis are well recognized as potential complications of high doses of cumulative radiation to uninvolved normal tissue, there are no specific data to suggest overall dose guidelines. Therefore, from a practical standpoint, every effort should be taken to minimize such exposure, and advanced external-beam radiation techniques utilizing image guidance, intensity modulation, and particle therapy may prove beneficial (Weber et al. 2007). Additionally, there are preliminary data from UCLA that preoperative hypofractionated radiation (28 Gy at 3.5 Gy/fraction) combined with intra-arterial chemotherapy is effective.

3.2 Brachytherapy

Whether utilized in combination with external-beam radiotherapy or alone, brachytherapy should represent a closely coordinated effort between the surgery and radiation oncology teams with thorough advanced planning. At the time of resection, the tumor bed should be marked with radiopaque surgical clips. In the operating room, afterloading brachytherapy catheters should be placed with 1-cm spacing within a single plane on the tumor bed with the goal of achieving radial coverage of 1–2 cm. The parallel orientation of the catheters should be secured with absorbable sutures or mesh. The catheters may be anchored to the skin with either sutures or latex balls on both ends. In general, catheters are oriented perpendicular to the incision. However, if a major nerve runs through the surgical bed, catheters may be placed parallel to the nerve to allow an arrangement that keeps the dose to the nerve sheath under 50 Gy.

Depending on the spare tissue, wounds may be closed either by primary means or with unirradiated autologous tissue. Some clinicians are investigating the use of temporary negative-pressure wound therapy to decrease potential radiation injury to the mobilized skin flaps or the plastic surgical flap reconstruction (Torres et al. 2007). The negative-pressure dressing eliminates potential movement of the catheters while the patient is in hospital, and the bulk of the dressing displaces the edges of the surgical wound, limiting their exposure to radiation.

Following confirmation of parallel catheter orientation on X-ray or fluoroscopy, Ir-192 insertion should commence between days 5–7 to allow appropriate wound healing. The prescribed dose rate may range from 40 to 80 cGy/h with the dose specified at 0.5 cm from the plane of the implant. Ideally, the dose variation should not be more than 5–10% across the plane of the implant. Using modern treatment planning techniques, dose prescriptions can be made to a target volume (such as the clinical target volume delineated as a structure with a 5-mm expansion from the operative bed encompassed by at least 90% of the prescription dose) (Cambeiro et al. 2015). For patients being reirradiated with brachytherapy alone, the target dose should be 45–50 Gy. In patients who undergo preoperative external-beam radiation in combination with brachytherapy, the brachytherapy boost dose is 15–20 Gy, and catheters may be loaded within 48 h of surgery (Dalton et al. 1996).

3.3 IOERT

Similar to brachytherapy, IOERT mandates advanced planning and coordination between the surgery and radiation oncology teams. Applicator size should be selected to encompass the entire surgical bed. If the surgical bed is very large and exceeds the size of available applicators, the option is to either use abutting fields (with risk of overdose) or treat only the high-risk areas, such as the surgical tumor bed closer to the resection margin. If the percentage of tissue overlapped exceeds a few millimeters, the risk of necrosis may be unacceptable. The selection of electron-beam energy depends upon the amount of residual tumor: 4- to 9-MeV beams may be used for clinical high-risk areas or microscopic residual disease, while 12–15 MeV may be necessary for macroscopic residual. Because IOERT is performed during surgery, it is always given as a single radiation fraction. Although the biologic effectiveness of this single fraction is not completely understood, it is estimated to be biologically equivalent to at least a dose factor of two to three times greater than that delivered by conventional fractionation (Okunieff et al. 1999; Willett et al. 2007). Thus, 10–20 Gy administered by IOERT has been estimated to have the cell-killing equivalence of 20–60 Gy given by conventional external-beam radiation. Therefore, the recommended IOERT reirradiation dose is between 10 and 20 Gy depending on the margin status and peripheral nerve proximity. If the nerves cannot be physically displaced or if there is a risk of devitalizing the structure, then the IOERT nerve dose should be limited to 10 Gy, and an attempt should be made to protect the nerves with pliable lead sheets for the remaining component of the IOERT dose (Azinovic et al. 2003). A tissue bolus may also be used to protect critical structures beyond the depth of the tumor bed. Prescription doses are often prescribed to the 85–90 % isodose line (Tinkle et al. 2015).

4 Surgery Alone

Questions regarding both the effectiveness of salvage therapy and its treatment-related morbidity have led some clinicians to advocate for surgery alone for patients with recurrent STS. Some clinicians recommended radical surgery in the form of amputation (Shiu et al. 1975; Essner et al. 1991; Singer et al. 1992); however, conservative surgery alone may be an option. Torres et al. reported the outcomes and treatment toxicity after wide local re-excision, with or without additional radiation therapy, for patients with an isolated first local recurrence of soft tissue sarcoma. This study was a retrospective analysis of 62 patients treated at MDACC between 1991 and 2004. All patients had undergone surgery and external-beam radiation at the time of their initial diagnosis. For their recurrent disease, 25 patients were treated with wide local excision alone, and 37 patients were treated with wide local excision and additional radiation (45–64 Gy). In the majority of the reirradiated patients (33 of 37 patients), the radiation was delivered via Ir-192 brachytherapy in a manner analogous to that described above. Reirradiation was not associated with statistically significant improved local control with 5-year actuarial local control rates of 58 % with radiotherapy and 39 % without ($p = 0.4$). Similarly, disease-specific survival and distant metastasis-free survival did not differ between groups. Yet complications requiring outpatient or surgical management were more common in patients who had undergone reirradiation (with a 5-year actuarial complication rate of 80 % vs. 17 %; $p < 0.001$). Amputation rate was also higher in the subgroup of patients who underwent extremity reirradiation (35 % with radiation vs. 11 % without; $p = 0.05$), although only 1 amputation was performed to resolve a treatment-related complication. Although selection biases and a small cohort size confounded the retrospective analysis, the authors concluded that local treatment intensification with additional brachytherapy does not clearly improve outcome after surgical excision alone and is associated with an increase in complications. However, it is important to acknowledge that these comparative outcomes contradict data from other investigators (Catton et al. 1996).

5 Future Directions

As with other recurrent malignancies, patient selection is paramount in determining who will benefit from aggressive salvage therapy for recurrent STS. To properly guide management, more data are needed to determine who will most benefit from reirradiation. To improve the therapeutic ratio in those patients who require a second course of radiation, several important questions must be considered as part of the treatment algorithm. The following questions remain the focus of ongoing research:

1. What is the relationship between time interval for recurrences and disease control? How does the interval between radiation courses influence normal tissue effects of reirradiation?

2. How do we optimally define the target volume? Is it necessary to irradiate the entire initial tumor bed and the entire recurrent tumor bed? What is the optimal target margin and might new imaging modalities help focus our efforts on areas of particularly high risk?
3. What is the role of chemotherapies or targeted agents for radiosensitization in tumor cells that have demonstrated radioresistence?
4. What is the ideal total dose and fractionation schedule (hypofractionation versus standard fractionation)? Does hyperfractionation reduce the risk of late tissue toxicity?
5. What is the ideal modality to effectively address recurrence and limit unnecessary normal tissue reirradiation: brachytherapy, IOERT, IMRT, tomotherapy, proton therapy, carbon ion therapy, or a combination thereof?

As we continue to refine the selection criteria for those who are most likely to benefit from limited surgery and reirradiation for locally recurrent STS, we will better be able to design appropriate studies to address the persistent questions outlined above. Improved prognostic indices, selection criteria, and comparative studies will be critical in advancing the field.

Conclusion

The optimal management of locally recurrent STS must be individualized and depends on prior therapy, the location of the recurrence, and the feasibility of conservative surgery. The likelihood of ultimate local control ranges from 37 to 100%. As with de novo sarcomas, factors for local control of recurrent STS are impacted by well-known risk factors, including the number of previous recurrences, tumor grade, margin status/extent of resection, deep location, and non-extremity tumor site (Pearlstone et al. 1999; Ramanathan et al. 2001; Moureau-Zabotto et al. 2004; Torres et al. 2007; Sabolch et al. 2012). Options for treatment include a wide local re-excision followed by a variety of reirradiation techniques, each with the potential for significant side effects. It is critical to consider overall patient prognosis in the treatment algorithm. The nature of the local recurrence, rather than its presence per se, is the most useful guide to prognosis, and studies exist to help determine an individual's risk index (Ramanathan et al. 2001). For select patients, repeat irradiation may be unnecessary.

References

Azinovic I, Martinez Monge R, Javier Aristu J, Salgado E, Villafranca E, Fernandez Hidalgo O et al (2003) Intraoperative radiotherapy electron boost followed by moderate doses of external beam radiotherapy in resected soft-tissue sarcoma of the extremities. Radiother Oncol 67(3):331–337

Cambeiro M, Aristu JJ, Moreno Jimenez M, Arbea L, Ramos L, San Julian M et al (2015) Salvage wide resection with intraoperative electron beam therapy or HDR brachytherapy in the management of isolated local recurrences of soft tissue sarcomas of the extremities and the superficial trunk. Brachytherapy 14(1):62–70

Casson AG, Putnam JB, Natarajan G, Johnston DA, Mountain C, McMurtrey M et al (1992) Five-year survival after pulmonary metastasectomy for adult soft tissue sarcoma. Cancer 69(3):662–668

Catton C, Davis A, Bell R, O'Sullivan B, Fornasier V, Wunder J et al (1996) Soft tissue sarcoma of the extremity. Limb salvage after failure of combined conservative therapy. Radiother Oncol 41(3):209–214

Crago AM, Brennan MF (2015) Principles in management of soft tissue sarcoma. Adv Surg 49:107–122

Dalton RR, Lanciano RM, Hoffman JP, Eisenberg BL (1996) Wound complications after resection and immediate postoperative brachytherapy in the management of soft-tissue sarcomas. Ann Surg Oncol 3(1):51–56

Essner R, Selch M, Eilber FR (1991) Reirradiation for extremity soft tissue sarcomas. Local control and complications. Cancer 67(11):2813–2817

Garcia Franco CE, Algarra SM, Ezcurra AT, Guillen-Grima F, San-Julian M, Mindan JP et al (2009) Long-term results after resection for soft tissue sarcoma pulmonary metastases. Interact Cardiovasc Thorac Surg 9(2):223–226

Giuliano AE, Eilber FR, Morton DL (1982) The management of locally recurrent soft-tissue sarcoma. Ann Surg 196(1):87–91

Graham JD, Robinson MH, Harmer CL (1992) Re-irradiation of soft-tissue sarcoma. Br J Radiol 65(770):157–161

Horner MJ, Ries LAG, Krapcho M, Neyman N, Aminou R, Howlader N, et al (1975–2006) SEER Cancer Statistics Review. National Cancer Institute. Bethesda, MD. http://seer.cancer.gov/csr/1975_2006/

Indelicato DJ, Meadows K, Gibbs CP Jr, Morris CG, Scarborough MT, Zlotecki RA (2009) Effectiveness and morbidity associated with reirradiation in conservative salvage management of recurrent soft-tissue sarcoma. Int J Radiat Oncol Biol Phys 73(1):267–272

Karakousis CP, Emrich LJ, Rao U, Krishnamsetty RM (1986) Feasibility of limb salvage and survival in soft tissue sarcomas. Cancer 57(3):484–491

Kinsella TJ, Loeffler JS, Fraass BA, Tepper J (1983) Extremity preservation by combined modality therapy in sarcomas of the hand and foot: an analysis of local control, disease free survival and functional result. Int J Radiat Oncol Biol Phys 9(8):1115–1119

Lindberg RD, Martin RG, Romsdahl MM, Barkley HT Jr (1981) Conservative surgery and postoperative radiotherapy in 300 adults with soft-tissue sarcomas. Cancer 47(10):2391–2397

Moureau-Zabotto L, Thomas L, Bui BN, Chevreau C, Stockle E, Martel P et al (2004) Management of soft tissue sarcomas (STS) in first isolated local recurrence: a retrospective study of 83 cases. Radiother Oncol 73(3):313–319

Mundt AJ, Awan A, Sibley GS, Simon M, Rubin SJ, Samuels B et al (1995) Conservative surgery and adjuvant radiation therapy in the management of adult soft tissue sarcoma of the extremities: clinical and radiobiological results. Int J Radiat Oncol Biol Phys 32(4):977–985

National Comprehensive Cancer Network (2016) NCCN clinical practice guidelines in oncology. Soft tissue sarcomas. Fort Washington, PA. http://www.nccn.org/professionals/physician_gls/f_guidelines.asp

Nori D, Schupak K, Shiu MH, Brennan MF (1991) Role of brachytherapy in recurrent extremity sarcoma in patients treated with prior surgery and irradiation. Int J Radiat Oncol Biol Phys 20(6):1229–1233

Okunieff P, Sundararaman S, Chen Y (1999) Biology of large dose per fraction radiation therapy. In: Gunderson LL, Willett CG, Harrison LB, Calvo FA (eds) Intraoperative irradiation. Humana Press, Inc, Totowa, pp 25–46

Pearlstone DB, Janjan NA, Feig BW, Yasko AW, Hunt KK, Pollock RE et al (1999) Re-resection with brachytherapy for locally recurrent soft tissue sarcoma arising in a previously radiated field. Cancer J Sci Am 5(1):26–33

Pisters PW, Harrison LB, Leung DH, Woodruff JM, Casper ES, Brennan MF (1996) Long-term results of a prospective randomized trial of adjuvant brachytherapy in soft tissue sarcoma. J Clin Oncol 14(3):859–868

Ramanathan RC, A'Hern R, Fisher C, Thomas JM (2001) Prognostic index for extremity soft tissue sarcomas with isolated local recurrence. Ann Surg Oncol 8(4):278–289

Rehders A, Hosch SB, Scheunemann P, Stoecklein NH, Knoefel WT, Peiper M (2007) Benefit of surgical treatment of lung metastasis in soft tissue sarcoma. Arch Surg 142(1):70–75; discussion 6

Rosenberg SA, Tepper J, Glatstein E, Costa J, Baker A, Brennan M et al (1982) The treatment of soft-tissue sarcomas of the extremities: prospective randomized evaluations of (1) limb-sparing surgery plus radiation therapy compared with amputation and (2) the role of adjuvant chemotherapy. Ann Surg 196(3):305–315

Sabolch A, Feng M, Griffith K, Rzasa C, Gadzala L, Feng F et al (2012) Risk factors for local recurrence and metastasis in soft tissue sarcomas of the extremity. Am J Clin Oncol 35(2):151–157

Shiu MH, Castro EB, Hajdu SI, Fortner JG (1975) Surgical treatment of 297 soft tissue sarcomas of the lower extremity. Ann Surg 182(5):597–602

Siegel RL, Miller KD, Jemal A (2016) Cancer statistics, 2016. CA Cancer J Clin 66(1):7–30

Singer S, Antman K, Corson JM, Eberlein TJ (1992) Long-term salvageability for patients with locally recurrent soft-tissue sarcomas. Arch Surg 127(5):548–553; discussion 53–54

Spencer SA, Harris J, Wheeler RH, Machtay M, Schultz C, Spanos W et al (2008) Final report of RTOG 9610, a multi-institutional trial of reirradiation and chemotherapy for unresectable recurrent squamous cell carcinoma of the head and neck. Head Neck 30(3):281–288

Stojadinovic A, Jaques DP, Leung DH, Healey JH, Brennan MF (2001) Amputation for recurrent soft tissue sarcoma of the extremity: indications and outcome. Ann Surg Oncol 8(6):509–518

Suit HD, Mankin HJ, Wood WC, Proppe KH (1985) Preoperative, intraoperative, and postoperative radiation in the treatment of primary soft tissue sarcoma. Cancer 55(11):2659–2667

Tinkle CL, Weinberg V, Braunstein SE, Wustrack R, Horvai A, Jahan T et al (2015) Intraoperative radiotherapy in the management of locally recurrent extremity soft tissue sarcoma. Sarcoma 2015:913565

Torres MA, Ballo MT, Butler CE, Feig BW, Cormier JN, Lewis VO et al (2007) Management of locally recurrent soft-tissue sarcoma after prior surgery and radiation therapy. Int J Radiat Oncol Biol Phys 67(4):1124–1129

Valentini V, Morganti AG, Gambacorta MA, Mohiuddin M, Doglietto GB, Coco C et al (2006) Preoperative hyperfractionated chemoradiation for locally recurrent rectal cancer in patients previously irradiated to the pelvis: a multicentric phase II study. Int J Radiat Oncol Biol Phys 64(4):1129–1139

van Geel AN, Pastorino U, Jauch KW, Judson IR, van Coevorden F, Buesa JM et al (1996) Surgical treatment of lung metastases: the European Organization for Research and Treatment of Cancer-Soft Tissue and Bone Sarcoma Group study of 255 patients. Cancer 77(4):675–682

Verazin GT, Warneke JA, Driscoll DL, Karakousis C, Petrelli NJ, Takita H (1992) Resection of lung metastases from soft-tissue sarcomas. A multivariate analysis. Arch Surg 127(12):1407–1411

Weber DC, Rutz HP, Bolsi A, Pedroni E, Coray A, Jermann M et al (2007) Spot scanning proton therapy in the curative treatment of adult patients with sar-

coma: the Paul Scherrer institute experience. Int J Radiat Oncol Biol Phys 69(3):865–871
Willett CG, Czito BG, Tyler DS (2007) Intraoperative radiation therapy. J Clin Oncol 25(8):971–977
Wood WC, Suit HD, Mankin HJ, Cohen AM, Proppe K (1984) Radiation and conservative surgery in the treatment of soft tissue sarcoma. Am J Surg 147(4):537–541
Yang JC, Chang AE, Baker AR, Sindelar WF, Danforth DN, Topalian SL et al (1998) Randomized prospective study of the benefit of adjuvant radiation therapy in the treatment of soft tissue sarcomas of the extremity. J Clin Oncol 16(1):197–203
Zagars GK, Ballo MT, Pisters PW, Pollock RE, Patel SR, Benjamin RS (2003) Prognostic factors for disease-specific survival after first relapse of soft-tissue sarcoma: analysis of 402 patients with disease relapse after initial conservative surgery and radiotherapy. Int J Radiat Oncol Biol Phys 57(3):739–747
Zelefsky MJ, Nori D, Shiu MH, Brennan MF (1990) Limb salvage in soft tissue sarcomas involving neurovascular structures using combined surgical resection and brachytherapy. Int J Radiat Oncol Biol Phys 19(4):913–918

Re-irradiation for Recurrent Skin Cancer

Michael J. Veness and Puma Sundaresan

Contents

The original version of this chapter was revised. An erratum to this chapter can be found at 10.1007/978-3-319-41825-4_78.

M.J. Veness (✉) • P. Sundaresan
Department of Radiation Oncology, Crown Princess Mary Cancer Centre, Westmead Hospital, Westmead, NSW 2145, Australia

University of Sydney, Sydney, NSW, Australia
e-mail: michael.veness@health.nsw.gov.au

Abstract

Radiotherapy has an important role in the management of patients with cutaneous malignancy. Non-melanoma skin cancer (NMSC) is the most frequent malignancy worldwide, and as such the absolute number of patients receiving radiotherapy each year is high. An often and well-documented scenario is the development of a second NMSC, if not within a previous radiotherapy field, certainly in close proximity to a previous radiotherapy field, and therefore there may be a requirement to consider overlapping any new radiotherapy field with previously irradiated tissue, if other options are not considered. Published evidence for cutaneous re-irradiation is sparse especially as other options such as surgery are often available. Despite this select patients may be considered for re-irradiation, be that local or occasionally regional, especially where other options are not feasible.

1 Introduction

1.1 Non-melanoma Skin Cancer

Non-melanoma skin cancer (NMSC) is the most frequent malignancy worldwide usually arising in fair-skinned Caucasians, especially males. Australians experience the highest incidence of NMSC in the world (Perera et al. 2015). Most

Med Radiol Radiat Oncol (2016)
DOI 10.1007/174_2016_37, © Springer International Publishing Switzerland
Published Online: 13 Apr 2016

patients are older (60–70 years), and 75–80 % will have a basal cell carcinoma (BCC) with the remainder (20–25 %) having a squamous cell carcinoma (SCC). The sun-exposed head and neck (HN), especially the midface, are the most frequently involved area (70–80 %) followed by the extremities and trunk. Collectively, BCC and SCC comprise 95 % of all NMSC.

Radiotherapy (RT) is an important nonsurgical modality that is frequently utilized in the definitive, adjuvant or palliative settings in select patients with cutaneous malignancies (Veness 2008). Of note, patients diagnosed with one NMSC are at risk of developing metachronous lesions with this risk estimated at 10 times that of the general population (Marcil and Stern 2000). New primary lesions may be close enough (5–10 mm) to a previous RT field to limit further RT as a first choice option without the risk of overlapping RT fields.

Merkel cell carcinoma (MCC) is an uncommon small cell (neuroendocrine) cutaneous malignancy typically arising in elderly white patients and characterized by high rates of relapse. MCC is a very radioresponsive malignancy where RT also plays an important role (Hruby et al. 2013).

1.2 Malignant Melanoma

Malignant melanoma (MM) accounts for ~5 % of skin malignancies and is the third most common cancer in Australia with over 10,000 cases diagnosed annually with an increasing incidence worldwide. The role of RT in the management of primary MM is less well defined compared with that in NMSC but is expanding as supportive evidence is published (Hong and Fogarty 2012).

Patients presenting with recurrent or new skin cancers are not uncommon and pose particular difficulties in the HN region, if re-irradiation is a consideration. The literature describing this clinical scenario is sparse, and the level of evidence to support the management of these patients is of low level and often limited to the expert opinion of experienced clinicians.

2 Primary Lesion Treatment

2.1 Primary Treatment of Squamous Cell and Basal Cell Carcinoma

Definitive RT is an option where the outcome, i.e. cosmetic (e.g. nasal BCC), and/or function is considered better with RT compared to surgery. Typically older patients with midface lesions where complex surgery (graft or local flap) is required are better treated with RT. The cosmetic result from well-fractionated (2–3 Gy fraction sizes) RT is excellent. In general, the local control rate for 1–2 cm BCC/SCC treated with various modalities is 80–90 %, and therefore additional factors such as availability, cost and patient comorbidity need to be considered during treatment decisions (Cognetta et al. 2012). Older patients of poor performance status can be effectively treated with 5–6 larger fractions (5–6 Gy) often receiving 2–3 fractions per week (Ferro et al. 2015).

2.2 Adjuvant Radiotherapy for Squamous Cell and Basal Cell Carcinoma

Adjuvant local RT is an effective option when excision is inadequate and re-excision is not possible. The aim of adjuvant RT is to reduce the risk of recurrence by sterilizing residual microscopic disease. A retrospective institutional study of patients with lower lip SCC documented a 37 % local recurrence rate in excised patients not receiving adjuvant RT (27 % close/positive margins) vs. 6 % local recurrence rate in patients treated with surgery and adjuvant RT (94 % close/positive margins) (Babington et al. 2003).

2.3 Primary Treatment of Merkel Cell Carcinoma

Excision is the initial treatment in most patients with operable MCC and will establish a diagnosis. However, achieving wide excision margins (2–3 cm), noting also that intradermal lymphatic vessel spread is well documented in MCC, is difficult in the HN. Most studies support a benefit in locoregional control and survival with the addition of adjuvant RT. RT field margins in MCC are usually wider (3–4 cm) compared with NMSC (1–2 cm) and the RT dose often lower.

In medically or technically inoperable patients, RT alone offers potential cure with one study of 43 inoperable patients (median lesion size 30 mm) documenting an 85 % infield control rate and a 5-year overall survival of 40 % (Veness and Howle 2015).

2.4 Primary Treatment of Malignant Melanoma

Primary melanoma should be treated with wide local excision ± sentinel lymph node biopsy (SLNB). Definitive RT has no role unless surgery is refused or not possible. Patients with lentigo maligna (in situ melanoma) can be offered definitive RT with excellent infield control rates of 90–100 % (Fogarty et al. 2014).

3 Regional Treatment

3.1 Regional Treatment of Squamous Cell Carcinoma

Patients with SCC can develop nodal metastases although only a minority (2–3 %) do so. High-risk patients with SCC have a higher incidence (10–20 %) of developing nodal metastases, with most developing 6–12 months following treatment of the primary. The role of elective RT in high-risk patients is investigational, but patients with clinical nodal metastases should undergo dissection and adjuvant RT (Porceddu et al. 2015).

3.2 Regional Treatment of Merkel Cell Carcinoma

Patients with MCC are at high risk (30–50 %) of harbouring subclinical regional metastases. SLNB will improve the ability to detect subclinical nodal metastases, and patients with a positive SLNB should undergo regional RT. Patients unable to undergo a SLNB should receive prophylactic regional RT (Gunaratne et al. 2015).

3.3 Regional Treatment of Malignant Melanoma

Therapeutic nodal dissection is recommended in patients with biopsy-proven clinical nodal metastases. After surgery the risk of regional (and systemic) recurrence may justify adjuvant RT (48 Gy in 20 fractions) with a recent multicentre randomized study ($n=250$) from Australia confirming a significant reduction in regional recurrence from 31 to 19 % (HR 1.77; 1.02–3.08, $p=0.041$) in patients randomized to surgery and adjuvant RT (Henderson et al. 2015).

4 Recurrent Skin Cancer After Radiotherapy

4.1 Previous Radiotherapy

Previous RT may preclude re-irradiation as an option for retreatment although cases need to be considered individually. Important factors that need to be considered in re-irradiating include the previous RT field and degree of overlap with current field, the dose fractionation schedule prescribed, the modality utilized and the time interval since the RT. An estimation of the dose received at the skin surface and at depth, and the structures irradiated, is important. Converting total doses to a 2 Gy biological equivalent dose (BED) using equivalence tables allows an estimation of the potential risk of re-irradiating, although the clinical data to support this is limited (Barton 1995).

Patients may have received RT, often hypofractionated, many years previously and have poor recollection of details. Similarly, obtaining relevant technical details may be difficult or impossible. The presence of late RT infield changes, such as telangiectasia and hypo- (most common) or hyperpigmentation, may be helpful to delineate the treatment field and assess clinically the degree of late RT-induced changes. There may be variability in late RT changes based on patient factors such as skin type and ongoing solar damage.

Re-irradiation may also be considered in the adjuvant setting in cases of patients undergoing extensive salvage surgery with removal of previously irradiated tissues (Fig. 1a, b). It is not uncommon that patients will exhibit unfavourable pathology and be recommended adjuvant RT to reduce the risk of recurrence.

4.2 Infield Recurrence After Radiotherapy for Non-melanoma Skin Cancer

Infield recurrence after RT for NMSC is not common. A typical scenario for infield recurrence when it does occur is local recurrence of a midface BCC after previous definitive RT. A clinical scenario such as this, particularly in the setting of a deep recurrence located in the midface, can pose a difficult management problem (Smith and Grande 1991), and patients may be better approached with salvage surgery rather than further RT.

Presentations of new NMSC adjacent to a previously irradiated site are a more common scenario as are recurrences at the edge of a previously treated RT field (marginal recurrence). These patients may be candidates for further RT, and ideally the details of previous treatment including the prescribed dose/fractionation schedule should be obtained, but are not always available.

Clinical assessment is very important, and patients exhibiting obvious late RT changes such as infield cutaneous hypo- (or hyper)pigmentation, telangiectasia, epidermal atrophy or fibrosis (Fig. 2) are not optimal candidates for re-irradiation.

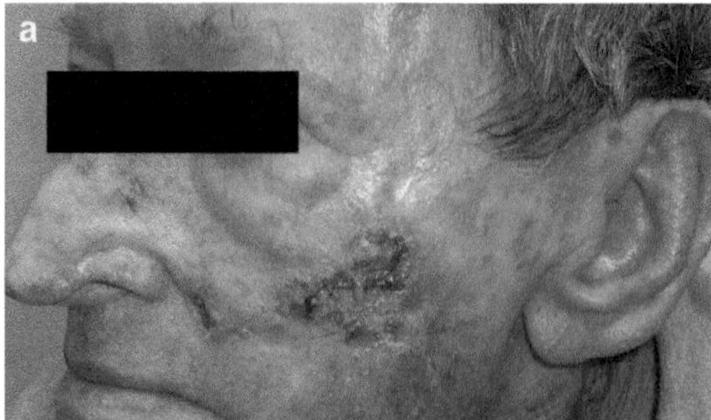

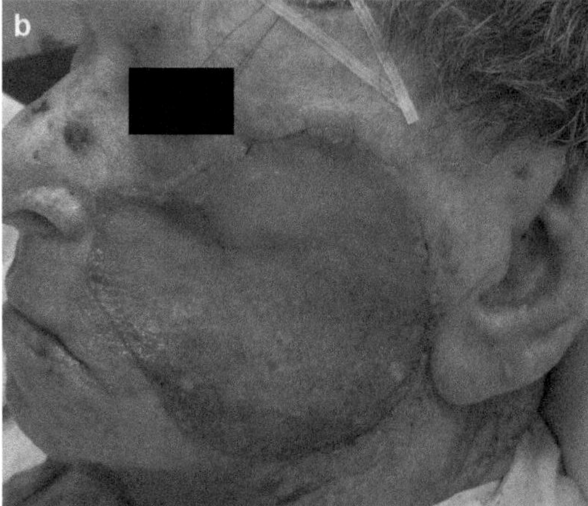

Fig. 1 (**a**) A 75-year-old Caucasian male who previously received 50 Gy in 20 daily fractions using superficial energy photons in the setting of a squamous cell carcinoma. Note the infield hypopigmentation and epidermal atrophy delineating his radiotherapy field. Anterior to this the patient now has a biopsy-proven new cutaneous squamous cell carcinoma which encroaches over the previous field. The need to overlap any further radiotherapy field meant the patient was recommended surgery. (**b**) The patient underwent wide excision and free tissue graft reconstruction. Despite this the pathology was unfavourable with a close deep excision margin and the presence of perineural invasion. The patient was recommended adjuvant radiotherapy to a dose of 50 Gy in 20 daily fractions using orthovoltage energy photons. Because of the removal of the previously irradiated tissue, the risk of re-irradiation was deemed negligible

4.3 Local Re-irradiation

There is limited preclinical animal data to suggest a retreatment tolerance of >90 % for late dermal necrosis after an 18 Gy single dose and further RT (Simmonds et al. 1989). However, extrapolating this data to the human subject following fractionated cutaneous RT needs to be done with caution. We therefore do not recommend re-local irradiation as a first option but may be considered in select patients.

There is sparse evidence documenting re-irradiation as an alternate option to surgery in the setting of infield (or marginal) recurrence. In a small series of 17 irradiated patients with

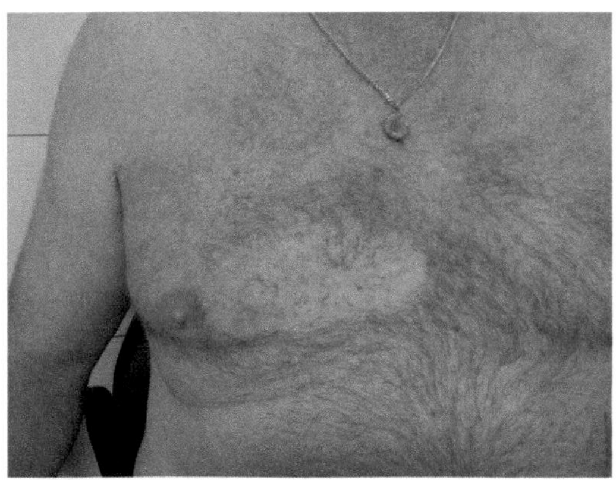

Fig. 2 A 55-year-old male previously diagnosed with a Merkel cell carcinoma located on his right side chest wall and receiving 55 Gy in 25 daily fractions using superficial energy photons following excision. The radiotherapy field is well delineated by hypopigmentation, loss of body hair and telangiectasia. Patients manifesting this degree of late radiotherapy cutaneous changes are poor candidates to receive further radiotherapy

recurrent HN NMSC (eight BCCs, nine SCCs), all were re-irradiated to a cumulative median surface BED of 103 Gy (range 48.78 Gy–143.5 Gy) and median 108 Gy at 5 mm depth, with 10/17 (59 %) achieving local control and two developing subsequent skin defects (Chao et al. 1995). Median interval from the initial RT was 4 years. The authors concluded that patients receiving an initial BED of <55 Gy at 5 mm depth and a cumulative BED of no >110 Gy at the skin surface had the best outcome, with retreatment fraction sizes limited to 2 Gy to further reduce late tissue reactions. Therefore, the BED of the initial RT and the re-irradiation should not exceed 110 Gy. Interestingly on review of the initial RT details, the authors documented suboptimal initial treatment in 10 of the 17 patients further re-enforcing the need for optimal upfront treatment as a means to reduce the risk of recurrence.

In contrast to the aforementioned series, five lesions were re-irradiated by a Spanish group (no details available) and three recurred with the authors suggesting a benefit in only select patients (Hernandez-Machin et al. 2007).

In a case study of a patient with recurrent auricular SCC previously treated with multiple operations and adjuvant RT, the authors utilized stereotactic body radiotherapy (SBRT) as a means to deliver high-dose (50 Gy in five fractions) re-irradiation and spare surrounding normal tissues. The previous dose fractionation schedule was 60 Gy in 21 fractions. By limiting the treated volume to 2 mm beyond gross tumour, the patient experienced complete clinical regression with no late complications, although the interval from re-irradiation to assessment was not documented. The authors hypothesized that SBRT by delivering large doses per fraction (>10 Gy) may provide a higher likelihood of achieving local control. Of note the 2 Gy BED re-irradiation dose was 100 Gy. This approach is counterintuitive and differs to what many radiation oncologists would recommend when re-irradiating a patient but does indicate that modern techniques of delivering RT such as SBRT and intensity-modulated radiotherapy (IMRT) require further investigation (Brotherston and Poon 2015).

In contrast to re-irradiating using large fractions of RT, 14 patients with secondary-induced angiosarcomas of the breast were re-irradiated utilizing hyperfractionated and accelerated re-irradiation (HART). Multiple abutting electron fields with bolus (post-operatively) or tangential photon fields (preoperatively) were used, and all except one patient received 1 Gy three times daily (4 h interfraction break) with doses varying between 45 and 75 Gy. Previously most patients had received 60 Gy. The authors documented minimal late side effects (four patients with rib fractures) and mild-moderate limb lymphedema with 79 % achieving disease control. In these patients the authors concluded that using a small retreatment fraction of 1 Gy was likely to minimize late normal tissue side effects (Smith et al. 2014).

4.4 Regional Re-irradiation

Regional recurrence after RT, usually adjuvant (i.e. parotid and/or neck metastatic SCC, MCC or MM), poses a more difficult problem, as patients will usually have had a large volume (e.g. ipsilateral parotid ± hemi-neck) of normal tissue (e.g. mandible, soft tissue, brainstem/spinal cord, nerves, carotid artery) irradiated to 50–60 Gy. Following appropriate restaging operable patients should proceed to surgery. For inoperable patients the evidence available for re-irradiation relates predominantly to treating mucosal HNSCC patients. In this analogous setting, recent evidence has emerged supporting the use of highly conformal IMRT (Duprez et al. 2009). Patients retreated with IMRT are likely to have a better outcome (improved locoregional control and decreased severe late effects) compared with conventional 3D conformal re-irradiation. The best results are achieved with radical re-irradiation doses of ~60–70 Gy in 2 Gy daily fractions and retreatment volumes limited to ~2 cm around gross disease or the resection bed. The spine, brainstem and optic chiasm should receive a limited retreatment dose (15–25 Gy) if previously irradiated to tolerance. Of note, even when utilizing IMRT, serious late toxicity and treatment-related deaths are reported in around 20 % of patients. The addition of concurrent chemotherapy to re-irradiation has also been recommended in select patients with mucosal SCC. The role of re-irradiating after salvage nodal surgery is less well defined, but in patients with unfavourable pathology (i.e. close/positive excision margins, extranodal spread), it may be considered.

4.5 Radiotherapy Techniques

Patients considered candidates for local re-irradiation should have treatment limited to the site of recurrence with appropriate field margins to encompass subclinical extension. A not uncommon scenario is that of the need to irradiate the lateral nose when the opposite side has previously been irradiated. In this situation the midline nasal septum may have received a dose of RT at depth from one side and therefore may also receive further RT from the contralateral RT. An estimate should be made based on delivery angles, the use (or not) of septal shields or packing and the beam used as to whether there is any risk to the cartilage from the overlapping beams (Fig. 3). The selection of an appropriate energy superficial/orthovoltage photon beam should aim to ensure adequate coverage of deep tumour involvement, but also respecting the dose delivered to noninvolved deeper tissue.

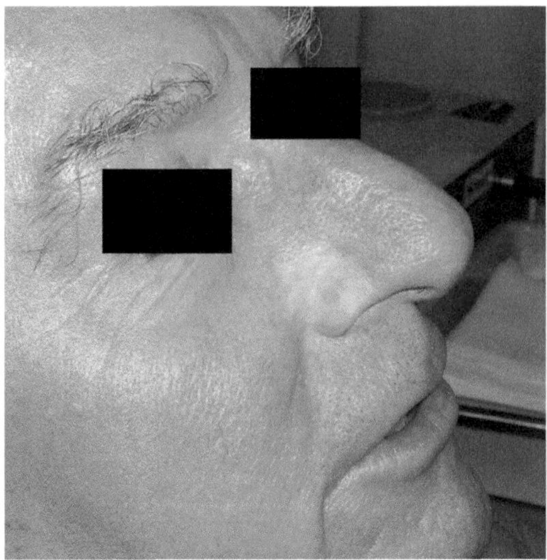

Fig. 3 A 72-year-old male with obvious late changes many years after receiving radiotherapy to his right side lower/posterior nose. The patient was unable to recall details of his treatment which had taken place at another hospital. He presents now with a basal cell carcinoma located on his left side lower nose and declined excision in favour of radiotherapy. Treatment was delivered with superficial energy photons with nasal packing and a left nasal shield inserted to minimize dose to the nasal septum

Electron beam RT is an alternative technique; however, using small field low-energy (5–6 MeV) electron beams raises issues of skin sparing and the need to add tissue-equivalent bolus. Considerations using electron beam RT include the issues of wider treatment field penumbra, dose constriction and rapid drop-off at depth (van Hezewijk et al. 2010). Patients in some circumstances may be able to undergo CT simulation and planning with isodose curves calculated to estimate the RT dose delivered at depth.

Tomotherapy is a type of IMRT utilizing a helical system of delivery and CT scan image verification. This delivery of highly conformal megavoltage RT has been used in the setting of advanced NMSC and may be an option, if available, to limit the volume of tissue irradiated, which could potentially be of benefit in the retreatment setting (Kramkimel et al. 2014).

Despite some contrary evidence, we recommend RT fraction sizes be limited to 1.8–2 Gy to further reduce the risk of late tissue changes. With very limited evidence to guide clinicians, it is recommended that retreatment total doses be also limited to ~50–55 Gy at 5 mm depth and that the cumulative skin dose does not exceed ~110 Gy. The role of hyperfractionation using 1.1–1.3 Gy fractions twice daily in this setting as a means to reduce the risk of late effects is potentially another approach.

Re-irradiating nodal basins carries a greater risk of late complications because of the increased volume of tissue and the number of structures re-irradiated. In keeping with data from the HN mucosal SCC literature, retreatment volumes should be limited to the operative bed or to gross disease with 2–3 cm margins and using IMRT- or CT-planned conformal treatment. Elective nodal treatment should be avoided. The treatment toxicity will be greater than with local site re-irradiation, and patients should therefore be of good performance status.

4.6 Brachytherapy

Brachytherapy uses radioactive emitting sources (e.g. iridium-192) to treat skin cancers by direct contact, be that using surface moulds or interstitial needles. Its role is well established in the primary treatment of NMSC with excellent cure rates of 90–95 % and minimal complications. The concept of brachytherapy is appealing in the retreatment of suitable infield RT local recurrences because of the limited retreatment of surrounding tissue. Despite this, data to support this approach as an option is lacking, and therefore brachytherapy remains an option only in centres with the expertise to deliver this (Gauden et al. 2013).

Conclusion

The evidence to guide clinicians for re-irradiating skin cancer patients is limited. Whilst RT plays an important role in the definitive and adjuvant treatment of many patients, the role of re-irradiation is less clear, especially as surgical salvage is often considered the appropriate treatment. Despite this select patients may benefit from re-irradiation particularly if further surgery is associated with unacceptable cosmetic and functional consequences or a patient's performance status and co-morbidities preclude surgery.

References

Babington S, Veness MJ, Cakir B, Gebski V, Morgan G (2003) Squamous cell carcinoma of the lip: does adjuvant radiotherapy improve local control following incomplete or inadequate excision? ANZ J Surg 73: 621–625

Barton M (1995) Tables of equivalent dose in 2 Gy fractions: a simple application of the linear quadratic formula. Int J Radiat Oncol Biol Phys 31:371–378

Brotherston D, Poon I (2015) SBRT treatment of multiple recurrent auricular squamous cell carcinoma following surgical and conventional radiation treatment failure. Cureus 7, e325

Chao CKS, Gerber RM, Perez CA (1995) Reirradiation of recurrent skin cancer of the face. Cancer 75: 2351–2355

Cognetta AB, Howard BM, Heaton HP et al (2012) Superficial x-ray in the treatment of basal and squamous cell carcinomas: a viable option in select patients. J Am Acad Dermatol 67:1235–1241

Duprez F, Madani I, Bonte K et al (2009) Intensity-modulated radiotherapy for recurrent and second primary head and neck cancer in previously irradiated territory. Radiol Oncol 93:563–569

Ferro M, Deodata F, Macchia G et al (2015) Short-course radiotherapy in elderly patients with early stage non-melanoma skin cancer: A phase 2 study. Cancer Invest 33:34–38

Fogarty GB, Hong A, Scolyer RA et al (2014) Radiotherapy for lentigo maligna: a literature review and recommendations for treatment. Br J Dermatol 170:52–58

Gauden R, Pracy M, Avery AM et al (2013) HDR brachytherapy for superficial non-melanoma skin cancers. JMIRO 57:212–217

Gunaratne D, Howle J, Veness MJ (2016) Sentinel lymph node biopsy in Merkel cell carcinoma: a 15 year institutional experience and statistical analysis of 721 reported cases. BJD 174:273–281

Henderson MA, Burmeister BH, Ainslie J et al (2015) Adjuvant lymph-node field radiotherapy versus observation only in patients with melanoma at high risk of further lymph-node field relapse after lymphadenectomy (ANZMTG 01.02/TROG 02.01): 6-year follow-up of a phase 3, randomised controlled trial. Lancet Oncol 16:1049–1060

Hernandez-Machin B, Borrego L, Gil-Garcia M, Hernandez BH (2007) Office-based radiation therapy

for cutaneous carcinoma: evaluation of 710 treatments. Int J Dermatol 46:453–459
Hruby G, Scolyer RA, Thompson JF (2013) The important role of radiation treatment in the management of Merkel cell carcinoma. Br J Dermatol 169:975–982
Hong A, Fogarty G (2012) Role of radiation therapy in cutaneous melanoma. Cancer J 18:203–207
Kramkimel N, Dendal R, Bolle S, Zefkili S, Fourquet A, Kirova YM (2014) Management of advanced non-melanoma skin cancers using helical tomotherapy. JEADV 28:641–650
Marcil I, Stern RS (2000) Risk of developing a subsequent nonmelanoma skin cancer in patients with a history of nonmelanoma skin cancer: a critical review of the literature and meta-analysis. Arch Dermatol 136:1524–1530
Perera E, Gnaneswaran N, Staines C, Win AK, Sinclair R (2015) Incidence and prevalence of non-melanoma skin cancer in Australia: a systematic review. Austral J Dermatol 56:258–267
Porceddu S, Veness M, Guminski A (2015) Non-melanoma cutaneous head and neck cancer and Merkel cell carcinoma – Current concepts, advances and controversies. J Clin Oncol 33:3338–3345
Simmonds RH, Hopewell JW, Robbins ME (1989) Residual radiation-induced injury in dermal tissue: implications for retreatment. Br J Radiol 62:915–920
Smith SP, Grande DJ (1991) Basal cell carcinoma recurring after radiotherapy: a unique, difficult treatment subclass of recurrent basal cell carcinoma. J Dermatol Surg Oncol 17:26–10
Smith TL, Morris CG, Mendenhall NP (2014) Angiosarcoma after breast-conserving therapy: Long-term disease control and late effects with hyperfractionated accelerated re-irradiation (HART). Acta Oncol 53:235–241
Van Hezewijk M, Creutzberg CL, Putter H et al (2010) Efficacy of a hypofractionated schedule in electron beam radiotherapy for epithelial skin cancer: analysis of 434 cases. Radiol Oncol 95:245–249
Veness MJ (2008) The important role of radiotherapy in patients with non-melanoma skin cancer and other cutaneous entities. JMIRO 52:278–286
Veness M, Howle J (2015) Radiotherapy alone in patients with Merkel cell carcinoma: the Westmead hospital experience of 41 patients. Australas J Dermatol 56:19–24

Leukemia and Lymphoma

Chris R. Kelsey and Grace J. Kim

Contents

Abstract

Leukemias and lymphomas comprise a diverse collection of malignancies with unique clinical behavior. Radiation therapy plays an integral role in the definitive, adjuvant, and palliative management of these hematologic malignancies. As opposed to most epithelial and mesenchymal malignancies, hematologic malignancies typically require lower doses of radiation therapy. Most can be controlled with 24–40 Gy, well within the tolerance of most normal tissues. In the palliative setting, exceptionally low doses (e.g., 4 Gy) are often sufficient. This characteristic of hematologic malignancies allows for re-treatment, when necessary, in most circumstances. In this chapter, we will review the major histologic subtypes of hematologic malignancies and discuss the settings where re-irradiation is sometimes encountered in clinical practice.

Abbreviations

ABVD	Doxorubicin, bleomycin, vinblastine, dacarbazine
GHSG	German Hodgkin Study Group
ICE	Ifosfamide, carboplatin, etoposide
R-CHOP	Rituximab, cyclophosphamide, doxorubicin, vincristine, and prednisone
MALT	Mucosa-associated lymphoid tissue
CNS	Central nervous system

The original version of this chapter was revised. An erratum to this chapter can be found at 10.1007/978-3-319-41825-4_78.

C.R. Kelsey, MD (✉) • G.J. Kim, MD, PhD
Department of Radiation Oncology,
Duke University Medical Center, Durham, NC, USA
e-mail: christopher.kelsey@duke.edu

Med Radiol Radiat Oncol (2016)
DOI 10.1007/174_2016_32, © Springer International Publishing Switzerland
Published Online: 21 Apr 2016

TBI	Total body irradiation
RT	Radiation therapy
PET-CT	Positron emission tomography-computed tomography

1 Introduction

Leukemias and lymphomas comprise a diverse collection of malignancies with unique clinical behavior. Radiation therapy plays an integral role in the definitive, adjuvant, and palliative management of these hematologic malignancies. In some histologies, particularly for localized, low-grade diseases such as follicular lymphoma and marginal zone lymphoma, radiation therapy alone is typically the definitive treatment. For other subtypes treated primarily with chemotherapy, radiation therapy is used in the consolidation setting to decrease the risk of relapse and improve survival. This would include Hodgkin lymphoma and diffuse large B-cell lymphoma. Total body irradiation is often utilized in the conditioning regimen prior to allogeneic stem cell transplant for acute leukemias and occasionally lymphomas. Finally, a short course of radiation therapy can be utilized in all histologic subtypes to palliate symptoms related to uncontrolled local disease.

As opposed to most epithelial and mesenchymal malignancies, hematologic malignancies typically require lower doses of radiation therapy. Compared to 50–70 Gy, which is often required in the definitive setting for solid tumors, most hematologic malignancies can be controlled with 24–40 Gy, well within the tolerance of most normal tissues. In the palliative setting, exceptionally low doses (e.g., 4 Gy) are often sufficient. This characteristic of hematologic malignancies allows for re-treatment, when necessary, in most circumstances.

In this chapter, we will review the major histologic subtypes of hematologic malignancies and discuss the settings where re-irradiation is sometimes encountered in clinical practice.

2 Hodgkin Lymphoma

Early-stage (I-II) Hodgkin lymphoma is managed primarily with combination chemotherapy, mostly commonly ABVD (doxorubicin, bleomycin, vinblastine, dacarbazine). Consolidation radiation therapy, directed at originally involved sites, decreases the risk of recurrence (Herbst et al. 2010) and may improve overall survival (Olszewski et al. 2015). For patients with favorable disease, two cycles of ABVD followed by 20 Gy of radiation are an established standard based on the German Hodgkin Study Group (GHSG) HD10 trial (Engert et al. 2010). For patients with unfavorable disease (three or more sites of disease, large mediastinal adenopathy, extranodal disease, and/or an unfavorable B-symptom/erythrocyte sedimentation rate profile), four cycles of ABVD followed by 30 Gy of radiation are utilized, based on GHSG HD11 (Eich et al. 2010). When more intense chemotherapy regimens are utilized (Eich et al. 2010), or more cycles of ABVD are administered (Torok et al. 2015), doses of 20 Gy seem sufficient, even for unfavorable disease. With combined modality therapy, relapse occurs in ~10–15 % of patients.

The role of consolidation radiation therapy in advanced Hodgkin lymphoma is controversial but often pursued for bulky disease, limited presentations, and when less than a complete response is achieved with chemotherapy.

There are several circumstances where a second course of radiation therapy may be appropriate in patients with relapsed Hodgkin lymphoma. One scenario is a patient with a localized relapse who refuses or is not a good candidate for further intense systemic therapy, including transplant. The GHSG reported on 100 patients with relapsed disease who were treated with salvage radiation therapy (Josting et al. 2005). At first diagnosis, 38 % had early-stage disease and 68 % had received radiation therapy. At relapse, 87 % of the patients had localized (stage I–II) disease. Salvage radiotherapy most commonly involved treatment to an involved field (37 %) or mantle field (42 %), with a median dose of 40 Gy. The actuarial 5-year

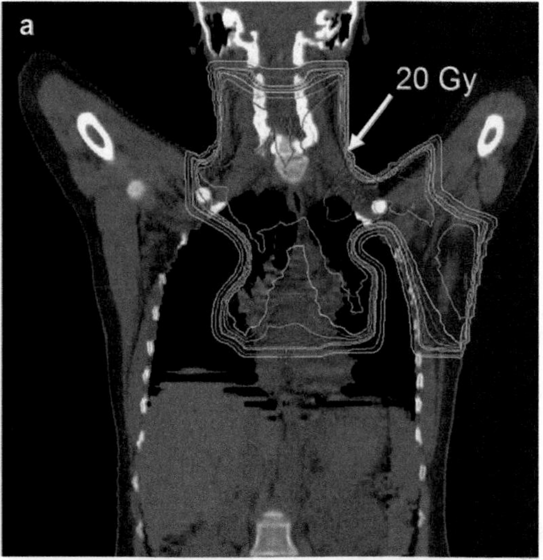

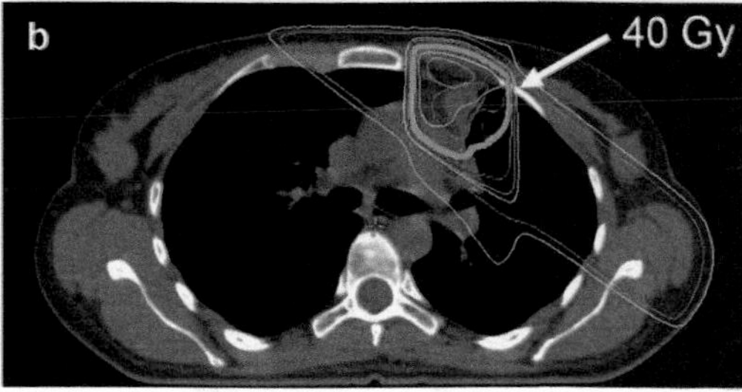

Fig. 1 A 36-year-old female presented with early-stage, unfavorable Hodgkin lymphoma and was treated with combined modality therapy consisting of six cycles of ABVD followed by low-dose (20 Gy) consolidation RT (panel **a**). Her disease recurred in the mediastinum (panel **b**, *red contour*) within the RT field. She received three cycles of ICE followed by high-dose chemotherapy and autologous stem cell transplant. One year later, she was found to have recurrence at the same site in the mediastinum. She declined further chemotherapy. A definitive course of RT (40 Gy) was given (panel **b**, *green* contour). She remains without evidence of recurrence 4 years after completing salvage re-irradiation

freedom from a second failure and overall survival were 28 % and 51 %, respectively. Thus, while high-dose chemotherapy and autologous stem cell transplant remain the preferred treatment for relapsed Hodgkin lymphoma, definitive radiation therapy for select patients, particularly those with localized relapses, is appropriate (Fig. 1).

Another circumstance is relapsed disease within the transplant setting. Investigators from Memorial Sloan Kettering Cancer Center reported on 65 patients with relapsed/refractory Hodgkin lymphoma, 60 % of whom had received prior radiation therapy (Moskowitz et al. 2001). The treatment program began with two cycles of ICE (ifosfamide, carboplatin, etoposide). If a satisfactory response was achieved, then accelerated fractionation, involved-field radiation therapy was pursued to patients with disease ≥5 cm at relapse or who had residual disease after ICE (1.8 Gy bid to 18–36 Gy, depending on disease status and prior radiation therapy). Upon completion of involved-field radiation therapy, patients proceeded with total lymphoid irradiation (1.8 Gy bid to 18 Gy). This was followed by further chemotherapy and autologous stem cell transplant. At a median follow-up of 43 months, the 5-year event-free survival was 58 %. Re-irradiation only to involved sites, without total lymphoid irradiation, may also be an appropriate strategy in select patients with relapsed disease after combined modality therapy. Low doses (~20 Gy) may be appropriate depending on the clinical circumstances.

Finally, radiation therapy can be utilized to palliate local symptoms in patients with refractory Hodgkin lymphoma. Durable responses can be achieved in the majority of patients with 20–30 Gy (Kaplan 1972). Such doses are rarely associated with significant side effects and can be safely given, using modern techniques, even when prior radiation therapy has been administered (Fig. 2).

3 Diffuse Large B-cell Lymphoma

As with Hodgkin lymphoma, early-stage (I-II) diffuse large B-cell lymphoma is often managed with a combination of systemic therapy and radiation therapy. This typically consists of three to six cycles of immunochemotherapy, most commonly R-CHOP (rituximab, cyclophosphamide, doxorubicin, vincristine, and prednisone), followed by consolidation radiation therapy. The

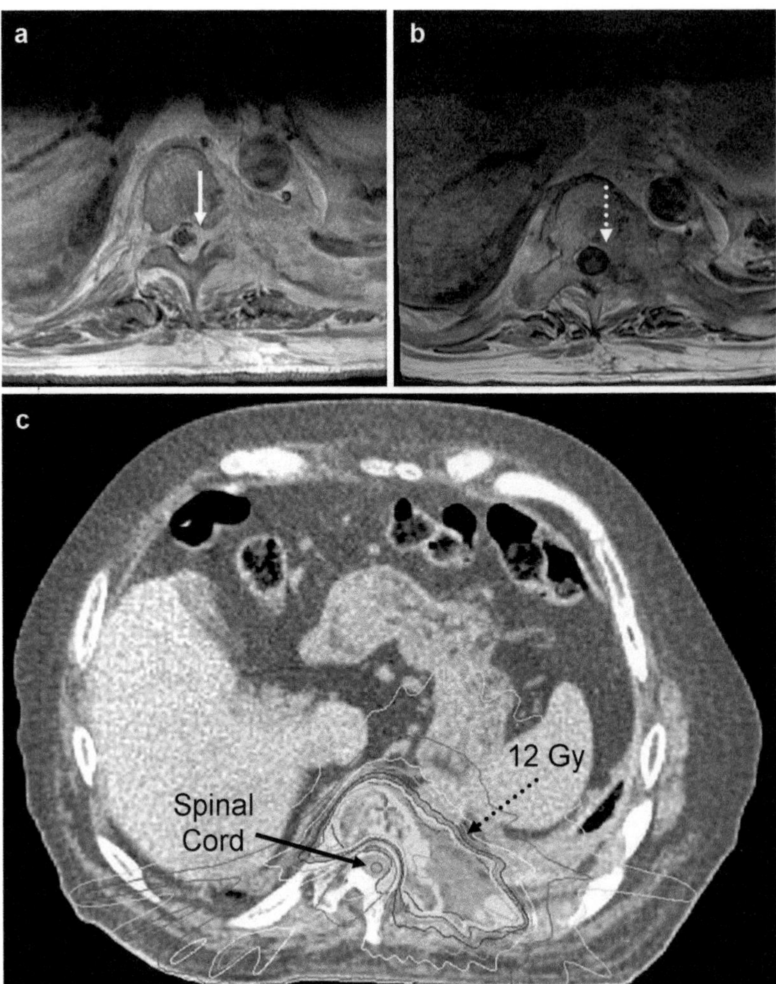

Fig. 2 A 51-year-old male with refractory Hodgkin lymphoma, who had previously been treated with multiple courses of RT to the chest and abdomen, presented with paralysis due to epidural disease in the lower thoracic spine (*white solid arrow*, panel **a**). Due to prior RT to that area that approached spinal cord tolerance, he received 14 Gy with conventional RT which cleared the disease in the epidural space (*white dashed arrow*, panel **b**). Due to persistent disease in the surrounding bone and soft tissues, he received a stereotactic body radiation therapy boost with sparing of the spinal cord (*black solid arrow*, panel **c**) consisting of 12 Gy in 3 fractions (*yellow contour*, *black dashed arrow*, panel **c**). Thus, the total dose to gross disease in the spine was 26 Gy. Over the course of several months his lower extremity strength improved, he became ambulatory with the assistance of a walker and returned to work

Eastern Cooperative Oncology Group study 1484 demonstrated that consolidation radiation therapy after eight cycles of CHOP was associated with reduced rates of local failure (4 % vs. 16 %, p = 0.06) and improved 6-year disease-free survival (73 % vs. 56 %, p = 0.05), the primary endpoint of the study (Horning et al. 2004). A dose of 30 Gy is typically utilized after a complete response to immunochemotherapy is achieved. Higher doses (≥40 Gy) may be necessary in the setting of a partial response or with refractory disease.

Patients with advanced disease (III-IV) are generally treated with immunochemotherapy alone. Radiation therapy is utilized in select patients. Indications for radiation therapy include bulky disease (Held et al. 2014), partial response to systemic therapy (Dorth et al. 2011; Sehn et al. 2013), and limited skeletal involvement (Held et al. 2013). Select patients with technically advanced

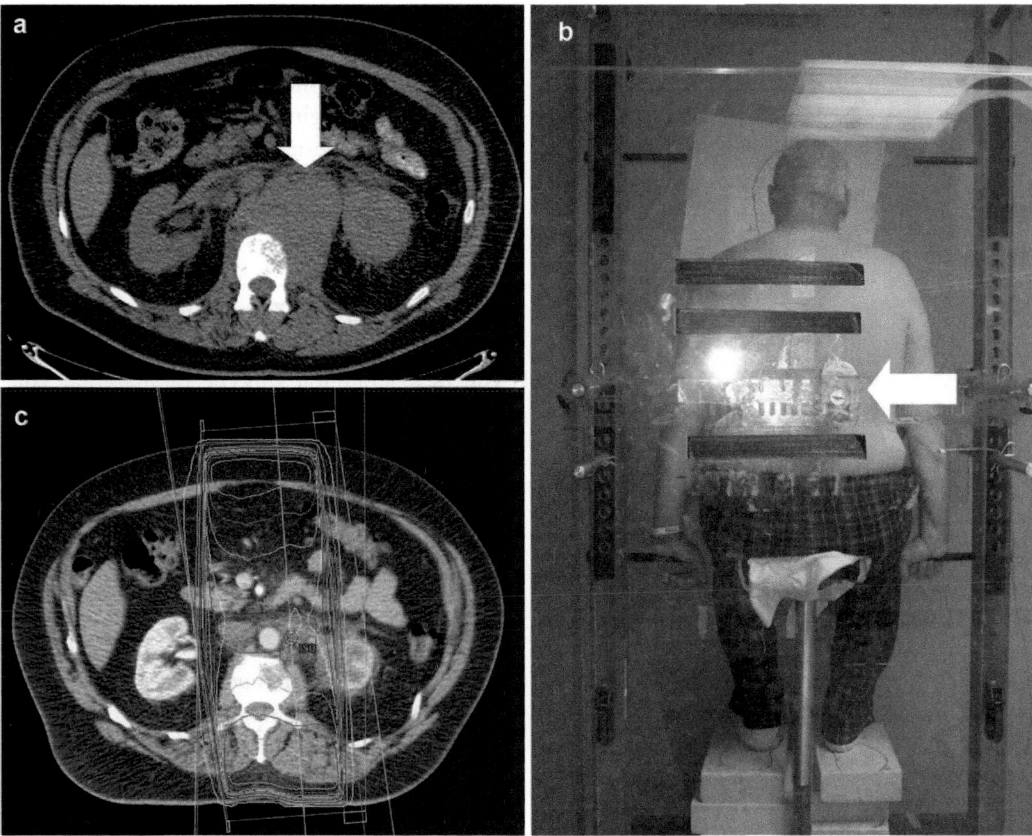

Fig. 3 A 52-year-old male presented with low back pain and found to have a retroperitoneal mass (*white arrow*, panel **a**). Biopsy showed DLBCL, and positron emission tomography-computed tomography (PET-CT) imaging showed diffuse adenopathy with bulky retroperitoneal disease invading adjacent vertebral bodies and obstructing the left ureter leading to kidney dysfunction. He received six cycles of R-CHOP, achieving a complete response by PET-CT, followed by 30 Gy consolidation RT to the intra-abdominal disease (panel **b**). One year later, he was found to have diffuse disease progression confirmed with biopsy. He only achieved a partial response to three different salvage chemotherapy regimens. With refractory disease, a myeloablative allogeneic stem cell transplant was recommended utilizing a TBI-based regimen with custom shielding of the right kidney (*white arrow*, panel **c**)

disease but limited presentations may also benefit from consolidation radiation therapy. In advanced stages, as more chemotherapy cycles are generally used with more widespread disease (and thus larger field sizes), lower doses such as 20 Gy seem reasonable (Dorth et al. 2012).

About a third of patients with diffuse large B-cell lymphoma will suffer a relapse. First-line treatment at relapse for appropriate candidates is non-cross-reactive chemotherapy followed by high-dose chemotherapy and autologous hematopoietic cell transplantation. Further radiation therapy must be tailored to the individual circumstances. Factors that must be considered include the prior dose of radiation utilized, field treated, interval between initial treatment and relapse, extent of relapse, response to salvage chemotherapy, etc.

Total body irradiation may be utilized, in select circumstances, in the relapsed setting as part of the conditioning regimen (Fig. 3). As doses of 12–14 Gy are required for transplant, this is usually feasible without significant risk. A second course of localized radiation therapy in the salvage setting may also be feasible depending on the circumstances. Finally, in those patients who are nonresponders to high-dose chemotherapy, fail transplant, or have a poor performance status, palliative radiation therapy can be considered. Radiation can be used in this setting to relieve symptomatic areas. As in Hodgkin lymphoma, re-treatment is generally possible due to the lower consolidation radiation doses needed for lymphoma. Response rates have been reported to be as high as 50–80 % with doses as low as 4 Gy (Murthy et al. 2008; Haas et al. 2005). Such doses can be utilized in almost all patients. If this is unsuccessful, more conventional palliative doses can be pursued (20–24 Gy).

4 Follicular Lymphoma

Approximately 20 % of patients with follicular lymphoma present with localized (stage I or contiguous stage II) disease. The optimal treatment for these patients is controversial as no randomized studies have compared radiation therapy alone (the traditional standard) with more modern approaches such as immunochemotherapy, with or without radiation therapy (Friedberg et al. 2012), or observation. Large database studies suggest that radiation therapy improves survival in this setting (Vargo et al. 2015; Pugh et al. 2010). With radiation therapy alone, approximately 50 % of patients have long-term disease control. When the disease does relapse, the predominant pattern of failure is distant (i.e., originally uninvolved lymph node sites).

The majority of patients with follicular lymphoma present with advanced (stage III–IV) disease. Systemic therapy, consisting of both immunotherapy (e.g., rituximab) and chemotherapy, is the foundation of follicular lymphoma management. Radiation therapy can be beneficial in a number of circumstances. For example, in settings where there is localized disease progression or poor response to systemic therapy, especially if symptoms are present that require palliation, radiation therapy may be appropriately employed. Depending upon the clinical circumstances, it is often prudent to treat with a low-dose approach (2 Gy × 2). A total dose of 4 Gy is almost always well tolerated, and response rates exceed 80–90 % (Haas et al. 2003; Russo et al. 2013).

Local control with conventional doses of radiation therapy is very high (24–30 Gy). The most common re-irradiation scenario is in patients receiving 2 Gy × 2 for palliation who either fail to respond or subsequently relapse in field. In this circumstance, it is almost always feasible to give a more protracted regimen (20–30 Gy) which invariably leads to the desired response (Fig. 4) or, in the instance of relapsing patients, to give another 4 Gy.

5 Marginal Zone Lymphoma

The most common subtype of marginal zone lymphoma encountered by radiation oncologists is extranodal marginal zone lymphoma of mucosa-associated lymphoid tissue (MALT lymphoma). These lymphomas most commonly arise within the stomach, orbital adnexa, parotid gland, skin, thyroid gland, and lung. The majority of patients present with localized disease. While an initial trial of antibiotics is appropriate for localized *Helicobacter pylori*-positive gastric MALT lymphoma, definitive radiation therapy is the preferred treatment for most other presentations. Complete responses to low-dose radiation therapy (24–30 Gy) are the norm (>95 %). Local failure is extraordinarily rare. In a recent large series from the Princess Margaret and Memorial Sloan Kettering Hospitals, failure within the radiation field occurred in 3–5 % of patients (Goda et al. 2010; Teckie et al. 2015). The dominant pattern of failure is at distant sites, typically in areas that are commonly involved by MALT. Thus, the need for radiation therapy for a previously irradiated area is unusual. In such circumstances, low-dose (2 Gy × 2) radiation could be used for palliative purposes (Russo et al. 2013). In select circumstances, depending upon initial dose and location, it may be possible to pursue a second definitive (~24–30 Gy) course of therapy. The more common circumstance is treating a new area for a localized distant relapse (Fig. 5).

6 Plasma Cell Neoplasms

The most common plasma cell neoplasms that radiation oncologists encounter are solitary plasmacytomas and multiple myeloma. Only

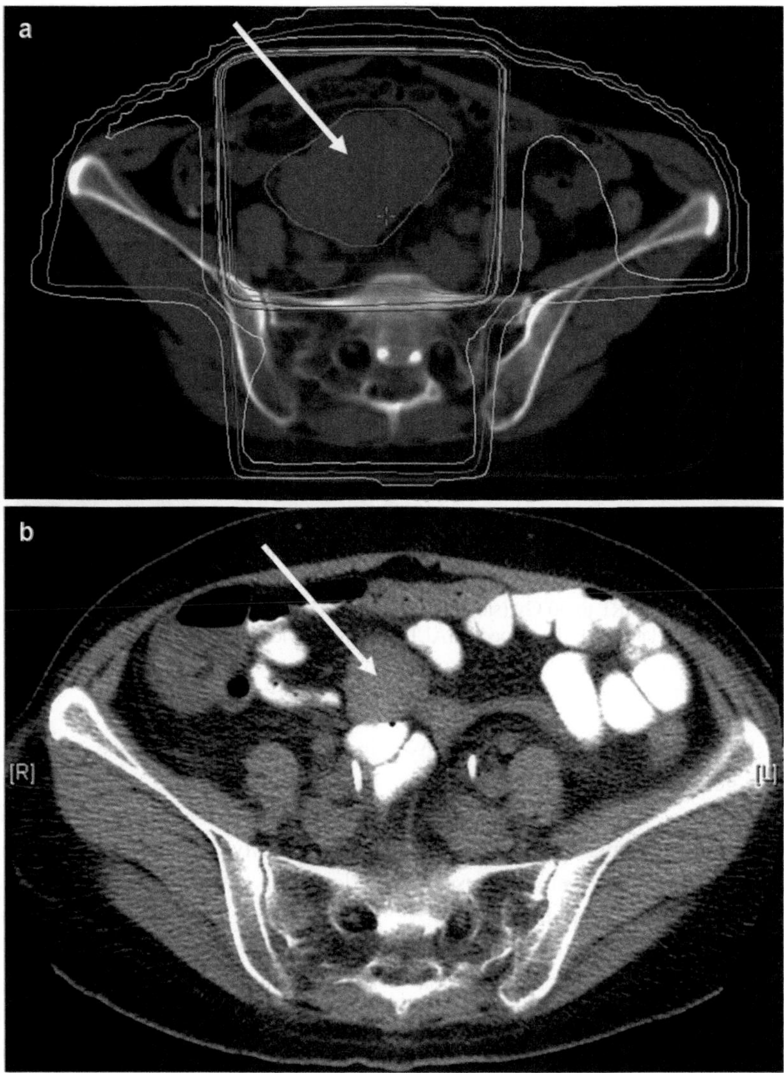

Fig. 4 A 63-year-old female was diagnosed with stage III, low-grade, follicular lymphoma at age 53. She was initially treated with chemotherapy. Four years later, the disease recurred in the abdomen and she was treated with rituximab. Upon progression she received RT (4 Gy × 1) without response. The mass was re-biopsied and confirmed to be grade 2 follicular lymphoma. As she had a single site of active disease (8 cm), a more protracted course of RT was pursued (2 Gy qd to 30 Gy) (panel **a**, *white arrow*). She tolerated RT well and achieved a partial response at 1 year (panel **b**, *white arrow*)

5 % of plasma cell neoplasms are solitary lesions, which can develop at either osseous sites or in extramedullary locations, the latter most commonly in the head and neck region. For both, the preferred treatment is definitive radiation therapy to a dose of 40–45 Gy. Local control is largely determined by size of the primary tumor with larger tumors having a higher risk of local recurrence (Ozsahin et al. 2006; Tsang et al. 2001). The dominant pattern of failure is systemic progression to multiple myeloma. For osseous and extramedullary plasmacytomas, the 10-year risk of developing multiple myeloma is approximately 70 % and 35 %, respectively (Ozsahin et al. 2006). The majority of patients diagnosed with a plasma cell neoplasm have multiple myeloma. Painful lytic lesions are a common complica-

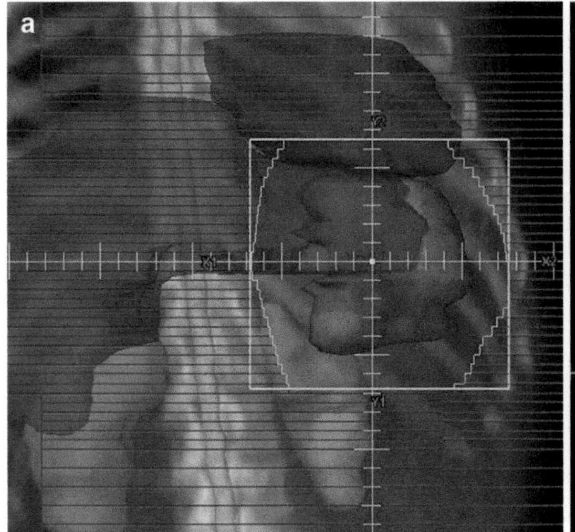

Fig. 5 A 68-year-old male was diagnosed with *Helicobacter pylori*-negative gastric MALT lymphoma and achieved a durable complete remission with RT to 30 Gy (stomach in *red*, panel **a**). Four years later, he developed MALT lymphoma along the mandibular alveolar ridge. Most of the disease was removed at the time of biopsy. He received RT to 24 Gy (original extent of disease in *red*, panel **b**) and is without evidence of recurrence 3 years later

tion which a short course of radiation therapy can palliate. In general, doses of 8–24 Gy are recommended.

It is unusual for a solitary plasmacytoma to fail locally without evidence of systemic progression. In such cases, a second course of radiation therapy could be considered. There have been anecdotal reports of long-term disease control in such circumstances (Mendenhall et al. 1980). The location of the original disease and ability to avoid critical normal regional structures would dictate whether re-irradiation is feasible. Similarly, it is typically unnecessary to repeat a course of radiation therapy for myeloma. However, in circumstances where pain recurs and there is obvious radiographic or pathologic evidence of persistent disease, a second course of radiation is almost always feasible given the relatively low doses that are sufficient to palliate pain (Fig. 6).

7 CNS Lymphoma

Primary central nervous system (CNS) lymphoma is a relatively rare subtype of non-Hodgkin lymphoma. The most important treatment component is high-dose methotrexate, typically given in conjunction with other systemic agents including rituximab (Morris and Abrey 2009). The role of consolidation radiation therapy is controversial, primarily due to the risk of neurotoxicity in older adults after systemic high-dose methotrexate (Abrey et al. 1998). In the presence of a complete response, low-dose (23.4 Gy) whole brain radiation therapy is often utilized and seems to be associated with favorable clinical outcomes, including a low risk of subsequent failure in the brain and a low risk of neurotoxicity (Morris et al. 2013).

Secondary CNS lymphoma occurs when systemic disease secondarily involves the CNS. Current regimens in fit patients utilize a similar approach as primary CNS lymphoma, often in conjunction with high-dose chemotherapy and autologous stem cell transplant. The role of radiation therapy in secondary CNS lymphoma is not established.

Generally, repeat whole brain radiation therapy is not recommended in primary or secondary CNS lymphoma. Stereotactic radiosurgery, in which a tumor is treated with a single, high-dose conformal treatment, has been employed in the setting of limited intracranial progression after whole brain radiation therapy for CNS lymphomas (Kumar et al. 2015; Matsumoto et al. 2007;

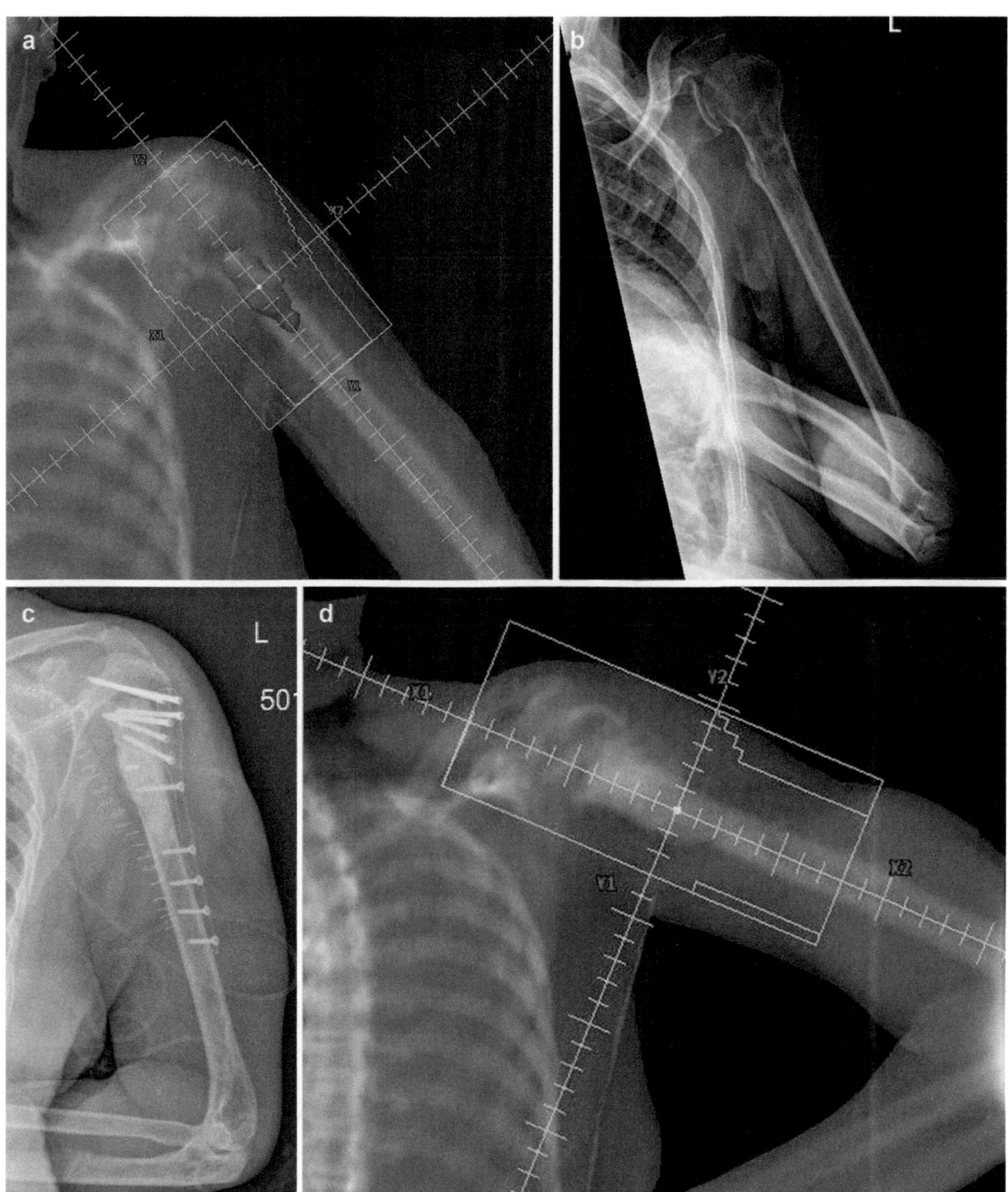

Fig. 6 An 86-year-old female was treated for a painful left humeral lytic lesion with palliative RT (20 Gy in 4 Gy fractions) (panel **a**). Her pain improved but approximately 18 months later she developed a nondisplaced pathologic fracture of the proximal humeral metadiaphysis at the site of the original lytic lesion (panel **b**). She underwent open reduction and internal fixation with cement reconstruction (panel **c**). Biopsy confirmed myeloma. Due to persistent pain, she underwent a second course of RT using the same total dose but a higher dose per fraction (20 Gy in 5 Gy fractions) with subsequent improvement in pain (panel **d**)

Kenai et al. 2006) (Fig. 7). Doses of 12–18 Gy have been utilized with overall response rates of ~85 %. Median survival, in heterogeneous populations of patients, is reported to be 10–17 months. As expected, radiosurgery is well tolerated without significant complications. However, distant brain failures are common after stereotactic radiosurgery (Matsumoto et al. 2007), presumably given the multifocality of intracranial disease.

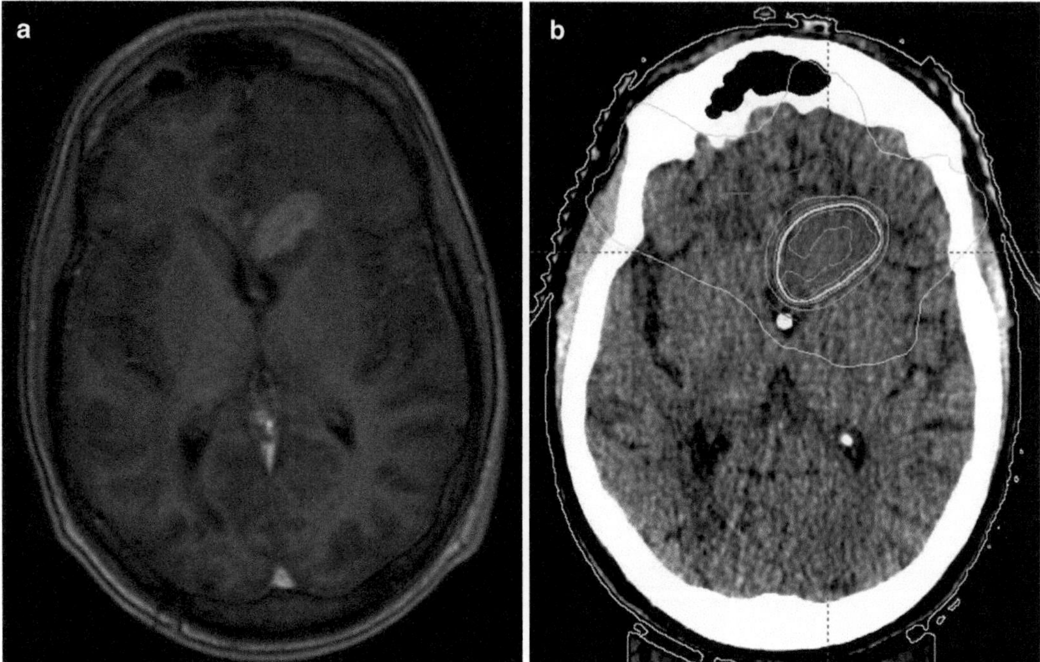

Fig. 7 A 26-year-old male was treated for stage II DLBCL with eight cycles of R-CHOP but subsequently failed with two parenchymal lesions in the brain. He received further chemotherapy followed by an autologous stem cell transplant. As part of the preparative regimen, he received TBI (13.5 Gy) in addition to a boost to the brain (10 Gy). About 1 year later, he developed a new parenchymal brain lesion distant from his previous intracranial disease (panel **a**). Given the prior whole brain radiation therapy, this was treated with stereotactic radiosurgery (panel **b**, *yellow contour* is 15 Gy isodose line)

8 Cutaneous Lymphomas

Cutaneous lymphomas consist of both T-cell and B-cell histologies. The most common T-cell histologies are mycosis fungoides and CD30-positive lymphoproliferative disorders, which include lymphomatoid papulosis and primary cutaneous anaplastic large cell lymphoma. The B-cell histologies include primary cutaneous follicle center lymphoma, marginal zone lymphoma, and diffuse large B-cell lymphoma, leg type.

Mycosis fungoides is the most common cutaneous lymphoma and radiation therapy plays an integral role in its management. For the rare patient with unilesional disease, definitive radiation therapy can lead to long-term remission and potential cures (Wilson et al. 1998; Micaily et al. 1998; Piccinno et al. 2009). Local control in this setting is ~95 %. For the vast majority of patients, however, who present with widespread patch/plaque disease or with cutaneous tumors, the goal of therapy is palliative. Radiation therapy is particularly advantageous for those with thick plaques or tumors. Local radiation therapy, using doses of 7–20 Gy, leads to response rates of ~90 % (Thomas et al. 2013; Neelis et al. 2009). Unfortunately, with time, many lesions will progress and re-irradiation becomes necessary. Such low doses allow for re-irradiation, sometimes more than once, without difficulty. Acute and long-term risks of local radiation therapy, utilizing the relatively low doses mentioned above, are minimal. Pigmentation changes and alopecia, both from the disease and the treatment, are most common.

Total skin electron beam therapy is advantageous for patients with generalized disease, particularly for those with thick plaques, tumors, or whose disease is refractory to other modalities. Complete response rates range from 75 to 85 % for those with patch/plaque (T2) disease (Jones et al. 2002; Ysebaert et al. 2004; Navi et al. 2011) and

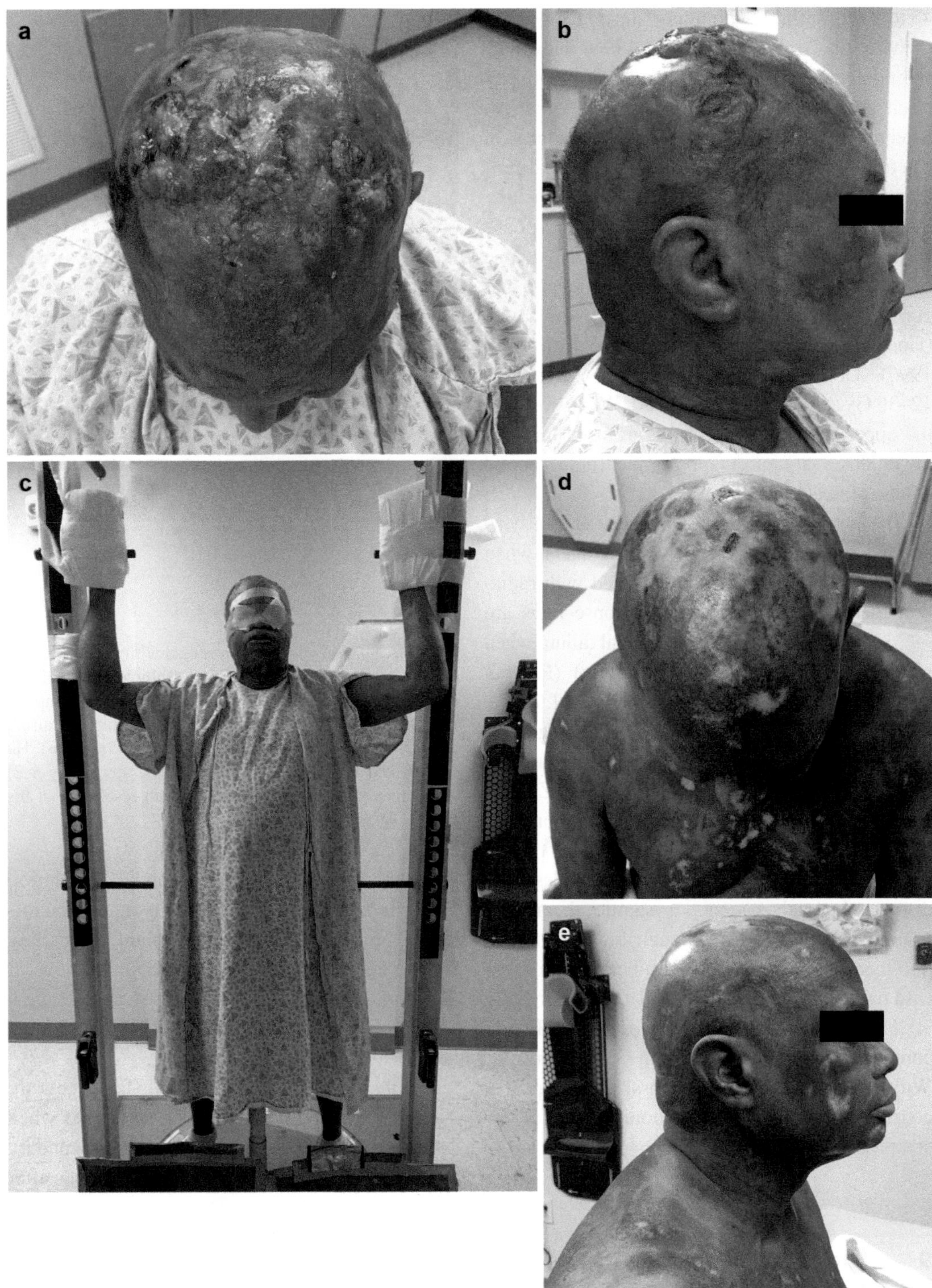

Fig. 8 A 59-year-old male was diagnosed with mycosis fungoides at age 52. He was treated with numerous modalities for patch/plaque stage (T2) disease and ultimately underwent total skin electron beam therapy (36 Gy) for refractory tumor-stage (T3) disease. Over the next 2 years, he received local radiation therapy (10–20 Gy) to multiple sites for symptomatic disease. He presented with widespread tumors and plaques, especially on the face (panels **a**, **b**). Preparatory to an allogeneic stem cell transplant, a second course of total skin electron beam therapy was pursued in an attempt to clear the cutaneous disease (panel **c**). He received 24 Gy with selective boosts. He achieved a good response (panels **d**, **e**) and proceeded with an allogeneic stem cell transplant

45 to 80% for those with tumor-stage (T3) disease (Navi et al. 2011; Quiros et al. 1996). However, essentially all patients relapse and re-irradiation is often necessary. As mentioned above, local re-irradiation is rarely problematic. Even total skin electron beam therapy can be repeated. Ideal candidates for repeat total skin electron beam therapy include those who achieved a good initial response and reasonable response duration to the first course of therapy, failure of subsequent treatments, and generalized symptomatic skin involvement (Hoppe 2003; Becker et al. 1995; Wilson et al. 1996). Given clinical circumstances, doses of 12–36 Gy are typically prescribed. When doses on the upper end of this spectrum are used initially, lower doses are most appropriate for a second course of treatment (Fig. 8).

The low-grade primary cutaneous B-cell lymphomas (marginal zone and follicle center), when localized, are most commonly treated with radiation therapy alone. Complete response rates are ~99% with a very low chance of local failure when given conventional doses (24–36 Gy) (Pashtan et al. 2013; Senff et al. 2007; Hamilton et al. 2013). Such patients are at high risk of developing additional sites of disease, but relapses are usually localized to the skin (Senff et al. 2007; Zinzani et al. 2006), and a second course of radiation therapy can be employed quite easily. Rarer is the patient who presents or relapses with widespread disease. In such patients, systemic therapy is usually most appropriate though low-dose radiation therapy (e.g., 2 Gy × 2) can be useful for disease palliation (Neelis et al. 2009). Approximately 90% of lesions will regress with low-dose RT, with complete responses observed in ~75% (Fig. 9). With such low doses, it is possible to repeat a course of radiation therapy more than once for symptomatic relief.

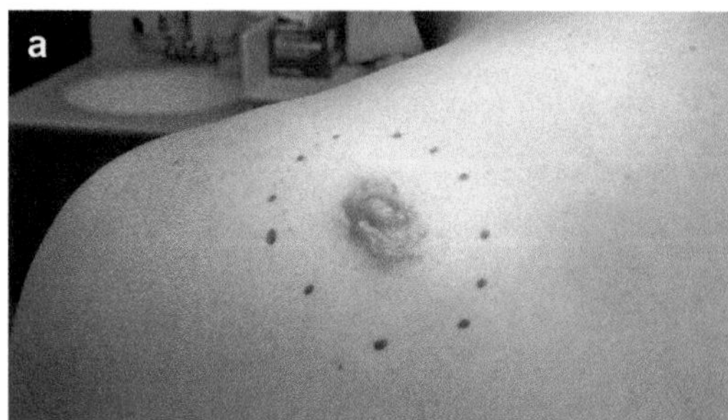

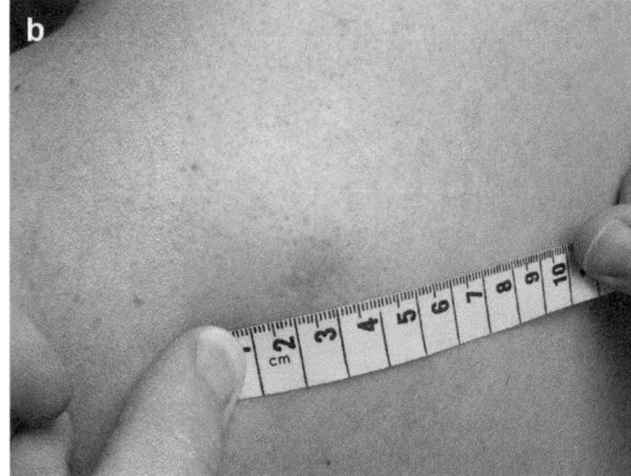

Fig. 9 A 39-year-old male presented with multifocal primary cutaneous B-cell lymphoma (follicle center histology). He was treated with rituximab with a complete response at all sites of disease except a pruritic, raised, erythematous lesion on his upper left back (panel **a**). He was treated with low-dose radiation therapy (2 Gy × 2) and achieved a complete response with resolution of his pruritis (panel **b**)

9 Total Body Irradiation

Allogeneic stem cell transplantation is often recommended for patients with high-risk or relapsed acute leukemias and some lymphomas including diffuse large B-cell lymphoma and Hodgkin lymphoma. Total body irradiation (TBI) is an established modality in the conditioning regimen prior to transplant, especially for the acute leukemias. While a single dose of 8 Gy was used historically, most centers now use fractionated regimens, typically 12–14 Gy administered in 6–9 fractions.

While rare, patients occasionally fail to engraft. This is classified as primary graft failure when donor cells fail to engraft altogether or secondary graft failure when there is loss of donor cells after an initial engraftment. The prognosis of such patients is poor, even with second transplantation (Schriber et al. 2010). Regimens incorporating low-dose TBI (2 Gy × 1) have been reported with successful engraftment. TBI can play an important role by eradicating residual host immune cells facilitating a successful engraftment (Gyurkocza et al. 2009; Sumi et al. 2010; Shimizu

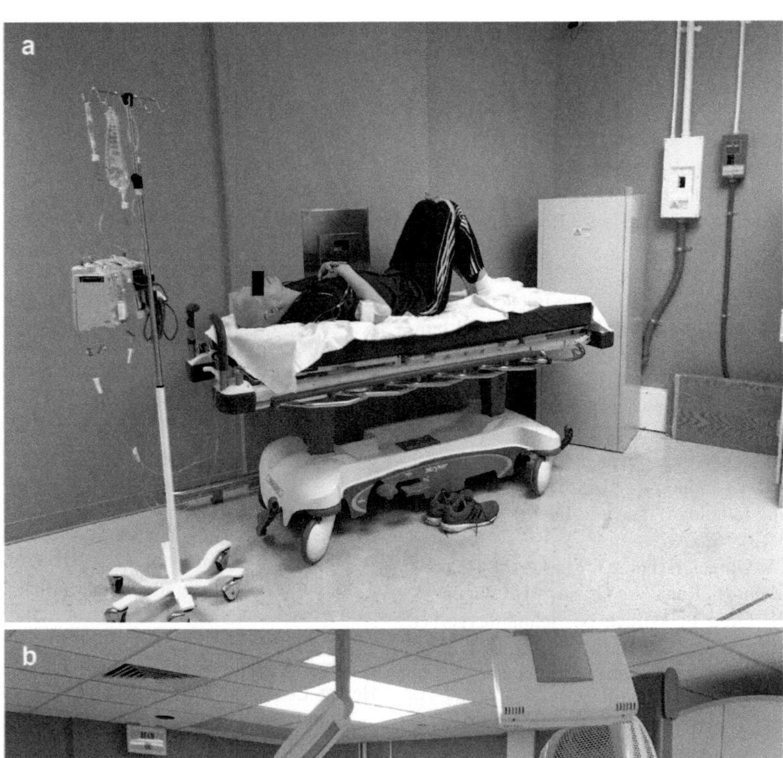

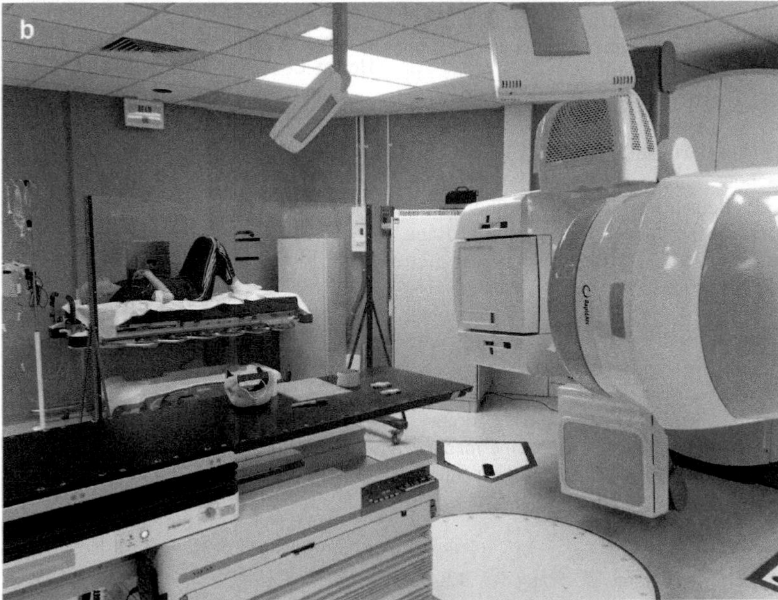

Fig. 10 This 19-year-old male was diagnosed with acute lymphocytic leukemia with CNS involvement. After achieving remission with induction chemotherapy and intrathecal methotrexate, he underwent myeloablative conditioning with TBI (1.5 Gy bid to 13.5 Gy) with a boost to the testicles and craniospinal axis. His conditioning also included high-dose fludarabine followed by a dual cord stem cell transplant. He failed to engraft and underwent a one-day preparative regimen consisting of fludarabine, cyclophosphamide, alemtuzumab, and additional TBI (2 Gy × 1) followed by another cord blood stem transplant which resulted in successful engraftment. Panel **a** shows the patient positioned in a lateral position. Panel **b** demonstrates placement of the patient in comparison with the linear accelerator with the spoiler in position

et al. 2009), even in patients previously receiving a myeloablative TBI-based regimen (Sumi et al. 2010; Shimizu et al. 2009) (Fig. 10).

Acknowledgment The authors would like to thank Leonard R. Prosnitz, M.D., for his thoughtful comments that improved the quality of the chapter.

References

Abrey LE, DeAngelis LM, Yahalom J (1998) Long-term survival in primary CNS lymphoma. J Clin Oncol 16(3):859–863

Becker M, Hoppe RT, Knox SJ (1995) Multiple courses of high-dose total skin electron beam therapy in the management of mycosis fungoides. Int J Radiat Oncol Biol Phys 32(5):1445–1449

Dorth JA, Chino JP, Prosnitz LR, Diehl LF, Beaven AW, Coleman RE, Kelsey CR (2011) The impact of radiation therapy in patients with diffuse large B-cell lymphoma with positive post-chemotherapy FDG-PET or gallium-67 scans. Ann Oncol 22(2):405–410

Dorth JA, Prosnitz LR, Broadwater G, Diehl LF, Beaven AW, Coleman RE, Kelsey CR (2012) Impact of consolidation radiation therapy in stage III-IV diffuse large B-cell lymphoma with negative post-chemotherapy radiologic imaging. Int J Radiat Oncol Biol Phys 84(3):762–767

Eich HT, Diehl V, Gorgen H, Pabst T, Markova J, Debus J, Ho A, Dorken B, Rank A, Grosu AL, Wiegel T, Karstens JH, Greil R, Willich N, Schmidberger H, Dohner H, Borchmann P, Muller-Hermelink HK, Muller RP, Engert A (2010) Intensified chemotherapy and dose-reduced involved-field radiotherapy in patients with early unfavorable Hodgkin's lymphoma: final analysis of the German Hodgkin Study Group HD11 trial. J Clin Oncol 28(27):4199–4206

Engert A, Plutschow A, Eich HT, Lohri A, Dorken B, Borchmann P, Berger B, Greil R, Willborn KC, Wilhelm M, Debus J, Eble MJ, Sokler M, Ho A, Rank A, Ganser A, Trumper L, Bokemeyer C, Kirchner H, Schubert J, Kral Z, Fuchs M, Muller-Hermelink HK, Muller RP, Diehl V (2010) Reduced treatment intensity in patients with early-stage Hodgkin's lymphoma. New Engl J Med 363(7):640–652

Friedberg JW, Byrtek M, Link BK, Flowers C, Taylor M, Hainsworth J, Cerhan JR, Zelenetz AD, Hirata J, Miller TP (2012) Effectiveness of first-line management strategies for stage I follicular lymphoma: analysis of the National LymphoCare Study. J Clin Oncol 30(27):3368–3375

Goda JS, Gospodarowicz M, Pintilie M, Wells W, Hodgson DC, Sun A, Crump M, Tsang RW (2010) Long-term outcome in localized extranodal mucosa-associated lymphoid tissue lymphomas treated with radiotherapy. Cancer 116(16):3815–3824

Gyurkocza B, Cao TM, Storb RF, Lange T, Leisenring W, Franke GN, Sorror M, Hoppe R, Maloney DG, Negrin RS, Shizuru JA, Sandmaier BM (2009) Salvage allogeneic hematopoietic cell transplantation with fludarabine and low-dose total body irradiation after rejection of first allografts. Biol Blood Marrow Transplant 15(10):1314–1322

Haas RL, Poortmans P, de Jong D, Aleman BM, Dewit LG, Verheij M, Hart AA, van Oers MH, van der Hulst M, Baars JW, Bartelink H (2003) High response rates and lasting remissions after low-dose involved field radiotherapy in indolent lymphomas. J Clin Oncol 21(13):2474–2480

Haas RL, Poortmans P, de Jong D, Verheij M, van der Hulst M, de Boer JP, Bartelink H (2005) Effective palliation by low dose local radiotherapy for recurrent and/or chemotherapy refractory non-follicular lymphoma patients. Eur J Cancer 41(12):1724–1730

Hamilton SN, Wai ES, Tan K, Alexander C, Gascoyne RD, Connors JM (2013) Treatment and outcomes in patients with primary cutaneous B-cell lymphoma: the BC Cancer Agency experience. Int J Radiat Oncol Biol Phys 87(4):719–725

Held G, Zeynalova S, Murawski N, Ziepert M, Kempf B, Viardot A, Dreyling M, Hallek M, Witzens-Harig M, Fleckenstein J, Rube C, Zwick C, Glass B, Schmitz N, Pfreundschuh M (2013) Impact of rituximab and radiotherapy on outcome of patients with aggressive B-cell lymphoma and skeletal involvement. J Clin Oncol 31(32):4115–4122

Held G, Murawski N, Ziepert M, Fleckenstein J, Poschel V, Zwick C, Bittenbring J, Hanel M, Wilhelm S, Schubert J, Schmitz N, Loffler M, Rube C, Pfreundschuh M (2014) Role of radiotherapy to bulky disease in elderly patients with aggressive B-cell lymphoma. J Clin Oncol 32(11):1112–1118

Herbst C, Rehan FA, Brillant C, Bohlius J, Skoetz N, Schulz H, Monsef I, Specht L, Engert A (2010) Combined modality treatment improves tumor control and overall survival in patients with early stage Hodgkin's lymphoma: a systematic review. Haematologica 95(3):494–500

Hoppe RT (2003) Mycosis fungoides: radiation therapy. Dermatol Ther 16(4):347–354

Horning SJ, Weller E, Kim K, Earle JD, O'Connell MJ, Habermann TM, Glick JH (2004) Chemotherapy with or without radiotherapy in limited-stage diffuse aggressive non-Hodgkin's lymphoma: Eastern Cooperative Oncology Group study 1484. J Clin Oncol 22(15):3032–3038

Jones GW, Kacinski BM, Wilson LD, Willemze R, Spittle M, Hohenberg G, Handl-Zeller L, Trautinger F, Knobler R (2002) Total skin electron radiation in the management of mycosis fungoides: Consensus of the European Organization for Research and Treatment of Cancer (EORTC) Cutaneous Lymphoma Project Group. J Am Acad Dermatol 47(3):364–370

Josting A, Nogova L, Franklin J, Glossmann JP, Eich HT, Sieber M, Schober T, Boettcher HD, Schulz U, Muller RP, Diehl V, Engert A (2005) Salvage radiotherapy in patients with relapsed and refractory Hodgkin's lymphoma: a retrospective analysis from the German Hodgkin Lymphoma Study Group. J Clin Oncol 23(7):1522–1529

Kaplan H (1972) Hodgkin's disease, vol 1. Harvard University Press, Cambridge, MA

Kenai H, Yamashita M, Nakamura T, Asano T, Momii Y, Nagatomi H (2006) Gamma Knife surgery for primary central nervous system lymphoma: usefulness as palliative local tumor control. J Neurosurg 105(Suppl):133–138

Kumar R, Laack N, Pollock BE, Link M, O'Neill BP, Parney IF (2015) Stereotactic radiosurgery in the treatment of recurrent CNS lymphoma. World Neurosurg 84(2):390–397

Matsumoto Y, Horiike S, Fujimoto Y, Shimizu D, Kudo-Nakata Y, Kimura S, Sato M, Nomura K, Kaneko H, Kobayashi Y, Shimazaki C, Taniwaki M (2007) Effectiveness and limitation of gamma knife radiosurgery for relapsed central nervous system lymphoma: a retrospective analysis in one institution. Int J Hematol 85(4):333–337

Mendenhall CM, Thar TL, Million RR (1980) Solitary plasmacytoma of bone and soft tissue. Int J Radiat Oncol Biol Phys 6(11):1497–1501

Micaily B, Miyamoto C, Kantor G, Lessin S, Rook A, Brady L, Goodman R, Vonderheid EC (1998) Radiotherapy for unilesional mycosis fungoides. Int J Radiat Oncol Biol Phys 42(2):361–364

Morris PG, Abrey LE (2009) Therapeutic challenges in primary CNS lymphoma. Lancet Neurol 8(6): 581–592

Morris PG, Correa DD, Yahalom J, Raizer JJ, Schiff D, Grant B, Grimm S, Lai RK, Reiner AS, Panageas K, Karimi S, Curry R, Shah G, Abrey LE, DeAngelis LM, Omuro A (2013) Rituximab, methotrexate, procarbazine, and vincristine followed by consolidation reduced-dose whole-brain radiotherapy and cytarabine in newly diagnosed primary CNS lymphoma: final results and long-term outcome. J Clin Oncol 31(31):3971–3979

Moskowitz CH, Nimer SD, Zelenetz AD, Trippett T, Hedrick EE, Filippa DA, Louie D, Gonzales M, Walits J, Coady-Lyons N, Qin J, Frank R, Bertino JR, Goy A, Noy A, O'Brien JP, Straus D, Portlock CS, Yahalom J (2001) A 2-step comprehensive high-dose chemoradiotherapy second-line program for relapsed and refractory Hodgkin disease: analysis by intent to treat and development of a prognostic model. Blood 97(3):616–623

Murthy V, Thomas K, Foo K, Cunningham D, Johnson B, Norman A, Horwich A (2008) Efficacy of palliative low-dose involved-field radiation therapy in advanced lymphoma: a phase II study. Clin Lymphoma Myeloma 8(4):241–245

Navi D, Riaz N, Levin YS, Sullivan NC, Kim YH, Hoppe RT (2011) The Stanford University experience with conventional-dose, total skin electron-beam therapy in the treatment of generalized patch or plaque (T2) and tumor (T3) mycosis fungoides. Arch Dermatol 147(5):561–567

Neelis KJ, Schimmel EC, Vermeer MH, Senff NJ, Willemze R, Noordijk EM (2009) Low-dose palliative radiotherapy for cutaneous B- and T-cell lymphomas. Int J Radiat Oncol Biol Phys 74(1):154–158

Olszewski AJ, Shrestha R, Castillo JJ (2015) Treatment selection and outcomes in early-stage classical Hodgkin lymphoma: analysis of the National Cancer Data Base. J Clin Oncol 33(6):625–633

Ozsahin M, Tsang RW, Poortmans P, Belkacemi Y, Bolla M, Dincbas FO, Landmann C, Castelain B, Buijsen J, Curschmann J, Kadish SP, Kowalczyk A, Anacak Y, Hammer J, Nguyen TD, Studer G, Cooper R, Sengoz M, Scandolaro L, Zouhair A (2006) Outcomes and patterns of failure in solitary plasmacytoma: a multicenter Rare Cancer Network study of 258 patients. Int J Radiat Oncol Biol Phys 64(1):210–217

Pashtan I, Mauch PM, Chen YH, Dorfman DM, Silver B, Ng AK (2013) Radiotherapy in the management of localized primary cutaneous B-cell lymphoma. Leukemia Lymphoma 54(4):726–730

Piccinno R, Caccialanza M, Percivalle S (2009) Minimal stage IA mycosis fungoides. Results of radiotherapy in 15 patients. J Dermatolog Treat 20(3):165–168

Pugh TJ, Ballonoff A, Newman F, Rabinovitch R (2010) Improved survival in patients with early stage low-grade follicular lymphoma treated with radiation: a surveillance, epidemiology, and end results database analysis. Cancer 116(16):3843–3851

Quiros PA, Kacinski BM, Wilson LD (1996) Extent of skin involvement as a prognostic indicator of disease free and overall survival of patients with T3 cutaneous T-cell lymphoma treated with total skin electron beam radiation therapy. Cancer 77(9):1912–1917

Russo AL, Chen YH, Martin NE, Vinjamoori A, Luthy SK, Freedman A, Michaelson EM, Silver B, Mauch PM, Ng AK (2013) Low-dose involved-field radiation in the treatment of non-hodgkin lymphoma: predictors of response and treatment failure. Int J Radiat Oncol Biol Phys 86(1):121–127

Schriber J, Agovi MA, Ho V, Ballen KK, Bacigalupo A, Lazarus HM, Bredeson CN, Gupta V, Maziarz RT, Hale GA, Litzow MR, Logan B, Bornhauser M, Giller RH, Isola L, Marks DI, Rizzo JD, Pasquini MC (2010) Second unrelated donor hematopoietic cell transplantation for primary graft failure. Biol Blood Marrow Transplant 16(8):1099–1106

Sehn LH, Klasa R, Shenkier T, Villa D, Slack GW, Gascoyne RD, Benard F, Wilson D, Morris J, Parsons C, Pickles T, Connors JM, Savage KJ (2013) Long-term experience with PET-guided consolidation radiation therapy (XRT) in patient with advanced stage diffuse large B-cell Lymphoma (DLBCL) treated with R-CHOP. Hematol Oncol 31(S1):96–150

Senff NJ, Hoefnagel JJ, Neelis KJ, Vermeer MH, Noordijk EM, Willemze R, Dutch Cutaneous Lymphoma G (2007) Results of radiotherapy in 153 primary cutaneous B-Cell lymphomas classified according to the WHO-EORTC classification. Arch Dermatol 143(12):1520–1526

Shimizu I, Kobayashi H, Nasu K, Otsuki F, Ueki T, Sumi M, Ueno M, Ichikawa N, Nakao S (2009) Successful engraftment of cord blood following a one-day reduced-intensity conditioning regimen in two patients suffering primary graft failure and sepsis. Bone Marrow Transplant 44(9):617–618

Sumi M, Shimizu I, Sato K, Ueki T, Akahane D, Ueno M, Ichikawa N, Nakao S, Kobayashi H (2010) Graft failure in cord blood transplantation successfully treated with short-term reduced-intensity conditioning regimen and second allogeneic transplantation. Int J Hematol 92(5):744–750

Teckie S, Qi S, Lovie S, Navarrett S, Hsu M, Noy A, Portlock C, Yahalom J (2015) Long-term outcomes and patterns of relapse of early-stage extranodal marginal zone lymphoma treated with radiation therapy with curative intent. Int J Radiat Oncol Biol Phys 92(1):130–137

Thomas TO, Agrawal P, Guitart J, Rosen ST, Rademaker AW, Querfeld C, Hayes JP, Kuzel TM, Mittal BB (2013) Outcome of patients treated with a single-fraction dose of palliative radiation for cutaneous T-cell lymphoma. Int J Radiat Oncol Biol Phys 85(3):747–753

Torok JA, Wu Y, Prosnitz LR, Kim GJ, Beaven AW, Diehl LF, Kelsey CR (2015) Low-dose consolidation radiation therapy for early stage unfavorable Hodgkin lymphoma. Int J Radiat Oncol Biol Phys 92(1):54–59

Tsang RW, Gospodarowicz MK, Pintilie M, Bezjak A, Wells W, Hodgson DC, Stewart AK (2001) Solitary plasmacytoma treated with radiotherapy: impact of tumor size on outcome. Int J Radiat Oncol Biol Phys 50(1):113–120

Vargo JA, Gill BS, Balasubramani GK, Beriwal S (2015) What is the optimal management of early-stage low-grade follicular lymphoma in the modern era? Cancer 121(18):3325–3334

Wilson LD, Quiros PA, Kolenik SA, Heald PW, Braverman IM, Edelson RL, Kacinski BM (1996) Additional courses of total skin electron beam therapy in the treatment of patients with recurrent cutaneous T-cell lymphoma. J Am Acad Dermatol 35(1):69–73

Wilson LD, Kacinski BM, Jones GW (1998) Local superficial radiotherapy in the management of minimal stage IA cutaneous T-cell lymphoma (Mycosis Fungoides). Int J Radiat Oncol Biol Phys 40(1): 109–115

Ysebaert L, Truc G, Dalac S, Lambert D, Petrella T, Barillot I, Naudy S, Horiot JC, Maingon P (2004) Ultimate results of radiation therapy for T1-T2 mycosis fungoides (including reirradiation). Int J Radiat Oncol Biol Phys 58(4):1128–1134

Zinzani PL, Quaglino P, Pimpinelli N, Berti E, Baliva G, Rupoli S, Martelli M, Alaibac M, Borroni G, Chimenti S, Alterini R, Alinari L, Fierro MT, Cappello N, Pileri A, Soligo D, Paulli M, Pileri S, Santucci M, Bernengo MG (2006) Prognostic factors in primary cutaneous B-cell lymphoma: the Italian Study Group for Cutaneous Lymphomas. J Clin Oncol 24(9): 1376–1382

Bone Metastases

Yvette van der Linden and Peter Hoskin

Contents

The original version of this chapter was revised. An erratum to this chapter can be found at 10.1007/978-3-319-41825-4_78.

Y. van der Linden (✉)
Department of Radiotherapy, Leiden University Medical Centre, Leiden, The Netherlands
e-mail: ymvanderlinden@lumc.nl

P. Hoskin
Department of Radiotherapy, Mount Vernon Hospital, London, UK

Abstract

The treatment of bone metastases comprises a large part of the radiotherapy daily practice. Palliative radiotherapy has proven to be successful in treating pain caused by metastatic lesions in any bone and in treating neurological complaints caused by compression of the spinal cord due to lesions in the spinal column. In most prospective randomized trials on radiotherapy for bone pain, responses up to 70 % were reported. However, when survival was prolonged, recurrent pain was reported in up to 50 % of patients. It is to be expected for the future, since patients are living longer with disseminated disease, that symptoms may recur and therefore retreatment of bone metastases for palliative reasons will increase. In this chapter, the evidence-based outcomes for response and duration of response to initial and subsequent radiotherapy will be presented. Guidelines will be formulated for retreatment in bone metastases, with a focus on timing, expected complications, and preferred radiotherapy techniques. More intensive radiation techniques like intensity-modulated and stereotactic radiotherapy will be discussed for their role in retreatment of bone metastases.

Med Radiol Radiat Oncol (2016)
DOI 10.1007/174_2016_72, © Springer International Publishing Switzerland
Published Online: 09 Aug 2016

1 Introduction

1.1 Epidemiology

In approximately half of all patients who are diagnosed with cancer from various sites, metastatic spread of tumor cells occurs during follow-up. For the patient this signifies a catastrophic event: it means that the malignant process is incurable and treatment is no longer directed toward cure. Only optimal palliation of disease-related symptoms is achievable. Bone is the third most frequent site of tumor metastasis, after the lung and liver. The malignant tumors that frequently metastasize to the skeleton are from common primary sites, in particular the breast, prostate, and lung. The incidence and prevalence of bone metastases in cancer patients are difficult to determine with accuracy, and the clinical incidence is lower than the true pathological rate. Studies report a frequency of 10–47 % of all patients with breast cancer developing metastases to the bone detected during their illness (Miller and Whitehill 1984; Kamby et al. 1987; Wedin et al. 2001), but in autopsy studies, more than 70 % of breast cancer patients had tumor deposits in the bone (Galasko 1981; Lee 1983).

Duration of survival after the clinical manifestation of bone metastases depends on whether the metastasis is a solitary lesion or multiple metastases exist throughout the skeleton. When the patient also has visceral metastases, the prognosis is generally worse. In addition, the type of primary tumor affects the disease outcome. Patients with breast cancer or prostate cancer may have a prolonged survival, sometimes stretching over several years. Improvements in systemic therapy and the relatively long clinical course of these primary tumors underline this observation. However, the majority of patients treated in palliative bone metastases trials die within 5–12 months after radiotherapy for bone metastases (Ratanatharathorn et al. 1999; van der Linden et al. 2006).

When considering radical treatment options, the probability of occult metastasis is a major factor for physicians when deciding which treatment to apply. When there is a high risk, then adjuvant systemic therapy or, in the case of bone metastases, bisphosphonates or RANKL inhibitors (Lipton et al. 2016) may take precedence over the use of potentially disabling surgical procedures. For the radiotherapy department and its employees, care for patients with painful bone metastases comprises 10–15 % of the daily workload.

1.2 Clinical Implications and Treatment Modalities

Bone metastases may cause a range of clinical complications, varying from mild to severe pain at the site of the metastasis, pathological fracture of bone, spinal cord compression (SCC) or nerve root compression syndromes, and hypercalcemia. The intensity of these symptoms is mostly dependent on the localization and extent of the lesion in the skeleton. A variety of palliative treatment modalities is available for bone metastases. The majority of treatments are directed toward optimum palliation with minimum treatment-related morbidity. Treatment choice is dependent on the symptoms and life expectancy of the patient and whether comorbidity exists that may increase the risk of a particular treatment. Other influencing factors are the localization of the metastasis in the skeleton and whether the metastasis is solitary or multiple.

1.2.1 Pain

The mechanisms that underlie the sensation of pain caused by metastasis are poorly understood. The presence of pain does not seem to be correlated with the type of tumor, location, and number or size of the metastases (Hoskin 1988; Vakaet and Boterberg 2004). It is thought that when tumor cells grow, the periosteum, which is the highly innervated connective tissue sheath that covers the external surface of the bone, is stretched. Pain receptors (nociceptors) are subsequently activated and may show sensitization, which is manifested as a decreased threshold of activation after injury and the emergence of spontaneous activity (Mercadante 1997; Payne 2003). This may explain why some lesions cause such a deep, dull, aching sensation without even the least contact (Coleman 1997). In addition, chemical mediators of pain such as prostaglandins are thought to play a role (Hoskin 1988). Treatment strategies are focused on these abovementioned mechanisms.

Analgesic drugs that inhibit certain pathways are available and relatively simple to administer. Bone pain may respond to simple analgesics and nonsteroidal anti-inflammatory drugs (NSAIDs) as well as strong opioids; titration using the principles of the analgesic ladder should be used. Adjuvant analgesics such as steroids and nerve sedatives, e.g., gabapentin and pregabalin, also have an important role. Depending on the type, quantity, and duration of analgesic intake, the patient may suffer from significant side effects. For example, opioids cause nausea, constipation, and drowsiness. Nonsteroidal anti-inflammatory drugs may cause gastrointestinal ulceration with subsequent bleeding. Steroids should be administered for as short a time as possible to minimize side effects such as water retention, insomnia, weight gain, and glucose intolerance.

For localized pain, radiotherapy is a well-accepted treatment modality with a 60–80 % likelihood of overall pain relief reported (Wu et al. 2003; Sze et al. 2003; Falkmer et al. 2003). The mechanism of the analgesic effect from radiotherapy remains unknown. Because the onset of pain relief is often rapid, within days, it is not likely to be dependent upon tumor shrinkage alone (Hoskin 1988). It is probable that a response mechanism through modification of chemical mediators such as prostaglandins is important.

The side effects of radiotherapy are dependent on the part of the body irradiated, treatment volume, and total radiotherapy dose. Transient side effects include tiredness, skin reactions, or gastrointestinal complaints such as nausea or diarrhea. Pain flare may also be seen in a small number of patients. If multiple bony sites causing diffuse pain are painful, then, instead of several smaller fields, a single wide-field radiotherapy may be considered with good results (Salazar et al. 2001; Berg et al. 2009). This technique may be associated with more acute side effects, particularly gastrointestinal symptoms and transient bone marrow depression. In general, palliative radiotherapy is a safe, well-tolerated treatment which can be repeated if required.

Surgery is another option for the local treatment of pain in weight-bearing long bones. For example, if a patient suffers from a painful osteolytic metastasis in the femur or humerus with cortical involvement and rising instability, osteosynthesis may cause immediate relief of pain and prevent pathological fracture. In a subgroup analysis of the Dutch Bone Metastasis Study, an axial cortical involvement of more than 30 mm gave rise to a 25 % chance of fracture during follow-up (van der Linden et al. 2003, 2004a). The treating physician should always weigh the morbidity of a surgical procedure against the beneficial stabilizing capability of prophylactic surgery. If a patient with a high-risk lesion is considered inoperable, local radiotherapy may be given and remineralization will occur, but may take 6–12 weeks for the bone to heal during which time the risk of fracture remains (Koswig and Budach 1999). Currently the use of computer finite element modeling, in place of subjective doctors' opinion based on clinical experience, is being tested in a large set of prospective CT scanning data of patients with femoral bone metastases to study whether accurate prediction of fracture can be improved (Tanck et al. 2009).

Minimally invasive procedures such as vertebroplasty in osteolytic spinal metastases may be considered for the treatment of back pain (Lieberman and Reinhardt 2003; Kallmes and Jensen 2003; Bartels et al. 2008) due to vertebral collapse. Vertebroplasty involves the injection of polymethyl methacrylate into the vertebra to immediately strengthen the affected bone. No prospective studies have been conducted so far to test the effectiveness of vertebroplasty versus radiotherapy for the treatment of pain.

A relatively new treatment for painful bone metastases is radiofrequency ablation (RFA), which utilizes a high-frequency alternating current that is passed from a needle electrode into surrounding tissue, resulting in frictional heating and necrosis. A decrease of pain in 95–100 % of treated patients has been reported with this technique (Goetz et al. 2004; Dupuy et al. 2010). No comparative studies are reported so far comparing this technique with the gold standard of local radiotherapy.

If a patient has diffuse pain arising from numerous metastases, and especially if visceral metastases are present too, a systemic treatment should be considered if available and effective alongside local treatment. This is particularly relevant for patients with breast cancer or prostate cancer in whom there can be a major benefit from these treatments. A variety of effective chemotherapeutic agents, hormonal therapies (Harvey 1997), and radionuclides (Quilty et al. 1994; Falkmer et al. 2003; Sartor et al. 2014) are available. In addition, regular infusions with potent inhibitors of osteoclastic bone resorption such as bisphosphonates or RANKL inhibitors decrease the number of skeletal related events in patients with breast cancer, myeloma, and prostate cancer (Hortobagyi et al. 1996; Rogers et al. 1997; Falkmer et al. 2003; Lipton 2003; Lipton et al. 2016), as well as in patients with lung cancer and other solid tumors (Rosen et al. 2004).

1.2.2 Spinal Cord or Nerve Root Compression Syndromes

Soft tissue extension of tumors in the vertebrae may compress nerve roots or the spinal cord causing neurological symptoms ranging from neuropathic pain and cauda equina syndromes with loss of sphincter control to total paraplegia. Pathological fracture of the vertebrae may result in bone fragments compressing nerve roots or the spinal cord causing the same symptoms. In general, if a patient presents with neurological symptoms, an emergency MRI should be obtained to identify possible spinal cord compression in order to start treatment as soon as possible (Rades et al. 2002; Bartels et al. 2008). The majority of cases arise either due to extradural compression or invasion of the spinal cord by metastases from an adjacent vertebral body. The physiology of the spinal cord and cauda equina damage is thought to relate initially to venous obstruction and edema rather than direct physical pressure causing the initial symptoms. Although a classification system based on clinical symptoms has been proposed to choose the appropriate treatment for each patient presenting with a spinal metastasis (Harrington 1986), there is no broad consensus on the most appropriate treatment or sequence of treatments for patients with spinal metastases. More recently, the Spinal Instability Neoplastic Score as a measure for spinal instability has been recommended to use as a tool to discuss indications for surgery, especially in patients without neurological symptoms (Fisher et al. 2010). Although its predictive power is under debate, the use of SINS helps radiation oncologists and spinal surgeons to discuss the most appropriate treatment options for individual patients.

In general, radiotherapy in combination with high-dose steroids can be effective treatment in spinal cord or nerve root compression syndromes. Decrease of symptoms after radiotherapy doses of 16–24 Gy was reported in 10–90 % of the patients, depending on the severity and duration of the pretreatment neurological symptoms (Maranzano and Latini 1995; Maranzano et al. 1997, 2005, 2009; Roos et al. 2000; Rades et al. 2002; Hoskin et al. 2003). Exceptions are patients with lymphoma or germ cell tumors where primary chemotherapy may be appropriate. A surgical procedure to the spine should be considered if bone fragments endanger the spinal cord, if neurological symptoms do not respond to radiotherapy, or if tolerance doses for the spinal cord with radiotherapy have been reached (Harrington 1986). Several surgical techniques have been developed ranging from minimally invasive methods such as palliative laminectomy to extensive procedures including radical en bloc resection and stabilization. The choice of surgical technique depends on expected survival, treatment-related morbidity, and outcome after treatment. In general, the more extensive the surgical technique, the more prolonged the palliative effect will be, but, also, the greater the treatment-related morbidity for the patient (Harrington 1986). A randomized trial in 101 patients with spinal cord compression studied surgery plus radiotherapy versus radiotherapy alone and showed a significant improvement in mobility for the combination arm (Patchell et al. 2005), predominantly confined to patients younger than 65 years (Chi et al. 2009). There is still debate about these results, however, because the patients were a highly selected group and accrued over a period of 10 years. In contrast a matched pair analysis by Rades et al. in 342 patients showed no significant differences in outcome after surgery plus radiotherapy vs. radiotherapy alone (Rades et al. 2010a). Groups were matched for 11 potential prognostic factors and compared for posttreatment motor function, ambulatory status, regaining ambulatory status, local control, and survival. Further randomized studies are required addressing the relative role of radiotherapy and surgery in metastatic spinal cord compression.

2 Radiotherapy for Pain from Bone Metastases

2.1 Initial Treatment for Pain

Different palliative radiotherapy schedules have been studied in numerous trials, ranging from a single fraction of 4, 6, or 8–20 Gy in 5 fractions, 24 Gy in 6 fractions, 30 Gy in 10 fractions, and even 40 Gy in 20 fractions (Tong et al. 1982; Madsen 1983; Price et al. 1986; Hirokawa et al. 1988; Okawa et al. 1988; Cole 1989; Kagei et al. 1990; Hoskin et al. 1992; Rasmusson et al. 1995; Niewald et al. 1996; Gaze et al. 1997; Jeremic et al. 1998; Nielsen et al. 1998; Koswig and Budach 1999; Steenland et al. 1999; Kirkbride et al. 2000a; Salazar et al. 2001; van der Linden et al. 2004b; Hartsell et al. 2005; Kaasa et al. 2006; Foro et al. 2008; Berg et al. 2009; Hoskin et al. 2015). No clear dose/effect relationship has been seen in any of these trials. Subsequently, three large meta-analyses have confirmed the equal effectiveness of a single-dose schedule compared to more protracted regimens (Wu et al. 2003; Wai Man et al. 2004; Chow et al. 2007a). A single fraction of 8 Gy is therefore considered to be the standard radiotherapy schedule for patients with uncomplicated bone pain, that is, for bone lesions without neurological complaints and without a high risk of pathological fracture (Wu et al. 2003; Wai Man et al. 2004; Chow et al. 2007a, b). In these trials, 3–4 weeks after treatment, 65–72 % of the patients had achieved a response, and in patients with a prolonged survival (>1 year), 80 % achieved durable benefit from single-dose radiotherapy with no advantage to a more protracted regimen (van der Linden et al. 2006). In patients with a survival of less than 12 weeks, a single fraction was effective in up to 50 % of the patients, again with no benefit to a higher total dose (Meeuse et al. 2010). Sixty percent of these poor-prognosis patients had persisting pain scores of five or higher (on a pain score ranging from 0 to 10), underlining the necessity of adequate pain management in these patients in addition to palliative radiotherapy. In a randomized study in 272 patients with neuropathic pain (i.e., the presence of a radiating cutaneous component in the distribution of one or more spinal nerves or peripheral nerves), a single dose was not inferior to 20 Gy in 5 fractions (Roos et al. 2005). Overall response rate and time to failure following a single dose were somewhat poorer (53 vs. 61 %), but the differences were not statistically significant. The authors recommend a single fraction for particular subsets of patients, such as those with a short expected survival. Although in patients with painful spinal metastases some authors advocate that pain is the herald of subsequent neurological symptoms, and therefore a higher initial dose is required, only 3 % of 342 patients with spinal metastases who were irradiated within a randomized prospective trial progressed to a spinal cord compression (van der Linden et al. 2005). A single fraction of 8 Gy is therefore considered a safe and effective dose for pain caused by uncomplicated spinal metastases.

Optimally, the simulation procedure and actual treatment with a single fraction can take place on the same day, a so-called one-stop treatment, which is most favorable for patients who usually have a deteriorating condition and a limited life expectancy. A single fraction diminishes the number of visits to the radiotherapy department and the discomfort caused by positioning on the treatment couch at each treatment session. Few, but mostly self-limiting side effects such as pain flare or nausea are reported in the trials. Some patients (24–44 %) may experience a pain flare shortly after single-dose or short-course radiotherapy (Loblaw et al. 2007; Hird et al. 2009a).

Retrospective studies reported that short courses of oral dexamethasone may prevent such a flare (Chow et al. 2007a, b; Hird et al. 2009b). Recently, Chow et al. reported the results of the first randomized trial on the role of dexamethasone in preventing pain flare (Chow et al. 2015). They found in 298 patients an absolute reduction in pain flare of 9 % (35 % in the placebo group vs. 26 % with 5 doses of 8 mg dexamethasone, $p = 0.05$). The second trial has currently reached its accrual in the Netherlands (Westhoff et al. 2014).

2.2 Response Definitions

Because most of the trials have used different end point definitions making comparison of trial results somewhat difficult, an International Bone Metastasis Consensus Working Party published in 2002 and 2012 a set of end point measurements to promote consistency in future bone metastasis trials (Chow et al. 2002, 2012). They recommended that response should be based on patient self-assessments of pain using a numerical rating score from 0 (= no pain) to 10 (= worst imaginable pain). Pain should be measured using a multidimensional pain questionnaire such as the Brief Pain Inventory (BPI), which also notes pain medication as well as quality of life issues. Frequent assessments, preferably weekly, are necessary to obtain usable data. Any changes in pain medication during follow-up should be accounted for in the response calculations to show the true effectiveness of radiotherapy:

- Response to treatment is calculated taking into account pain score and changes in the administration of opioids. A change from level 1 or 2 to level 3 analgesia is noted as an analgesic increase. If the patient has stopped using level 3 analgesics, this is noted as an analgesic decrease.
- Partial response (PR) is defined as (1) a decrease in the initial pain score by at least two points on the 11-point pain scale, without analgesic increase, or (2) analgesic decrease without an increase in pain.
- Complete response (CR) is defined as a decrease in the initial pain score to zero on the pain scale, without concomitant analgesic increase. When pain scores remain unaltered or when they increase, the patient is considered to be a nonresponder (NR).
- Progression after response is defined as (a) an increase in pain with return to the initial pain score or higher, without analgesic increase, or (b) analgesic increase irrespective of the pain score.

Response percentages should be calculated at 1, 2, and 3 months and noted with and without the effect of any possible retreatment during follow-up. In a validation study by Li et al., responses at 2 months seemed most appropriate because maximum pain relief is seen even after 4 weeks in some patients, and because at 3 months, patients may already have dropped out due to deteriorating condition or death (Li et al. 2008). In addition, response occurring after 3 months may reflect secondary interventions. With these straightforward end point definitions, the radiotherapy community as a whole has a powerful tool that enables it to work together at an international level and guide research toward improving optimal treatment.

In daily radiotherapy practice, patients should be asked to give repeat pain scores using the same multidimensional pain questionnaire as mentioned in the consensus manuscript. The patient should be asked whether the pain is present only when active or even at rest and also whether the pain is bothersome. In studies, reported pain severity cutoff points on the 11-point pain scale from 0 to 10 are 1–4 for mild pain, 5–6 for moderate pain, and 7–10 for severe pain (Li et al. 2007). Based on interference with functioning and quality of life, a recent paper suggests to adapt 1–4 for mild pain, 5–7 for moderate pain, and 8–10 for severe pain (Chow et al. 2016). A pain score above four or five is generally considered a threshold for active pain management. Meaningful changes in pain score have been studied from the patient's perspective. Patients perceived an improvement in their pain when their self-reported pain score decreased by at least two points, regardless of the initial height of the pain (Chow et al. 2005). Another way of measuring response is by reporting the duration of response, as a meaningful way to express durability of the treatment effect. Mean duration of response in the Dutch Bone Metastasis Trial was 24 weeks for patients with breast cancer, 18 weeks in patients with prostate cancer, and 11 weeks in patients with lung cancer or other types of cancer (van der Linden et al. 2004a, b). Another way of reporting duration of response is by calculating the Net Pain Relief (NPR), i.e., the time (in weeks) of pain response divided by the remaining lifetime (in weeks) (Ratanatharathorn et al. 1999). The NPR is not frequently used in the literature to evaluate effectiveness of palliative radiotherapy, but is a useful tool in more objectively addressing response duration. In order to calculate NPR, adequate follow-up is needed, with continuing pain score measurements even after a response has been reached. In one study which has used this approach in 160 patients receiving 8 Gy single fraction or 30 Gy in 10 fractions, no differences in NPR were observed: 68 % to SF vs. 71 % to MF (Foro et al. 2008).

2.3 Retreatment for Pain

There are three clinical situations where retreatment for pain caused by bone metastases may be considered:

1. Patients who experience no pain relief or even pain progression after initial radiotherapy
2. Patients who have a partial response with initial radiotherapy and hope to achieve further pain reduction with more radiotherapy
3. Patients with a partial or complete response with initial radiotherapy but subsequent recurrence of pain during follow-up

In the Dutch trial, almost 50 % of the patients who responded reported progressive pain, that is, pain intensity returning to the original pain score at baseline (van der Linden et al. 2004a, b). Most published trials have reported progression rates of between 28 and 61 % in patients who responded to initial radiotherapy (Ratanatharathorn et al. 1999). It is these patients who are most likely to benefit from a retreatment (Figs. 1a, b and 2). Because the response to initial treatment takes about 3–4 weeks to occur, it is recommended to consider reirradiation after a minimum interval of 4 weeks (Chow et al. 2002).

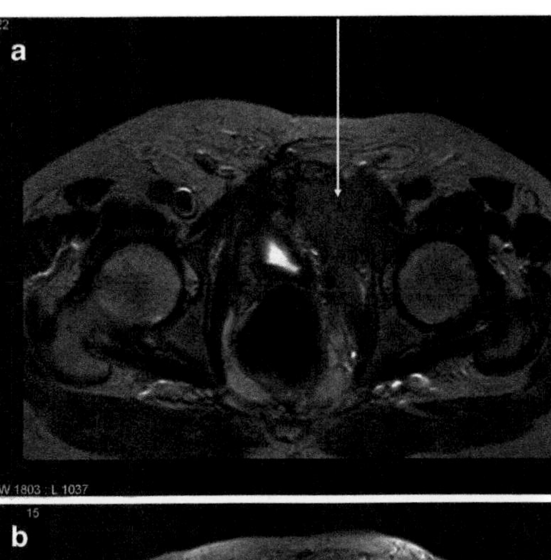

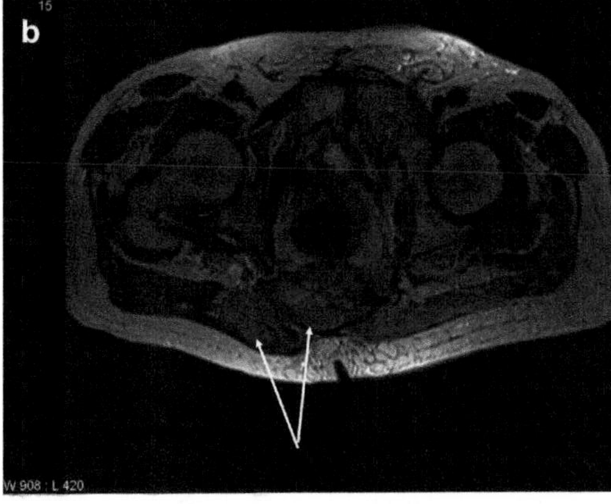

Fig. 1 (**a**, **b**) Magnetic resonance imaging (MRI) scans at initial presentation with skeletal metastases from prostate cancer in a 66-year-old man, previously treated with radical prostatectomy (**a**). The white arrow indicates a large, painful pubic bone metastasis. Due to public holidays in December 2008, treatment with a standard regimen of 30 Gy in 10 fractions was difficult to organize. Therefore, the patient was irradiated with 7 fractions of 4 Gy. Complete pain relief was obtained. In March 2010, increasing pain in the irradiated region and the lower back resulted in repeat MRI. A large new metastasis in the sacral bone with considerable soft tissue extension was found (**b**, *white arrow*). Taking into account performance status (ECOG 1) and life expectancy (more than 6 months), the patient was treated with two conventionally simulated fields encompassing both the previously irradiated and the new lesion (30 Gy in 10 fractions). Excellent pain response was obtained again

2.3.1 Retreatment Rates in Randomized Trials

Among the randomized trials comparing single versus multiple fractions for painful bone metastases, retreatment rates were consistently higher after the single-dose schedules. Percentages

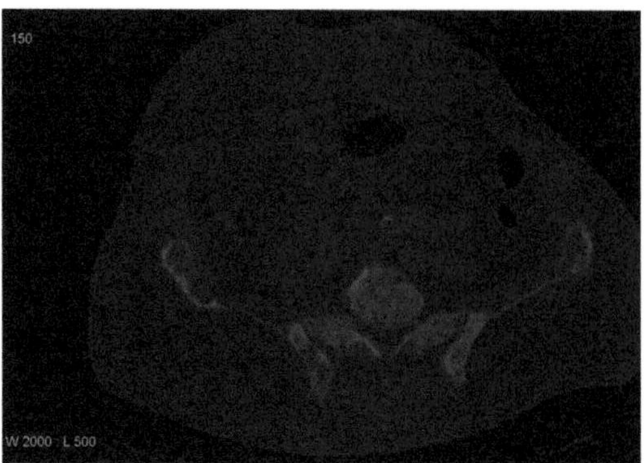

Fig. 2 Computed tomography scans in a 76-year-old man with known metastatic prostate cancer, treated with endocrine therapy and zoledronic acid. In November 2009, the disease was considered castration resistant. Palliative radiotherapy (8 Gy single fraction) was administered to the sacroiliac joints and os sacrum. Complete pain response was achieved. Chemotherapy was initiated, but later discontinued when disease progression occurred in June 2010. The patient was referred for local reirradiation to the same painful region. He received another single fraction (8 Gy) with complete response

varied from 11 to 42 % after a single fraction to 0–24 % after multiple fractions (Table 1). It has been proposed that because of the higher necessity for retreatment, the single-fraction regimen was not as effective as more protracted regimens when looking at durability of response. On the other hand, the retreatment percentages in the trials were most likely biased, since retreatment was done at the discretion of the treating radiation oncologists and patients, neither of whom were blinded to the initial treatment. Disbelief in the effectiveness of a single fraction, or the awareness that still more radiation was possible, may contribute to these percentages. The study protocols did not prescribe a minimum time interval between initial and retreatment, or a minimum pain score requirement, and the dose for retreatment was also not defined. In addition many patients with recurrent pain or poor response to initial radiation may have been lost to follow-up or may not be referred back to their

Table 1 Retreatment percentages in randomized trials on dose fractionation schedules for bone metastases

	Publication year	Number of randomized patients	Randomization arms	Retreatment (%)		*p*-value
				Low dose	High dose	
Trials comparing single-fraction versus multiple-fraction regimens						
RTOG	2005	898	8 Gy vs. 30 Gy/10#	18 %	9 %	<0.001
Foro Arnolot	2008	160	8 Gy vs. 30 Gy/10#	28 %	2 %	[a]
Kaasa	2006	376	8 Gy vs. 30 Gy/10#	27 %	9 %	0.002
BPTWP	1999	761	8 Gy vs. 20 Gy/5#	23 %	10 %	<0.001
DBMS	1999	1157	8 Gy vs. 24 Gy/6#	24 %	7 %	<0.001
Nielsen	1998	241	8 Gy vs. 20 Gy/5#	20 %	2 %	[a]
Cole	1989	29	8 Gy vs. 24 Gy/6#	25 %	0 %	[a]
Price	1986	288	8 Gy vs. 30 Gy/10#	11 %	3 %	[a]
Trials comparing different single-fraction regimens						
Jeremic	1998	327	4 Gy vs. 6 Gy vs. 8 Gy	42 %	38 %	NS
Hoskin	1992	270	4 Gy vs. 8 Gy	20 %	9 %	[a]
Trials comparing different multiple-fraction regimens						
Niewald	1996	100	20 Gy/5# vs. 30 Gy/15#	2 %	2 %	NS
Tong	1982	750	Single metastases 20 Gy/5# vs. 40 Gy/15# Multiple metastases 15 Gy/5# vs. 20 y/5# vs. 30 Gy/10#	24 % 23 %	11 % 12 %	[a]

[a]Not stated
NS not significant

radiation oncologist for consideration of retreatment. A reanalysis of the original database of the Dutch trial was completed using the consensus criteria for response with a closer look at specific reasons to retreat (Chow et al. 2002; van der Linden et al. 2004a, b). After 8 Gy single fraction, 24 % of the patients were retreated versus only 6 % after 24 Gy in six fractions ($p<0.001$). Response to initial treatment without the effect of retreatment was 71 % after SF vs. 73 % after MF ($p=0.84$). Retreatment raised the response rate to 75 % for SF; MF response rates remained unaltered ($p=0.54$). The response status after initial treatment did not predict for retreatment: 35 % SF vs. 8 % MF nonresponders, and 22 % SF vs. 10 % MF patients with progressive pain were retreated. After progressive pain was observed, mean time to retreatment was 7 weeks in SF patients versus 10 weeks in MF patients. The preceding mean pain score was 7.5 in SF patients and 7.8 in MF patients. In conclusion, it appeared that physicians were more reluctant to retreat initial MF patients than initial SF patients.

2.3.2 Effectiveness

Until 2014, responses to retreatment have been reported only in retrospective and nonrandomized prospective studies. Price et al. reported on seven patients who, after failure to respond to the initial single 4 Gy fraction, were given a second radiotherapy within 8 weeks (Price et al. 1986). Four of them received a single 8 Gy and the other three a fractionated course with a higher total dose. No significant pain relief was achieved by the second radiotherapy treatment in any of these seven patients (Price et al. 1988). Cole reported in 42 patients that retreatment of patients after initial single- or multiple-fraction treatment was not successful in most patients, and 50 % needed supplementary stronger analgesics (Cole 1989). Hoskin et al. randomized patients in a prospective study to either 4 or 8 Gy single dose for the initial treatment of metastatic bone pain. During the 12-week study period, 28 patients randomized to 4 Gy were retreated with radiotherapy to the same site compared to 12 randomized to 8 Gy. 12/17 (71 %) evaluable patients responded to retreatment in the 4 Gy arm and 4/9 (44 %) responded in the 8 Gy arm (Hoskin et al. 1992). Uppelschoten et al. reported that after long intervals from initial single 6 Gy of radiation, retreatment with another 6 Gy was able to reduce pain in 13 out of 18 patients (72 %) (Uppelschoten et al. 1995). Mithal et al. published a retrospective analysis of 105 consecutive patients treated with palliative radiotherapy for painful bone metastases. A total of 280 individual treatment sites were identified, of which 57 were retreated once and eight were retreated twice. The overall response rate to initial treatment was 84 % for pain relief, and to retreatment the response rate was 87 %. 7/8 (88 %) patients retreated for a second time also achieved pain relief. No relation to radiation dose, primary tumor type, or site was observed (Mithal et al. 1994). Jeremic et al. investigated the effectiveness of a single fraction of 4 Gy given for retreatment of bone metastasis after initial single-fraction radiotherapy. Of 135 patients retreated, 109 patients were retreated because of pain relapsing, and 80 (74 %) patients responded (complete response (CR)=31 %, partial response (PR)=42 %). Among the 26 patients that initially did not respond, 46 % responded. The authors concluded that the lack of response to an initial single fraction should not deter repeat irradiation. The same group also reported the efficacy of a second single 4 Gy retreatment for painful bone metastases following two previous single fractions. The overall response rate of 25 patients (19 responders and six nonresponders) was 80 %, with both complete response and partial response being 40 % (Jeremic et al. 2002). In Radiation Therapy Oncology Group (RTOG) studies that involved wide-field or hemibody radiotherapy, patients who relapsed after wide-field irradiation were reported to tolerate local irradiation within that field with success (Quasim 1981; Salazar et al. 1986). Van der Linden et al. studied 173 patients who were retreated within the randomized Dutch Bone Metastasis Study ($n=1157$) (van der Linden et al. 2004a, b). In 137 retreated SF patients, 33 % received a second SF and 67 % received MFs. In 36 retreated initial MF patients, 25 % received second MF and 75 % received a SF. To evaluate whether response to initial treatment influenced the choice for the second treatment schedule, the response status before retreatment was studied. There was no correlation between the initial response status and the retreatment schedule. In total, 63 % of retreated patients responded to retreatment: 66 % of retreated SF patients responded compared with 46 % of MF patients ($p=0.12$, HR 1.6 (0.9–3.0)). After retreatment, time to response was not different for initial SF and MF patients, but the mean duration of remission was substantially longer in initial SF patients, 16 weeks vs. only 8 weeks in initial MF patients. For SF patients, response to retreatment was irrespective of the initial response: 66 %, 67 %, and 70 % of initial nonresponders, responders, and progressive patients, respectively, responded to retreatment. Although more initial SF than MF nonresponding patients responded to retreatment, due to small numbers, this difference was not significant (66 vs. 33 %, respectively, $p=0.13$, HR 3.0 (0.7–12.7)). Of nonresponders to an initial SF, 88 % responded to a second SF and 53 % to MF. Of the latter, 10 % of responses were due to a decrease in analgesic intake. Overall, no major differences in mean time to response after retreatment were reported. Mean duration of remission ranged from 4 weeks in initial MF nonresponders to 25 weeks in initial SF nonresponders. Patients with prostate cancer had the lowest success rate: 20 % of initial nonresponding patients responded, and only 19 % of patients with progression responded again. Patients with breast cancer had the highest response percentages for nonresponders and progressive patients (82 % and 89 %, respectively). Mean duration of remission was longest in initial nonresponding breast cancer patients (23 weeks). Van Helvoirt et al. actively contacted 298 consecutive patients 4 weeks after initial single-fraction therapy to evaluate response and, if necessary, to offer retreatment (van Helvoirt and Bratelli 2008). Seventy-five percent of the patients were satisfied with their pain response, and 75 % of the non-satisfied patients requested retreatment. Of these, 87 % responded after a second single fraction. In 37 patients with recurrent pain, 83 % responded to a second single fraction. In 2012, Huisman et al. performed a systematic review on ten articles and a meta-analysis on seven (Huisman et al. 2012). Of the 2,694 patients initially treated for metastatic bone pain, 527 (20 %) patients underwent reirradiation. Overall, a pain response after reirradiation was achieved in 58 % of patients (pooled overall response rate 0.58, 95 % confidence interval = 0.49–0.67). There was a substantial between-study heterogeneity ($I^2=63.3$ %, $p=0.01$) because of clinical and methodological differences between studies. In 2014, the results from the international randomized trial on retreatment in painful bone metastases were published (Chow et al. 2014a, b). A total of 850 patients were randomized between a single fraction of 8 or 20 Gy in 5 fractions for retreatment. In the intention-to-treat population, 118 (28 %) patients allocated to 8 Gy and 135 (32 %) allocated to 20 Gy had an overall pain response to treatment ($p=0.21$, response difference of 4·00 % [upper limit of the 95 % CI 9·2, less than the prespecified non-inferiority margin of 10 %]). In the per-protocol population, 116 (45 %) of 258 patients and 134 (51 %) of 263 patients, respectively, had an overall pain response to treatment ($p=0.17$, response difference 6·00 % [upper limit of the 95 % CI 13·2, greater than the prespecified non-inferiority margin of 10 %]). They concluded that for retreatment, 8 Gy in a single fraction seemed to be non-inferior and less toxic than 20 Gy in multiple fractions.

In patients with longer life expectancies, a second or even third retreatment may be considered if earlier radiotherapy treatments have given satisfactory pain responses. Cumulative total doses should be calculated taking into account nearness of critical radiosensitive organs, such as the spinal cord, kidney, bowel, or skin. No clear-cut answer is yet available to guide which dose schedules should be used for a first retreatment, second retreatment, or even third retreatment.

3 Radiotherapy for Bone Metastases: Spinal Cord Compression (SCC)

3.1 Initial Treatment for Spinal Cord Compression

There is no standard fractionation schedule for the treatment of spinal cord compression. Rades et al. have published several papers based on a large retrospective database (Rades et al. 2002, Rades et al. 2005a, 2006, 2008a, b, 2009, 2010a, b, c).

In general, radiotherapy is most effective in improving motor function when neurological complaints have developed over a longer period of time (>14 days), in patients with a longer interval from primary diagnosis to SCC, who are ambulatory before radiotherapy, with a good performance status, or with favorable histologies like myeloma and lymphoma (Rades et al. 2005a). In their series they showed that both short-course (single fraction of 8 or 20 Gy in 5 fractions) and long-course treatments (30–40 Gy in 10–20 fractions) resulted in the same functional outcome in patients with breast cancer ($n=335$), prostate cancer ($n=281$), non-small cell lung cancer ($n=252$), or renal cell carcinoma ($n=87$). An exception was the treatment of myeloma patients ($n=172$). Functionally, they fared better with long-course radiotherapy with improvements of motor function reported at 12 months in 74 versus 40 % after short-course radiotherapy ($p=0.003$) (Rades et al. 2006).

In addition to functional outcome, however, significantly more in-field recurrences appeared after short-course radiotherapy than after long-course schedules (at 1 year, 18 vs. 5 % recurrence, $p<0.001$) (Rades et al. 2005a, b). This effect was most prevalent in patients with breast cancer (1-year local control 96 % after long course vs. 84 % after short course) and prostate cancer (94 vs. 77 %). If patients have an expected good prognosis, a long-course schedule should therefore be considered.

Three randomized trials have been published on the relative effectiveness of different schedules for SCC in patients with a life expectancy of less than 6 months. The first compared in 276 patients 16 Gy in 2 fractions with a split-course treatment of 15 Gy in 3 fractions followed after an interval by 15 Gy in 5 fractions (Maranzano et al. 2005). After treatment, 68 and 71 % were able to walk with no difference between both arms. Median survival was 4 months and median duration of improvement was 3.5 months for both arms. In the second trial by the same group, 303 patients were randomized between 16 Gy in 2 fractions and a single fraction of 8 Gy (Maranzano et al. 2009). No difference in response was found between the two RT schedules adopted. Median duration of response was 5 and 4.5 months for short-course and single-dose RT ($p=0.4$), respectively. The median overall survival was 4 months for all cases. The more recent randomized SCORE 2 trial has shown that 20 Gy in 5 fractions is equivalent to 30 Gy in 10 fractions for patients with intermediate and poor life expectancy using motor function and ambulatory status as end points (Rades et al. 2016). Currently in the UK, the randomized SCORAD trial is studying the effectiveness of 8 Gy single fraction versus 20 Gy in 5 fractions in patients with spinal cord compression and a minimum life expectancy of 2 months.

In order to make an appropriate decision for treatment in individual patients with SCC, a number of scoring systems can be used, all based upon prognostic factors for survival and outcome (Chow et al. 2006; Rades et al. 2008a, b). Important prognostic factors are the performance status of the patient, the number of spinal metastases, the presence of visceral metastases, and the type of primary tumor.

In conclusion, based on the available literature, the common practice in most Western countries is to deliver 20 Gy in 5 fractions in patients with a minimum life expectancy of 3 months or 30 Gy in 10 fractions in patients with a more prolonged life expectancy (minimum 1 year). A shorter schedule of 1 or 2 × 8 Gy is perhaps the optimal schedule in patients with a prognosis less than 3 months.

Oral dexamethasone is usually combined with radiotherapy to diminish any surrounding edema and should be started as soon as possible, preferably before the first radiation fraction can be delivered. The appropriate dose of dexamethasone is still a matter of debate. High doses of dexamethasone (96–100 mg/day) seem more effective than low-dose dexamethasone (10–16 mg/day), but are associated with significantly more serious adverse effects (Vecht et al. 1989; Heimdal et al. 1992; Sorensen et al. 1994). Moderate doses of dexamethasone (16–32 mg/day) have proven to be effective and safe and are therefore advocated. If the neurological situation improves after palliative radiotherapy, a reducing schedule of dexamethasone should be started. If the neurological situation deteriorates despite adequate doses of dexamethasone and radiotherapy, and no surgical intervention is possible, or if paraplegia persists, a reduction schedule should be started to prevent disabling side effects from long-term use of high-dose steroids.

3.2 Retreatment for Spinal Cord Compression

Responses to retreatment in patients with spinal cord compression have been reported so far only in retrospective studies (Rades et al. 2005b, 2008c). Outcome after retreatment with 1 xx 8 Gy ($n=48$), 5 × 3 Gy ($n=29$), 5 × 4 Gy ($n=30$), 7 × 3 Gy ($n=3$), 10–12 × 2 Gy ($n=11$), or 17 × 1.8 Gy ($n=3$) was published in a series of 124 patients. Cumulative biologically effective dose (BED) (first course of RT plus re-RT) ranged from 77.5–142.6 Gy2 and was ≤120 Gy2 in 114 (92 %) patients. Motor function improved in 45 (36 %) patients, was stable in another 62 (50 %) patients, and deteriorated in 17 (14 %) patients, with no difference between the radiation doses. Multivariate analysis found the effect of retreatment on motor function was significantly associated with the response to the first course of radiotherapy ($p=0.048$), performance status ($p=0.020$), time to development of motor deficits before retreatment ($p=0.002$), and visceral metastases ($p<0.001$). Within the limitations of these retrospective study and the relatively short follow-up after retreatment, spinal retreatment appeared to be effective and safe when the cumulative BED was ≤120 Gy2.

4 Toxicity

4.1 Acute and Late Toxicity

If repeated radiotherapy for bone metastases is considered, toxicity will depend on the previously applied dose, time between initial and second treatment, and localization within the body in relation to sensitive organs in the vicinity. Toxicity in the study by Jeremic et al. using 4 Gy as retreatment dose was low and only gastrointestinal (Jeremic et al. 1999). Grade 1 or 2 diarrhea (RTOG acute toxicity criteria) was observed in 25/135 (19 %) patients. No acute toxicity > grade 3 was reported. Pathological fractures were reported in 3/135 (2 %) patients and spinal cord compression in 3/135 (2 %) patients in their series. In 25 patients retreated with a second retreatment dose of 4 Gy from the same group, no acute or late high-grade toxicity (>3) was observed (Jeremic et al. 2002). No pathological fractures or spinal cord compression were seen in any of these patients during the follow-up. Within the Dutch Bone Metastasis Study, toxicity 1 month after retreatment was scored in approximately 73 % of the 173 retreated patients (van der Linden et al. 2004a, b). No major differences in nausea, vomiting, itching, painful skin, or tiredness were reported between initial SF or MF patients. Most SF and MF patients reported none or only mild nausea and vomiting. Nausea score 4 (very bad) was reported in 12 % of MF patients vs. 6 % of SF patients ($p=0.39$). Vomiting score 4 (very bad) was reported in one MF patient and two SF patients ($p=0.49$). Significant skin reaction defined by itching score 4 (very bad) was seen in two SF patients. One SF patient reported a painful skin score 4 (very bad). Severe tiredness was reported in 18 % of SF patients and 27 % of MF patients ($p=0.41$). After retreatment in the study by Rades et al. in 124 patients with SCC, acute toxicity was mild, and late toxicity, such as radiation myelopathy, was not observed (Rades et al. 2008c).

4.2 Risk of Myelopathy

Radiation-induced myelopathy is a late complication after radiotherapy and can occur months to years after treatment. The exact pathogenesis of myelopathy remains obscure. Although significant recovery of the spinal cord after elective small doses is possible (Ang et al. 2001; Kirkpatrick et al. 2010), when applying higher radiotherapy doses, larger doses per fraction, and when previous exposure to radiation is the case, a higher probability of developing radiation-induced myelopathy will be present. Experimental data indicate that the total dose of the first and second radiotherapy, interval to retreatment, length of the irradiated spinal cord, and age of the treated animals influence the risk of radiation-induced myelopathy. An experimental study based upon the available literature concluded that the (extrapolated) probability of myelopathy at 45 Gy is 0.03 % and at 50 Gy, 0.2 % (Schultheiss 2008). The dose for a 5 % myelopathy rate is 59.3 Gy. Graphical analysis indicates that the sensitivity of the thoracic cord is less than that of the cervical cord.

There is extensive literature on the use of single fractions of 8 or 10 Gy for uncomplicated spinal metastases, none of which has identified a detectable risk of myelopathy. A retrospective analysis of 465 patients treated for spinal cord compression identified only one possible case of myelopathy in a patient receiving 16 Gy in 2 fractions, becoming symptomatic 19 months after initial presentation (Maranzano et al. 2001). In addition the estimated risk of radiation myelopathy from palliative radiotherapy for non-small cell lung cancer was calculated using over 1000 patients taking part in a series of Medical Research Council (MRC) trials (Macbeth et al. 1996). These patients will have had similar doses of radiotherapy to the spinal cord. Only five patients were reported as having radiation myelopathy, two who had received 17 Gy in 2 fractions and three who had 39 Gy in 13 fractions; there were no cases in patients who received a single fraction of 10 Gy. The overall cumulative risk was estimated as 0.8 % at 1 year and 1.5 % at 2 years. The risk of radiation myelopathy therefore appears negligible after a single fraction. Nieder et al. studied the cumulative doses in 78 patients (Nieder et al. 2005, 2006). On the basis of the literature data included in their analysis, the risk of myelopathy appeared small after a cumulative biologically equivalent dose of 135.5 Gy2 when the interval was not shorter than 6 months and the dose of each course was <98 Gy2. In more detail, risk points were given to cumulative BED (0=<120 Gy2, 1=120–130 Gy2, 2=130–140 Gy2, 3=140–150 Gy2, 4=150–160 Gy2, 5=160–170 Gy2, 6=170–180 Gy2, 7=180–190 Gy2, 8=190–200 Gy2, 9=>200 Gy2), highest BED of all treatment series in a particular individual (if one course>= 102 Gy2=4.5 points), and interval between initial and second treatment (if <6 months, 4.5 points). In low-risk patients (≤3 points), chance of radiation-induced myelopathy was 3 %, in intermediate-risk patients (4–6 points) 25 %, and in high-risk patients (>6 points) even 90 %. Stereotactic body radiotherapy (SBRT) in spinal metastases, if given at least 5 months after conventional palliative radiotherapy with a reirradiation thecal sac maximum dose of 20–25 Gy2, appears to be safe provided the total maximum dose does not exceed approximately 70 Gy2, and the SBRT thecal sac maximum dose comprises no more than approximately 50 % of the total dose in Gy2 (Sahgal et al. 2012).

5 Radiotherapy Techniques

5.1 Dose Planning, Patient Positioning Verification

At the simulation procedure, usually, there is no need of fixation of the affected limb or, in case of spinal metastases, the torso of the patient. For lesions in the skull or head and neck, a mask can be made. Preferably, a computed tomography (CT) scan is used to optimally review the area at which the patient points out the origin of the pain (Haddad et al. 2006). Markers can be placed on the skin. Then, the painful area of the patient is scanned widely. Ideally, patients can wait after the simulation procedure for a short while and receive the radiotherapy treatment at the same visit, a so-called one-stop treatment. For bone metastases in long bones, where no vital organs are in the way, usually a straightforward planning technique using two parallel-opposed fields is used, and optimal target coverage is readily achieved. For metastases in the spine, especially in lower thoracic and lumbar vertebra with bowel, stomach, and/or kidneys in the proximity of the painful vertebra, there is an increased risk of toxicity when these organs at risk receive a large dose of radiation, especially in single-dose regimens. Most vertebrae lie virtually in the midbody, and therefore, the radiotherapeutic option with the most optimal dose coverage is a two-field parallel-opposed technique (Barton et al. 2002). Unfortunately, with this approach a large dose is applied to the ventral lying organs at risk, and a single posterior field may therefore be preferred prescribed at a dose depth to cover the vertebral body with the 80 % isodose at the ventral side of the vertebra. Six to ten MV beams should be used to reduce the area of high dose in the subcutaneous tissues dorsally and/or bowel ventrally. When large fields are used for extensive lesions in the bone, prophylactic antiemetic drugs and steroids should be given 15–30 min before treatment to prevent toxicity (Sykes et al. 1997; Kirkbride et al. 2000b).

If the patient has considerable pain which interferes with achieving comfortable supine position on the treatment couch, it is possible that the position of the patient will shift during treatment delivery resulting in a geographical miss; to avoid this, the treatment fields should not be too small and should have adequate margin. Optimally, online patient positioning verification is used, using either megavoltage images (MVIs) with an electronic portal imaging device and a matching procedure or, if present, cone beam CT (Letourneau et al. 2007; Haas et al. 2013). If an online imaging protocol is not available, then, at least, off-line MVIs should be taken, to check whether the target bone has been irradiated as planned. If pain does not respond, the doctors must be able to verify that initial treatment has been given accurately.

5.2 IMRT, Stereotactic Radiotherapy, and VMAT

Retrospective publications have reported on the effectiveness of newer, sophisticated radiation techniques in spinal metastases, with about 85 % relief of pain reported using intensity-modulated radiotherapy (IMRT), stereotactic radiotherapy, or volumetric-modulated arc radiotherapy (VMAT) (Ryu et al. 2003; Chang et al. 2007; Gerszten et al. 2007; Gibbs et al. 2007; Jin et al. 2007; Mancosu et al. 2010). These techniques make it possible to deliver higher radiation doses safely; however, they require a high standard of precision in targeting the beam to the tumor shape and exact location (Fig. 3). Therefore, these techniques are highly time-consuming and costly when compared with conventional radiotherapy. The most important potential value of these techniques when treating bone metastases is in enabling irradiation of the spine without

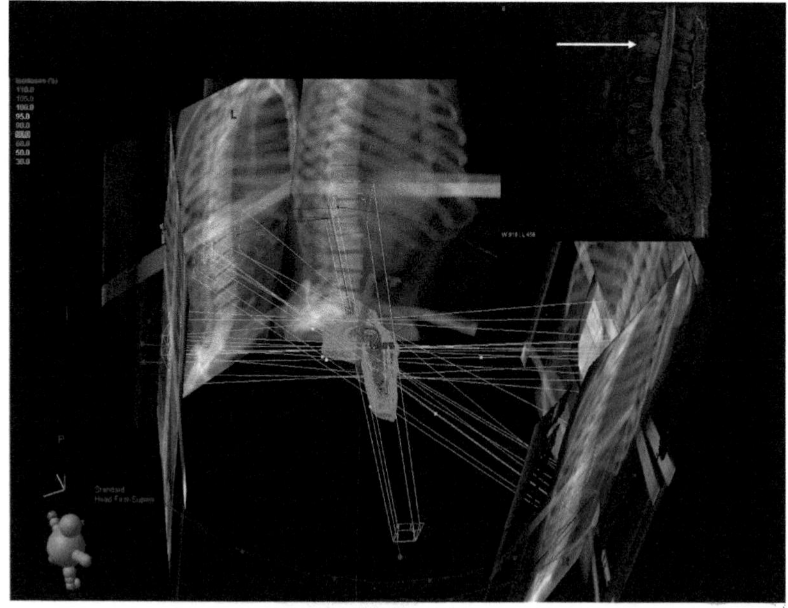

Fig. 3 Reirradiation of vertebral body metastasis (*white arrow*, upper right corner) might require advanced planning and high-precision delivery techniques such as stereotactic and intensity-modulated radiotherapy with image guidance, resulting in steep dose gradients if the dose to the spinal cord is to be kept within safe limits

treating the spinal cord, which is often the major limiting factor for high-dose radiation because of its intrinsic radiosensitivity (Ryu et al. 2007; Mancosu et al. 2010). After maximum spinal radiation tolerance has been reached, complications such as radiation-induced spinal cord injury may occur. These advanced techniques provide the possibility to reirradiate the spine in already heavily pretreated patients. In addition, smaller radiation fields may be used focusing on the affected bone alone. In the study by Jin and colleagues, 270 lesions in 196 patients were treated. The preliminary results of 49 patients were reported (Jin et al. 2007). The single doses were increased with increasing experience from 10 to 16 Gy. The average treatment duration, including setup, position localization and verification, and radiation delivery, was 50 min. Although pain relief was achieved in 85 % of the patients, functional outcome was not reported. Dose-related spinal cord complications were presented in another publication by the same group (Ryu et al. 2007). Two hundred and thirty radiosurgically treated lesions in 177 patients were included with up to three circumscriptive lesions (up to two adjacent vertebrae) treated. The median survival was 4.2 months. In this series, patients received a single fraction ranging from 8 to 18 Gy per lesion. Only one instance (0.4 %) of a dose-related myelopathy occurred in a patient who received 16 Gy.

In a cohort of 500 histologically proven metastases to the spine in 344 patients undergoing spinal radiosurgery, 86 % of the patients had long-term improvement of pain (Gerszten et al. 2007). Median follow-up was 21 months (range 3–53 months). Radiation-induced spinal cord injury did not occur. About 70 % of the patients had received conventional radiotherapy at the involved level before radiosurgery. Although patients with a neurologic deficit were excluded from treatment, as were those with overt spinal instability, in 35 cases, progressive neurologic deficit was reported before the start of the treatment. Of these, 85 % experienced some improvement. The average duration of the treatment (including setup, position localization and verification, and radiation delivery) was 90 min. In another prospective cohort of 74 patients harboring 102 metastatic lesions, 83.9 % of the patients reported relief or improvement of the symptoms (pain and neurologic deficit) (Gibbs et al. 2007). Only patients who did not present with paralysis, spinal instability, or lesions extending more than two adjacent vertebral segments were treated radiosurgically. A detailed analysis was not provided, but three patients (4 %) were mentioned who developed symptoms due to a radiation-induced myelopathy. In a dose planning study, VMAT technology was used to demonstrate optimal target coverage while avoiding damage to the adjacent spinal cord in ten hypothetical cases of patients with spinal metastases (Mancosu et al. 2010).

Although not proven in a randomized trial, these studies suggest that IMRT, stereotactic radiotherapy, and VMAT are effective treatment options for selected patients with spinal metastases. Two randomized studies on SBRT are currently accruing patients, RTOG 0631 (Ryu et al. 2014) and the Dutch RACOST study. The theoretical advantages are obvious, and the clinical results are promising, but it should be emphasized that worldwide, conventional external beam radiotherapy is still the gold standard for spinal metastases. Availability and costs prohibit widespread use of advanced techniques for these palliative indications. Further long-term studies and cost-effectiveness studies are needed before widespread use of advanced-technique treatments can be justified (Bhattacharya and Hoskin 2015).

6 Remarks

Bone metastases are very common in patients with disseminated cancer. Although, in general, small lesions give few symptoms and large lesions may cause severe problems, there is no consistent correlation between size of the metastasis and severity of the symptoms. It is therefore important to monitor patients carefully and choose diagnostic imaging tools and subsequent treatments individualized for each patient. In addition, patients and their relatives should be informed of the symptoms of bone metastases and the possibilities of local treatment which can be repeated. During their illness, many patients receive one or more different treatments, sometimes concomitantly or consecutively. Ideally, the treating physicians and healthcare workers will cooperate in a multidisciplinary setting and discuss the best choice of treatment for each patient, taking into account life expectancy and expected outcome after any palliative treatment. Radiotherapy for symptomatic bone metastases is a valuable treatment option for the palliation of cancer patients and, where indicated, retreatment is possible and effective.

References

Ang KK, Jiang GL, Feng Y, Stephens LC, Tucker SL, Price RE (2001) Extent and kinetics of recovery of occult spinal cord injury. Int J Radiat Oncol Biol Phys 50:1013–1020

Bartels RH, van der Linden YM, van der Graaf WT (2008) Spinal extradural metastasis: review of current treatment options. CA Cancer J Clin 58:245–259

Barton R, Robinson G, Gutierrez E, Kirkbride P, McLean M (2002) Palliative radiation for vertebral metastases: the effect of variation in prescription parameters on the dose received at depth. Int J Radiat Oncol Biol Phys 52:1083–1091

Berg RS, Yilmaz MK, Hoyer M, Keldsen N, Nielsen OS, Ewertz M (2009) Half body irradiation of patients with multiple bone metastases: a phase II trial. Acta Oncol 48:556–561

Bhattacharya IS, Hoskin PJ (2015) Stereotactic body radiotherapy for spinal and bone metastases. Clin Oncol (R Coll Radiol) 27:298–306

Bone Pain Trial Working Party (1999) 8 Gy single fraction radiotherapy for the treatment of metastatic skeletal pain: randomised comparison with a multifraction schedule over 12 months of patient follow-up. Radiother Oncol 52(2):111–121

Chang EL, Shiu AS, Mendel E, Mathews LA, Mahajan A, Allen PK et al (2007) Phase I/II study of stereotactic body radiotherapy for spinal metastasis and its pattern of failure. J Neurosurg Spine 7:151–160

Chi JH, Gokaslan Z, McCormick P, Tibbs PA, Kryscio RJ, Patchell RA (2009) Selecting treatment for patients with malignant epidural spinal cord compression-does age matter? Results from a randomized clinical trial. Spine (Phila Pa 1976) 34:431–435

Chow E, Wu J, Hoskin P, Coia L, Bentzen S, Blitzer P (2002) International consensus on palliative radiotherapy endpoints for future clinical trials in bone metastases. Radiother Oncol 64:275–280

Chow E, Ling A, Davis L, Panzarella T, Danjoux C (2005) Pain flare following external beam radiotherapy and meaningful change in pain scores in the treatment of bone metastases. Radiother Oncol 75:64–69

Chow E, Harris K, Fung K (2006) Successful validation of a survival prediction model in patients with metastases in the spinal column. Int J Radiat Oncol Biol Phys 65:1522–1527

Chow E, Harris K, Fan G, Tsao M, Sze WM (2007a) Palliative radiotherapy trials for bone metastases: a systematic review. J Clin Oncol 25:1423–1436

Chow E, Loblaw A, Harris K, Doyle M, Goh P, Chiu H et al (2007b) Dexamethasone for the prophylaxis of radiation-induced pain flare after palliative radiotherapy for bone metastases: a pilot study. Support Care Cancer 15:643–647

Chow E, Hoskin P, Mitera G, Zeng L, Lutz S, Roos D et al; International Bone Metastases Consensus Working Party (2012) Update of the international consensus on palliative radiotherapy endpoints for future clinical trials in bone metastases. Int J Radiat Oncol Biol Phys 82:1730–1737

Chow E, van der Linden YM, Roos D, Hartsell WF, Hoskin P, Wu JS et al (2014a) Single versus multiple fractions of repeat radiation for painful bone metastases: a randomised, controlled, non-inferiority trial. Lancet Oncol 15:164–171

Chow E, Meyer RM, Chen BE, van der Linden YM, Roos D, Hartsell WF et al (2014b) Impact of reirradiation of painful osseous metastases on quality of life and function: a secondary analysis of the NCIC CTG SC.20 randomized trial. J Clin Oncol 32:3867–3873

Chow E, Meyer RM, Ding K, Nabid A, Chabot P, Wong P et al (2015) Dexamethasone in the prophylaxis of radiation-induced pain flare after palliative radiotherapy for bone metastases: a double-blind, randomised placebo-controlled, phase 3 trial. Lancet Oncol 16: 1463–1472

Chow E, Ding K, Parulekar WR, Wong RK, van der Linden YM, Roos D et al (2016) Revisiting classification of pain from bone metastases as mild, moderate, or severe based on correlation with function and quality of life. Support Care Cancer 24:1617–1623

Cole DJ (1989) A randomized trial of a single treatment versus conventional fractionation in the palliative radiotherapy of painful bone metastases. Clin Oncol (R Coll Radiol) 1:59–62

Coleman RE (1997) Skeletal complications of malignancy. Cancer 80(8 Suppl):1588–1594

Dupuy DE, Liu D, Hartfeil D, Hanna L, Blume JD, Ahrar K et al (2010) Percutaneous radiofrequency ablation of painful osseous metastases: a multicenter American College of Radiology Imaging Network trial. Cancer 116:989–997

Falkmer U, Jarhult J, Wersall P, Cavallin-Stahl E (2003) A systematic overview of radiation therapy effects in skeletal metastases. Acta Oncol 42:620–633

Fisher CG, DiPaola CP, Ryken TC, Bilsky MH, Shaffrey CI, Berven SH et al (2010) A novel classification system for spinal instability in neoplastic disease: an evidence-based approach and expert consensus from the Spine Oncology Study Group. Spine (Phila Pa 1976) 35:E1221–E1229

Foro AP, Fontanals AV, Galceran JC, Lynd F, Latiesas XS, de Dios NR et al (2008) Randomized clinical trial with two palliative radiotherapy regimens in painful bone metastases: 30 Gy in 10 fractions compared with 8 Gy in single fraction. Radiother Oncol 89:150–155

Galasko CS (1981) The anatomy and pathways of bone metastases. In: Weiss L, Gilbert A (eds) Bone metastases. GK Hall, Boston, pp 49–63

Gaze MN, Kelly CG, Kerr GR, Cull A, Cowie VJ, Gregor A et al (1997) Pain relief and quality of life following radiotherapy for bone metastases: a randomised trial of two fractionation schedules. Radiother Oncol 45:109–116

Gerszten PC, Burton SA, Ozhasoglu C, Welch WC (2007) Radiosurgery for spinal metastases: clinical experience in 500 cases from a single institution. Spine (Phila Pa 1976) 32:193–199

Gibbs IC, Kamnerdsupaphon P, Ryu MR, Dodd R, Kiernan M, Chang SD et al (2007) Image-guided robotic radiosurgery for spinal metastases. Radiother Oncol 82:185–190

Goetz MP, Callstrom MR, Charboneau JW, Farrell MA, Maus TP, Welch TJ et al (2004) Percutaneous image-guided radiofrequency ablation of painful metastases involving bone: a multicenter study. J Clin Oncol 22:300–306

Haas RL, Betgen A, Wolfrat M, Panneman C, Remeijer P (2013) Cone beam CT assisted irradiation of painful vertebral metastases without prior virtual simulation: a quick and patient friendly procedure. Radiother Oncol 106:375–377

Haddad P, Cheung F, Pond G, Easton D, Cops F, Bezjak A et al (2006) Computerized tomographic simulation compared with clinical mark-up in palliative radiotherapy: a prospective study. Int J Radiat Oncol Biol Phys 65:824–829

Harrington KD (1986) Metastatic disease of the spine. J Bone Joint Surg Am 68:1110–1115

Hartsell WF, Konski AA, Scott CB, Bruner DW, Scarantino CW, Ivker RA et al (2005) Randomized trial of short- versus long-course radiotherapy for palliation of painful bone metastases. J Natl Cancer Inst 97:798–804

Harvey HA (1997) Issues concerning the role of chemotherapy and hormonal therapy of bone metastases from breast carcinoma. Cancer 80(8 Suppl):1646–1651

Heimdal K, Hirschberg H, Slettebo H, Watne K, Nome O (1992) High incidence of serious side effects of high-dose dexamethasone treatment in patients with epidural spinal cord compression. J Neurooncol 12:141–144

Hird A, Chow E, Zhang L, Wong R, Wu J, Sinclair E et al (2009a) Determining the incidence of pain flare following palliative radiotherapy for symptomatic bone metastases: results from three Canadian cancer centers. Int J Radiat Oncol Biol Phys 75:193–197

Hird A, Zhang L, Holt T, Fairchild A, Deangelis C, Loblaw A et al (2009b) Dexamethasone for the prophylaxis of radiation-induced pain flare after palliative radiotherapy for symptomatic bone metastases: a phase II study. Clin Oncol (R Coll Radiol) 21:329–335

Hirokawa Y, Wadasaki K, Kashiwado K (1988) A multi-institutional prospective randomized study of radiation therapy of bone metastases (Japanese). Nippon Igaku Hoshasen Gakkai Zasshi 48:1425–1431

Hortobagyi GN, Theriault RL, Porter L, Blayney D, Lipton A, Sinoff C et al (1996) Efficacy of pamidronate in reducing skeletal complications in patients with breast cancer and lytic bone metastases. Protocol 19 Aredia Breast Cancer Study Group. N Engl J Med 335:1785–1791

Hoskin PJ (1988) Scientific and clinical aspects of radiotherapy in the relief of bone pain. Cancer Surv 7:69–86

Hoskin PJ, Price P, Easton D, Regan J, Austin D, Palmer S et al (1992) A prospective randomised trial of 4 Gy or 8 Gy single doses in the treatment of metastatic bone pain. Radiother Oncol 23:74–78

Hoskin P, Grover A, Bhana R (2003) Metastatic spinal cord compression: radiotherapy outcome and dose fractionation. Radiother Oncol 68:175–180

Hoskin P, Rojas A, Fidarova E, Jalali R, Mena Merino A, Poitevin A et al (2015) IAEA randomised trial of optimal single dose radiotherapy in the treatment of painful bone metastases. Radiother Oncol 116:10–14

Huisman M, van den Bosch MA, Wijlemans JW, van Vulpen M, van der Linden YM, Verkooijen HM (2012) Effectiveness of reirradiation for painful bone metastases: a systematic review and meta-analysis. Int J Radiat Oncol Biol Phys 84:8–14

Jeremic B, Shibamoto Y, Acimovic L, Milicic B, Milisavljevic S, Nikolic N et al (1998) A randomized trial of three single-dose radiation therapy regimens in the treatment of metastatic bone pain. Int J Radiat Oncol Biol Phys 42:161–167

Jeremic B, Shibamoto Y, Igrutinovic I (1999) Single 4 Gy re-irradiation for painful bone metastasis following single fraction radiotherapy. Radiother Oncol 52:123–127

Jeremic B, Shibamoto Y, Igrutinovic I (2002) Second single 4 Gy reirradiation for painful bone metastasis. J Pain Symptom Manage 23:26–30

Jin JY, Chen Q, Jin R, Rock J, Anderson J, Li S et al (2007) Technical and clinical experience with spine radiosurgery: a new technology for management of localized spine metastases. Technol Cancer Res Treat 6:127–133

Kaasa S, Brenne E, Lund JA, Fayers P, Falkmer U, Holmberg M et al (2006) Prospective randomised multicenter trial on single fraction radiotherapy (8 Gy x 1) versus multiple fractions (3 Gy x 10) in the treatment of painful bone metastases. Radiother Oncol 79:278–284

Kagei K, Suyuki K, Sherato H (1990) Prospective randomized trial of single high dose versus multiple fraction radiation therapy for the treatment of bone metastasis. Gan No Rinsho 36:2553–2558

Kallmes DF, Jensen ME (2003) Percutaneous vertebroplasty. Radiology 229:27–36

Kamby C, Vejborg I, Daugaard S, Guldhammer B, Dirksen H, Rossing N et al (1987) Clinical and radiologic characteristics of bone metastases in breast cancer. Cancer 60:2524–2531

Kirkbride P, Warde P, Panzarella A (2000a) A randomised trial comparing the efficacy of single fraction radiation therapy plus ondansetron with fractionated radiation therapy in the palliation of skeletal metastases (Abstract). Int J Radiat Oncol Biol Phys 48(3 Suppl):185

Kirkbride P, Bezjak A, Pater J, Zee B, Palmer MJ, Wong R et al (2000b) Dexamethasone for the prophylaxis of radiation-induced emesis: a National Cancer Institute of Canada Clinical Trials Group phase III study. J Clin Oncol 18:1960–1966

Kirkpatrick JP, van der Kogel AJ, Schultheiss TE (2010) Radiation dose-volume effects in the spinal cord. Int J Radiat Oncol Biol Phys 76(3 Suppl):S42–S49

Koswig S, Budach V (1999) Remineralization and pain relief in bone metastases after different radiotherapy fractions (10 times 3 Gy vs. 1 time 8 Gy). A prospective study. Strahlenther Onkol 175:500–508

Lee YT (1983) Breast carcinoma: pattern of metastasis at autopsy. J Surg Oncol 23:175–180

Letourneau D, Wong R, Moseley D, Sharpe MB, Ansell S, Gospodarowicz M et al (2007) Online planning and delivery technique for radiotherapy of spinal metastases using cone-beam CT: image quality and system performance. Int J Radiat Oncol Biol Phys 67:1229–1237

Li KK, Harris K, Hadi S, Chow E (2007) What should be the optimal cut points for mild, moderate, and severe pain? J Palliat Med 10:1338–1346

Li KK, Hadi S, Kirou-Mauro A, Chow E (2008) When should we define the response rates in the treatment of bone metastases by palliative radiotherapy? Clin Oncol (R Coll Radiol) 20:83–89

Lieberman I, Reinhardt MK (2003) Vertebroplasty and kyphoplasty for osteolytic vertebral collapse. Clin Orthop (415 Suppl):S176–S186

Lipton A (2003) Bisphosphonates and metastatic breast carcinoma. Cancer 97(3 Suppl):848–853

Lipton A, Fizazi K, Stopeck AT, Henry DH, Smith MR, Shore N et al (2016) Effect of denosumab versus zoledronic acid in preventing skeletal-related events in patients with bone metastases by baseline characteristics. Eur J Cancer 53:75–83

Loblaw DA, Wu JS, Kirkbride P, Panzarella T, Smith K, Aslanidis J et al (2007) Pain flare in patients with bone metastases after palliative radiotherapy–a nested randomized control trial. Support Care Cancer 15:451–455

Macbeth FR, Wheldon TE, Girling DJ, Stephens RJ, Machin D, Bleehen NM et al (1996) Radiation myelopathy: estimates of risk in 1048 patients in three randomized trials of palliative radiotherapy for non-small cell lung cancer. The Medical Research Council Lung Cancer Working Party. Clin Oncol (R Coll Radiol) 8:176–181

Madsen EL (1983) Painful bone metastasis: efficacy of radiotherapy assessed by the patients: a randomized trial comparing 4 Gy X 6 versus 10 Gy X 2. Int J Radiat Oncol Biol Phys 9:1775–1779

Mancosu P, Navarria P, Bignardi M, Cozzi L, Fogliata A, Lattuada P et al (2010) Re-irradiation of metastatic spinal cord compression: a feasibility study by volumetric-modulated arc radiotherapy for in-field recurrence creating a dosimetric hole on the central canal. Radiother Oncol 94:67–70

Maranzano E, Latini P (1995) Effectiveness of radiation therapy without surgery in metastatic spinal cord compression: final results from a prospective trial. Int J Radiat Oncol Biol Phys 32:959–967

Maranzano E, Latini P, Perrucci E, Beneventi S, Lupatelli M, Corgna E (1997) Short-course radiotherapy (8Gy x 2) in metastatic spinal cord compression: an effective and feasible treatment. Int J Radiat Oncol Biol Phys 38:1037–1044

Maranzano E, Bellavita R, Floridi P, Celani G, Righetti E, Lupattelli M et al (2001) Radiation-induced myelopathy in long-term surviving metastatic spinal cord compression patients after hypofractionated radiotherapy: a clinical and magnetic resonance imaging analysis. Radiother Oncol 60:281–288

Maranzano E, Bellavita R, Rossi R, De Angelis V, Frattegiani A, Bagnoli R et al (2005) Short-course versus split-course radiotherapy in metastatic spinal cord compression: results of a phase III, randomized, multicenter trial. J Clin Oncol 23:3358–3365

Maranzano E, Trippa F, Casale M, Costantini S, Lupattelli M, Bellavita R et al (2009) 8Gy single-dose radiotherapy is effective in metastatic spinal cord compression: results of a phase III randomized multicentre Italian trial. Radiother Oncol 93:174–179

Meeuse JJ, van der Linden YM, van Tienhoven G, Gans RO, Leer JW, Reyners AK (2010) Efficacy of radiotherapy for painful bone metastases during the last 12 weeks of life: results from the Dutch Bone Metastasis Study. Cancer 116:2716–2725

Mercadante S (1997) Malignant bone pain: pathophysiology and treatment. Pain 69:1–18

Miller F, Whitehill R (1984) Carcinoma of the breast metastatic to the skeleton. Clin Orthop 184:121–127

Mithal NP, Needham PR, Hoskin PJ (1994) Retreatment with radiotherapy for painful bone metastases. Int J Radiat Oncol Biol Phys 29:1011–1014

Nieder C, Grosu AL, Andratschke NH, Molls M (2005) Proposal of human spinal cord reirradiation dose based on collection of data from 40 patients. Int J Radiat Oncol Biol Phys 61:851–855

Nieder C, Grosu AL, Andratschke NH, Molls M (2006) Update of human spinal cord reirradiation tolerance based on additional data from 38 patients. Int J Radiat Oncol Biol Phys 66:1446–1449

Nielsen OS, Bentzen SM, Sandberg E, Gadeberg CC, Timothy AR (1998) Randomized trial of single dose versus fractionated palliative radiotherapy of bone metastases. Radiother Oncol 47:233–240

Niewald M, Tkocz HJ, Abel U, Scheib T, Walter K, Nieder C et al (1996) Rapid course radiation therapy vs. more standard treatment: a randomized trial for bone metastases. Int J Radiat Oncol Biol Phys 36:1085–1089

Okawa T, Kita M, Goto M, Nishijima H, Miyaji N (1988) Randomized prospective clinical study of small, large and twice-a-day fraction radiotherapy for painful bone metastases. Radiother Oncol 13:99–104

Patchell R, Tibbs PA, Regine WF, Payne R (2005) Direct decompressive surgical resection in the treatment of spinal cord compression caused by metastatic cancer: a randomised trial. Lancet 366:643–648

Payne R (2003) Mechanisms and management of bone pain. Cancer 80:1608–1613

Price P, Hoskin PJ, Easton D, Austin D, Palmer SG, Yarnold JR (1986) Prospective randomised trial of single and multifraction radiotherapy schedules in the treatment of painful bony metastases. Radiother Oncol 6:247–255

Price P, Hoskin PJ, Easton D, Austin D, Palmer S, Yarnold JR (1988) Low dose single fraction radiotherapy in the treatment of metastatic bone pain: a pilot study. Radiother Oncol 12:297–300

Quasim M (1981) Half body irradiation in metastatic carcinomas. Clin Radiol 32:215–219

Quilty PM, Kirk D, Bolger JJ (1994) A comparison of the palliative effects of strontium-89 and external beam radiotherapy in metastatic prostate cancer. Radiother Oncol 31:33–40

Rades D, Heidenreich F, Karstens JH (2002) Final results of a prospective study of the prognostic value of the time to develop motor deficits before irradiation in metastatic spinal cord compression. Int J Radiat Oncol Biol Phys 53:975–979

Rades D, Stalpers L, Veninga T (2005a) Evaluation of five radiation schedules and prognostic factors for metastatic spinal cord compression in a series of 1304 patients. J Clin Oncol 23:3366–3375

Rades D, Stalpers LJ, Veninga T, Hoskin PJ (2005b) Spinal reirradiation after short-course RT for metastatic spinal cord compression. Int J Radiat Oncol Biol Phys 63:872–875

Rades D, Hoskin PJ, Stalpers LJ, Schulte R, Poortmans P, Veninga T et al (2006) Short-course radiotherapy is not optimal for spinal cord compression due to myeloma. Int J Radiat Oncol Biol Phys 64:1452–1457

Rades D, Dunst J, Schild S (2008a) The first score predicting overall survival in patients with metastatic spinal cord compression. Cancer 112:157–161

Rades D, Rudat V, Veninga T, Stalpers LJ, Basic H, Karstens JH et al (2008b) A score predicting posttreatment ambulatory status in patients irradiated for metastatic spinal cord compression. Int J Radiat Oncol Biol Phys 72:905–908

Rades D, Rudat V, Veninga T, Stalpers LJ, Hoskin PJ, Schild SE (2008c) Prognostic factors for functional outcome and survival after reirradiation for in-field recurrences of metastatic spinal cord compression. Cancer 113:1090–1096

Rades D, Lange M, Veninga T, Rudat V, Bajrovic A, Stalpers LJ et al (2009) Preliminary results of spinal cord compression recurrence evaluation (score-1) study comparing short-course versus long-course radiotherapy for local control of malignant epidural spinal cord compression. Int J Radiat Oncol Biol Phys 73:228–234

Rades D, Huttenlocher S, Dunst J, Bajrovic A, Karstens JH, Rudat V et al (2010a) Matched pair analysis comparing surgery followed by radiotherapy and radiotherapy alone for metastatic spinal cord compression. J Clin Oncol 28:3597–3604

Rades D, Douglas S, Veninga T, Stalpers LJ, Hoskin PJ, Bajrovic A et al (2010b) Validation and simplification of a score predicting survival in patients irradiated for metastatic spinal cord compression. Cancer 116:3670–3673

Rades D, Douglas S, Huttenlocher S, Rudat V, Veninga T, Stalpers LJ et al (2011a) Validation of a score predicting post-treatment ambulatory status after radiotherapy for metastatic spinal cord compression. Int J Radiat Oncol Biol Phys 79:1503–1506

Rades D, Freundt K, Meyners T, Bajrovic A, Basic H, Karstens JH et al (2011b) Dose escalation for metastatic spinal cord compression in patients with relatively radioresistant tumors. Int J Radiat Oncol Biol Phys 80:1492–1497

Rades D, Šegedin B, Conde-Moreno AJ, Garcia R, Perpar A, Metz M et al (2016) Radiotherapy with 4 Gy×5 versus 3 Gy×10 for metastatic epidural spinal cord compression: final results of the SCORE-2 trial (ARO 2009/01). J Clin Oncol 34:597–602

Rasmusson B, Vejborg I, Jensen AB, Andersson M, Banning AM, Hoffmann T et al (1995) Irradiation of bone metastases in breast cancer patients: a randomized study with 1 year follow-up. Radiother Oncol 34:179–184

Ratanatharathorn V, Powers WE, Moss WT, Perez CA (1999) Bone metastasis: review and critical analysis of random allocation trials of local field treatment. Int J Radiat Oncol Biol Phys 44:1–18

Rogers MJ, Watts DJ, Russell RG (1997) Overview of bisphosphonates. Cancer 80(8 Suppl):1652–1657

Roos DE, O'Brien PC, Smith JG, Spry NA, Hoskin PJ, Burmeister BH et al (2000) A role for radiotherapy in neuropathic bone pain: preliminary response rates from a prospective trial (Trans-tasman radiation oncology group, TROG 96.05) [published erratum appears in Int J Radiat Oncol Biol Phys 2000;47:545]. Int J Radiat Oncol Biol Phys 46:975–981

Roos DE, Turner SL, O'Brien PC, Smith JG, Spry NA, Burmeister BH et al (2005) Randomized trial of 8 Gy in 1 versus 20 Gy in 5 fractions of radiotherapy for neuropathic pain due to bone metastases (Trans-Tasman Radiation Oncology Group, TROG 96.05). Radiother Oncol 75:54–63

Rosen LS, Gordon D, Simon Tchekmedyian N, Yanagihara R, Hirsh V, Krzakowski M et al (2004) Long term efficacy and safety of Zoledronic acid in the treatment of skeletal metastases in patients with non-small cell lung carcinoma and other solid tumors. A randomized, phase III, double-blind, placebo-controlled trial. Cancer 100:2613–2621

Ryu S, Fang YF, Rock J, Zhu J, Chu A, Kagan E et al (2003) Image-guided and intensity-modulated radiosurgery for patients with spinal metastasis. Cancer 97:2013–2018

Ryu S, Jin JY, Jin R, Rock J, Ajlouni M, Movsas B et al (2007) Partial volume tolerance of the spinal cord and complications of single-dose radiosurgery. Cancer 109:628–636

Ryu S, Pugh SL, Gerszten PC, Yin FF, Timmerman RD, Hitchcock YJ et al (2014) RTOG 0631 phase 2/3 study of image guided stereotactic radiosurgery for localized (1-3) spine metastases: phase 2 results. Pract Radiat Oncol 4:76–81

Sahgal A, Ma L, Weinberg V, Gibbs IC, Chao S, Chang UK et al (2012) Reirradiation human spinal cord tolerance for stereotactic body radiotherapy. Int J Radiat Oncol Biol Phys 82:107–116

Salazar OM, Rubin P, Hendrickson FR, Komaki R, Poulter C, Newall J et al (1986) Single-dose half-body irradiation for palliation of multiple bone metastases from solid tumors. Final Radiation Therapy Oncology Group report. Cancer 58:29–36

Salazar OM, Sandhu T, da Motta NW, Escutia MA, Lanzos-Gonzales E, Mouelle-Sone A et al (2001) Fractionated half-body irradiation (HBI) for the rapid palliation of widespread, symptomatic, metastatic bone disease: a randomized Phase III trial of the International Atomic Energy Agency (IAEA). Int J Radiat Oncol Biol Phys 50:765–775

Sartor O, Coleman R, Nilsson S, Heinrich D, Helle SI, O'Sullivan JM et al (2014) Effect of radium-223 dichloride on symptomatic skeletal events in patients with castration-resistant prostate cancer and bone metastases: results from a phase 3, double-blind, randomised trial. Lancet Oncol 15:738–746

Schultheiss TE (2008) The radiation dose-response of the human spinal cord. Int J Radiat Oncol Biol Phys 71:1455–1459

Sorensen S, Helweg-Larsen S, Mouridsen H, Hansen HH (1994) Effect of high-dose dexamethasone in carcinomatous metastatic spinal cord compression treated with radiotherapy: a randomised trial. Eur J Cancer 30A:22–27

Steenland E, Leer JW, van Houwelingen H, Post WJ, van den Hout WB, Kievit J et al (1999) The effect of a single fraction compared to multiple fractions on painful bone metastases: a global analysis of the Dutch Bone Metastasis Study. Radiother Oncol 52:101–109

Sykes AJ, Kiltie AE, Stewart AL (1997) Ondansetron versus a chlorpromazine and dexamethasone combination for the prevention of nausea and vomiting: a prospective, randomised study to assess efficacy, cost effectiveness and quality of life following single-fraction radiotherapy. Support Care Cancer 5:500–503

Sze WM, Shelley MD, Held I, Wilt TJ, Mason MD (2003) Palliation of metastatic bone pain: single fraction versus multifraction radiotherapy. A systematic review of randomised trials. Clin Oncol (R Coll Radiol) 15:345–352

Sze WM, Shelley M, Held I, Mason M (2004) Palliation of metastatic bone pain: single fraction versus multifraction radiotherapy – a systematic review of the randomised trials. Cochrane Database Syst Rev (2):CD004721

Tanck E, van Aken JB, van der Linden YM, Schreuder HW, Binkowski M, Huizenga H et al (2009) Pathological fracture prediction in patients with metastatic lesions can be improved with quantitative computed tomography based computer models. Bone 45:777–783

Tong D, Gillick L, Hendrickson FR (1982) The palliation of symptomatic osseous metastases: final results of the Study by the Radiation Therapy Oncology Group. Cancer 50:893–899

Uppelschoten JM, Wanders SL, de Jong JM (1995) Single-dose radiotherapy (6 Gy): palliation in painful bone metastases. Radiother Oncol 36:198–202

Vakaet LA, Boterberg T (2004) Pain control by ionizing radiation of bone metastasis. Int J Dev Biol 48:599–606

van der Linden YM, Kroon HM, Dijkstra PD, Lok JJ, Noordijk EM, Leer JWH et al (2003) Simple radiographic parameter predicts fracturing in metastatic femoral bone lesions: results from a randomized trial. Radiother Oncol 69:21–31

van der Linden YM, Dijkstra PD, Kroon HM, Lok JJ, Noordijk EM, Leer J et al (2004a) Comparative analysis of risk factors for pathological fracture with femoral metastases. Results based on a randomised trial of radiotherapy. J Bone Joint Surg Br 86:566–573

van der Linden YM, Lok JJ, Steenland E, Martijn H, Houwelingen JC, Leer JWH et al (2004b) Single fraction radiotherapy is efficacious: a further analysis of the Dutch Bone Metastasis Study controlling for the influence of retreatment. Int J Radiat Oncol Biol Phys 59:528–537

van der Linden YM, Dijkstra PDS, Vonk EJA, Marijnen CAM, Leer JWH (2005) Prediction of survival in patients with metastases in the spinal column. Cancer 103:320–328

van der Linden YM, Steenland E, van Houwelingen H, Post WJ, Oei B, Marijnen CAM et al (2006) Patients with a favourable prognosis are equally palliated with single and multiple fraction radiotherapy: results on survival in the Dutch Bone Metastasis Study. Radiother Oncol 48:245–253

van Helvoirt R, Bratelli K (2008) Both immediate and late retreatment with single fraction radiotherapy are effective in palliating patients with painful skeletal metastases: a prospective cohort analysis. Radiother Oncol 88(Suppl):S51

Vecht CJ, Haaxma-Reiche H, van Putten WL, de Visser M, Vries EP, Twijnstra A (1989) Initial bolus of conventional versus high-dose dexamethasone in metastatic spinal cord compression. Neurology 39:1255–1257

Wedin R, Bauer H, Rutqvist LE (2001) Surgical treatment for skeletal breast cancer metastases. A population-based study of 641 patients. Cancer 92:257–262

Westhoff PG, de Graeff A, Geerling JI, Reyners AK, van der Linden YM (2014) Dexamethasone for the prevention of a pain flare after palliative radiotherapy for painful bone metastases: a multicenter double-blind placebo-controlled randomized trial. BMC Cancer 14:347

Wu JS, Wong R, Johnston M, Bezjak A, Whelan T (2003) Meta-analysis of dose-fractionation radiotherapy trials for the palliation of painful bone metastases. Int J Radiat Oncol Biol Phys 55:594–605

Brain Metastases

Carsten Nieder, Anca L. Grosu,
and Minesh P. Mehta

Contents

The original version of this chapter was revised.
An erratum to this chapter can be found at
10.1007/978-3-319-41825-4_78.

C. Nieder, MD (✉)
Department of Oncology and Palliative Medicine,
Nordland Hospital, Prinsensgate 164,
Bodø 8092, Norway
e-mail: Carsten.Nieder@nordlandssykehuset.no

A.L. Grosu, MD
Department of Radiation Oncology, University
Hospital Freiburg, Robert Koch Str. 3,
Freiburg 79106, Germany

M.P. Mehta, MD
Department of Radiation Oncology, University of
Maryland School of Medicine, Baltimore, MD, USA

Abstract

In many patients with brain metastases, the primary therapeutic aim is symptom palliation and maintenance of neurologic function, but in a small selected cohort, long-term survival and even cure are possible. Central nervous system failures might develop after initial treatment, either locally (regrowth of a previously treated lesion), regionally (elsewhere in the brain parenchyma), or even in the form of leptomeningeal dissemination, the latter carrying the worst prognosis. Some of these failures will not require local therapy because they develop in the terminal phase of general cancer progression where active brain metastasis treatment is neither expected to prolong survival nor improve the patient's quality of life. At the other end of the spectrum, patients with limited, brain-only, relapse require effective intracranial disease control as a prerequisite for extended survival. The present chapter reviews reirradiation with brachytherapy, stereotactic radiosurgery, fractionated stereotactic radiotherapy and whole-brain radiotherapy.

1 Outcome and Relapse Rates After First-Line Radiotherapy

Patients with brain metastases present with a variable number, size, and location of brain metastases, with different patterns and activity of

Med Radiol Radiat Oncol (2016)
DOI 10.1007/174_2016_58, © Springer International Publishing Switzerland
Published Online: 21 Apr 2016

extracranial disease and with a wide range of comorbidities and performance status. Therefore, they represent a heterogeneous group with large variations in survival, often influenced by the molecular characteristics, and the availability of targeted therapies for the underlying neoplasm. The number of available treatment options has increased since the era of corticosteroids and 2-D radiotherapy, now including but not limited to resection, whole-brain radiotherapy (WBRT), radiosurgery, chemotherapy, targeted agents, and immune checkpoint inhibitors. In general, for the vast majority, the primary therapeutic aim is symptom palliation and maintenance of neurologic function, but in a small selected cohort, long-term survival and even cure are possible. Commonly used first-line approaches include short-course palliative WBRT, stereotactic radiosurgery (SRS) with or without additional WBRT, and surgical resection with or without postoperative WBRT or focal radiotherapy including SRS to the resection cavity or even delivered preoperatively, prior to resection. Specific histologic and molecularly defined types of tumors do respond to systemic chemotherapy or targeted agents, the role of which is evolving. Immune checkpoint inhibitors, either singly, or in combination with SRS are also being used, currently mostly in melanoma, but with likely application in non-small cell lung cancer as well. Central nervous system failures might develop after each of these approaches, either locally (regrowth of a previously treated lesion), regionally (elsewhere in the brain parenchyma), or even in the form of leptomeningeal dissemination, the latter carrying the worst prognosis. Some of these failures will not require local therapy because they develop in the terminal phase of general cancer progression where active brain metastasis treatment is neither expected to prolong survival nor improve the patient's quality of life (Ammirati et al. 2010). In other words, patients in poor general condition and with untreatable and life-threatening extracranial disease will typically be managed by best supportive care. At the other end of the spectrum, patients with limited brain-only relapse require effective intracranial disease control as a prerequisite for extended survival (Nieder et al. 2015).

In the first-line setting, prospective data on the efficacy of palliative WBRT were generated by the Radiation Therapy Oncology Group (RTOG) in the trials 69-01 and 73-61. Their reports suggested that the median survival of patients treated with WBRT is longer (3–6 months) than that of patients managed with steroids without radiotherapy (1–2 months). The Medical Research Council (MRC) has recently completed a large-scale randomized trial of steroids/best supportive care alone versus the same treatment plus WBRT in patients with primary non-small cell lung cancer, which is awaiting publication. The aforementioned RTOG studies described that 43–64 % of patients experienced neurologic response by week 2 (Borgelt et al. 1980, 1981). More recently, various groups have reported responses in the same range. For example, after 30 Gy WBRT, Antoniou et al. reported benefit in 38 % of patients (Antoniou et al. 2005); Sundstrom et al. reported symptomatic relief allowing steroid dose reduction in 66 % of patients after ≥25 Gy irradiation (Sundstrom et al. 1998), and Nieder et al. reported radiographic responses in comparable proportions of patients (Nieder et al. 1997).

Radiographic responses after WBRT with 30 Gy in 10 fractions are more likely in brain metastases from lung and breast cancer (Stea et al. 2006). Responders were found to have significantly longer overall survival in many series. WBRT-induced tumor shrinkage correlated with better survival and neurocognitive function preservation in a cohort of 135 patients from a phase III trial of WBRT plus the sensitizing agent motexafin gadolinium (Li et al. 2007). Previous RTOG data also suggest that patients with controlled brain metastases after WBRT tend to experience stable mini-mental status examination (MMSE) scores, while those with uncontrolled lesions had an average drop of 6 points by 3 months (Regine et al. 2001). Overall, no correlation between radiation dose and palliation could be established in the trials that compared different fractionation schedules (Gelber et al. 1981; Chatani et al. 1994).

The WBRT dosing/fractionation question was recently addressed in a AANS/CNS Guidelines Analysis (Gaspar et al. 2010). Twenty-three studies met the eligibility criteria for this question, and of these, 17 were unique. The 17 unique studies fell into three evidence class categories as follows: ten class I studies (nine randomized controlled trials and one randomized phase I/II trial), six class II studies (retrospective cohort studies), and one class III study (prospective cohort study with historical controls). The radiation dosages were expressed in terms of Gy_{10} biologically effective doses (BED), and no correction for accelerated repopulation was attempted. The analysis was stratified by low or high dose versus control dose. The control group consisted of patients treated with 30 Gy in 10 fractions for a BED = 39 Gy_{10} (therefore assigning the low-dose regimens as a BED <39 Gy_{10} and high-dose regimens as a BED >39 Gy_{10}). None of the trials demonstrated a meaningful improvement in any endpoint relative to dose; specifically, survival was not improved. There was considerable overlap in terms of survival even at the same dose level in different trials, underscoring the significance of host-specific variables in determining survival. There was no difference in the relative risk (RR) of mortality at 6 months in the low-dose (BED <39 Gy_{10}) group compared to that in the WBRT control group (BED = 39 Gy_{10}) (6 month mortality (RR 1.05; 95 % CI 0.90, 1.23; $p = 0.52$)). When the high-dose (BED >39 Gy_{10}) group was compared to the WBRT control group (BED = 39 Gy_{10}), no difference in 6-month mortality (RR 1.05; 95 % CI 0.94, 1.18; $p = 0.39$) was identified. Similar comparisons were made for overall survival and neurologic function, and no dose-effect was identified for either endpoint. In view of this lack of a clear dose-effect relationship, recent multi-institutional analyses are in accordance with previous recommendations of short-course treatment, e.g., 5 fractions of 4 Gy, for patients with limited life expectancy (Rades et al. 2007c), or 10 fractions of 3 Gy or 15 fractions of 2.5 Gy for patients with longer life expectancy.

Estimation of prognosis is possible by using the RTOG recursive partitioning analysis (RPA) classes, first described by Gaspar et al. 1997 (Table 1) and the newly described graded prognostic assessment (GPA) score including its diagnosis-specific variant developed by Sperduto et al. 2010 (Table 2). Recent refinements of the GPA now incorporate molecular markers for breast and non-small cell lung cancer, and a similar analysis for melanoma is underway. The impact of histology also needs to be considered. After a standard WBRT course (30 Gy in 10 fractions over 2 weeks), all metastases from squamous cell carcinoma and adenocarcinoma (primary breast cancer excluded) visible on contrast-enhanced CT scans eventually relapsed or progressed within a time period of 14 months (Nieder et al. 1997). Better results were obtained in small cell carcinoma and primary breast cancer in whom less than 50 % of the WBRT-treated brain metastases relapsed or progressed. The risk of local progression after WBRT is higher in large-volume lesions, compared to smaller lesions (≥1 cc versus <1 cc), though not to a statistically significant degree. The implication here is that in patients in whom long-term survival is anticipated, the modest doses delivered by WBRT alone are inadequate for long-term control,

Table 1 Prognostic value of recursive partitioning analysis (RPA) classes

Reference	Number of patients	RPA class I	RPA class II	RPA class III
Gaspar et al. (1997)	1,200	7.1	4.2	2.3
Lutterbach et al. (2002)	916	8.2	4.9	1.8 (IIIA 3.2)
Nieder et al. (2000)	528	10.5	3.5	2.0
Agboola et al. (1998)	125 (resected brain met.)	14.8	9.9	6.0
Tendulkar et al. (2006)	271 (resected single brain met.)	21.4	9.0	8.9
Lorenzoni et al. (2004)	110 (RS)	27.6	10.7	2.8
Sneed et al. (2002)	268 (RS only)	14.0	8.2	5.3
	301 (RS + WBRT)	15.2	7.0	5.5

Median survival in months from different publications
RPA class I age <65 years, Karnofsky performance status ≥70, controlled primary tumor, no extracranial metastases, *RPA class II* all other patients, *RPA class III* Karnofsky performance status <70

Table 2 Overview of results with the graded prognostic assessment (GPA) score

Study	Median survival class I	Median survival class II	Median survival class III	Median survival class IV
Sperduto et al. (2008a) 1,960 patients who participated in clinical trials	11.0	8.9	3.8	2.6
Nieder et al. (2009) 232 patients treated outside of clinical trials	10.3	5.6	3.5	1.9
Nieder et al. (2008) 64 patients treated with surgery and WBRT	18.9	9.8	5.5	3.7
Sperduto et al. (2008b) 140 patients treated outside of clinical trials[a]	21.7	17.5	5.9	3.0

Median survival in months from different publications
In the GPA system, 3 different values (0, 0.5, or 1) are assigned for each of these 4 parameters: age (≥60; 50–59; <50), KPS (<70; 70–80; 90–100), number of brain metastases (>3; 2–3; 1), and extracranial metastases (present; not applicable; none). Patients in class I have a sum of 3.5–4 points, those in class II have 3 points, those in class III have 1.5–2.5 points, and those in class IV have 0–1 points. Note that diagnosis-specific scores might better predict the outcome of patients with primary malignant melanoma, renal cell cancer, and various breast cancer subtypes (Sperduto et al. 2010). A nomogram derived from this data has also been published (Barnholtz-Sloan et al. 2012)
WBRT whole-brain radiotherapy
[a]Several patients were treated with radiosurgery alone or radiosurgery plus WBRT

especially for larger lesions, and squamous and non-breast adenocarcinoma histologies.

Focal treatment such as SRS improves the local control observed with WBRT. In a small randomized study, patients with two to four brain metastases (all ≤25 mm diameter) either received WBRT alone (30 Gy in 12 fractions) or WBRT plus SRS (Kondziolka et al. 1999). The rate of local failure at 1 year was 100 % after WBRT alone but only 8 % in patients who had boost SRS. Median survival was 7.5 vs. 11 months for patients who received WBRT vs. WBRT plus SRS ($p=0.22$). A randomized study by the RTOG enrolled 333 patients with one to three brain metastases (Andrews et al. 2004). WBRT dose was 37.5 Gy in 15 fractions in both groups. SRS boost dose was adjusted to lesion size (15 Gy in lesions larger than 3 cm, 24 Gy in those up to 2 cm, and 18 Gy in others). Median survival was significantly better after SRS boost in patients with single brain metastasis. By post hoc multivariate analysis, survival was also improved in RPA class I patients. SRS-treated patients were more likely to have a stable or improved performance status at 6 months (43 vs. 27 %, $p=0.03$). Central imaging review showed higher response rates at 3 months and better 1-year control of the SRS-treated lesions, $p=0.01$. The risk of developing a local recurrence was 43 % greater with WBRT alone.

The risk of serious toxicity after WBRT appears rather low, even if prospective studies have demonstrated variable degrees of neurocognitive deficits during extended follow-up (Aoyama et al. 2007; Chang et al. 2009). Furthermore one must acknowledge that any type of cancer treatment might cause measurable neurocognitive decline, including SRS alone (Rugo and Ahles 2003; Heflin et al. 2005; Chang et al. 2009) and that some post-radiation symptoms might be caused by certain drugs rather than radiation itself (Nieder et al. 1999; Klein et al. 2002).

Local control of a limited number (mostly one to three) of brain metastases can effectively be achieved by surgical resection or SRS with or without adjuvant WBRT (Table 3). Recent data suggest that local control can also be achieved with SRS in patients with more numerous metastases, for example, ten or more (Yamamoto et al. 2014). The number of patients dying from uncontrolled brain metastases despite intensive local treatment ranges from 20 to 30 %. In general,

Table 3 Results of surgery and stereotactic radiosurgery (SRS) for brain metastases

Reference	*n* (patients and lesions)	Prescribed dose (median; range [Gy])[a]	Median OS	1-year PFS (%)
Patchell et al. (1990)	25/25	Surgery	9.5	80
Patchell et al. (1998)	49/49	Surgery	11.0	82
Pirzkall et al. (1998)	236/311	20; 10–30	5.5	89
Cho et al. (1998)	73/136	17.5; 6–50	7.8	80
Kocher et al. (1998)	106/157	20; 12–25	8.0	85
Sneed et al. (1999)	62/118[b] 43/117[c]	18; 15–22 17.5; 15–22	11.3 11.1	80 86
Varlotto et al. (2003)	137/208	16; 12–25	Not given	90
Andrews et al. (2004)	164/269[d]	Not given; 15–24	6.5	82
Bhatnagar et al. (2007)	205/4–18 lesions each[e]	16; 12–20	8.0	71

OS overall survival in months, *PFS* progression-free survival
[a]Prescription isodose or point varied; some series included SRS plus WBRT
[b]SRS only
[c]SRS plus WBRT (no significant difference in OS and PFS between both groups)
[d]SRS plus WBRT
[e]SRS plus/minus WBRT

SRS doses have varied with lesion size although it is counterintuitive to treat larger tumors with lower doses of radiation. While small lesions typically receive minimum doses of 20–24 Gy to the margin of the lesion, those that measure between 2 and 3 cm are treated with 18–20 Gy and those that measure between 3 and 4 cm with 15–16 Gy and sometimes with doses as low as 12 Gy, based on location. A retrospective analysis of 375 lesions suggests that 1-year local control after 18 Gy or less is in the range of 45–49 % as opposed to 85 % after 24 Gy (Vogelbaum et al. 2006). In the Japanese SRS study of 132 patients treated with lower SRS doses, discussed in greater detail below, only 4 patients (3 %) developed radionecrosis (Aoyama et al. 2006). Prognosis of SRS patients might be estimated either by RPA classes, DS-GPA, or the score index for radiosurgery (SIR) (Weltman et al. 2001; Lorenzoni et al. 2004). The most favorable SIR group contains patients with age ≤50 years, Karnofsky performance status (KPS) >70 %, no evidence of systemic disease at the time of SRS, limited number of brain lesions, and largest SRS-treated lesion <13 ml. After many years of controversy about the role of combining WBRT with SRS and considerable variation in practice, comparable to the discussion around WBRT after surgical resection of brain metastases, four randomized trials and a meta-analysis have attempted to address the issue (Aoyama et al. 2006; Chang et al. 2009; Kocher et al. 2011; Sahgal et al. 2015; Brown et al. 2015). The Japanese prospective randomized multicenter phase III study of SRS alone vs. SRS and WBRT (Aoyama et al. 2006) was designed with the primary endpoint of survival, with an overly generous expected difference of 30 %. The trial included adult patients with Karnofsky performance score >60 % and a maximum of four brain metastases, none exceeding 3 cm diameter. WBRT was given in 10 fractions of 3 Gy. SRS dose varied with size of the lesion (up to 2 cm, 22–25 Gy; >2 cm, 18–20 Gy margin dose) and was reduced by 30 % if WBRT was given. The combined arm contained 65 patients, the SRS arm 67 patients. Almost 50 % of patients had a single lesion. Median survival was 7.5 months after SRS plus WBRT and 8 months after SRS alone. One-year survival in the combined treatment arm was actually relatively increased by 36 %, but this did not reach statistical significance due to low patient numbers (38.5 vs. 28.4 %, $p > 0.05$). After SRS alone, 2 patients developed serious late complications (radionecrosis and grade 4 seizures, respectively). After SRS plus WBRT, 3 patients developed a radionecrosis, and 3 showed signs of leukoencephalopathy. The trial revealed statistically significant differences in local control. The rate of actuarial failure at 1 year was 47 % after combined treatment but significantly greater at 76 % after SRS alone (relative increase of 62 %; $p<0.001$). New lesions developed in 42 vs. 64 % (of SRS alone patients) ($p=0.003$). WBRT reduced the risk of failure at the site of SRS from 27 to 11 % after 1 year ($p=0.002$).

A recent reanalysis of this trial has further fueled the survival debate. Based on a handful of retrospective reviews, substantially underpowered prospective trials, and a meta-analysis based on these underpowered trials, it has been widely concluded that omission of WBRT does not decrease overall survival (OS), primarily because salvage therapies are effective, and systemic progression is the key competing cause of mortality (Sahgal et al. 2015). This assertion may perhaps be true, but diligent review of the available data would caution against jumping to such a conclusion on the basis of the relative weakness of the supporting data, as well as the recent emergence of contradictory data from the aforementioned Japanese trial. An analysis of three pieces of data in the literature should induce a degree of interpretive caution. As early as 1998, Pirzkall et al. reported a single-institution 236-patient retrospective experience of SRS with or without WBRT, demonstrating a trend for superior survival (OS) in favor of WBRT (1- and 2-year OS of 30 vs. 19 and 14 vs. 8 %), but much more impressive was the recognition that in patients without extracranial disease, i.e., in those in whom systemic progression as a competing cause of mortality is largely diminished, the median survival was impressively different at 15.4 vs. 8.3 months, in favor of WBRT (reaching only borderline significance because of the small numbers). This allows one to posit the very reasonable hypothesis that a certain proportion of patients with brain metastases are destined to succumb to intracranial progression (after all we see such compartmental progression as a cause of death in other organs such as the lungs, liver, etc.) and enhanced control of intracranial progression will lengthen their survival.

Finally, a recent reanalysis of the randomized Japanese JROSG-99 trial, using the validated graded prognostic assessment (GPA) stratification model and applied to all non-small cell lung cancer patients on the trial, reveals a median survival of 16.7 versus 10.6 months in favor of the WBRT+SRS arm (vs. SRS alone, $p=0.03$) for the favorable (GPA = 2.5–4) subgroup, without demonstrating an advantage for the inferior prognosis group, providing further support that intracranial control matters and one accepts a lower rate at the potential peril of diminishing overall survival (Aoyama et al. 2006).

A European phase III trial (EORTC 22952-26001) included 359 patients, 199 underwent SRS, and 160 underwent surgery (Kocher et al. 2011). In the SRS group, 100 patients were allocated to observation, and 99 were allocated to WBRT. After surgery, 79 patients were allocated to observation, and 81 were allocated to adjuvant WBRT. The median time to WHO performance status more than 2 was 10.0 months (95 % CI, 8.1–11.7 months) after observation and 9.5 months (95 % CI, 7.8–11.9 months) after WBRT ($p=0.7$). Overall survival was similar in the two arms (median, 10.9 vs. 10.7 months, $p=0.9$). WBRT reduced the 2-year relapse rate both at initial sites (surgery, 59–27 %, $p<0.001$; SRS, 31–19 %, $p=0.04$) and at new sites (surgery, 42–23 %, $p=0.008$; SRS, 48–33 %, $p=0.02$). Salvage therapies were used more frequently after observation than after WBRT. Intracranial progression caused death in 44 % of patients in the observation arm and in 28 % of patients in the WBRT arm.

The randomized trial from the M.D. Anderson Cancer Center re-emphasized patient selection issues as critical for overall survival. In this trial, patients with one to three newly diagnosed brain metastases were randomly assigned to SRS plus WBRT or SRS alone, and over an almost 7-year time frame, 58 patients were recruited and stratified by RPA class, number of brain metastases, and histology (Chang et al. 2009). The primary endpoint was neurocognitive function: measured as a 5-point drop compared with baseline in Hopkins Verbal Learning Test-Revised (HVLT-R) total recall at 4 months. An interim analysis showed that there was a high probability (96 %) that patients assigned to receive SRS plus WBRT were more likely to show a decline in learning and memory function at 4 months than patients assigned to receive SRS alone. Further, at 4 months there were four deaths (13 %) in the group that received SRS alone, and eight deaths (29 %) in the group that received SRS plus WBRT, and 73 % of patients in the SRS plus WBRT group were free from CNS recurrence at 1 year, compared with 27 % of patients who received SRS alone ($p=0.0003$). These differences in early death bring into question the generalizability of the HVLT-R score results; it is well known that a general disease-related decline due to progression, especially in the preterminal phase, will cause a significant drop in neurocognitive function, and its attribution to a single component, such as WBRT, can be misleading. Early deaths in neuro-oncology are almost invariably consequential to systemic progression of disease in this setting. In fact, there were several differences in patient characteristics between the two cohorts which could explain both the early deaths and the differences in 4-month HVLT-R scores. When the constellation of prognostic factors is evaluated collectively, the SRS alone group, compared to SRS plus WBRT, had far more favorable characteristics, such as more female patients (60 vs. 39 %), fewer patients with multiple brain metastases (40 vs. 46 %), lower intracranial disease burden (1.4 vs. 2.3 cc), superior RPA (23 vs. 11 % RPA Class 1) and GPA (10 vs. 3.5 % GPA score 3.5) distribution, fewer patients with liver metastases (7 vs. 18 %), etc.; the small patient numbers precluded any of these factors from individually reaching statistical significance, but taken collectively, the prognostic variables were substantially skewed in favor of the SRS group. As would be expected from the use of WBRT, the 1-year local tumor control rate was 67 % for patients in the SRS group but considerably superior at 100 % for patients in the SRS plus WBRT group, and additionally, the 1-year distant brain tumor control rate was 45 % for patients in the SRS group and 73 % for patients in the SRS plus WBRT group. The 1-year freedom from CNS recurrence was 27 % (95 % CI 14–51) for SRS alone and 73 % (46–100) for SRS plus WBRT. This trial therefore emphasizes three crucial points when evaluating brain metastases data:

1. Local control as well as distant control in the brain is significantly improved by WBRT as an adjunct to focal therapies.
2. Patient selection variables can significantly skew neurocognitive and survival outcomes, and small trials are unlikely to statistically pick up these differences in patient prognostic variables.
3. Early decline in some neurocognitive functions, such as memory recall as measured by HVLT-R, can be impacted by several variables, including WBRT, and the early decline is suggestive of an "early-responding" cell population.

2 Reirradiation: Whole-Brain Radiotherapy

The key issues guiding clinicians in the first-line setting remain important in selecting appropriate management options for patients who relapse after brain irradiation (Table 4). However, few prospective clinical studies formally addressing the role of reirradiation for brain metastases have been published. Salvage WBRT after previous SRS is a common treatment option with survival results indistinguishable from those of first-line WBRT, i.e., usually 3–6 months median survival (Khuntia et al. 2006). A repeat course of WBRT is less commonly employed due to concerns about lack of efficacy and the potential for neurocognitive deficits. Historical experience with WBRT dates back to a retrospective study by Shehata et al. (1974) and another study by Kurup et al. (1980), which will not be reviewed in greater detail. Both are limited by the fact that they date back to the pre-CT era and few systemic treatment options existed at that time. Thus, rapid progression of systemic disease was an even bigger problem than it is now. The first study extending into the CT era, but pre-dating the advent of SRS salvage for recurrence, was reported in 1988 (Hazuka and Kinzie 1988). It included 44 patients (34 % with non-small cell and 20 % with small cell lung cancer), all of

Table 4 Key questions when selecting between the different treatment options for recurrent brain metastases

Is the patient's performance status after initiation of steroid treatment at a level that justifies initiation of radiation therapy?
Do laboratory tests point to advanced extracranial disease status and poor tolerability/efficacy of the planned therapy?
Are extracranial disease sites absent or controlled, and if so, does one expect continued extracranial disease control?
Will systemic treatment be offered or are there no more options left?
Will brain control impact on the survival of the patient or is treatment focused on palliation of symptoms?
Will surgical intervention lead to rapid symptom improvement or effective local control, if comorbidity and other factors allow for consideration of invasive measures? Could the same goals be achieved without surgery?
Might the cumulative radiation dose to critical normal tissue structures result in serious toxicity in patients with expect prolonged survival?
What would be the functional consequence of treatment-induced injury?
How did the lesion(s) respond to initial radiotherapy and how long is the interval?

whom had previously received WBRT for brain metastases. The reasons for retreatment with WBRT (and in a small number of patients, large-volume partial brain reirradiation) were the appearance of new intracranial lesions (47 %), new lesions plus progression of pre-existing metastases (10 %), and local progression of pre-existing metastases only (43 %). The median interval between initial WBRT and reirradiation was 8 months, with a minimum of 8 weeks. The median initial dose was 30 Gy in 10 fractions of 3 Gy, and the median retreatment dose was 25 Gy (range 6–36 Gy, dose per fraction 2–4 Gy). Median survival after repeat WBRT was only 8 weeks. Partial neurological improvement was observed in 27 % of patients. Two patients most likely died as a direct consequence of brain necrosis (brain necropsy result). Both were treated to rather high cumulative doses, especially if one calculates biologically equivalent doses. In one case, WBRT to 32 Gy in 8 fractions of 4 Gy was followed by WBRT to 30 Gy in 10 fractions of 3 Gy (necrosis after 20 weeks from reirradiation). In the other case, WBRT to 30 Gy in 10 fractions of 3 Gy was followed by partial brain RT to 33 Gy in 10 fractions of 3 Gy (necrosis after 11 weeks from reirradiation). The reirradiation tolerance of the human brain is reviewed in detail in other chapters of this book.

Limited, but more recent experience with 2 courses of WBRT in 72 patients, the majority with primary lung cancers suggests that 31 % of patients experienced a partial clinical response after reirradiation (Sadikov et al. 2007). In responders, the mean duration of response was 5.1 months. The median survival after reirradiation was 4.1 months. One patient was reported as having memory impairment and pituitary insufficiency after 5 months of progression-free survival. However, assessment of toxicity in this and other similar series is hampered by their retrospective nature and the poor performance status of most patients. The most frequent dose used for the initial radiotherapy was 20 Gy in 5 fractions. The most common reirradiation schema were 25 Gy in 10 fractions, 20 Gy in 10 fractions, and 15 Gy in 5 fractions. Median interval between the two courses of brain radiation was 9.6 months, with a minimum 8 weeks. The typical patient had a performance status of 1 or 2. Patients with better performance status experienced significantly longer survival after reirradiation, comparable to the study by Aktan et al. (2015; median 2.2 months if KPS ≤70; 5.3 months for all 34 patients). In initial nonresponders, median survival was only 0.9 months after reirradiation, implying that this might be a crucial variable to consider. Surprisingly, the interval between the two courses had no impact on survival.

In another retrospective series of 52 patients, a slightly better clinical response rate (42 %) as well as better median overall survival (almost 5 months) was reported (Cooper et al. 1990). The major difference and potential explanation were that patients were offered reirradiation only if they maintained good general condition for at least 4 months after initial WBRT (median 30 Gy in 10 fractions of 3 Gy), excluding nonresponders, and patients experiencing early decline. The most common reirradiation regimen was 25 Gy in 10 fractions of 2.5 Gy.

Another series, published in 1996 by Wong et al. (86 reirradiated patients including 18 with partial brain fields), included an equal number of lung and breast cancer patients (31 each). The median dose of initial WBRT was 30 Gy, usually given in 10 fractions. The median interval to reirradiation was 7.6 months, with a minimum of 6 weeks. The median dose of reirradiation was 20 Gy, with a maximum 30.6 Gy. Complete or partial symptomatic neurological improvement was observed in 27 and 43 % of patients, respectively. The median response duration was 2.8 months. Median survival was 4 months. The only significant prognostic factor for survival was the absence of extracranial metastases. Scharp et al. (2014) analyzed 134 patients, of whom 60 were treated with initial prophylactic WBRT (87 % had lung cancer). The median interval was 13 months (minimum 3) and the median doses 30 plus 20 Gy, both in 2-Gy fractions. Median survival was 2.8 months, and clinical improvement was observed in 39 % of patients. Significantly shorter survival was seen in patients with small cell lung cancer, KPS <70, or progressive primary tumor. A series of 49 patients was reported from Guo et al. (2014). Median interval was 11.5 months (minimum 1.5 months), median initial dose 30 Gy, and median repeat dose 20 Gy. Median KPS was 70. Improved symptoms were reported in 27 %, and median survival was 3 months. Comparable results were reported by Ozgen et al. (2013); median survival in 28 patients was 3 months and symptomatic response rate 39 %.

Minniti et al. (2014) combined reirradiation (25 Gy, 10 fractions) with concurrent temozolomide (75 mg/m^2). They treated 27 patients whose median age was 54 years. Minimum KPS was 60. Eighteen patients had lung cancer. Median survival was 6.2 months. Seventeen patients (63 %) had improved symptoms. Severe toxicity was not observed. Survival was significantly longer in patients with stable or absent extracranial disease. Survival was slightly better than in other studies, but interstudy comparison is hampered by the heterogeneity of the different study populations. Without randomized trials, the role of temozolomide is difficult to define.

Overall, the studies reviewed here reported median survival of 2–6.2 months (median 4.0) and improvement of symptoms in 27–70 % of patients (median 35 %). Shorter survival was seen in patients with KPS <70, progressive primary tumor, or extracranial metastases.

Helical tomotherapy can also be utilized in patients who develop multiple brain metastases in spite of previous WBRT (Sterzing et al. 2009). Both patients treated with this technique had previously received 40 Gy in 20 fractions of 2 Gy. The whole-brain reirradiation dose was limited to 15 Gy, while the enhancing lesions plus a 2-mm margin received 30 Gy in 10 fractions of 3 Gy. In the first case, 8 metastases from breast cancer were present 18 months after first-line WBRT. With a follow-up of 12 months, local control was achieved. In the second case, 11 metastases from non-small cell lung cancer were present 18 months after initial WBRT. With a follow-up of 6 months, local control was achieved. No serious toxicity was recorded. In Fig. 1, we show an example of a patient with multiple recurrent brain metastases from breast cancer treated with tomotherapy. The patient had received two prior courses of WBRT, initially 30 Gy in 10 fractions and then 25 Gy in 10 fractions both achieving complete responses; five subsequent individual recurrences were treated with two courses of SRS, also resulting in complete response; the tomotherapy IMRT plan was utilized for 9 new lesions, and the dose was 30 Gy in 15 fractions; most of the normal brain was kept below 10 Gy, and the patient has sustained local control more than 8 months after this course of therapy and for over 42 months since initial presentation with brain metastases. The case illustrates that with modern and advanced radiotherapy techniques, innovative salvage options become possible, and anecdotally, in selected patients, local control and durable survival are achieved. Figures 2, 3, and 4 provide treatment details regarding three other patients at one of the authors' institutions, utilizing other unique radiotherapy approaches.

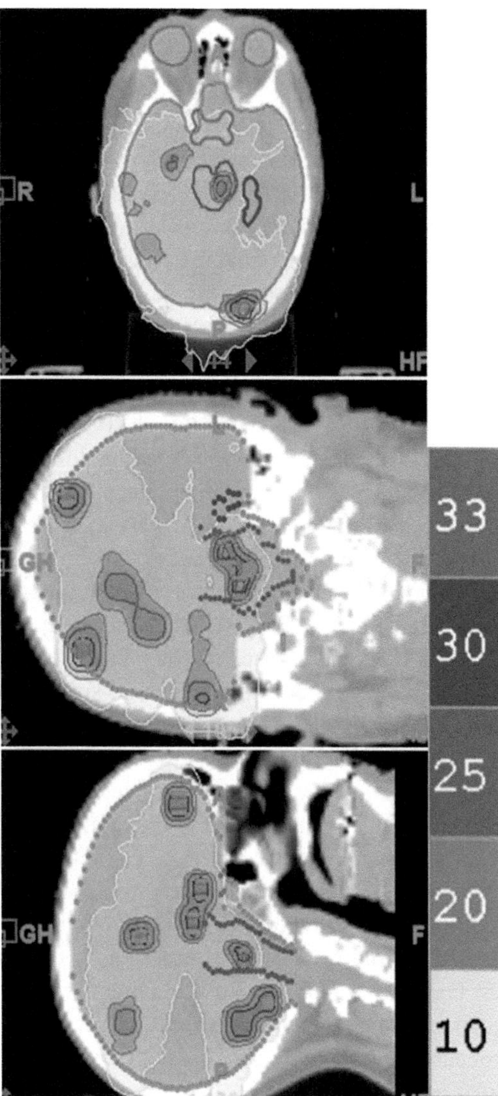

Fig. 1 An example of a patient with multiple recurrent brain metastases from breast cancer treated with tomotherapy. The patient had received two prior courses of WBRT, initially 30 Gy in 10 fractions and then 25 Gy in 10 fractions both achieving complete responses; five subsequent individual recurrences were treated with two courses of radiosurgery, also resulting in complete response; the tomotherapy IMRT plan was utilized for nine new lesions, and the dose was 30 Gy in 15 fractions; most of the normal brain was kept below 10 Gy, and the patient has sustained local control more than 8 months after this course of therapy and for over 42 months since initial presentation with brain metastases

3 Reirradiation: Stereotactic Radiosurgery

The potential advantages of SRS as salvage treatment after WBRT were realized early during the development of this technique (Loeffler et al. 1990). Several series published in the early 1990s included some patients reirradiated with SRS (Adler et al. 1992; Engenhart et al. 1993). Their results lead to recommendations that patients with recurrent lesions should be treated with stereotactic high-precision techniques. The RTOG embarked on a prospective phase I clinical trial of SRS in recurrent, previously irradiated primary brain tumors and brain metastases, one of few prospective studies in the field. RTOG study 90-05 was a dose escalation trial, which included 100 patients with brain metastases and 56 with primary brain tumors. The brain metastasis patients were included after prior WBRT to a median dose of 30 Gy (Shaw et al. 1996, 2000). SRS could be administered with a linear accelerator or Gamma Knife. Eligible patients had received first-line radiotherapy at least 3 months prior to study entry, and in the study, the actual median interval was 17 months. Their KPS was ≥60 and life expectancy ≥3 months. Seventy-eight percent had single lesions. Dose was determined by the maximum diameter of the tumor. Initial doses were 18 Gy for lesions ≤20 mm, 15 Gy for lesions measuring 21–30 mm, and 12 Gy for lesions measuring 31–40 mm. Dose was prescribed to the 50–90% isodose line, which was to encompass the entire enhancing target volume. The dose was escalated in 3 Gy increments providing there was not an excess of unacceptable toxicity. The trial eventually defined the maximum acutely tolerable SRS dose in this setting, except for lesions ≤20 mm where the dose was not escalated beyond 24 Gy because of investigators' reluctance. While small lesions ≤20 mm can be treated with up to 24 Gy to the margin of the lesion, those that measure between 21 and 30 mm might receive 18 Gy and those that measure between 31 and 40 mm 15 Gy.

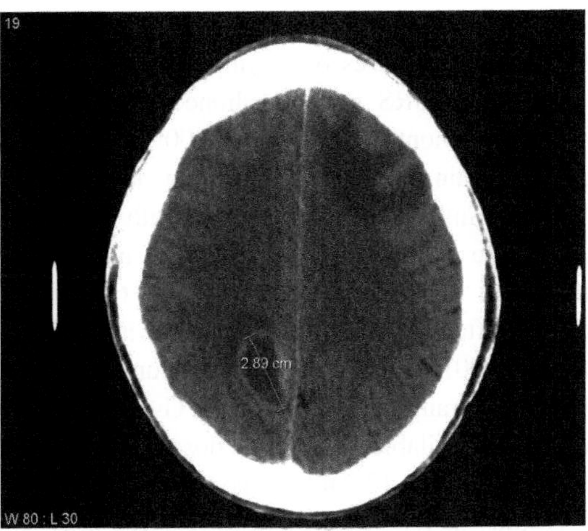

Fig. 2 An illustrative case from one of the authors' institutions (Nordland Hospital Bodø, Norway). A 63-year-old male patient was diagnosed with squamous cell lung cancer stage III B in December 2007. He received systemic platinum-based chemotherapy and thoracic radiotherapy. In November 2008, the patient collapsed, and a computed tomography (CT) scan of the brain revealed four brain metastases, maximum diameter 3.1 cm. No extracranial metastases were detected; all laboratory tests were unremarkable. The intrathoracic status was judged to be ongoing partial remission. The patients Karnofsky performance status (KPS) at that time was 70. Whole-brain radiotherapy (WBRT) was administered (10 fractions of 3 Gy). Three months later, CT scans of the brain showed partial remission of all four lesions. However, another 3 months later, all 4 lesions had increased in size. No additional new brain metastases were detected. The patient was referred for salvage treatment. When considering the key questions presented in Table 4, the following statements could be made.

Is the patient's performance status after initiation of steroid treatment at a level that justifies initiation of radiation therapy? Yes, the KPS at the time of progression was 70.

Do laboratory tests point to advanced extracranial disease status and poor tolerability/efficacy of the planned therapy? No, the only abnormal finding was slight anemia.

Are extracranial disease sites absent or controlled, and if so, does one expect continued extracranial disease control? No extracranial metastases were detected, but the primary tumor had increased slightly (less than 25 %, no clinical symptoms).

Will systemic treatment be offered, or are there no more options left? Second-line chemotherapy in case of symptomatic progression of the lung tumor was an option.

Will brain control impact on the survival of the patient or is treatment focused on palliation of symptoms? The biggest threat at that time was death from uncontrolled brain metastases.

Will surgical intervention lead to rapid symptom improvement or effective local control, if comorbidity and other factors allow for consideration of invasive measures? Could the same goals be achieved without surgery? No surgical candidate based on the number of brain metastases. None of them caused hydrocephalus or other immediately threatening complications.

Might the cumulative radiation dose to critical normal tissue structures result in serious toxicity in patients with expect prolonged survival? The probability of long-term survival was considered low.

What would be the functional consequence of treatment-induced injury? Not applicable.

How did the lesion(s) respond to initial radiotherapy and how long is the interval? All 4 metastases had initially responded, the interval of 6 months did permit reirradiation.

The image above shows the second largest brain metastasis (diameter 2.9 cm, cystic lesion) and the contralateral edema indicating the presence of another lesion, which was slightly larger. When deciding between stereotactic radiosurgery (SRS) and other options in this case, the following facts were considered. Based on number and size of the lesions as well as the limited survival expectation after second-line chemotherapy in patients with relapsed non-small cell lung cancer, the patient was not an ideal candidate for SRS. Repeat WBRT was not necessary as no new lesions were present and the 4 metastases could be covered by a quite simple 3-dimensional conformal radiotherapy technique with two isocenters and two non-overlapping pairs of opposing fields, each covering two of the metastases. A dose of 30 Gy in 10 fractions of 3 Gy was given. As after the first course (30 Gy WBRT), a partial remission was obtained. The patient did not develop serious acute or late toxicity. He died without obvious neurological deficits 6.3 months after reirradiation as a result of pneumonia, which was considered a complication of the primary lung cancer

Median survival was 7.5 months. A 1-year survival rate of 26 % was observed. Some cases of further local progression in spite of SRS were observed, mainly within the first 6 months after SRS. Long-term toxicity data for brain metastasis patients are available only from the initial publication (Shaw et al. 1996). They are based on 64 patients. Four patients developed radionecrosis requiring operation 5–14 months after SRS. From the final report (Shaw et al. 2000), combined radionecrosis data on patients with brain metastases and primary brain tumors are available. The actuarial incidence was 8 and 11 % at 12 and 24 months, respectively. This study therefore provides tentative evidence that retreatment with SRS can produce local control in a certain proportion of brain metastases patients, but the approximate 10 % incidence of necrosis must be factored in. Several options can be considered to either lower this rate or possibly manage necrosis, including fractionated stereotactic radiotherapy and the recent use of bevacizumab, which might improve symptoms and imaging findings resulting from radionecrosis (Gonzalez et al. 2007; Torcuator et al. 2009; Boothe et al. 2013).

Linear accelerator-based SRS was used in 54 patients with 97 metastases (recurrent after WBRT) in another study (Noël et al. 2001). The patients' KPS was 60-100. The median interval was 9 months, with a minimum of 2 months. The median tumor volume was 1.2 cc. A median minimal dose of 16.2 Gy was prescribed, while the median maximal dose was 21.2 Gy. No serious side effects were reported with this dose prescription. Only 5 metastases recurred after salvage SRS. The 1-year survival rate was 31 %. RPA class was a significant prognostic factor for overall survival. Comparable outcomes were achieved in a retrospective series that included 111 patients (Chao et al. 2008). SRS doses were usually prescribed according to the RTOG 90-05 guidelines. Median survival was 9.9 months. Twenty-five percent of patients devel-

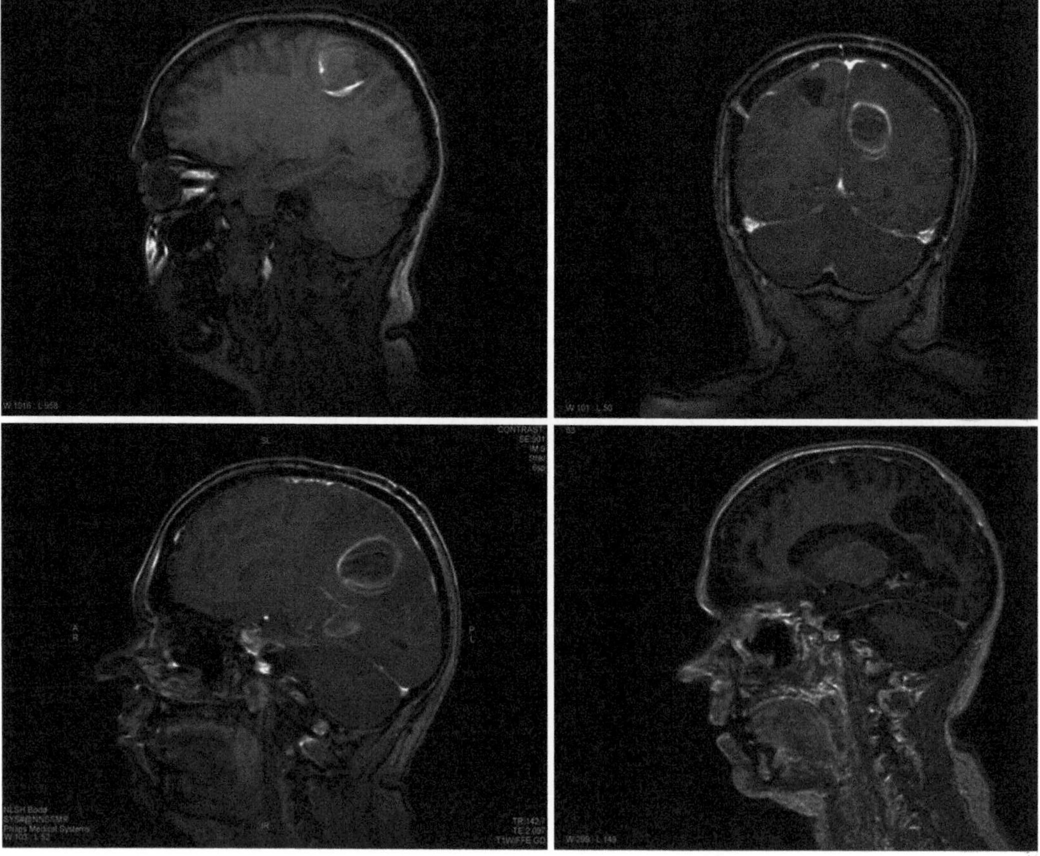

oped further local progression in spite of salvage SRS. Poorer local control was observed in lesions >2 cm, which usually had been treated with lower radiation doses. Gwak et al. treated 46 patients with 100 recurrent metastases with CyberKnife radiosurgery (2009). The average dose was 23 Gy in 1–3 fractions. The median interval from WBRT was 5 months. The mean volume was 12.4 cc. Median survival was 10 months, but 1-year progression-free survival was only 57 %. In these patients with quite large metastases, e.g., compared to the abovementioned series by Noël et al. (2001), acute toxicity was observed in 22 % of patients. Toxicity after >6 months occurred in 21 %.

More recent data were derived from a retrospective review of 106 patients irradiated for a median of 2 metastases (range, 1–12) with a median dose of 21 Gy (range, 12–24) prescribed to the 50 % isodose (Kurtz et al. 2014). With a median follow-up of 10.5 months, local control was 83 % at 6 months and 60 % at 1 year. Median progression-free survival was 6.2 months. Median overall survival was 11.7 months from salvage SRS and 22 months from initial diagnosis. Caballero et al. (2012) analyzed 310 patients. The median number of brain metastases was 3 and interval from WBRT to SRS 8 months. The median survival was 8.4 months overall and 12.0 vs. 7.9 months for single vs. multiple lesions ($p=0.001$). There was no relationship between number of lesions and survival after excluding patients with single metastases. Retrospective population-based data from Canada suggested that salvage SRS after WBRT was not associated with compromised survival compared to immediate boost SRS (Hsu et al. 2013).

A large analysis of 2200 metastases treated with Gamma Knife SRS also included a subgroup of 72 lesions that were reirradiated with a second SRS (Sneed et al. 2015). Prescribed dose was chosen primarily based on treatment volume or location in the brainstem, not taking into account prior WBRT or SRS. After prior SRS, the median dose was

Fig. 3 An illustrative case from one of the authors' institutions (Nordland Hospital Bodø, Norway). The patient is a 45-year-old female. In October 2004, she had noted a few days of hypesthesia in her left leg, followed by slight hemiparesis and a seizure resulting in hospitalization. A magnetic resonance imaging (MRI) scan of the brain revealed a tumor in the right parietal lobe, presumably representing a glioma. In November 2004, a partial resection (because of the proximity to the motor cortex) was performed. Histology demonstrated a malignant melanoma metastasis. Staging including examinations of the eyes, head, and neck mucosa and total skin, gynecological evaluation, bone scintigraphy, and computed tomography (CT) scans showed an enlarged left adrenal gland as the only pathological finding. The adrenal mass was removed completely by laparoscopic surgery, and histology corresponded to that of the brain metastasis. Treatment proceeded with postoperative whole-brain radiotherapy (WBRT), 10 fractions of 3 Gy, without boost. In February 2005, the patient noted headaches and a decreasing general condition. A MRI scan disclosed two new brain metastases in the left parietal and temporal lobe, respectively (see image below: previous resection cavity in the right parietal lobe, new lesions in the left hemisphere). While the parietal tumor could be resected completely, the temporal lesion was treated with Gamma Knife radiosurgery (SRS). The peripheral minimum dose was 15 Gy.

In March 2005, the patient developed abdominal symptoms, and a CT scan showed a right abdominal mass presumably representing inflammation in and around the vermiform appendix and ovary. Surgery including ovarectomy and appendectomy was performed, and the histology demonstrated again the same type of malignant melanoma. The tumor was limited to the vermiform appendix without spread to peritoneum or lymph nodes and was judged to be removed completely. After a symptom-free interval, routine MRI evaluation in November 2005 disclosed progression of the unresectable SRS-treated temporal lesion, and a second Gamma Knife procedure was performed. The interval to the previous SRS was approximately 8 months. Since then, the patient returned to repeated follow-up examinations including MRI and CT scans. The last one was performed in March 2015, i.e., more than 10 years after the first neurosurgical resection. No potential signs of disease were detectable. The patient has a Karnofsky performance status (KPS) of 80 % resulting from slight concentration and endurance problems. No radionecrosis or other serious complication was recorded in this unusual case, which illustrates the potential impact of aggressive local management in highly selected patients. Of course, the potential diagnosis of radiation necrosis after SRS must be excluded by appropriate imaging methods such as positron emission tomography (PET) with an amino acid tracer, e.g., ^{11}C-methionine, or newer MRI techniques incl. spectroscopy before proceeding to further radiation treatment. In some cases, a histopathological diagnosis of recurrent metastasis might be required. Further information on differentiation between radionecrosis and recurrent tumor can be found in the following studies and reviews: Sundgren 2009 (MR spectroscopy), Barajas et al. 2009 (dynamic susceptibility-weighted contrast-enhanced perfusion MRI), Dequesada et al. 2008 (MRI), Terakawa et al. 2008 and Chung et al. 2002 (PET), Serizawa et al. 2005 (single photon emission computed tomography), Walker et al. 2014 (overview)

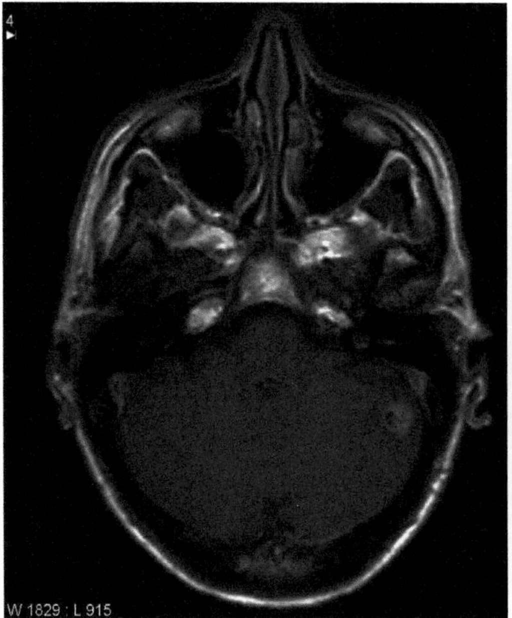

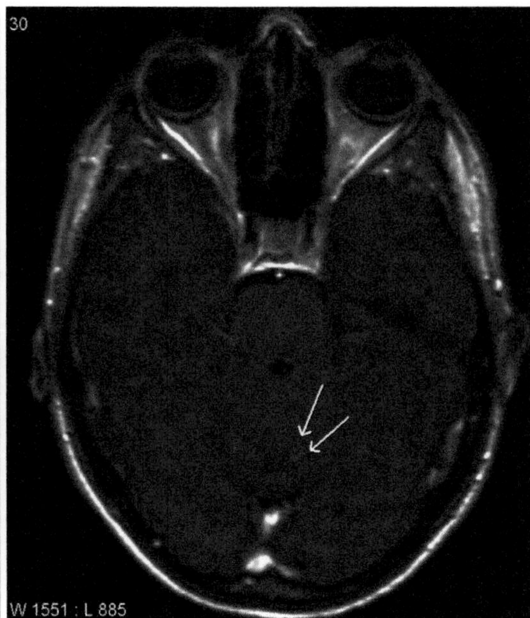

Fig. 4 An illustrative case from one of the authors' institutions (Nordland Hospital Bodø, Norway). The patient is a 46-year-old female with triple-negative breast cancer stage T1 N0 M0. Two years after the initial diagnosis and breast conserving treatment, headaches led to magnetic resonance imaging (MRI) diagnosis of a single 7-mm-large cerebellar metastasis. Pulmonary metastases were detected at the same time. *Arrows* are needed to indicate where the lesion is located

Treatment consisted of stereotactic radiosurgery and systemic chemotherapy (two different lines, anthracycline based and taxanes). Nine months later, four new brain metastases were found (supra- and infratentorial; one example is shown above).

The pulmonary metastases progressed at the same time. The patients Karnofsky performance status was 70. She received palliative whole-brain radiotherapy (WBRT), 30 Gy in 10 fractions of 3 Gy. She then started third-line chemotherapy with capecitabine. A partial remission of all 4 brain metastases was achieved, but the pulmonary disease progressed further. The patient died 5 months after WBRT from progressive pulmonary metastases with pleural and pericardiac effusions

18 Gy and the median target volume size 0.94 cc. Adverse radiation effects were judged on serial MRI scans. The 1-year cumulative incidence was 20 % for symptomatic and 37 % for overall adverse radiation effects. Compared to SRS without any prior or concomitant further radiotherapy, the hazard ratio for adverse radiation effects after re-SRS was 3.7 (95 % confidence interval 1.3–10.8; multivariate analysis). Efficacy results were not reported.

4 Reirradiation: Fractionated Stereotactic Radiotherapy (FSRT)

A normal brain tissue dose recommendation in SRS planning is to limit the volume receiving 10 Gy or more to 10–12 cc. For larger tumors, or those in proximity to critical sensitive structures, fractionated high-precision treatment with stereotactic localization and mask fixation of the head might offer a solution (Fig. 5). Only relatively small patient series are available to assess the outcomes with this approach. A Japanese series included seven patients with previously irradiated brain metastases (Tokuuye et al. 1998). The patient characteristics are comparable to those from other SRS series, but lesion size was larger. Fractionation was individualized, e.g., 33 Gy in 11 fractions of 3 Gy or 24 Gy in 4 fractions of 6 Gy. In these selected patients, results comparable to those of the RTOG SRS trial were found. In a Canadian study, SRS was used in smaller lesions ($n=35$, maximum diameter 3 cm for supratentorial and 2 cm for posterior fossa metastases, dose of 22.5 Gy prescribed to the 90 % isodose), while a split dose was used in larger ones (29.7 Gy at the 90 % isodose surface

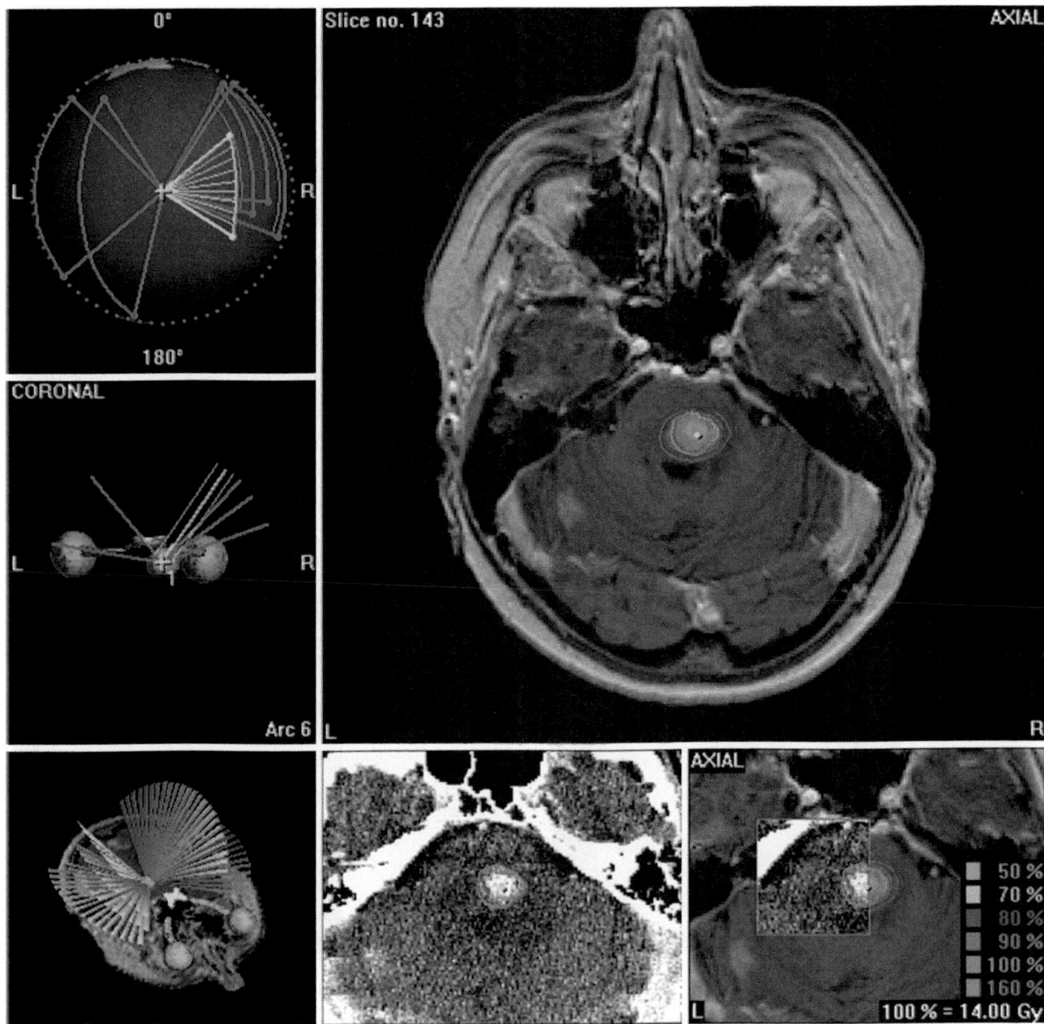

Fig. 5 A hypothetical case with a rather large metastasis in the brain stem where the therapeutic ratio of stereotactic radiosurgery is small. The long-term tumor control probability with a margin dose of 14 Gy, as displayed here, is not satisfactory. Under such circumstances, fractionated stereotactic radiotherapy might be considered

in 2 fractions, $n = 69$) (Davey et al. 2007). A total of 180 metastases were treated in these 104 patients. The median time from WBRT to SRS was 7.6 months, and from WBRT to fractionated treatment, it was 6 months. Median survival after retreatment was 4 months after SRS and 6 months after 2 fractions.

The results of FSRT after SRS in 43 patients with 47 lesions were reported by Minniti et al. (2016). The patients received three daily fractions of 7–8 Gy. The 1-year survival rate was 37 % and the 1-year local control rate 70 %. Compared to NSCLC and breast cancer metastases, those from malignant melanoma were significantly less likely to be locally controlled. Better KPS and stable extracranial disease predicted for longer survival. The risk of radiological changes suggestive of radionecrosis was 34 % at 1 year (crude rate 19 % or 9/47 lesions). Fourteen percent of patients had associated neurological deficits RTOG grade 2 or 3. Figure 6 shows examples of amino acid (MET and FET) positron emission tomography (PET) after SRS.

As reported by Holt et al. (2015), surgical resection is often favored after initial SRS because it provides pathological characterization of any

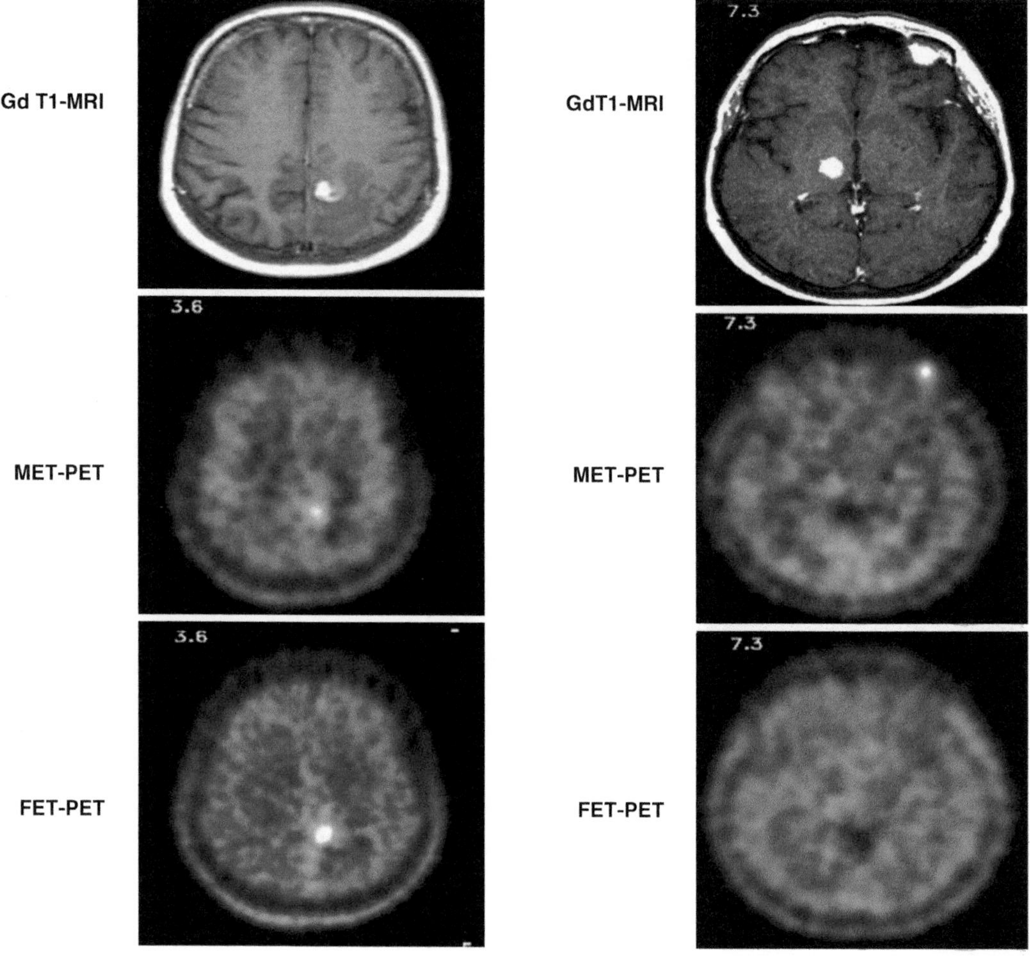

Fig. 6 After stereotactic radiosurgery for brain metastases, amino acid (MET and FET) positron emission tomography (*PET*) may facilitate differentiation between local recurrence (**a**) and radiation-induced toxicity (**b**)

residual tumor. Their experience with SRS followed by surgery and further FSRT or SRS to the tumor bed relates to 15 lesions in 13 patients. Ten lesions received adjuvant radiotherapy; the remaining 5 were treated after additional local tumor growth was detected. Malignant melanoma was the prevailing primary diagnosis (60 %). The median interval was 6 months and the median follow-up after reirradiation 9 months. Initial SRS was given to a median dose of 21 Gy (range 18–27; median size 4.3 cc). The median reirradiation dose was 21 Gy (range 16–30 in 1–3 fractions; median size 9.4 cc). Eight patients received further radiotherapy for new metastases during the disease trajectory, WBRT or SRS. Local control at 1 year was 75 %. One-year survival rate was 43 %. One patient developed grade 2 radionecrosis with grade 3 seizures and another patient grade 3 radionecrosis.

Kim et al. (2013) analyzed outcomes in patients without prior WBRT who were treated with a second course of SRS/FSRT for locally or regionally recurrent metastases, $n=32$. Multivariate analysis showed that upon retreatment, local recurrences were more likely to fail than regional recurrences (hazard ratio 8.8, $p=0.02$). Median survival for all patients from first SRS/FSRT was 14.6 and 7.9 months from second SRS/FSRT. Thirty-eight percent of patients ultimately received WBRT as salvage therapy after the second SRS/FSRT.

5 Reirradiation: Brachytherapy

The majority of reports on brachytherapy for recurrent brain metastases were published in the 1980s and 1990s, i.e., before SRS and FSRT became widely available. They are reviewed very briefly. The retrospective study from Freiburg, Germany, included 21 patients with recurrent brain metastases after previous radiotherapy with or without surgery (Ostertag and Kreth 1995). Interstitial 125-iodine implants were used. Median survival was 6 months. A Canadian series reported on 10 patients with local recurrences after surgery and WBRT (Bernstein et al. 1995). The median interval to 125-iodine brachytherapy was 8 months. Five patients died of further local progression. Median survival was almost 11 months. Two reports from the University of California San Francisco also describe the role of brachytherapy. In 1989, this group published the results of 14 patients with progressive brain metastases (13 had been treated with WBRT) (Prados et al. 1989). Twenty years later, a new report including 21 such patients was published (Huang et al. 2009). These 21 patients were treated between 1997 and 2003, i.e., approximately 3.5 patients per year. Median survival in the most recent study was 7.3 months. The 1-year local freedom from progression probability was 86%. The brain freedom from progression probability was lower, i.e., 43%, as a result of new lesions. Radiation necrosis might develop more often after brachytherapy than after SRS, but no randomized head-to-head comparison in patients with recurrent brain metastases is available.

References

Adler JR, Cox RS, Kaplan I, Martin DP (1992) Stereotactic radiosurgical treatment of brain metastases. J Neurosurg 76:444–449

Agboola O, Benoit B, Cross P et al (1998) Prognostic factors derived from recursive partitioning analysis (RPA) of Radiation Therapy Oncology Group (RTOG) brain metastases trials applied to surgically resected and irradiated brain metastatic cases. Int J Radiat Oncol Biol Phys 42:155–159

Aktan K, Koc M, Kanyilmaz G, Tezcan Y (2015) Outcomes of reirradiation in the treatment of patients with multiple brain metastases of solid tumors: a retrospective analysis. Ann Transl Med 3:325

Ammirati M, Cobbs CS, Linskey ME et al (2010) The role of retreatment in the management of recurrent/progressive brain metastases: a systematic review and evidence-based clinical practice guideline. J Neurooncol 96:85–96

Andrews DW, Scott CB, Sperduto PW et al (2004) Whole brain radiation therapy with or without stereotactic radiosurgery boost for patients with one to three brain metastases: phase III results of the RTOG 9508 randomised trial. Lancet 363:1665–1672

Antoniou D, Kyprianou K, Stathopoulos GP et al (2005) Response to radiotherapy in brain metastases and survival of patients with non-small cell lung cancer. Oncol Rep 14:733–736

Aoyama H, Shirato H, Tago M et al (2006) Stereotactic radiosurgery plus whole-brain radiation therapy vs stereotactic radiosurgery alone for treatment of brain metastases. A randomized controlled trial. JAMA 295:2483–2491

Aoyama H, Tago M, Kato N et al (2007) Neurocognitive function of patients with brain metastasis who received either whole brain radiotherapy plus stereotactic radiosurgery or radiosurgery alone. Int J Radiat Oncol Biol Phys 68:1388–1395

Barajas RF, Chang JS, Sneed PK et al (2009) Distinguishing recurrent intra-axial metastatic tumor from radiation necrosis following gamma knife radiosurgery using dynamic susceptibility-weighted contrast-enhanced perfusion MR imaging. AJNR Am J Neuroradiol 30:367–372

Barnholtz-Sloan JS, Yu C, Sloan AE et al (2012) A nomogram for individualized estimation of survival among patients with brain metastasis. Neuro Oncol 14:910–918

Bernstein M, Cabantog A, Laperriere N et al (1995) Brachytherapy for recurrent single brain metastasis. Can J Neurol Sci 22:13–16

Bhatnagar AK, Kondziolka D, Lunsford LD, Flickinger JC (2007) Recursive partitioning analysis of prognostic factors for patients with four or more intracranial metastases treated with radiosurgery. Technol Cancer Res Treat 6:153–160

Boothe D, Young R, Yamada Y et al (2013) Bevacizumab as a treatment for radiation necrosis of brain metastases post stereotactic radiosurgery. Neuro Oncol 15:1257–1263

Borgelt B, Gelber R, Larson M et al (1980) The palliation of brain metastases: final results of the first two studies of the Radiation Therapy Oncology Group. Int J Radiat Oncol Biol Phys 6:1–9

Borgelt B, Gelber R, Kramer S et al (1981) Ultra-rapid high dose irradiation scheduled for the palliation of brain metastases. Int J Radiat Oncol Biol Phys 7:1633–1638

Brown PD, Asher AL, Ballman KV et al. (2015) NCCTG N0574 (Alliance): A phase III randomized trial of whole brain radiation therapy (WBRT) in addition to radiosurgery (SRS) in patients with 1 to 3 brain metastases. J Clin Oncol 33, (suppl; abstr LBA4).

Caballero JA, Sneed PK, Lamborn KR et al (2012) Prognostic factors for survival in patients treated with stereotactic radiosurgery for recurrent brain metastases after prior whole brain radiotherapy. Int J Radiat Oncol Biol Phys 83:303–309

Chang EL, Wefel JS, Hess KR et al (2009) Neurocognition in patients with brain metastases treated with radiosurgery or radiosurgery plus whole-brain irradiation: a randomised controlled trial. Lancet Oncol 10:1037–1044

Chao ST, Barnett GH, Vogelbaum MA et al (2008) Salvage stereotactic radiosurgery effectively treats recurrences from whole-brain radiation therapy. Cancer 113:2198–2204

Chatani M, Matayoshi Y, Masaki N, Inoue T (1994) Radiation therapy for brain metastases from lung carcinoma. Prospective randomized trial according to the level of lactate dehydrogenase. Strahlenther Onkol 170:155–161

Cho KH, Hall WA, Gerbi BJ et al (1998) Patient selection criteria for the treatment of brain metastases with stereotactic radiosurgery. J Neurooncol 40:73–86

Chung JK, Kim YK, Kim SK et al (2002) Usefulness of 11C-methionine PET in the evaluation of brain lesions that are hypo- or isometabolic on 18F-FDG PET. Eur J Nucl Med Mol Imaging 29:176–182

Cooper J, Steinfeld A, Lerch I (1990) Cerebral metastases: value of reirradiation in selected patients. Radiology 174:883–885

Davey P, Schwartz ML, Scora D et al (2007) Fractionated (split dose) radiosurgery in patients with recurrent brain metastases: implications for survival. Br J Neurosurg 21:491–495

Dequesada IM, Quisling RG, Yachnis A, Friedman WA (2008) Can standard magnetic resonance imaging reliably distinguish recurrent tumor from radiation necrosis after radiosurgery for brain metastases? A radiographic-pathological study. Neurosurgery 63:898–903

Engenhart R, Kimmig BN, Höver KH et al (1993) Long-term follow-up for brain metastases treated by percutaneous stereotactic single high-dose irradiation. Cancer 71:1353–1361

Gaspar L, Scott C, Rotman M et al (1997) Recursive partitioning analysis (RPA) of prognostic factors in three Radiation Therapy Oncology Group (RTOG) brain metastases trials. Int J Radiat Oncol Biol Phys 37:745–751

Gaspar LE, Mehta MP, Patchell RA et al (2010) The role of whole brain radiation therapy in the management of newly diagnosed brain metastases: a systematic review and evidence-based clinical practice guideline. J Neurooncol 96(1):17–32; available as epub online

Gelber RD, Larson M, Borgelt BB, Kramer S (1981) Equivalence of radiation schedules for the palliative treatment of brain metastases in patients with favorable prognosis. Cancer 48:1749–1753

Gonzalez J, Kumar AJ, Conrad CA, Levin VA (2007) Effect of bevacizumab on radiation necrosis of the brain. Int J Radiat Oncol Biol Phys 67:323–326

Guo S, Balagamwala EH, Reddy C et al (2014) Clinical and radiographic outcomes from repeat whole-brain radiation therapy for brain metastases in the age of stereotactic radiosurgery. Am J Clin Oncol, epub

Gwak HS, Yoo HJ, Youn SM et al (2009) Radiosurgery for recurrent brain metastases after whole-brain radiotherapy: factors affecting radiation-induced neurological outcome. J Korean Neurosurg Soc 45:275–283

Hazuka MB, Kinzie JJ (1988) Brain metastases: results and effects of re-irradiation. Int J Radiat Oncol Biol Phys 15:433–437

Heflin LH, Meyerowitz BE, Hall P et al (2005) Cancer as a risk factor for long-term cognitive deficits and dementia. J Natl Cancer Inst 97:854–856

Holt DE, Gill BS, Clump DA et al (2015) Tumor bed radiosurgery following resection and prior stereotactic radiosurgery for locally persistent brain metastasis. Front Oncol 5:84

Hsu F, Kouhestani P, Nguyen S et al (2013) Population-based outcomes of boost versus salvage radiosurgery for brain metastases after whole brain radiotherapy. Radiother Oncol 108:128–131

Huang K, Sneed PK, Kunwar S et al (2009) Surgical resection and permanent iodine-125 brachytherapy for brain metastases. J Neurooncol 91:83–93

Khuntia D, Brown P, Li J, Mehta MP (2006) Whole-brain radiotherapy in the management of brain metastasis. J Clin Oncol 24:1295–1304

Kim DH, Schultheiss TE, Radany EH et al (2013) Clinical outcomes of patients treated with a second course of stereotactic radiosurgery for locally or regionally recurrent brain metastases after prior stereotactic radiosurgery. J Neurooncol 115:37–43

Klein M, Heimans JJ, Aaronson NK et al (2002) Effect of radiotherapy and other treatment-related factors on mid-term to long-term cognitive sequelae in low-grade gliomas: a comparative study. Lancet 360:1361–1368

Kocher M, Voges J, Müller RP et al (1998) Linac radiosurgery for patients with a limited number of brain metastases. J Radiosurg 1:9–15

Kocher M, Soffietti R, Abacioglu U et al (2011) Adjuvant whole-brain radiotherapy versus observation after radiosurgery or surgical resection of one to three cerebral metastases: results of the EORTC 22952-26001 study. J Clin Oncol 29:134–141

Kondziolka D, Patel A, Lunsford LD et al (1999) Stereotactic radiosurgery plus whole brain radiotherapy versus radiotherapy alone for patients with multiple brain metastases. Int J Radiat Oncol Biol Phys 45:427–434

Kurtz G, Zadeh G, Gingras-Hill G et al (2014) Salvage radiosurgery for brain metastases: prognostic factors to consider in patient selection. Int J Radiat Oncol Biol Phys 88:137–142

Kurup P, Reddy S, Hendrickson FR (1980) Results of re-irradiation for cerebral metastases. Cancer 46:2587–2589

Li J, Bentzen SM, Renschler M et al (2007) Regression after whole-brain radiation therapy for brain metastases correlates with survival and improved neurocognitive function. J Clin Oncol 25:1260–1266

Loeffler JS, Kooy HM, Wen PY et al (1990) The treatment of recurrent brain metastases with stereotactic radiosurgery. J Clin Oncol 8:576–582

Lorenzoni J, Devriendt D, Massager N et al (2004) Radiosurgery for treatment of brain metastases: estimation of patient eligibility using three stratification systems. Int J Radiat Oncol Biol Phys 60:218–224

Lutterbach J, Bartelt S, Stancu E, Guttenberger R (2002) Patients with brain metastases: hope for recursive partitioning analysis (RPA) class 3. Radiother Oncol 63:339–345

Minniti G, Scaringi C, Lanzetta G et al (2014) Whole brain reirradiation and concurrent temozolomide in patients with brain metastases. J Neurooncol 118:329–334

Minniti G, Scaringi C, Paolini S et al (2016) Repeated stereotactic radiosurgery for patients with progressive brain metastases. J Neurooncol 126(1):91–97

Nieder C, Berberich W, Schnabel K (1997) Tumor-related prognostic factors for remission of brain metastases after radiotherapy. Int J Radiat Oncol Biol Phys 39:25–30

Nieder C, Nestle U, Motaref B et al (2000) Prognostic factors in brain metastases: should patients be selected for aggressive treatment according to recursive partitioning analysis (RPA) classes? Int J Radiat Oncol Biol Phys 46:297–302

Nieder C, Geinitz H, Molls M (2008) Validation of the graded prognostic assessment index for surgically treated patients with brain metastases. Anticancer Res 28:3015–3017

Nieder C, Marienhagen K, Geinitz H et al (2009) Validation of the graded prognostic assessment index for patients with brain metastases. Acta Oncol 48:457–459

Nieder C, Leicht A, Motaref B, Nestle U, Niewald M, Schnabel K (1999) Late radiation toxicity after whole brain radiotherapy: the influence of antiepileptic drugs. Am J Clin Oncol. 22(6):573–9

Nieder C, Oehlke O, Hintz M, Grosu AL (2015) The challenge of durable brain control in patients with brain-only metastases from breast cancer. Springerplus 4:585

Noël G, Proudhom MA, Valery CA et al (2001) Radiosurgery for reirradiation of brain metastases: results in 54 patients. Radiother Oncol 60:61–67

Ostertag CB, Kreth FW (1995) Interstitial iodine-125 radiosurgery for cerebral metastases. Br J Neurosurg 9:593–603

Ozgen Z, Atasoy BM, Kefeli AU et al (2013) The benefit of whole brain reirradiation in patients with multiple brain metastases. Radiat Oncol 8:186

Patchell RA, Tibbs PA, Walsh JW et al (1990) A randomized trial of surgery in the treatment of single metastases to the brain. N Engl J Med 322:494–500

Patchell RA, Tibbs PA, Regine WF et al (1998) Postoperative radiotherapy in the treatment of single metastases to the brain: a randomized trial. JAMA 280:1485–1489

Pirzkall A, Debus J, Lohr F et al (1998) Radiosurgery alone or in combination with whole-brain radiotherapy for brain metastases. J Clin Oncol 16:3563–3569

Prados M, Leibel S, Barnett CM, Gutin P (1989) Interstitial brachytherapy for metastatic brain tumors. Cancer 63:657–660

Rades D, Pluemer A, Veninga T et al (2007a) A boost in addition to whole-brain radiotherapy improves patient outcome after resection of 1 or 2 brain metastases in recursive partitioning analysis class 1 and 2 patients. Cancer 110:1551–1559

Rades D, Bohlen G, Pluemer A et al (2007b) Stereotactic radiosurgery alone versus resection plus whole-brain radiotherapy for 1 or 2 brain metastases in recursive partitioning analysis class 1 and 2 patients. Cancer 109:2515–2521

Rades D, Haatanen T, Schild SE, Dunst J (2007c) Dose escalation beyond 30 grays in 10 fractions for patients with multiple brain metastases. Cancer 110: 1345–1350

Regine WF, Scott C, Murray K, Curran W (2001) Neurocognitive outcome in brain metastases patients treated with accelerated-fractionation vs. accelerated-hyperfractionated radiotherapy: an analysis from Radiation Therapy Oncology Group Study 91-04. Int J Radiat Oncol Biol Phys 51:711–717

Rugo HS, Ahles T (2003) The impact of adjuvant therapy for breast cancer on cognitive function: current evidence and directions for research. Semin Oncol 30:749–762

Sadikov E, Bezjak A, Yi QL et al (2007) Value of whole brain re-irradiation for brain metastases – single centre experience. Clin Oncol (R Coll Radiol) 19:532–538

Sahgal A, Aoyama H, Kocher M et al (2015) Phase 3 trials of stereotactic radiosurgery with or without whole-brain radiation therapy for 1 to 4 brain metastases: individual patient data meta-analysis. Int J Radiat Oncol Biol Phys 91:710–717

Scharp M, Hauswald H, Bischof M et al (2014) Re-irradiation in the treatment of patients with cerebral metastases of solid tumors: retrospective analysis. Radiat Oncol 9:4

Serizawa T, Saeki N, Higuchi Y et al (2005) Diagnostic value of thallium-201 chloride single-photon emission computerized tomography in differentiating tumor recurrence from radiation injury after gamma knife surgery for metastatic brain tumors. J Neurosurg 102(Suppl):266–271

Shaw E, Scott C, Souhami L et al (1996) Radiosurgery for the treatment of previously irradiated recurrent primary brain tumors and brain metastases: initial report of RTOG protocol 90-05. Int J Radiat Oncol Biol Phys 34:647–654

Shaw E, Scott C, Souhami L et al (2000) Single dose radiosurgical treatment of recurrent previously irradiated primary brain tumors and brain metastases: final report of RTOG protocol 90-05. Int J Radiat Oncol Biol Phys 47:291–298

Shehata WM, Hendrickson FR, Hindo WA (1974) Rapid fractionation technique and re-treatment of cerebral metastases by irradiation. Cancer 34:257–261

Sneed PK, Lamborn KR, Forstner JM et al (1999) Radiosurgery for brain metastases: is whole brain radiotherapy necessary? Int J Radiat Oncol Biol Phys 43:549–558

Sneed PK, Suh JH, Goetsch SJ et al (2002) A multi-institutional review of radiosurgery alone vs. radiosurgery with whole brain radiotherapy as the initial management of brain metastases. Int J Radiat Oncol Biol Phys 53:519–526

Sneed PK, Mendez J, Vemer van den Hoek J et al (2015) Adverse radiation effect after stereotactic radiosurgery for brain metastases: incidence, time course, and risk factors. J Neurosurg 123:373–386

Sperduto PW, Berkey B, Gaspar LE et al (2008a) A new prognostic index and comparison to three other indices for patients with brain metastases: an analysis of 1,960 patients in the RTOG database. Int J Radiat Oncol Biol Phys 70:510–514

Sperduto CM, Watanabe Y, Mullan J et al (2008b) A validation study of a new prognostic index for patients with brain metastases: the Graded Prognostic Assessment. J Neurosurg 109(Suppl):87–89

Sperduto PW, Chao ST, Sneed PK et al (2010) Diagnosis-specific prognostic factors, indexes, and treatment outcomes for patients with newly diagnosed brain metastases: a multi-institutional analysis of 4,259 patients. Int J Radiat Oncol Biol Phys 77:655–661

Stea B, Suh JH, Boyd AP et al (2006) Whole-brain radiotherapy with or without efaproxiral for the treatment of brain metastases: determinants of response and its prognostic value for subsequent survival. Int J Radiat Oncol Biol Phys 64:1023–1030

Sterzing F, Welzel T, Sroka-Perez G et al (2009) Reirradiation of multiple brain metastases with helical tomotherapy. Strahlenther Onkol 185:89–93

Sundgren PC (2009) MR spectroscopy in radiation injury. AJNR Am J Neuroradiol 30:1469–1476

Sundstrom JT, Minn H, Lertola KK et al (1998) Prognosis of patients treated for intracranial metastases with whole-brain irradiation. Ann Med 30:296–299

Tendulkar RD, Liu SW, Barnett GH et al (2006) RPA classification has prognostic significance for surgically resected single brain metastasis. Int J Radiat Oncol Biol Phys 66:810–817

Terakawa Y, Tsuyuguchi N, Iwai Y et al (2008) Diagnostic accuracy of 11C-methionine PET for differentiation of recurrent brain tumors from radiation necrosis after radiotherapy. J Nucl Med 49:694–699

Tokuuye K, Akine Y, Sumi M et al (1998) Reirradiation of brain and skull base tumors with fractionated stereotactic radiotherapy. Int J Radiat Oncol Biol Phys 40:1151–1155

Torcuator R, Zuniga R, Mohan YS et al (2009) Initial experience with bevacizumab treatment for biopsy confirmed cerebral radiation necrosis. J Neurooncol 94:63–68

Varlotto JM, Flickinger JC, Niranjan A et al (2003) Analysis of tumor control and toxicity in patients who have survived at least one year after radiosurgery for brain metastases. Int J Radiat Oncol Biol Phys 57:452–464

Vogelbaum MA, Angelov L, Lee SY et al (2006) Local control of brain metastases by stereotactic radiosurgery in relation to dose to the tumor margin. J Neurosurg 104:907–912

Walker AJ, Ruzevick J, Malayeri AA et al (2014) Postradiation imaging changes in the CNS: how can we differentiate between treatment effect and disease progression? Future Oncol 10:1277–1297

Weltman E, Salvajoli JV, Brandt RA et al (2001) Radiosurgery for brain metastases: who may not benefit? Int J Radiat Oncol Biol Phys 51:1320–1327

Wong WW, Schild SE, Sawyer TE, Shaw EG (1996) Analysis of outcome in patients reirradiated for brain metastases. Int J Radiat Oncol Biol Phys 34:585–590

Yamamoto M, Serizawa T, Shuto T et al (2014) Stereotactic radiosurgery for patients with multiple brain metastases (JLGK0901): a multi-institutional prospective observational study. Lancet Oncol 15:387–395

Erratum to: Re-Irradiation: New Frontiers

Carsten Nieder and Johannes Langendijk

The original version of the book has been revised: The chapter source lines of all the chapters has been updated to Medical Radiology – Radiation Oncology

The updated original online version for this chapter can be found at

DOI 10.1007/174_2016_59

DOI 10.1007/174_2016_60

DOI 10.1007/174_2016_34

DOI 10.1007/174_2016_62

DOI 10.1007/174_2016_55

DOI 10.1007/174_2016_71

DOI 10.1007/174_2016_66

DOI 10.1007/174_2016_33

C. Nieder, MD (✉)
Department of Oncology and Palliative Medicine,
Nordland Hospital, Bodø, Norway
e-mail: Carsten.Nieder@nordlandssykehuset.no

J. Langendijk, MD
Department of Radiation Oncology, University
Medical Center Groningen/University of Groningen,
Groningen, The Netherlands

Med Radiol Radiat Oncol (2017)
DOI 10.1007/978-3-319-41825-4_78, © Springer International Publishing Switzerland

DOI 10.1007/174_2016_76

DOI 10.1007/174_2016_48

DOI 10.1007/174_2016_61

DOI 10.1007/174_2016_77

DOI 10.1007/174_2016_75

DOI 10.1007/174_2016_56

DOI 10.1007/174_2016_67

DOI 10.1007/174_2016_47

DOI 10.1007/174_2016_57

DOI 10.1007/174_2016_37

DOI 10.1007/174_2016_32

DOI 10.1007/174_2016_72

DOI 10.1007/174_2016_58

DOI 10.1007/978-3-319-41825-4

Index

Med Radiol Radiat Oncol (2016)
DOI 10.1007/978-3-319-41825-4, © Springer International Publishing Switzerland